PARK'S
PEDIATRIC CARDIOLOGY
FOR PRACTITIONERS

Seventh Edition

PARK'S
PEDIATRIC
CARDIOLOGY
FOR PRACTITIONERS

Myung K. Park, *MD, FAAP, FACC*

Professor Emeritus (Pediatrics)
Former Director of Pediatric Cardiology
Former Director of Preventive Cardiology and Weight Management Clinic
University of Texas Health Science Center
San Antonio, Texas

Mehrdad Salamat, *MD, FAAP, FACC*

Clinical Associate Professor of Pediatrics
Texas A & M University Health Science Center
Bryan, Texas

Attending Cardiologist
Driscoll Children's Hospital
Corpus Christi, Texas

ELSEVIER

Elsevier
1600 John F. Kennedy Blvd.
Ste 1800
Philadelphia, PA 19103-2899

PARK'S PEDIATRIC CARDIOLOGY FOR PRACTITIONERS, SEVENTH EDITION   ISBN: 978-0-323-68107-0

Previous editions copyrighted 2014, 2008, 2002, 1996, 1988, and 1984

International Standard Book Number: 978-0-323-68107-0

Content Strategist: Sarah Barth
Content Development Specialist: Ann Ruzycka Anderson
Publishing Services Manager: Shereen Jameel
Project Manager: Aparna Venkatachalam
Designer: Ryan Cook

Printed in India

Last digit is the print number: 9 8 7 6 5 4 3

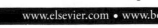

To my wife Issun,
our sons (Douglas, Christopher, and Warren),
daughters-in-law (Bomin and Soyeon), and
grandchildren (Natalie, Audrey, and Madeleine).

Myung K. Park, MD

In memory of my father,
whose love for reading was contagious,
whose love for education will remain eternal.

Mehrdad Salamat, MD

PREFACE

Since the publication of the sixth edition of *Park's Pediatric Cardiology for Practitioners* in 2014, important advances have been made not only in the diagnosis but also in the medical and surgical management of children with congenital and acquired heart diseases. These advances make it necessary to update this book. Extensive updating and revisions have been made throughout the book at the level that is appropriate for cardiology fellows, primary care physicians, residents, medical students, and other health care providers. This comprehensive book will also serve as a quick review for practicing cardiologists. Any health care provider who is interested in learning about pediatric cardiology topics will also find this book very informative. Despite extensive revision, the book maintains its original goal of providing practitioners with fundamental and practical information for the management of children with cardiac problems. Thus, the general layout of the book has been preserved to serve as a small reference book, avoiding excessive theoretical and sometimes controversial discussions or detailed surgical descriptions commonly found in subspecialty textbooks.

Although every topic and chapter has been updated, certain topics were given more revision than others. *Moderate revisions* were made to the following topics: non-invasive imaging techniques, device management of certain heart conditions, management of selected congenital heart defects, infective endocarditis, acute rheumatic fever, cardiomyopathies, cardiac arrhythmias, congestive heart failure, pulmonary hypertension, ambulatory blood pressure (BP) monitoring, and syncope in children. *Major revisions* were made to the following topics: pulse oximetry, Kawasaki disease, long and short QT syndromes, pediatric preventive cardiology, and athletes' sports participation. The neonatal pulse oximetry screening was extensively revised with inclusion of scientific background of the technique along with recommended algorithm by the American Academy of Pediatrics. Kawasaki disease was extensively updated, including evaluation of suspected incomplete Kawasaki disease with a recommended algorithm. Cardiac arrhythmias, especially supraventricular tachycardia, long QT syndrome, and short QT syndrome, received significant amount of revision. A new chapter on pediatric preventive cardiology was added to discuss metabolic syndrome, cardiovascular risk factors, dyslipidemia screening, obesity, and smoking to emphasize the need for practitioners' efforts in the prevention of heart disease during childhood. Eligibility recommendations for athletic participation have been updated based on the new 14-point evaluation, new classification of sports, and recommendations for specific heart conditions based on a recent American Heart Association and American College of Cardiology Joint Scientific Statement.

Sections dealing with BP and systemic hypertension have been expanded because the normal BP standards based on the age and height percentile published by the National High Blood Pressure Education Program (HBPEP) are not only scientifically and logically unsound but also impractical for busy practitioners to follow. This is an important issue because the consequences of the diagnosis and management of hypertension based on scientifically unsound BP standards are immense. As such, this important topic is discussed in depth, and borderline blood pressure levels that require physicians' attention are presented with data from the San Antonio Children's Blood Pressure Study. The data by the HBPEP are presented in the Appendix only for the sake of completeness. In addition, often neglected basic knowledge of BP measurement in clinical practice has been reviewed in some detail. The new 2017 classification of BP levels for children and adults are presented along with the revised recommendations.

I am very pleased to report that my long-time friend, Dr. Mehrdad Salamat, has accepted my invitation to become a coauthor of this book and to become the primary author of the future editions of the book. Dr. Salamat is an ardent teacher of pediatric cardiology, beloved by medical students, residents, pediatricians, nursing staff, and his peers. His participation as the coauthor has made this revision more objective and balanced. I am certain that Dr. Salamat will continue to maintain the original goal of this book in the future. I wish him the best in carrying out the paramount responsibility.

Myung K. Park, MD
San Antonio, Texas

FREQUENTLY USED ABBREVIATIONS

AR	aortic regurgitation
AS	aortic stenosis
ASA	atrial septal aneurysm
ASD	atrial septal defect
AV	atrioventricular
BDG	bidirectional Glenn operation
BP	blood pressure
BT	Blalock-Taussig
BVH	biventricular hypertrophy
CAD	coronary artery disease
CHD	congenital heart disease (or defect)
CHF	congestive heart failure
COA	coarctation of the aorta
CV	cardiovascular
DCM	dilated cardiomyopathy
DORV	double-outlet right ventricle
D-TGA	D-transposition of the great arteries
ECD	endocardial cushion defect
echo	echocardiography or echocardiographic
EF	ejection fraction
FS	fractional shortening
HCM	hypertrophic cardiomyopathy
HOCM	hypertrophic obstructive cardiomyopathy
HLHS	hypoplastic left heart syndrome
ICD	implantable cardioverter–defibrillator
IRBBB	incomplete right bundle branch block
IVC	inferior vena cava
LA	left atrium
LAD	left axis deviation
LAH	left atrial hypertrophy
LBBB	left bundle branch block
LPA	left pulmonary artery
L-TGA	L-transposition of the great arteries
LV	left ventricle or ventricular
LVH	left ventricular hypertrophy
LVOT	left ventricular outflow tract
MAPCAs	multiple aortopulmonary collateral arteries
MPA	main pulmonary artery
MR	mitral regurgitation
MS	mitral stenosis
MVP	mitral valve prolapse
PA	pulmonary artery or arterial
PAC	premature atrial contraction
PAPVR	partial anomalous pulmonary venous return
PBF	pulmonary blood flow
PDA	patent ductus arteriosus
PFO	patent foramen ovale
PPHN	persistent pulmonary hypertension of newborn
PR	pulmonary regurgitation
PS	pulmonary stenosis
PVC	premature ventricular contraction
PVOD	pulmonary vascular obstructive disease
PVR	pulmonary vascular resistance
RA	right atrium
RAD	right axis deviation
RAH	right atrial hypertrophy
RBBB	right bundle branch block
RPA	right pulmonary artery
RV	right ventricle or ventricular
RVH	right ventricular hypertrophy
RVOT	right ventricular outflow tract
S1	first heart sound
S2	second heart sound
S3	third heart sound
S4	fourth heart sound
SBE	subacute bacterial endocarditis
SEM	systolic ejection murmur
SVC	superior vena cava
SVR	systemic vascular resistance
SVT	supraventricular tachycardia
TAPVR	total anomalous pulmonary venous return
TGA	transposition of the great arteries
TOF	tetralogy of Fallot
TR	tricuspid regurgitation
TS	tricuspid stenosis
VSD	ventricular septal defect
VT	ventricular tachycardia
WPW	Wolff-Parkinson-White

CONTENTS

PART 1

Basic Tools in Routine Evaluation of Cardiac Patients

The initial office evaluation of a child with possible cardiac abnormalities is usually accomplished by history taking; physical examination that includes inspection, palpation, and auscultation; electrocardiography (ECG); and sometimes chest radiography.

The weight of the information gained from these different techniques varies with the type and severity of the disease. For example, if a mother had diabetes during her pregnancy, infants with macrosomia have an increased chance of having cardiac problems. In these infants, the prevalence of congenital heart disease (CHD) increases to three to four times that found in the general population. Ventricular septal defect (VSD), transposition of the great arteries (TGA), and coarctation of the aorta (COA) are more common defects. Congenital malformations of all types are increased in these infants. Hypertrophic cardiomyopathy with or without obstruction of the left ventricular outflow tract occurs in 10% to 20% of these infants, and they also have an increased risk of persistent pulmonary hypertension of the newborn. The physician should look for these defects when examining the child.

Auscultation may be the most important source of information in the diagnosis of acyanotic heart disease such as VSD or PDA. However, auscultation is rarely diagnostic in cyanotic CHD such as TGA, in which heart murmur is often absent. Careful palpation of the peripheral pulses is more important than auscultation in the detection of COA. Measurement of blood pressure is the most important diagnostic tool in the detection of hypertension. ECG and chest radiography have strengths and weaknesses in their ability to assess the severity of heart disease. ECG detects hypertrophy well and therefore detects conditions of pressure overload, but it is less reliable at detecting dilatation from volume overload. Chest radiography is most reliable in establishing volume overload, but it poorly demonstrates hypertrophy without dilatation.

The next four chapters discuss these basic tools (history, physical examination, ECG, chest radiography) in depth.

1

History Taking

As in the evaluation of any other system, history taking is a basic step in cardiac evaluation. Maternal history during pregnancy is often helpful in the diagnosis of congenital heart disease (CHD) because certain prenatal events are known to be teratogenic. Past history, including the immediate postnatal period, provides more direct information relevant to the cardiac evaluation. Family history also helps link a cardiac problem to other medical problems that may be prevalent in the family. Box 1.1 lists important aspects of history taking for children with potential cardiac problems.

GESTATIONAL AND NATAL HISTORY

Infections, medications, and excessive alcohol intake may cause CHD, especially if they occur early in pregnancy.

Infections

1. Maternal rubella infection during the first trimester of pregnancy commonly results in multiple anomalies, including cardiac defects.
2. Infections by cytomegalovirus, herpesvirus, and coxsackievirus B are suspected to be teratogenic if they occur in early pregnancy. Infections by these viruses later in pregnancy may cause myocarditis.
3. Human immunodeficiency virus infection has been associated with infantile cardiomyopathy.

Medications, Alcohol, and Smoking

1. Several medications are suspected teratogens.
   a. Amphetamines have been associated with ventricular septal defect (VSD), patent ductus arteriosus (PDA),

atrial septal defect (ASD), and transposition of the great arteries (TGA).
   b. Anticonvulsants are suspected of causing CHD. Phenytoin (Dilantin) has been associated with pulmonary stenosis (PS), aortic stenosis (AS), coarctation of the aorta (COA), and PDA. Trimethadione (Tridione) has been associated with TGA, tetralogy of Fallot (TOF), and hypoplastic left heart syndrome (HLHS).
   c. Angiotensin-converting enzyme (ACE) inhibitors (captopril, enalapril, lisinopril) and angiotensin II receptor antagonists (losartan) taken during the first trimester have been reported to cause congenital malformations of multiple systems, including cardiac defects (e.g., ASD, VSD, PDA, and PS).
   d. Lithium has been associated with Ebstein's anomaly.
   e. Retinoic acid may cause conotruncal anomalies.
   f. Valproic acid may be associated with various heart defects such as ASD, VSD, aortic stenosis, pulmonary atresia with intact ventricular septum, and COA.
   g. Other medications suspected of causing CHD (VSD, TOF, TGA) include progesterone and estrogen.
2. Excessive alcohol intake during pregnancy has been associated with VSD, PDA, ASD, and TOF (fetal alcohol syndrome).
3. Although cigarette smoking has not been proved to be teratogenic, it does cause intrauterine growth retardation.

Maternal Conditions

1. There is a high incidence of cardiomyopathy in infants born to mothers with diabetes. In addition, these babies have a higher incidence of structural heart defects (e.g., TGA, VSD, PDA, ECD, COA, HLHS).

BOX 1.1 Selected Aspects of History Taking

Gestational and Natal History
Infections, medications, excessive smoking, or alcohol intake during pregnancy
Birth weight

Postnatal, Past, and Present History
Weight gain, development, and feeding pattern
Cyanosis, "cyanotic spells," and squatting
Tachypnea, dyspnea, puffy eyelids
Frequency of respiratory infection
Exercise intolerance
Heart murmur
Chest pain
Syncope
Palpitation
Joint symptoms
Neurologic symptoms
Medications

Family History
Hereditary disease
Congenital heart defect
Rheumatic fever
Sudden unexpected death
Diabetes mellitus, arteriosclerotic heart disease, hypertension, dyslipidemia, and so on

2. Maternal lupus erythematosus and mixed connective tissue disease have been associated with a high incidence of congenital heart block in offspring secondary to placental crossing of maternal anti-Ro and anti-La antibodies.
3. The incidence of CHD increases from about 1% in the general population to as much as 15% if the mother has CHD, even if it is postoperative (see Table A.2 in Appendix A).

Birth Weight

Birth weight provides important information about the nature of the cardiac problem.
1. If an infant is small for gestational age, it may indicate intrauterine infections or use of chemicals or drugs by the mother. Rubella syndrome and fetal alcohol syndrome are typical examples.
2. Infants with high birth weight, often seen in offspring of mothers with diabetes, show a higher incidence of cardiac anomalies. Infants with TGA often have birth weights higher than average; these infants have cyanosis.

POSTNATAL HISTORY

Weight Gain, Development, and Feeding Pattern

Weight gain and general development may be delayed in infants and children with congestive heart failure (CHF) or severe cyanosis. Weight is affected more significantly than height. If weight is severely affected, physicians should suspect a more general dysmorphic condition. Poor feeding of recent onset may be an early sign of CHF in infants, especially if the poor feeding is the result of fatigue and dyspnea.

Cyanosis, "Cyanotic Spells," and Squatting

The presence of cyanosis should be assessed. If the parents think that their child has cyanosis, the physician should ask them about the onset (e.g., at birth, several days after birth), severity of cyanosis, permanent or paroxysmal nature, parts of the body that were cyanotic (e.g., fingers, toes, lips), and whether the cyanosis becomes worse after feeding. Evanescent acrocyanosis is normal in neonates.

A "cyanotic spell" is seen most frequently in infants with TOF and requires immediate attention, although it has become less frequent because most surgical repairs are done in early infancy. Physicians should ask about the time of its appearance (e.g., in the morning on awakening, after feeding), duration of the spells, and frequency of the spells. Most important is whether infants were breathing *fast* and *deep* during the spell or were holding their breath. This helps differentiate between a true cyanotic spell and a breath-holding spell.

The physician should ask whether the child squats when tired or has a favorite body position (e.g., knee–chest position) when tired. Squatting strongly suggests cyanotic heart disease, particularly TOF. Fortunately, squatting is extremely rare now with early surgical repair of cyanotic CHDs.

Tachypnea, Dyspnea, and Puffy Eyelids

Tachypnea, dyspnea, and puffy eyelids are signs of CHF. Left-sided heart failure produces tachypnea with or without dyspnea. Tachypnea becomes worse with feeding and eventually results in poor feeding and poor weight gain. A sleeping respiratory rate of more than 40 breaths/min is noteworthy. A rate of more than 60 breaths/min is abnormal, even in a newborn.

Wheezing or persistent cough at night may be an early sign of CHF. Puffy eyelids and sacral edema are signs of systemic venous congestion. Ankle edema, which is commonly seen in adults, is not found in infants.

Frequency of Respiratory Infections

Congenital heart diseases with large left-to-right shunt and increased pulmonary blood flow predispose to lower respiratory tract infections. Frequent upper respiratory tract infections are not related to CHD, although children with vascular rings may sound as if they have a chronic upper respiratory tract infection.

Exercise Intolerance

Decreased exercise tolerance may result from any significant heart disease, including large left-to-right shunt lesions, cyanotic defects, valvular stenosis or regurgitation, and arrhythmias. Obese children may be inactive and have decreased exercise tolerance in the absence of heart disease. A good assessment of exercise tolerance can be obtained by asking the following questions: Does the child keep up with other children? How many blocks can the child walk or run? How many flights of stairs can the child climb without fatigue? Does the weather or the time of day influence the child's exercise tolerance?

With infants who do not walk or run, an estimate of exercise tolerance can be gained from the infant's history of feeding pattern. Parents often report that the child takes naps; however, many normal children nap regularly.

Heart Murmur

If a heart murmur is the chief complaint, the physician should obtain information about the time of its first appearance and the circumstances of its discovery. A heart murmur heard within a few hours of birth usually indicates a stenotic lesion (AS, PS), atrioventricular (AV) valve regurgitation, or small left-to-right shunt lesions (VSD, PDA). The murmur of large left-to-right shunt lesions, such as VSD or PDA, may be delayed because of slow regression of pulmonary vascular resistance. In the case of stenotic lesion, the onset of the murmur is not affected by the pulmonary vascular resistance, and the murmur is usually heard shortly after birth. A heart murmur that is first noticed on a routine examination of a healthy-looking child is more likely to be innocent, especially if the same physician has been following the child's progress. A febrile illness is often associated with the discovery of a heart murmur.

Chest Pain

Chest pain is a common reason for referral and parental anxiety. If chest pain is the primary complaint, the physician asks whether the pain is activity related (e.g., Do you have chest pain only when you are active, or does it come even when you watch television?). The physician also asks about the duration (e.g., seconds, minutes, hours) and nature of the pain (e.g., sharp, stabbing, squeezing) and radiation to other parts of the body (e.g., neck, left shoulder, left arm). Chest pain of cardiac origin is not sharp; it manifests as a deep, heavy pressure or the feeling of choking or a squeezing sensation, and it is usually triggered by exercise. The physician should ask whether deep breathing improves or worsens the pain. Pain of cardiac origin, except for pericarditis, is not affected by respiration.

Cardiac conditions that may cause chest pain include severe AS (usually associated with activity), pulmonary hypertension or pulmonary vascular obstructive disease, and mitral valve prolapse (MVP). Chest pain in MVP is not necessarily associated with activity, but there may be a history of palpitation. There is increasing doubt about the relationship between chest pain and MVP in children. Less common cardiac conditions that can cause chest pain include severe PS, pericarditis of various causes, and current or history of Kawasaki's disease (in which stenosis or aneurysm of the coronary artery is common).

Most children complaining of chest pain do not have a cardiac condition (see Chapter 30); cardiac causes of chest pain are rare in children and adolescents. The three most common noncardiac causes of chest pain in children are costochondritis, trauma to the chest wall or muscle strain, and respiratory diseases with cough (e.g., bronchitis, asthma, pneumonia, pleuritis). The physician should ask whether the patient has experienced recent trauma to the chest or has engaged in activity that may have resulted in pectoralis muscle soreness.

Gastroesophageal reflux and exercise-induced asthma are other recognizable causes of noncardiac chest pain in children. Exercise-induced asthma (or bronchospasm) typically occurs 5 to 10 minutes into vigorous physical activities in a child with asthma or with inadequately treated asthma. It can occur in a child previously undiagnosed with asthma. A psychogenic cause of chest pain is also possible; parents should be asked whether there has been a recent cardiac death in the family.

Syncope

Syncope is a transient loss of consciousness and muscle tone that result from inadequate cerebral perfusion. Dizziness is the most common prodromal symptom of syncope. These complaints could represent a serious cardiac condition that may result in sudden death. It may also be due to noncardiac causes, such as benign vasovagal syncope, dehydration, metabolic abnormalities, or neuropsychiatric disorders. Dehydration or inadequate hydration is an important contributing factor.

A history of exertional syncope may suggest arrhythmias (particularly ventricular arrhythmias, such as seen in long QT syndrome, hypertrophic cardiomyopathy, or severe obstructive lesions, e.g., severe AS). Syncope provoked by exercise, that is accompanied by chest pain, or with a history of unoperated or operated heart disease suggests potential cardiac cause of syncope. Syncope while sitting down suggests arrhythmias or seizure disorders. Syncope while standing for a long time suggests vasovagal syncope (often in association with dehydration) without an underlying cardiac disease; this is the most common syncope in children (see Chapter 31 for further discussion). Hypoglycemia is a very rare cause of syncope occurring in the morning. Syncopal duration less than 1 minute suggests vasovagal syncope, hyperventilation, or syncope caused by another orthostatic mechanism. A longer duration of syncope suggests convulsive disorders, migraine, or cardiac arrhythmias.

Family history should include coronary heart disease risk factors, including history of myocardial infarction in family members younger than 30 years of age, cardiac arrhythmia, CHD, cardiomyopathies, long QT syndrome, seizures, metabolic and psychological disorders. A detailed discussion of this topic is presented in Chapter 31.

Palpitation

Palpitation is a subjective feeling of rapid heartbeats. Some parents and children report sinus tachycardia as palpitation. Paroxysms of tachycardia (e.g., supraventricular tachycardia) or single premature beats commonly cause palpitation (see Chapter 32). Children with hyperthyroidism or MVP may first be taken to the physician because of complaints of palpitation.

Joint Symptoms

When joint pain is the primary complaint, acute rheumatic arthritis or rheumatoid arthritis is a possibility, although the incidence of the former has dramatically decreased in recent years in the United States. The number of joints involved, duration of the symptom, and migratory or stationary nature of the pain are important. Arthritis of acute rheumatic fever typically involves large joints, either simultaneously or in succession, with a characteristic migratory nature. Pain in rheumatic joint is so severe that children refuse to walk. A history of recent sore throat (and throat culture results) or rashes suggestive of scarlet fever may be helpful. The physician also asks whether the joint was swollen, red, hot, or tender (see Chapter 20 for further discussion).

Neurologic Symptoms

A history of stroke suggests thromboembolism secondary to cyanotic CHD with polycythemia or infective endocarditis. In the absence of cyanosis, stroke can rarely be caused by paradoxical embolism of a venous thrombus through an ASD. Although very rare, primary hypercoagulable states should also be considered which include such conditions as factor V Leiden thrombophilia, antithrombin III deficiency, protein C deficiency, protein S deficiency, disorders of fibrinolytic system (e.g., hypoplasminogenemia, abnormal plasminogen, plasminogen activator deficiency), dysfibrinogenemia, factor XII deficiency, and lupus anticoagulant (Barger, 2000). A host of other conditions cause secondary hypercoagulable states. A history of headache may be a manifestation of cerebral hypoxia with cyanotic heart disease, severe polycythemia, or brain abscess in cyanotic children. Although it is claimed to occur in adults, hypertension with or without COA rarely causes headaches in children. Choreic movement strongly suggests rheumatic fever.

Medications

Physicians should note the name, dosage, timing, and duration of cardiac and noncardiac medications. Medications may be responsible for the chief complaint of the visit or certain physical findings. Tachycardia and palpitation may be caused by cold medications or antiasthmatic drugs.

A history of tobacco and illicit drug use, which could be the cause of chief complaints, should be obtained, preferably through a private interview with the child.

FAMILY HISTORY

Hereditary Disease

Some hereditary diseases may be associated with certain forms of CHD. For example, Marfan's syndrome is frequently associated with aortic aneurysm or with aortic or mitral insufficiency. Holt-Oram syndrome (ASD and limb abnormalities), long-QT syndrome (sudden death caused by ventricular arrhythmias), and idiopathic sudden death in the family should be inquired about. PS secondary to a dysplastic pulmonary valve is common in Noonan's syndrome. Lentiginous skin lesion (Noonan syndrome with multiple lentigines, formerly called LEOPARD syndrome) is often associated with PS and cardiomyopathy. Selected hereditary diseases in which cardiovascular disease is frequently found are listed in Table 2.1 along with other nonhereditary syndromes.

Congenital Heart Disease

The incidence of CHD in the general population is about 1% or, more precisely, 8 to 12 of 1000 live births. This does not include PDA in premature infants. The recurrence risk of CHD associated with inherited diseases or chromosomal abnormalities is related to the recurrent risk of the syndrome.

A history of CHD in close relatives increases the chance of CHD in a child. In general, when one child is affected, the risk of recurrence in siblings is about 3%, which is a threefold increase. Having a child with hypoplastic left heart syndrome (HLHS) increases the risk of CHD in subsequent child (to approximately 10%) and most centers perform fetal echocardiography. The risk of recurrence is related to the prevalence of particular defects. Whereas lesions with a higher prevalence (e.g., VSD) tend to have a higher risk of recurrence, lesions with a lower prevalence (e.g., tricuspid atresia, persistent truncus arteriosus) have a lower risk of recurrence. Table A.1 in Appendix A lists the recurrence risk figures for various CHDs, which can be used for counseling. The importance of cytoplasmic inheritance has recently been shown in some families based on the observation that the recurrence risk is substantially higher if the mother is the affected parent (see Table A.2 in Appendix A).

Rheumatic Fever

Rheumatic fever frequently occurs in more than one family member. There is a higher incidence of the condition among relatives of children with rheumatic fever. Although the knowledge of genetic factors involved in rheumatic fever is incomplete, it is generally agreed that there is an inherited susceptibility to acquiring rheumatic fever.

Hypertension and Atherosclerosis

Essential hypertension and coronary artery disease show a strong familial pattern. Therefore, when a physician suspects hypertension in a young person, it is important to obtain family history of hypertension. Atherosclerosis results from a complex process in which hereditary and environmental factors interact. The most important risk factor for atherosclerosis is the positive family history with coronary heart disease occurring before age 55 years in one's father or grandfather and before age 65 years in one's mother or grandmother. Clustering of cardiovascular risk factors occur frequently in the same individual (metabolic syndrome), which calls for investigation for other risk factors when one risk factor is found. Detailed discussion of cardiovascular risk factors is presented in Chapter 33.

2

Physical Examination

As with the examination of any child, the order and extent of the physical examination of infants and children with potential cardiac problems should be individualized. The more innocuous procedures, such as inspection, should be done first, and the more frightening or uncomfortable parts should be delayed until later in the examination.

Supine is the preferred position for examining patients in any age group. However, if older infants and young children between 1 and 3 years of age refuse to lie down, they can be examined initially while sitting on their mothers' laps.

GROWTH PATTERN

Growth impairment is frequently observed in infants with congenital heart diseases (CHDs). The growth chart should reflect height and weight in terms of absolute values and in percentiles. Accurate plotting and following of the growth curve are essential parts of the initial and follow-up evaluations of a child with significant heart problems. In overweight children, acanthosis nigricans should be checked in the neck, armpits, and abdomen.

Different patterns of growth impairment are seen in different types of CHD.

1. Cyanotic patients have disturbances in both height and weight.
2. Acyanotic patients, particularly those with large left-to-right shunts, tend to have more problems with weight gain than with linear growth. The degree of growth impairment is proportional to the size of the shunt.
3. Acyanotic patients with pressure overload lesions without intracardiac shunt grow normally.

Poor growth in a child with mild cardiac anomaly or failure of catch-up weight gain after repair of the defect may be caused by failure to recognize certain syndromes, inadequate calorie intake, or the underlying genetic predisposition.

INSPECTION

Much information can be gained by simple inspection without disturbing a sleeping infant or frightening a child with a stethoscope. Inspection should include the following: general appearance and nutritional state; any obvious syndrome or chromosomal abnormalities; color (i.e., cyanosis, pallor, jaundice); clubbing; respiratory rate, dyspnea, and retraction; sweat on the forehead; and chest inspection.

General Appearance and Nutritional State

The physician should note whether the child is in distress, well-nourished or undernourished, and happy or cranky. Obesity should also be noted; besides being associated with other cardiovascular risk factors such as dyslipidemia, hypertension, and hyperinsulinemia, obesity is also an independent risk factor for coronary artery disease.

Chromosomal Syndromes

Obvious chromosomal abnormalities known to be associated with certain congenital heart defects should be noted by the physician. For example, about 40% to 50% of children with Down syndrome have a congenital heart defect; the two most common defects are endocardial cushion defect (ECD) and ventricular septal defect (VSD). A newborn with trisomy 18 syndrome usually has a congenital heart defect. Table 2.1 shows cardiac defects associated with selected chromosomal abnormalities along with other hereditary and nonhereditary syndromes.

Hereditary and Nonhereditary Syndromes and Other Systems Malformations

Congenital cardiovascular anomalies are associated with a number of hereditary or nonhereditary syndromes and malformations of other systems. For example, a child with a missing thumb or deformities of a forearm may have an atrial septal defect (ASD) or VSD (e.g., Holt-Oram syndrome [cardio-limb syndrome]). Newborns with CHARGE (*c*oloboma, *h*eart defects, choanal *a*tresia, growth or mental *r*etardation, *g*enitourinary anomalies, *e*ar anomalies) association show a high prevalence of conotruncal abnormalities (e.g., tetralogy of Fallot [TOF], double-outlet right ventricle [RV], persistent truncus arteriosus). A list of cardiac anomalies in selected hereditary and nonhereditary syndromes is given in Table 2.1. Certain congenital malformations of other organ systems are associated with an increased prevalence of congenital heart defects (Table 2.2).

Color

The physician should note whether the child is cyanotic, pale, or jaundiced. In cases of cyanosis, the degree and distribution should be noted (e.g., throughout the body, only on the lower or upper half of the body). Mild cyanosis is difficult to detect. The arterial saturation is usually 85% or lower before cyanosis is detectable in patients with normal hemoglobin levels (see Chapter 11).

Cyanosis is more noticeable in natural light than in artificial light. Cyanosis of the lips may be misleading, particularly in children who have deep pigmentation. The physician should also check the tongue, nail beds, and conjunctiva. When in doubt, the use of pulse oximetry is confirmatory. Children with cyanosis do not always have cyanotic congenital heart defects. Cyanosis may result from respiratory diseases or central nervous system disorders. Cyanosis that is associated with arterial desaturation is called *central cyanosis*. Cyanosis associated with normal arterial saturation is called *peripheral cyanosis*. Even mild cyanosis in a newborn requires thorough investigation (see Chapter 14).

Peripheral cyanosis may be noticeable in newborns who are exposed to cold and those with congestive heart failure (CHF) because, in both conditions, peripheral blood flow is sluggish, losing more oxygen to peripheral tissues. Cyanosis is also seen in polycythemic patients with normal O_2 saturation (see Chapter 11 for the relationship between cyanosis and hemoglobin levels). Circumoral cyanosis, cyanosis around the mouth, is found in normal children with fair skin. Isolated circumoral cyanosis is not significant. Acrocyanosis is a bluish or red discoloration of the fingers and toes of normal newborns in the presence of normal arterial oxygen saturation.

Pallor may be seen in infants with vasoconstriction from CHF or circulatory shock or in severely anemic infants. Newborns with severe CHF and those with congenital hypothyroidism may have prolonged physiologic jaundice. Patent ductus arteriosus (PDA) and pulmonary stenosis (PS) are common in newborns with congenital hypothyroidism. Hepatic disease with jaundice may cause arterial desaturation because of the development of pulmonary arteriovenous fistula (e.g., arteriohepatic dysplasia).

Clubbing

Long-standing arterial desaturation (usually longer than 6 months' duration), even if too mild to be detected by an inexperienced person, results in clubbing of the fingernails and toenails. Clubbing from cyanotic CHD is almost not seen in the United States because of early surgical repairs of the defect. When fully developed, clubbing is characterized by a widening and thickening of the ends of the fingers and toes, as well as by convex fingernails and loss of the angle between the nail and nail bed (Fig. 2.1). Reddening and shininess of the terminal phalanges are seen in the early stages of clubbing. Clubbing appears earliest and most noticeably in the thumb. Clubbing may also be associated with lung disease (e.g., abscess), cirrhosis of the liver, and subacute bacterial endocarditis. Occasionally, clubbing occurs in normal people, such as in *familial clubbing*.

Respiratory Rate, Dyspnea, and Retraction

The physician should note the respiratory rate of every infant and child. If the infant breathes irregularly, the physician should count for a whole minute. The respiratory rate is faster in children who are crying, upset, eating, or feverish. The most reliable respiratory rate is that taken during sleep. After finishing a bottle of formula, an infant may breathe faster than normal for 5 to 10 minutes. A resting respiratory rate more than 40 breaths/min is unusual, and more than 60 breaths/min is abnormal at any age. Tachypnea, along with tachycardia, is the earliest sign of left-sided heart failure. If the child has dyspnea or retraction, this may be a sign of a more severe degree of left-sided heart failure or significant lung pathology.

Sweat on the Forehead

Infants with CHF often have a cold sweat on their foreheads. This is an expression of heightened sympathetic activity as a compensatory mechanism for decreased cardiac output.

TABLE 2.1   Major Syndromes Associated with Cardiovascular Abnormalities

Disorder	Cardiovascular Abnormalities: Frequency and Types	Major Features	Etiology
22q11.2 deletion syndrome (overlaps with and includes DiGeorge syndrome and velocardiofacial syndrome)	Frequent (74%); TOF (20%), VSD (14%), interrupted aortic arch (13%), truncus arteriosus (6%), vascular ring (6%), ASD (4%), others (10%)	Wide ranges of abnormalities of multiple organ systems, with each person having different manifestations; characteristic facies ("elfin facies," ptosis, hypertelorism, auricular abnormalities), cleft lip and other palatal abnormalities (69%), feeding problems, learning difficulties (90%), congenital heart defects (74%), hypocalcemia (50%), renal anomalies (31%), autoimmune disorders (77%), hearing loss, laryngoesophageal anomalies, growth hormone deficiency, seizures, autism (20%), psychiatric disorders (25% of adults), behavioral problems, and others	Most cases new mutations; otherwise AD; microdeletion of 22q11.2
Alagille syndrome (arteriohepatic dysplasia)	Frequent (85%); peripheral PA stenosis with or without complex cardiovascular abnormalities	Peculiar facies (95%) consisting of deep-set eyes; broad forehead; long, straight nose with flattened tip; prominent chin; and small, low-set malformed ears Paucity of intrahepatic interlobular bile duct with chronic cholestasis (91%), hypercholesterolemia Butterfly-like vertebral arch defects (87%) Growth retardation (50%) and mild mental retardation (16%)	AD 30%–50%; rest: new mutations; mostly mutations in 20p12.2(±)
CHARGE association	Common (65%); TOF, truncus arteriosus, aortic arch anomalies (e.g., vascular ring, interrupted aortic arch)	*C*oloboma, *h*eart defects, choanal *a*tresia, growth or mental *r*etardation, *g*enitourinary anomalies, *e*ar anomalies, genital hypoplasia	Most cases new mutations; 8q12.2
Carpenter syndrome	Frequent (50%); PDA, VSD, PS, TGA	Brachycephaly with variable craniosynostosis, mild facial hypoplasia, polydactyly and severe syndactyly ("mitten hands")	AR; 6p12.1-p11.2 19q13.2
Cockayne syndrome	Accelerated atherosclerosis	Senile-like changes beginning in infancy, dwarfing, microcephaly, prominent nose and sunken eyes, visual loss (retinal degeneration), and hearing loss	AR; 10q11.23 5q12.1
Cornelia de Lange (de Lange's) syndrome	Occasional (30%); VSD	Synophrys and hirsutism, prenatal growth retardation, microcephaly, anteverted nares, downturned mouth, mental retardation	AD; mutation in 5p13.2 (>50%)
Cri du chat syndrome (deletion 5p syndrome)	Occasional (25%); variable CHD (VSD, PDA, ASD)	Cat-like cry in infancy, microcephaly, downward slant of palpebral fissures	Partial deletion, short arm of chromosome 5
Crouzon disease (craniofacial dysostosis)	Occasional; PDA, COA	Ptosis with shallow orbits, premature craniosynostosis, maxillary hypoplasia	AD; mutation in 10q26.13
DiGeorge syndrome (part of 22q11.2 deletion syndrome)	Frequent; interrupted aortic arch, truncus arteriosus, VSD, PDA, TOF	Acronymically known as CATCH 22 syndrome: *c*ardiac defects, *a*bnormal facies (hypertelorism, short philtrum, cleft palate, downslanting eye), *t*hymic hypoplasia, *c*left palate, and *h*ypocalcemia resulting from 22q11 deletions.	AD; microdeletion of 22q11.2
Down syndrome (trisomy 21)	Frequent (40%–50%); ECD, VSD	Hypotonic, flat facies, slanted palpebral fissure, small eyes, mental deficiency, simian crease	Trisomy 21
Ehlers-Danlos syndrome (vascular Ehlers-Danlos syndrome [type 4])	Frequent; ASD, aneurysm of aorta and carotids, intracranial aneurysm, MVP	Hyperextensive joints, hyperelasticity, fragility and bruisability of skin, poor wound healing with thin scar	AD; mutation in 2q32.2

TABLE 2.1 Major Syndromes Associated with Cardiovascular Abnormalities—cont'd

Disorder	Cardiovascular Abnormalities: Frequency and Types	Major Features	Etiology
Ellis–van Creveld syndrome (chondroectodermal dysplasia)	Frequent (50%); ASD, single atrium	Short stature of prenatal onset, short distal extremities, narrow thorax with short ribs, polydactyly, nail hypoplasia, neonatal teeth	AR; mutation in 4p16.2
Fetal alcohol syndrome	Occasional (25%–30%); VSD, PDA, ASD, TOF	Prenatal growth retardation, microcephaly, short palpebral fissure, mental deficiency, irritable infant or hyperactive child	Ethanol or its byproducts
Fetal trimethadione syndrome	Occasional (15%–30%); TGA, VSD, TOF	Ear malformation, hypoplastic midface, unusual eyebrow configuration, mental deficiency, speech disorder	Exposure to trimethadione
Fetal warfarin syndrome	Occasional (15%–45%); TOF, VSD	Facial asymmetry and hypoplasia; hypoplasia or aplasia of the pinna with blind or absent external ear canal (microtia); ear tags; cleft lip or palate; epitubular dermoid; hypoplastic vertebrae	Exposure to warfarin
Friedreich ataxia	Frequent; hypertrophic cardiomyopathy progressing to heart failure	Late-onset ataxia, skeletal deformities	AR; mutation in 9q21.11
Goldenhar syndrome (craniofacial macrosomia)	Frequent (35%); VSD, TOF	Facial asymmetry and hypoplasia, microtia, ear tag, cleft lip or palate, hypoplastic vertebrae	Usually sporadic
Glycogen storage disease II (Pompe disease)	Very common; cardiomyopathy	Large tongue and flabby muscles, cardiomegaly; LVH and short PR interval on ECG, severe ventricular hypertrophy on echocardiogram; normal FBS and GTT	AR; mutation in 17q25.3
Holt-Oram syndrome (cardio-limb syndrome)	Frequent; ASD, VSD	Defects or absence of thumb or radius	AD mutations in 12q24.21
Homocystinuria	Frequent; medial degeneration of aorta and carotids, atrial or venous thrombosis	Subluxation of lens (usually by 10 yr), malar flush, osteoporosis, arachnodactyly, pectus excavatum or carinatum, mental defect	AR; mostly mutation in 21q22.3
Infant of diabetic mother	CHDs (3%–5%); TGA, VSD, COA; cardiomyopathy (10%–20%); PPHN	Macrosomia, hypoglycemia and hypocalcemia, polycythemia, hyperbilirubinemia, other congenital anomalies	Fetal exposure to high glucose levels
Kartagener syndrome (primary ciliary dyskinesia)	Dextrocardia (12%)	Situs inversus, chronic sinusitis and otitis media, bronchiectasis, abnormal respiratory cilia, immotile sperm	AR; different genes
LEOPARD syndrome (Noonan syndrome with multiple lentigines)	Very common; PS, HOCM, long PR interval on ECG	*L*entiginous skin lesion, *E*CG abnormalities, *o*cular hypertelorism, *p*ulmonary stenosis, *a*bnormal genitalia, *r*etarded growth, *d*eafness	AD; 85% mutation in 12q24.13
Long QT syndrome: Jervell and Lange-Nielsen syndrome (1) and Romano-Ward syndrome (2)	Very common; long QT interval on ECG, ventricular tachyarrhythmia	Congenital deafness (not in Romano-Ward syndrome), syncope resulting from ventricular arrhythmias, family history of sudden death (±)	Multiple mutations; AR (1), AD (2)
Marfan syndrome	Frequent; aortic aneurysm, aortic and/or mitral regurgitation; MVP	Arachnodactyly with hyperextensibility, subluxation of lens; pectus deformity, myopia	AD; mutation in 15q21.1
Mucopolysaccharidosis Hurler syndrome (type I) Hunter syndrome (type II) Morquio syndrome (type IV); types A and B	Frequent; aortic and/or mitral regurgitation, coronary artery disease	Coarse features, large tongue, depressed nasal bridge, kyphosis, retarded growth, hepatomegaly, corneal opacity (not in Hunter's syndrome), mental retardation; most patients die by 10 to 20 yr of age	AR (I) 4p16.3 XR (II) Xq28 AR (IV) 16q24.3 (A) 3p22.3 (B)

Continued

TABLE 2.1 Major Syndromes Associated with Cardiovascular Abnormalities—cont'd

Disorder	Cardiovascular Abnormalities: Frequency and Types	Major Features	Etiology
Muscular dystrophy (Duchenne type)	Frequent; cardiomyopathy, PVC	Waddling gait, "pseudohypertrophy" of calf muscle	XR; Xp21.2-p21.1
Neurofibromatosis (von Recklinghausen disease; NF type 1)	Occasional; PS, COA, pheo-chromocytoma	Cafe-au-lait spots, multiple neurofibroma, acoustic neuroma (type 2), variety of bone lesions	AD; 30%–50% new mutations; 17q11.2
Noonan syndrome (Turner-like syndrome)	Frequent; PS (dystrophic pulmonary valve), LVH (or anterior septal hypertrophy)	Similar to Turner syndrome but may occur both in males and females, without chromosomal abnormality	Usually sporadic; AD 12q24.13 (~50%)
Pierre Robin sequence	Occasional; VSD, PDA; less commonly ASD, COA, TOF	Micrognathia, glossoptosis, cleft soft palate	Usually sporadic
Osler-Rendu-Weber syndrome (hereditary hemorrhagic telangiectasia)	Occasional; pulmonary arteriovenous fistula	Hepatic involvement, telangiectases, hemangioma or fibrosis	AD
Osteogenesis imperfecta	Occasional; aortic dilatation, aortic regurgitation, MVP	Excessive bone fragility with deformities of skeleton, blue sclera, hyperlaxity of joints	AD or AR
Progeria (Hutchinson-Gilford syndrome)	Accelerated atherosclerosis	Alopecia, atrophy of subcutaneous fat, skeletal hypoplasia and dysplasia	Mutations in 1q22; AD
Rubella syndrome	Frequent (>95%); PDA and PA stenosis	Triad of the syndrome: deafness, cataract, and CHDs; others include intrauterine growth retardation, microcephaly, microphthalmia, hepatitis, neonatal thrombocytopenic purpura	Maternal rubella infection during the first trimester
Rubinstein-Taybi syndrome	Occasional (25%); PDA, VSD, ASD	Broad thumbs or toes; hypoplastic maxilla with narrow palate; beaked nose; short stature; mental retardation	Sporadic; 16p13.3 deletion
Smith-Lemli-Opitz syndrome	Occasional; VSD, PDA, others	Broad nasal tip with anteverted nostrils; ptosis of eyelids; syndactyly of second and third toes; short stature; mental retardation	AR; mutations in 11q13.4
Thrombocytopenia-absent radius (TAR) syndrome	Occasional (30%); TOF, ASD, dextrocardia	Thrombocytopenia, absent or hypoplastic radius, normal thumb; "leukemoid" granulocytosis and eosinophilia	AR; deletion of 1q21.1
Treacher Collins syndrome	Occasional; VSD, PDA, ASD	Underdeveloped lower jaw and zygomatic bone; defects of lower eyelids with downslanting palpebral fissure; malformation of auricle or ear canal defect; cleft palate	60% new mutation; AD
Trisomy 13 syndrome (Patau's syndrome)	Very common (80%); VSD, PDA, dextrocardia	Low birth weight, central facial anomalies, polydactyly, chronic hemangiomas, low-set ears, visceral and genital anomalies	Trisomy 13
Trisomy 18 syndrome (Edward syndrome)	Very common (90%); VSD, PDA, PS	Low birth weight, microcephaly, micrognathia, rocker-bottom feet, closed fist with overlapping fingers	Trisomy 18
Tuberous sclerosis	Frequent; rhabdomyoma	Triad of adenoma sebaceum (2–5 yr of age), seizures, and mental defect; cyst-like lesions in phalanges and elsewhere; fibrous-angiomatosus lesions (83%) with varying colors in nasolabial fold, cheeks, and elsewhere	AD; two thirds new mutations
Turner syndrome (XO syndrome)	Frequent (35%); COA, bicuspid aortic valve, AS; hypertension, aortic dissection later in life	Short female; broad chest with widely spaced nipples; congenital lymphedema with residual puffiness over the dorsum of fingers and toes (80%)	XO with 45 chromosomes
VATER association (VATER or VACTERL syndrome)	Common (>50%); VSD, other defects	Vertebral anomalies, anal atresia, congenital heart defects, tracheoesophageal (TE) fistula, renal dysplasia, limb anomalies (e.g., radial dysplasia)	Sporadic

TABLE 2.1   **Major Syndromes Associated with Cardiovascular Abnormalities—cont'd**

Disorder	Cardiovascular Abnormalities: Frequency and Types	Major Features	Etiology
Velocardiofacial syndrome (Sprintzen syndrome; part of 22q11.2 deletion syndrome)	Very common (85%); truncus arteriosus, TOF, pulmonary atresia with VSD, interrupted aortic arch type B, VSD, and TGA	Structural or functional palatal abnormalities, unique facial characteristics ("elfin facies" with auricular abnormalities, prominent nose with squared nasal root and narrow alar base, vertical maxillary excess with long face), hypernasal speech, conductive hearing loss, hypotonia, developmental delay and learning disability	AD; microdeletion of 22q11.2
Williams syndrome	Frequent; supravalvular AS, PA stenosis, renal artery stenosis	Varying degree of mental retardation, so-called "elfin" facies (consisting of some of the following: upturned nose, flat nasal bridge, long philtrum, flat malar area, wide mouth, full lips, widely spaced teeth, periorbital fullness); hypercalcemia of infancy?	Sporadic; 7q23 deletion
Zellweger syndrome (cerebro-hepato-renal syndrome)	Frequent; PDA, VSD or ASD	Hypotonia, high forehead with flat facies, hepatomegaly, albuminemia	AR; multiple genes

±, May or may not be present; *AD,* autosomal dominant; *AR,* autosomal recessive; *AS,* aortic stenosis; *ASD,* atrial septal defect; *CHD,* congenital heart disease; *COA,* coarctation of the aorta; *ECD,* endocardial cushion defect; *ECG,* electrocardiogram; *FBS,* fasting blood sugar; *GTT,* glucose tolerance test; *HOCM,* hypertrophic obstructive cardiomyopathy; *LVH,* left ventricular hypertrophy; *MVP,* mitral valve prolapse; *PA,* pulmonary artery; *PDA,* patent ductus arteriosus; *PPHN,* persistent pulmonary hypertension of newborn; *PS,* pulmonary stenosis; *TGA,* transposition of the great arteries; *TOF,* tetralogy of Fallot; *VSD,* ventricular septal defect; *XR,* sex-linked recessive.

TABLE 2.2   **Prevalence of Associated Congenital Heart Defects in Patients with Other System Malformation**

Organ System and Malformation	Frequency (Range) (%)	Specific Cardiac Defects
CENTRAL NERVOUS SYSTEM		
Hydrocephalus	6 (4.5–14.9)	VSD, ECD, TOF
Dandy-Walker syndrome	3 (2.5–4.3)	VSD
Agenesis of corpus callosum	15	No specific defects
Meckel-Gruber syndrome	14	No specific defects
THORACIC CAVITY		
TE fistula or esophageal atresia	21 (15–39)	VSD, ASD, TOF
Diaphragmatic hernia	11 (9.6–22.9)	No specific defects
GASTROINTESTINAL		
Duodenal atresia	17	No specific defects
Jejunal atresia	5	No specific defects
Anorectal anomalies	22	No specific defects
Imperforate anus	12	TOF, VSD
VENTRAL WALL		
Omphalocele	21 (19–32)	No specific defects
Gastroschisis	3 (0–7.7)	No specific defects
GENITOURINARY		
Renal agenesis		
Bilateral	43	No specific defects
Unilateral	17	No specific defects
Horseshoe kidney	39	No specific defects
Renal dysplasia	5	No specific defects

ASD, Atrial septal defect; *ECD,* endocardial cushion defect; *TE,* trachea-esophageal; *TOF,* tetralogy of Fallot; *VSD,* ventricular septal defect.
Modified from Copel JA, Kleinman CS: Congenital heart disease and extracardiac anomalies: association and indications for fetal echocardiography, *Am J Obstet Gynecol* 154:1121, 1986.

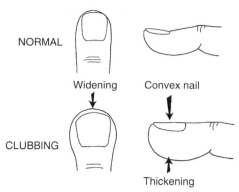

NORMAL

Widening   Convex nail

CLUBBING

Thickening

Fig. 2.1 Diagram of normal and clubbed fingers.

Acanthosis Nigricans

Acanthosis nigricans is a dark pigmentation of skin creases most commonly seen on the neck in the majority of obese children and those with type 2 diabetes. It is also found in the axillae, groins, and inner thighs and on the belt line of the abdomen. The affected skin can become thickened. This condition is associated with insulin resistance and it eventually causes type 2 diabetes. Rarely, acanthosis occurs in patients with Addison disease, Cushing syndrome, polycystic ovary syndrome (Stein-Leventhal syndrome), hypothyroidism, and hyperthyroidism. This condition is associated with insulin resistance and a higher risk of developing type 2 diabetes.

Inspection of the Chest

Precordial bulge, with or without actively visible cardiac activity, suggests chronic cardiac enlargement. Acute dilatation of the heart does not cause precordial bulge. Pigeon chest (pectus carinatum), in which the sternum protrudes on the midline, is usually not a result of cardiomegaly.

Pectus excavatum (undue depression of the sternum) rarely, if ever, causes significant cardiac embarrassment. Occasionally, it may be a cause of a pulmonary systolic murmur or a large cardiac silhouette on a posteroanterior view of a chest radiograph, which compensates for the diminished anteroposterior diameter of the chest. As a group, children with a significant pectus excavatum have a shorter endurance time than normal children.

Harrison's groove, a line of depression in the bottom of the rib cage along the attachment of the diaphragm, indicates poor lung compliance of long duration, such as that seen in large left-to-right shunt lesions.

PALPATION

Palpation should include the peripheral pulses (their presence or absence, the pulse rate, the volume of the pulses) and the precordium (the presence of a thrill, the point of maximal impulse [PMI], precordial hyperactivity). Although ordinarily palpation follows inspection, auscultation may be more fruitful on a sleeping infant who might wake up and become uncooperative.

Peripheral Pulses

1. The physician should count the pulse rate and note any irregularities in the rate and volume. The normal pulse rate varies with the patient's age and status. The younger the patient, the faster the pulse rate. Increased pulse rate may indicate excitement, fever, CHF, or arrhythmia. Bradycardia may mean heart block, effects of drugs, and so on. Irregularity of the pulse suggests arrhythmias, but sinus arrhythmia (an acceleration with inspiration) is normal.

2. The right and left arm and an arm and a leg should be compared for the volume of the pulse. Every patient should have palpable pedal pulses of the dorsalis pedis, tibialis posterior, or both. It is often easier to feel pedal pulses than femoral pulses. Attempts at palpating a femoral pulse often wake up a sleeping infant or upset a toddler. If a good pedal pulse is felt, coarctation of the aorta (COA) is effectively ruled out, especially if the blood pressure (BP) in the arm is normal.

3. Weak leg pulses and strong arm pulses suggest COA. If the right brachial pulse is stronger than the left brachial pulse, the cause may be COA occurring near the origin of the left subclavian artery or supravalvular aortic stenosis (AS). A weaker right brachial pulse than the left suggests aberrant right subclavian artery arising distal to the coarctation.

4. Bounding pulses are found in aortic run-off lesions such as PDA, aortic regurgitation (AR), large systemic arteriovenous fistula, or persistent truncus arteriosus (rarely). Pulses are bounding in premature infants because of the lack of subcutaneous tissue and because many have PDA.

5. Weak, thready pulses are found in cardiac failure or circulatory shock or in the leg of a patient with COA. A systemic-to-pulmonary artery (PA) shunt (either classic Blalock-Taussig shunt or modified Gore-Tex shunt) or subclavian flap angioplasty for repair of COA may result in an absent or weak pulse in the arm affected by surgery. Arterial injuries resulting from previous cardiac catheterization may cause a weak pulse in the affected limb.

6. Pulsus paradoxus (paradoxical pulse) is suspected when there is marked variation in the volume of arterial pulses with the respiratory cycle. The term *pulsus paradoxus* does *not* indicate a phase reversal; rather, it is an exaggeration of normal reduction of systolic pressure during inspiration. When arterial BP is being monitored through an indwelling arterial catheter, the presence of pulsus paradoxus is easily detected by a wide swing (>10 mm Hg) in arterial pressure. In a child without arterial pressure monitoring, accurate evaluation requires sphygmomanometry (Fig. 2.2). Pulsus paradoxus may be associated with cardiac tamponade secondary to pericardial effusion or constrictive pericarditis or to severe respiratory difficulties seen with asthma or pneumonia. It is also seen in patients who are on ventilators with high pressure settings, but in these cases, the BP increases with inflation.

The presence of pulsus paradoxus is confirmed by the use of a sphygmomanometer as described below.

a. The cuff pressure is raised about 20 mm Hg above the systolic pressure.

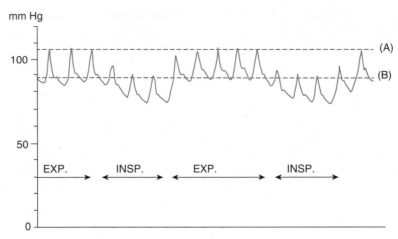

Fig. 2.2 Diagram of pulsus paradoxus. Note the reduction in systolic pressure of more than 10 mm Hg during inspiration. *EXP,* Expiration; *INSP,* inspiration.

b. The pressure is lowered slowly until Korotkoff sound 1 is heard for some but not all cardiac cycles, and the reading is noted (line A on Fig. 2.2).

c. The pressure is lowered further until systolic sounds are heard for all cardiac cycles, and the reading is noted (line B on Fig. 2.2).

d. If the difference between readings A and B is greater than 10 mm Hg, pulsus paradoxus is present.

Chest

One should palpate the following on the chest: apical impulse, PMI, hyperactivity of the precordium, and palpable thrill.

Apical Impulse

Palpation of the apical impulse is usually superior to percussion in the detection of cardiomegaly. Its location and diffuseness should be noted. Percussion in infants and children is inaccurate and adds little. The apical impulse is normally at the fifth intercostal space in the midclavicular line after age 7 years. Before this age, the apical impulse is in the fourth intercostal space just to the left of the midclavicular line. An apical impulse displaced laterally or downward suggests cardiac enlargement.

Point of Maximal Impulse

The PMI is helpful in determining whether the RV or left ventricle (LV) is dominant. With RV dominance, the impulse is maximal at the lower left sternal border or over the xiphoid process; with LV dominance, the impulse is maximal at the apex. Normal newborns and infants have RV dominance and therefore more RV impulse than older children. If the impulse is more diffuse and slow rising, it is called a *heave.* If it is well localized and sharp rising, it is called a *tap.* Heaves are often associated with volume overload. Taps are associated with pressure overload.

Hyperactive Precordium

The presence of a hyperactive precordium characterizes heart disease with volume overload, such as that seen in defects with large left-to-right shunts (e.g., PDA, VSD) or heart disease with severe valvular regurgitation (e.g., AR, mitral regurgitation [MR]).

Thrills

Thrills are vibratory sensations that represent palpable manifestations of loud, harsh murmurs. Palpation for thrills is often of diagnostic value. A thrill on the chest is felt better with the palm of the hand than with the tips of the fingers. However, the fingers are used to feel a thrill in the suprasternal notch and over the carotid arteries.

1. Thrills in the upper left sternal border originate from the pulmonary valve or PA and therefore are present in PS, PA stenosis, or PDA (rarely).
2. Thrills in the upper right sternal border are usually of aortic origin and are seen in AS.
3. Thrills in the lower left sternal border are characteristic of a VSD.
4. Thrills in the suprasternal notch suggest AS but may be found in PS, PDA, or COA.
5. The presence of a thrill over the carotid artery or arteries accompanied by a thrill in the suprasternal notch suggests diseases of the aorta or aortic valve (e.g., COA, AS). An isolated thrill in one of the carotid arteries without a thrill in the suprasternal notch may be a carotid bruit.
6. Thrills in the intercostal spaces are found in older children with severe COA and extensive intercostal collaterals.

BLOOD PRESSURE MEASUREMENT

Whenever possible, every child should have his or her BP measured as part of the physical examination. The status of the child at the time of BP measurement, such as moving, crying, or fighting, should be considered in the interpretation of obtained BP values before making any decision about the normalcy of the measurement. When BP is measured in a reasonably quiet situation, an average value of 2 or more BP values is compared with a set of normative BP standards to see if obtained BP values are normal or abnormal. Unfortunately, there have been multiples problems regarding the proper method of measuring BP as well as the normative BP standards for children.

Scientifically unsound methods of BP measurement using arm length-based BP cuffs, recommended by two previous National Institute of Health (NIH) Task Forces (of 1977 and 1987), have dominated the field and they have been the source of confusion for several decades. At this time, both the methodology and the BP standards recommended by the NIH Task Forces have been abandoned. An unfortunate part of these wrong recommendations was that most children's BP studies were carried out using wrong BP cuffs selected based on the length of the arm. In addition, the new sets of normative BP standards recommended by the Working Group of the National High Blood Pressure Education Program (NHBPEP) have major flaws scientifically and statistically and their usefulness has become debatable.

In this subsection, the following important issues in children's BP measurement will be discussed.

   a. What is the currently recommended BP measuring method?

   b. How good are BP standards recommended by the NHBPEP?

   c. Which normal BP standards should be used and why?

   d. How accurate are oscillometric BP measurements?

   e. Comparison of BP readings by oscillometric device and those by the auscultatory method

   f. How to interpret arm and leg BP values in children

   g. BP levels in neonates and small children

   h. How important is the concept of peripheral amplification of systolic pressure?

   i. Need for simplified BP tables

1. What is the currently recommended BP measuring method?

In the recent past, two Task Forces (1977 and 1987) of the NIH have recommended BP cuff selection based on the length of the arm, initially recommending the cuff width to be two thirds of the length of the arm and later changing it to three fourths of the length of the arm. The BP cuff selection based on the length of the arm is scientifically unsound and violates the physical principles underlying indirect BP measurement. The NIH Task Forces have provided normal BP standards based on these unscientific methods.

As early as 1901, von Recklinghausen recognized the importance of the width of the BP cuff in relation to the arm circumference. For adults, the correct BP cuff width has been settled as 40% of the circumference of the arm since 1951 by the recommendations of the American Heart Association (AHA) (Fig. 2.3). It made no sense to choose the BP cuff based on the arm length in children. Park and Guntheroth (1970) compared directly measured brachial artery pressure during cardiac catheterization and the arm BP measured using the cuff width 40% of the arm circumference and concluded that the same 40% arm circumference criterion was good for children. In 1988, the AHA's Special Task Force accepted the 40% cuff selection method for children, but the two past NIH Task Forces did not change their recommendations. In 2004, however, the Working Group of the NHBPEP has accepted the correct BP cuff selection method based on the arm circumference.

The following summarizes current views on BP measurement techniques recommended by the AHA and the NHBPEP.

   a. Both the AHA and the NHBPEP recommend the BP cuff width to be 40% of the circumference (equivalent to 125% of the diameter) of the arm with the cuff long enough to completely or nearly completely encircle the extremity. The cuff should be at least 40% of the arm circumference. When a 40% cuff is not available, it is better to choose one size bigger than the ideal one. One size smaller than the ideal cuff (i.e., 31%–35% arm circumference) gave readings much higher than the reference values (15 mm Hg higher for systolic pressure and 11 mm Hg higher for diastolic pressure). Conversely, one size larger cuff (i.e., 43%–48%) resulted in relatively smaller changes in BP readings (6 mm Hg lower for systolic pressure and 3 mm Hg lower for diastolic pressure) (Park et al, 1976).

   b. The NHBPEP recommends Korotkoff phase 5 (K5) as the diastolic pressure, but the AHA recommends K4 as the diastolic pressure; some earlier studies showed better agreement between K4 and direct intraarterial diastolic pressure in children.

   c. Both the AHA and the NHBPEP recommend averaging of 2 or more readings (because the averaged values are closer to the basal BP level and are more reproducible).

   d. Both the AHA and the NHBPEP recommend sitting position with the arm at the heart level.

2. How good are BP standards recommended by the NHB-PEP?

Normative BP standards recommended by the Working Group of the NHBPEP are not as good as it was made to believe; they have major flaws as described below.

   a. Although the Working Group recommended the BP cuff to be 40% of the circumference of the arm, the BP data comprising their standards were not obtained by the currently recommended method. The majority of the original data were obtained by the arm length–based cuff selection method. These values are also from single measurement, rather than the averages of 2 or more readings, as currently recommended. In other words, the original source of the elaborate BP standards of the Working Group is one that has been abandoned by the program itself.

   b. Expressing children's BP levels by age and height percentiles is statistically unsound. Height has no statistically important role in children's BP levels (Park, et al, 2001). Partial correlation analysis used in the San Antonio Children's Blood Pressure Study (the San Antonio Study) shows that when auscultatory BP levels were adjusted for age and weight, the correlation coefficient of systolic pressure with height was very small (r = 0.068 for boys; r = 0.072 for girls), but when adjusted for age and height, the correlation of systolic pressure with weight remained high (r = 0.343 for boys; r = 0.294 for girls). These findings indicate that the contribution of height to BP levels is negligible. The apparent

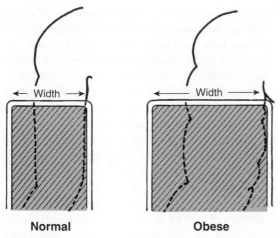

Fig. 2.3 Diagram showing a method of selecting an appropriate-sized blood pressure cuff based on the arm diameter. The cuff should be at least 40% (to 45%) of the arm circumference but less than 50%. The cuff width 125% of the arm diameter equals to 40% of the arm circumference: the cuff width approximately 140% of the arm diameter equals to 45% of the circumference. Therefore, one should aim for a cuff width between 125% and 140% of the arm diameter as shown.

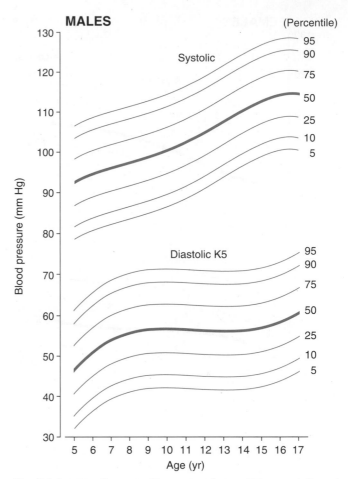

Fig. 2.4 Age-specific percentile curves of auscultatory systolic and diastolic (K5) pressures in boys 5 to 17 years of age. Blood pressure values are the average of three readings. The width of the blood pressure cuff was 40% (up to 50%) of the circumference of the arm. Percentile values for the figure are shown in Table B.3, Appendix B. (From Park MK, Menard SW, Yuan C: Comparison of blood pressure in children from three ethnic groups, *Am J Cardiol* 87:1305–1308, 2001.)

correlation of height to BP levels may all be secondary to a close correlation that exists between height and weight (r = 0.86). A similar conclusion was reached with oscillometric BP levels in the San Antonio study. Although weight is a very important contributor to BP, weight cannot be used as a second variable because this would interfere with detection of high BP in obese children. Thus, we found no rationale to use anything other than age and gender to express children's normative BP standards.

c. Requiring additional computations to find the height percentile of a child, especially on such highly variable office BP readings, is not only unreasonable and but also unjustified. Height has no statistical importance in children's BP readings.

d. The Working Group does not point out that the auscultatory and oscillometric BP readings are not interchangeable. The San Antonio Study, in which both auscultatory and oscillometric methods were used, found that oscillometric systolic pressures are significantly higher than auscultatory BP readings and thus they are not interchangeable (see later for further details). This finding is important in view of popular use of oscillometric device in BP measurements in pediatric practice.

3. Which normal BP standards should be used and why?

a. The BP standards of the NHBPEP are not acceptable standards because they are riddled with major flaws as discussed earlier. However, the NHBPEP's normative BP standards are presented in Appendix B for the sake of completeness (Tables B.1 and B.2, Appendix B).

b. Normative BP percentile values from the San Antonio Study are recommended as a better alternative to BP standards of the NHBPEP. The BP data from the San Antonio Study are the only available BP standards that have been obtained according to the currently recommended method. In the San Antonio Study, BP readings were obtained in more than 7000 school children of three ethnic groups (African American, Mexican American, and non-Hispanic white), enrolled in kindergarten through the 12th grade in the San Antonio, Texas, area. Both the auscultatory and oscillometric (model Dinamap 8100) methods were used in the study, and the data were the averages of three readings. No consistent ethnic difference was found among the three ethnic groups, but there were important gender differences. Therefore, auscultatory BP data were expressed according to age and gender (Park et al, 2001) (Figs. 2.4 and 2.5). Percentile BP values for these figures are presented in Appendix B (Tables B.3 and B.4).

c. When BP is measured using an oscillometric device, one should use a device-specific normative BP standards. The San Antonio Study found that the readings by auscultatory method and by Dinamap 8100 are

FEMALES

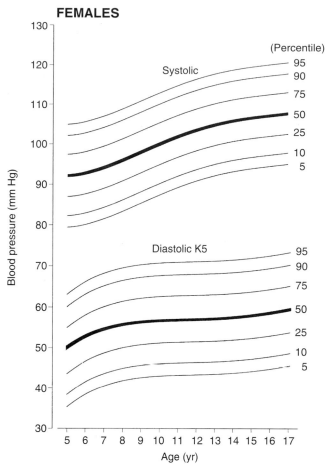

Fig. 2.5 Age-specific percentile curves of auscultatory systolic and diastolic (K5) pressures in girls 5 to 17 years of age. Blood pressure values are the average of three readings. The width of the blood pressure cuff was 40% (up to 50%) of the circumference of the arm. Percentile values for the figure are shown in Table B.4, Appendix B. (From Park MK, Menard SW, Yuan C: Comparison of blood pressure in children from three ethnic groups, *Am J Cardiol* 87:1305–1308, 2001.)

significantly different and thus are not interchangeable (Park et al, 2005) as will be described further. The San Antonio Study provides oscillometric specific BP standards for children. Percentile BP values by an oscillometric method (Dinamap 8100) are presented in Appendix B (Tables B.6 and B.7).

4. How accurate are oscillometric BP measurements?

The accuracy of indirect BP measurement by an oscillometric method (Dinamap Model 1846) has been demonstrated. In fact, oscillometric BP levels correlated better with intra-arterial pressures than the auscultatory method (Park et al, 1987). The oscillometric method also provides some advantages over auscultation; it eliminates observer-related variations, and it can be successfully used in infants and small children. Auscultatory BP measurement in small infants is not only difficult to obtain but also has not been shown to be accurate. Percentile values of normative oscillometric BPs in neonates and children up to 5 years of age are presented in Appendix B (Table B.5). Aside from the issue of accuracy, the oscillometric method is widely used in large pediatric and

pediatric cardiology practices and in the setting of emergency departments. One caution is that not all oscillometric devices in clinical use have been validated for their accuracy.

5. Comparison of BP readings by oscillometric device and those by the auscultatory method

In the San Antonio Study, we used both the auscultatory and oscillometric methods to obtain BP readings in children, alternating the device used, under exactly the same protocol. We found that BP levels obtained by the Dinamap (Model 8100) were on average 10 mm Hg higher than the auscultatory method for the systolic pressure and 5 mm Hg higher for the diastolic pressure (Park et al, 2001). This study, however, does not show superiority of any one of the devices but simply indicates that the indirect BP readings are different according to the sensitivity of the detection device used. It may imply that the detection of oscillation by the machine occurs earlier (at a higher level of systolic pressure) than sounds that human ears can hear. The gold standard remains an intraarterial BP reading. It is clear from this study that the auscultatory and the Dinamap BPs are not interchangeable. When oscillometric method is used, one must use oscillometric specific normative BP standards (Park et al, 2005). Dinamap 8100 specific BP standards are presented in Appendix B (Tables B.6 and B.7).

6. How to interpret arm and leg BP values in children

Four-extremity BP measurements are often obtained to rule out COA. The same cuff selection criterion (i.e., 40% of the circumference) applies for calf or thigh pressure determination, often requiring the use of a larger cuff for the lower extremity. The patient should be in supine position for BP measurements in the arm and leg. When using the auscultatory method, the thigh pressure is obtained with the stethoscope place in the popliteal fossa (over the popliteal artery) with the legs bent and in supine position. Calf BP is difficult to obtain by the auscultatory method.

How do BP levels in the arm and leg compare in normal children? Even when a considerably wider cuff is selected for the thigh, the Dinamap systolic pressure in the thigh or calf is about 5 to 10 mm Hg higher than that in the arm (Park et al, 1993). This partly reflects the peripheral amplification of systolic pressure (see later for further discussion). In newborns, however, the systolic pressures in the arm and the calf are the same (Park et al, 1989). The absence of a higher systolic pressure in the leg in newborns may be related to the presence of normally narrow segment of the aortic isthmus. Thus, the systolic pressure in the thigh (or calf) should be higher than or at least equal to that in the arm, except in newborns. If the systolic pressure is lower in the leg, COA may be present. Leg BP determinations are mandatory in a child with hypertension in the arm to rule out COA. The presence of a femoral pulse does not rule out a coarctation.

7. BP levels in neonates and small children

Blood pressure measurement is important in newborns and small children to diagnose COA, hypertension, or hypotension. In contrast to the recommendations of the NHBEP, the auscultatory method is difficult to apply in newborns and small children because of weak Korotkoff sounds in

TABLE 2.3	Normative Blood Pressure Levels by Dinamap Monitor in Children Age 5 Years and Younger[a]		
Age	Mean BP Levels (mm Hg)	90th Percentile	95th Percentile
1–3 days	64/41 (50)	75/49 (50)	78/52 (62)
1 mo–2 yr	95/58 (72)	106/68 (83)	110/71 (86)
2–5 yr	101/57 (74)	112/66 (82)	115/68 (85)

[a]Dinamap Model 1846SX was used. Blood pressure (BP) levels are systolic/diastolic, with the mean in parentheses.
Modified from Park MK, Menard SM: Normative oscillometric blood pressure values in the first 5 years in an office setting, *Am J Dis Child* 143:860, 1989.

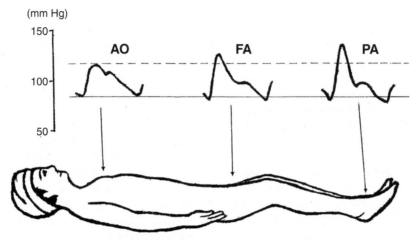

Fig. 2.6 Schematic diagram of pulse wave changes at different levels of the systemic arteries. *AO,* Aorta; *FA,* femoral artery; *PA,* pedal artery. (Modified from Geddes LA: *Handbook of Blood Pressure Measurement,* Clifton, NJ, 1991, Humana Press.)

these age groups, and thus normative standards are not reliable. Therefore, the oscillometric method is frequently used instead. Abbreviated normative Dinamap BP standards for newborns and small children (5 years of age and younger) are presented in Table 2.3. Full percentile values are presented in Appendix B (Table B.5).

8. How important is the concept of peripheral amplification of systolic pressure?

Many physicians incorrectly assume that peripherally measured BPs, such as those measured in the arm, reflect central aortic pressure. Some physicians also incorrectly think that the systolic pressure in the central aorta is higher than that in the brachial, radial, and pedal arteries. As shown schematically in Figure 2.6, systolic pressure becomes higher and higher as one moves farther peripherally, although the diastolic and mean pressures remain the same or decrease slightly (O'Rourke, 1968). This phenomenon is known as peripheral amplification of systolic pressure. If this is correct, how does blood flow distally? There is a change in the arterial pressure wave form with systolic peaking as one moves peripherally as shown in Figure 2.6, but the area under the curve decreases slightly in the peripheral sites, so that the blood flows peripherally.

The main purpose of measuring indirect BP is to estimate the pressure in the central aorta, the perfusing pressure for the brain and the heart. Systolic pressures measured, either by direct or indirect methods, do not always reflect the central aortic pressure. Peripherally obtained systolic pressures are usually higher than the central aortic pressure but the magnitude of difference is not easy to predict. Physicians should be aware of some clinically important situations, in which the peripheral amplification becomes more marked.

The following are some key points of the peripheral amplification of clinical significance.

1. The systolic amplification is greater in children (with more reactive arteries) than in older adults (who may have degenerative arterial disease).
   b. The amplification is more marked in vasoconstricted states, and many of them are clinically important, such as those seen (a) with impending circulatory shock from hemorrhage or dehydration, (b) in a child in CHF (in which generalized peripheral vasoconstriction is present), and (c) in patients receiving catecholamine infusion or other vasoconstrictors in the setting of critical care units.
   c. Reduced level of peripheral amplification of systolic pressure is noted in vasodilated states, such as those seen in subjects receiving vasodilators and after receiving a contrast dye (which has vasodilating effects) during cardiac catheterization.

At sites other than the upper arm, systolic pressure may be significantly higher than that in the central aorta. Although the systolic pressure in the arm tends to be slightly higher than that in the central aorta, the upper arm is the only place where the systolic amplification is smallest. Radial artery pressure is likely to be significantly higher than the brachial artery pressure. The following lists two clinically important examples.

a. Arm systolic pressure in subjects running on treadmill can be markedly higher than the central aortic pressure. A dramatic illustration of this phenomenon is shown in Figure 6.1 (in the section on exercise stress testing) in a young adult running on treadmill with catheters in the ascending aorta and the radial artery. At rest, the difference in systolic pressure between the two sites is about 30 mm Hg. At the last stage of the stress test, the difference increases further to 76 mm Hg, with the radial artery pressure reaching a state known as hypertensive emergency. Even in the setting of an intensive care unit, one should avoid using peripheral lines such as the radial artery if the pressure monitoring is the main purpose of the line; the mean pressure may be better than the systolic pressure in such a situation.

b. Nice-looking wrist BP devices are on the market. These devices are likely to give higher BP readings than the upper arm device, depending on the condition of the patient. Therefore, BP should not be obtained in the wrist.

9. Need for simplified BP tables

The main reason for measuring BP routinely is to identify those children with hypertension or those at risk of developing hypertension. Even though the BP standards from the San Antonio Study are simple enough to use, it is still time consuming to check the complete table in busy practice.

In 2009, Kaelber and Picket proposed a simple table of BP levels, without height percentiles, that may require attention or additional investigation being at "elevated blood pressure levels" (formerly called prehypertensive levels). Elevated BP is defined as BP levels between the 90th and 95th percentiles for children and 120 to 129 systolic and 80 mm Hg diastolic for adolescents (older than 13 years of age) and adults. We followed suit and developed similar tables of the 90th percentile values for both auscultatory and oscillometric BP for children based on the San Antonio Study (Table 2.4). It is interesting to find that the values suggested by Kaelber and Picket agree very closely with the 90th percentile values in the San Antonio Study. All one needs is this single page table posted on the wall of the BP room.

AUSCULTATION

Although auscultation of the heart requires more skill, it also provides more valuable information than other methods of physical examination. Whereas the bell-type chest piece is better suited for detecting low-frequency events, the diaphragm selectively picks up high-frequency events. When the bell is firmly pressed against the chest wall, it acts like the diaphragm by filtering out low-frequency sounds or murmurs and picking up high-frequency events. Physicians should ordinarily use both the bell and the diaphragm, although using the bell both lightly and firmly pressed against the chest may be equally effective, especially in sleeping infants. Using only the diaphragm may result in missing some important low-frequency murmurs or sounds, such as mid-diastolic rumble, pulmonary regurgitation (PR) murmur, and faint Still's innocent heart murmurs. One should not limit examination to the four traditional auscultatory areas. The entire precordium, as well as the sides and back of the chest, should be explored with the stethoscope. Systematic attention should be given to the following aspects:

1. Heart rate and regularity: Heart rate and regularity should be noted on every child. Extremely fast or slow heart rates

---

TABLE 2.4 The 90th Percentiles of Blood Pressure by Auscultatory and Oscillometric Methods from the San Antonio Study[a]

| | AUSCULTATORY | | | | | OSCILLOMETRIC | | | |
| Age (yr) | Male | | Female | | Age (yr) | Male | | Female | |
	SP	DP	SP	DP		SP	DP	SP	DP
5	103	60	102	60	5	115	68	114	68
6	105	64	103	63	6	117	68	115	68
7	107	66	104	65	7	118	69	116	69
8	108	68	106	67	8	119	70	118	70
9	109	68	108	67	9	121	70	119	70
10	111	68	110	68	10	122	71	121	71
11	113	68	112	68	11	124	71	122	71
12	116	68	113	68	12	126	71	123	71
13	118	68	115	68	13	129	71	125	71
14	120	68	116	68	14	131	72	125	72
15	120	69	117	69	15	133	72	126	72
16	120	71	117	69	16	134	72	126	72
17	120	73	118	70	17	134	72	126	72
≥18	120	73	120	70					

[a]The 90th percentiles of systolic pressure for males 14 years of age and older are higher than 120 mm Hg in the San Antonio Study, but 120 mm Hg is listed to be consistent with the definition of elevated blood pressure in adults.

DP, Diastolic pressure; *SP,* systolic pressure.

Values are from Park MK, Menard SW, Yuan C: Comparison of blood pressure in children from three ethnic groups, *Am J Cardiol* 87:1305–1308, 2001.

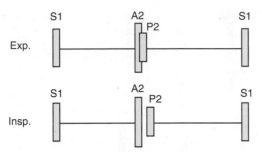

Fig. 2.7 Diagram showing the relative intensity of A2 and P2 and the respiratory variation in the degree of splitting of the S2 at the upper left sternal border (pulmonary area). *Exp,* Expiration; *Insp,* inspiration.

or irregularity in the rhythm should be evaluated by an electrocardiogram (ECG) and a long rhythm strip.

2. Heart sounds: Intensity and quality of the heart sounds, especially the second heart sound (S2), should be evaluated. Abnormalities of the first heart sound (S1) and the third heart sound (S3) and the presence of a gallop rhythm or the fourth sound (S4) should be noted. Muffled heart sounds should also be noted.

3. Systolic and diastolic sounds: An ejection click in early systole provides a clue to aortic or pulmonary valve stenosis. A midsystolic click provides important clues to the diagnosis of mitral valve prolapse (MVP). An opening snap in diastole (present in mitral stenosis [MS]) should be noted, but it is extremely rare in children.

4. Heart murmurs: Heart murmurs should be evaluated in terms of intensity, timing (systolic or diastolic), location, transmission, and quality.

Heart Sounds

The heart sound should be identified and analyzed before the analysis of heart murmurs (Fig. 2.7). Muffled and distant heart sounds are present in pericardial effusion and heart failure.

First Heart Sound

The S1 is associated with closure of the mitral and tricuspid valves. It is best heard at the apex or lower left sternal border. Splitting of the S1 may be found in normal children, but it is infrequent. Abnormally wide splitting of S1 may be found in right bundle branch block (RBBB) or Ebstein's anomaly. Splitting of S1 should be differentiated from ejection click or S4.

1. Ejection click is found in PS and bicuspid aortic valve. In patients with PS, it is easily audible at the upper left sternal border in PS. In bicuspid aortic valve, the click may be louder at the lower left sternal border or apex than at the upper right sternal border.

2. S4 is rare in children.

Second Heart Sound

The S2 in the upper left sternal border (i.e., pulmonary valve area) is of critical importance in pediatric cardiology. The S2 must be evaluated in terms of the degree of splitting and the intensity of the pulmonary closure component of the second

---

BOX 2.1   Summary of Abnormal S2

Abnormal Splitting
Widely split and fixed S2
  Volume overload (e.g., ASD, PAPVR)
  Pressure overload (e.g., PS)
  Electrical delay (e.g., RBBB)
  Early aortic closure (e.g., MR)
  Occasional normal child
Narrowly split S2
  Pulmonary hypertension
  AS
  Occasional normal child
Single S2
  Pulmonary hypertension
  One semilunar valve (e.g., pulmonary atresia, aortic atresia, persistent truncus arteriosus)
  P2 not audible (e.g., TGA, TOF, severe PS)
  Severe AS
  Occasional normal child
Paradoxically split S2
  Severe AS
  LBBB, WPW syndrome (type B)

Abnormal Intensity of P2
  Increased P2 (e.g., pulmonary hypertension)
  Decreased P2 (e.g., severe PS, TOF, TS)

AS, Aortic stenosis; *ASD,* atrial septal defect; *LBBB,* left bundle branch block; *MR,* mitral regurgitation; *PAPVR,* partial anomalous pulmonary venous return; *PS,* pulmonary stenosis; *RBBB,* right bundle branch block; *TGA,* transposition of the great arteries; *TOF,* tetralogy of Fallot; *TS,* tricuspid stenosis; *WPW,* Wolff-Parkinson-White.

---

heart sound (P2) in relation to the intensity of the aortic closure component of the second heart sound (A2). Although best heard with the diaphragm of a stethoscope, both components are readily audible with the bell. Abnormalities of splitting of the S2 and the intensity of the P2 are summarized in Box 2.1.

Splitting of the S2. In every normal child, with the exception of occasional newborns, two components of the S2 should be audible in the upper left sternal border. The first is the A2; the second is the P2. Both components are best heard at the pulmonary valve area (upper left sterna border). The A2 is *not* the second heart sound at the aortic area; rather, it is the first (or aortic closure) component of the second heart sound at the pulmonary area.

Normal Splitting of the S2. The degree of splitting of the S2 varies with respiration, increasing with inspiration and decreasing or becoming single with expiration (see Fig. 2.7). During inspiration, because of a greater negative pressure in the thoracic cavity, there is an increase in systemic venous return to the right side of the heart. This increased volume of blood in the RV prolongs the duration of RV ejection time, which delays the closure of the pulmonary valve, resulting in a wide splitting of the S2. The absence of splitting (i.e., single S2) or a widely split S2 usually indicates an abnormality.

Abnormal Splitting of the S2. Abnormal splitting may be in the form of wide splitting, narrow splitting, a single S2, or paradoxical splitting of the S2 (rarely).

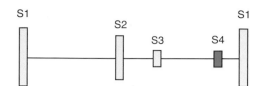

Fig. 2.8 Diagram showing the relative relationship of the heart sounds. The *filled bar* shows an abnormal sound.

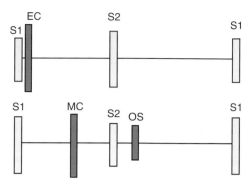

Fig. 2.9 Diagram showing the relative position of ejection click (EC), midsystolic click (MC), and diastolic opening snap (OS). *Filled bars* are abnormal sounds.

1. A widely split and fixed S2 is found in conditions that prolong the RV ejection time or that shorten the LV ejection. Therefore, it is found in:
   a. ASD or partial anomalous pulmonary venous return (PAPVR) (conditions in which the amount of blood ejected by the RV is increased; *volume overload)*
   b. PS (the valve stenosis prolongs the RV ejection time; *pressure overload)*
   c. RBBB (a delay in *electrical* activation of the RV) delays the completion of the RV ejection
   d. MR (a decreased forward output seen in this condition shortens the LV ejection time, causing aortic closure to occur earlier than normal)
   e. An occasional normal child, including "prolonged hangout time" seen in children with dilated PA (a condition called *idiopathic dilatation of the PA*). In dilated PA, the increased capacity of the artery produces less recoil to close the pulmonary valve, which delays closure.
2. A narrowly split S2 is found in conditions in which the pulmonary valve closes early (e.g., pulmonary hypertension) or the aortic valve closure is delayed (e.g., AS). This is occasionally found in a normal child.
3. A single S2 is found in the following situations:
   a. When only one semilunar valve is present (e.g., aortic or pulmonary atresia, persistent truncus arteriosus)
   b. When the P2 is not audible (e.g., transposition of the great arteries [TGA], TOF, severe PS)
   c. When aortic closure is delayed (e.g., severe AS)
   d. When the P2 occurs early (e.g., severe pulmonary hypertension)
   e. In an occasional normal child
4. *A paradoxically split S2* is found when the aortic closure (A2) follows the pulmonary closure (P2) and therefore is seen when the LV ejection is greatly delayed (e.g., severe AS, left bundle branch block [LBBB], sometimes Wolff-Parkinson-White [WPW] pre-excitation).

   Intensity of the P2. The *relative* intensity of the P2 compared with the A2 must be assessed in every child. In the pulmonary area, the A2 is usually louder than the P2 (see Fig. 2.7). Judgment as to normal intensity of the P2 is based on experience. There is no substitute for listening to the hearts of many normal children. Abnormal intensity of the P2 may suggest a pathologic condition. Increased intensity of the P2, compared with that of the A2, is found in pulmonary hypertension. Decreased intensity of the P2 is found in conditions with decreased diastolic pressure of the PA (e.g., severe PS, TOF, tricuspid atresia).

Third Heart Sound

The S3 is a somewhat low-frequency sound in early diastole and is related to rapid filling of the ventricle (Fig. 2.8). It is best heard at the apex or lower left sternal border. It is commonly heard in normal children and young adults. A loud S3 is abnormal and is audible in conditions with dilated ventricles and decreased ventricular compliance (e.g., large-shunt VSD or CHF). When tachycardia is present, it forms a "Kentucky" gallop.

Fourth Heart Sound or Atrial Sound

The S4 is a relatively low-frequency sound of late diastole (i.e., presystole) and is rare in infants and children (see Fig. 2.8). When present, it is always pathologic and is seen in conditions with decreased ventricular compliance or CHF. With tachycardia, it forms a "Tennessee" gallop.

Gallop Rhythm

A gallop rhythm is a rapid triple rhythm resulting from the combination of a loud S3, with or without an S4, and tachycardia. It generally implies a pathologic condition and is commonly present in CHF. A summation gallop represents tachycardia and a superimposed S3 and S4.

Systolic and Diastolic Sounds

1. An ejection click (or ejection sound) is usually caused by thickened semilunar valve leaflets and rarely dilated great arteries. It follows the S1 very closely and occurs at the time of the ventricular ejection's onset. Therefore, it sounds like a splitting of the S1. However, whereas it is usually audible at the base (either side of the upper sternal border), the split S1 is usually audible at the lower left sternal border (exception with an aortic click, discussed in a later section). If the physician hears what sounds like a split S1 at the upper sternal border, it may be an ejection click (Fig. 2.9). The pulmonary click is heard at the second and third left intercostal spaces and changes in intensity with respiration, being louder on expiration. The aortic click is best heard at the second right intercostal space but may be louder at the apex or mid-left sternal border. It usually does not change its intensity with respiration. The ejection click is most often associated with:

a. Stenosis of semilunar valves (e.g., PS or AS)

b. Dilated great arteries, which are seen in systemic or pulmonary hypertension, idiopathic dilatation of the PA, TOF (in which the aorta is dilated), and persistent truncus arteriosus

2. Midsystolic click with or without a late systolic murmur is heard at the apex in mitral valve prolapse (MVP) (see Fig. 2.9 and Chapter 21).

3. Diastolic opening snap is rare in children and is audible at the apex or lower left sternal border. It occurs somewhat earlier than the S3 during diastole and originates from a stenosis of the atrioventricular (AV) valve, such as MS (see Fig. 2.9).

Extracardiac Sounds

1. A pericardial friction rub is a grating, to-and-fro sound produced by friction of the heart against the pericardium. This sounds similar to sandpaper rubbed on wood. Such a sound usually indicates pericarditis. The intensity of the rub varies with the phase of the cardiac cycle rather than the respiratory cycle. It may become louder when the patient leans forward. Large accumulation of fluid (pericardial effusion) may result in disappearance of the rub.

2. A pericardial knock is an adventitious sound associated with chronic (i.e., constrictive) pericarditis. It rarely occurs in children.

Heart Murmurs

Each heart murmur must be analyzed in terms of intensity (grade 1 to 6), timing (systolic or diastolic), location, transmission, and quality (musical, vibratory, blowing, and so on).

Intensity

Intensity of the murmur is customarily graded from 1 to 6.

Grade 1: barely audible
Grade 2: soft but easily audible
Grade 3: moderately loud but not accompanied by a thrill
Grade 4: louder and associated with a thrill
Grade 5: audible with the stethoscope barely on the chest
Grade 6: audible with the stethoscope off the chest

The difference between grades 2 and 3 or grades 5 and 6 may be somewhat subjective. The intensity of the murmur may be influenced by the status of cardiac output. Thus, any factor that increases the cardiac output (e.g., fever, anemia, anxiety, exercise) intensifies any existing murmur or may even produce a murmur that is not audible at basal conditions.

Classification of Heart Murmurs

Based on the timing of the heart murmur in relation to the S1 and S2, the heart murmur is classified into systolic, diastolic, and AV.

Systolic Murmurs

Most heart murmurs are systolic in timing in that they occur between the S1 and S2. Systolic murmurs were classified by Aubrey Leatham in 1958 into two subtypes according to the time of onset: (1) ejection type and (2) regurgitant type (Fig. 2.10). Recently, Joseph Perloff classified systolic murmurs according to their time of onset and termination into four subtypes: (1) midsystolic (or ejection), (2) holosystolic, (3) early systolic, or (4) late systolic (Fig. 2.11). The holosystolic and early systolic murmurs of Perloff belong to the regurgitant murmur of Leatham. The types of murmurs (described earlier) and the location of the maximum intensity of the murmur are very important in the assessment of a systolic murmur. Transmission of the murmur to a particular direction and the quality of the murmur also help in deciding the cause of the murmur. These aspects are discussed in detail later.

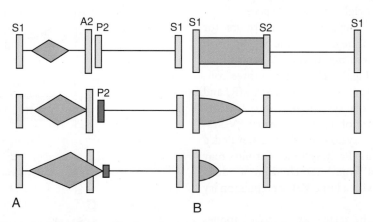

Fig. 2.10 Diagram of Leatham's classification of systolic murmurs. This classification is based primarily on the relationship of the S1 to the onset of the murmur. **A,** Ejection systolic murmurs. Short ejection-type murmur with the apex of the "diamond" in the early part of systole is found with mild stenosis of semilunar valves *(top)*. With increasing severity of stenosis, the murmur becomes louder and longer, and its apex moves toward the S2 *(middle)*. In severe pulmonary stenosis, the murmur is louder and may go beyond the A2 *(bottom)*. **B,** Regurgitant systolic murmurs. A regurgitant systolic murmur is most often caused by ventricular septal defect (VSD) and is usually holosystolic, extending all the way to the S2 *(top)*. The regurgitant murmur may end in middle or early systole (not holosystolic) in some children, especially in those with small-shunt VSD and in some neonates with VSD *(middle and bottom)*. Regardless of the length or intensity of the murmur, all regurgitant systolic murmurs are pathologic.

Types of Systolic Murmurs

1. **Midsystolic (or ejection systolic) murmurs.** A midsystolic murmur (or ejection type murmur) begins after S1 and ends before S2. Midsystolic murmurs coincide with turbulent flow through the semilunar valves and they occur in the following settings: (1) the flow of blood through stenotic or deformed semilunar valves (e.g., AS or PS); (2) accelerated systolic flow through normal semilunar valves, such as seen during pregnancy, fever, anemia, or thyrotoxicosis; and (3) innocent (normal) midsystolic murmurs (see Innocent Heart Murmurs later in this section). There is an interval between the S1 and the onset of the murmur, which coincides with the isovolumic contraction period. The intensity of the murmur increases toward the middle and then decreases during systole (crescendo–decrescendo or diamond shaped in contour). The murmur usually ends before the S2 (see Fig. 2.10A). The murmur may be short or long and is audible at the second left or second right intercostal space.

2. **Holosystolic murmurs.** Holosystolic murmurs begin with S1 and occupy all of systole up to the S2. No gap exists between the S1 and the onset of the murmur. Analysis of the presence or absence of a gap between the S1 and the onset of the systolic murmur is of utmost importance in distinguishing between midsystolic murmurs and holosystolic or early systolic murmurs. Holosystolic and early systolic murmurs of Perloff are regurgitant systolic murmurs of Leatham. The intensity of holosystolic murmurs usually plateaus all the way to the S2. Holosystolic murmurs are caused by the flow of blood from a chamber that is at a higher pressure throughout systole than the receiving chamber, and they usually occur while the semilunar valves are still closed. These murmurs are associated with *only* the following three conditions: VSD, MR, and tricuspid regurgitation (TR). None of these ordinarily occur at the base (i.e., second left or right intercostal space).

3. **Early systolic murmurs.** Early systolic murmurs (or short regurgitant murmurs) begin with the S1, diminish in decrescendo, and end well before the S2, generally at or before midsystole (see Fig. 2.11). Only the three conditions that cause holosystolic murmurs (VSD, MR, and TR) are the causes of an early systolic murmur. An early systolic murmur is a feature of TR with normal RV systolic pressure. When the RV systolic pressure is elevated, a holosystolic murmur results. Early systolic murmurs may occur in a neonate with a large VSD, children or adults with a very small VSD or with a large VSD and pulmonary hypertension.

4. **Late systolic murmurs.** The term "late systolic" applies when a murmur begins in mid- to late systole and proceeds up to the S2 (see Fig. 2.11). The late systolic murmur of mitral valve prolapse is prototypical (see Chapter 21).

Location of Systolic Murmurs

In addition to the type of systolic murmur, the location of maximal intensity of the murmur is important when diagnosing the heart murmur's origin. The following four locations are important: (1) upper left sternal border (pulmonary valve area), (2) upper right sternal border (aortic valve area), (3) lower left sternal border, and (4) apex. For example, a holosystolic murmur heard maximally at the lower left sternal border is characteristic of a VSD. A midsystolic murmur maximally audible at the second left intercostal space is usually pulmonary in origin. The location of the heart murmur often helps differentiate between a midsystolic murmur and a holosystolic murmur. For example, a long PS murmur may sound like the holosystolic murmur of a VSD; however, because the maximal intensity is at the upper left sternal border, it is unlikely that a VSD caused the murmur. Although rare, a subarterial infundibular VSD murmur may be maximally heard at the upper left sternal border. The differential diagnosis of systolic murmurs according to the location is discussed in detail in this section (Tables 2.5 to 2.8; Fig. 2.12).

Transmission of Systolic Murmurs

The transmission of systolic murmurs from the site of maximal intensity may help determine the murmur's origin. For example, an apical systolic murmur that transmits well to the left axilla and lower back is characteristic of MR, but one that radiates to the upper right sternal border and the neck is more likely to originate in the aortic valve. A systolic ejection murmur at the base that transmits well to the neck is more likely to be aortic in origin; one that transmits well to the back is more likely to be of pulmonary valve or PA origin.

Quality of Systolic Murmurs

The quality of a murmur may help diagnose heart disease. Systolic murmurs of MR or of a VSD have a uniform, high-pitched quality, often described as blowing. Midsystolic murmurs of AS or PS have a rough, grating quality. A common

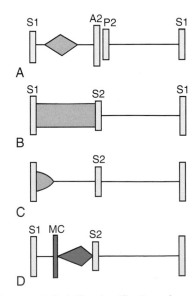

Fig. 2.11 Diagram of Perloff's classification of systolic murmurs. **A,** Midsystolic murmur is the same as ejection systolic murmur of Leatham. Holosystolic (**B**) and early systolic (**C**) murmurs are both regurgitant murmurs of Leatham. **D,** Late systolic murmur is typically audible with mitral valve prolapse.

TABLE 2.5 Differential Diagnosis of Systolic Murmurs at the Upper Left Sternal Border (Pulmonary Area)

Condition	Important Physical Findings	ECG Findings	Chest Radiography Findings
Pulmonary valve stenosis	SEM, grade 2 to 5 of 6 *Thrill (±) S2 may be split widely when mild *Ejection click (±) at 2LICS Transmit to the back	Normal if mild RAD *RVH RAH if severe	*Prominent MPA (poststenotic dilatation) Normal PVM
Atrial septal defect (ASD)	SEM, grade 2 to 3 of 6 *Widely split and fixed S2	RAD RVH *RBBB (rsR′ pattern)	*Increased PVM *RAE, RVE
Pulmonary flow murmur of new-born	SEM, grade 1 to 2 of 6 in newborns No thrill *Good transmission to the back and axilla	Normal	Normal
Pulmonary flow murmur of older children	SEM, grade 2 to 3 of 6 No thrill Poor transmission	Normal	Normal Occasional pectus excavatum or straight back
Pulmonary artery stenosis (PA stenosis)	SEM, grade 2 to 3 of 6 Occasional continuous murmur P2 may be loud *Transmits well to the back and both lung fields	RVH or Normal	Prominent hilar vessels (±)
Aortic stenosis (AS)	SEM, grade 2 to 5 of 6 *Also audible in 2RICS *Thrill (±) at 2RICS and/or SSN *Ejection click at apex, 3LICS, or 2RICS (±) Paradoxically split S2 if severe	Normal or LVH	Absence of prominent MPA Dilated aorta
Tetralogy of Fallot (TOF)	*Long SEM, grade 2 to 4 of 6, louder at MLSB Thrill (±) Loud, single S2 *Cyanosis, clubbing (±)	RAD *RVH or BVH RAH (±)	*Decreased PVM Normal heart size *Boot-shaped heart Right aortic arch (25%)
Coarctation of the aorta (COA)	SEM, grade 1 to 3 of 6 *Loudest at left interscapular area (back) *Weak or absent femorals Hypertension in arms Frequent associated aortic stenosis, bicuspid aortic valve, or MR	LVH in children RBBB (or RVH) in infants	*Classic "3" sign on plain film or "E" sign on barium esoph-agogram Rib notching (±)
Patent ductus arte-riosus (PDA)	*Continuous murmur at left infraclavicular area (grade 2 to 4 of 6) Occasional crescendic systolic only *Bonding pulses, if large Thrill (±)	Normal, LVH, or BVH	*Increased PVM *LAE, LVE
Total anomalous pulmonary venous return (TAPVR)	SEM, grade 2 to 3 of 6 Widely split and fixed S2 (±) *Quadruple or quintuple rhythm *Diastolic rumble at LLSB *Mild cyanosis (↓Po$_2$) and clubbing (±)	RAD RAH *RVH	*Increased PVM RAE and RVE Prominent MPA *"Snowman" sign
Partial anoma-lous pulmonary venous return (PAPVR)	Physical findings similar to those of ASD S2 not fixed unless associated with ASD	Same as in ASD	*Increased PVM *RAE and RVE "Scimitar" sign (±)

*Findings that are characteristic of the condition.

±, May or may not be present; *2LICS*, second left intercostal space; *2RICS*, second right intercostal space; *3LICS*, third left intercostal space; *BVH*, biventricular hypertrophy; *ECG*, electrocardiogram; *LAE*, left atrial enlargement; *LLSB*, lower left sternal border; *LVE*, left ventricular enlarge-ment; *LVH*, left ventricular hypertrophy; *MLSB*, mid-left sternal border; *MPA*, main pulmonary artery; *MR*, mitral regurgitation; *PA*, pulmonary artery; *PVM*, pulmonary vascular markings; *RAD*, right axis deviation; *RAE*, right atrial enlargement; *RAH*, right atrial hypertrophy; *RBBB*, right bundle branch block; *RVE*, right ventricular enlargement; *RVH*, right ventricular hypertrophy; *SEM*, systolic ejection murmur; *SSN*, suprasternal notch; *S2*, second heart sound.

TABLE 2.6 Differential Diagnosis of Systolic Murmurs at the Upper Right Sternal Border (Aortic Area)

Condition	Important Physical Findings	ECG Findings	Chest Radiography Findings
Aortic valve stenosis	SEM, grade 2 to 5 of 6, at 2RICS, may be louder at 3LICS *Thrill (±), URSB, SSN, and carotid arteries *Ejection click *Transmits well to neck S2 may be single	Normal or LVH with or without "strain"	Mild LVE (±) Prominent ascending aorta or aortic knob
Subaortic stenosis	SEM, grade 2 to 4 of 6 *AR murmur may be present in discrete stenosis No ejection click	Normal or LVH	Usually normal
Supravalvular aortic stenosis	SEM, grade 2 to 3 of 6 Thrill (±) No ejection click *Pulse and BP may be greater in right than left arm *Peculiar facies and mental deficiency (±) (Williams syndrome) Murmur may transmit well to the back (PA stenosis)	Normal, LVH, or BVH	Unremarkable

*Findings characteristic and important in the diagnosis of the condition.
+, May or may not be present; *2RICS,* second right intercostal space; *3LICS,* third left intercostal space; *AR,* aortic regurgitation; *BP,* blood pressure; *BVH,* biventricular hypertrophy; *ECG,* electrocardiogram; *LVE,* left ventricular enlargement; *LVH,* left ventricular hypertrophy; *PA,* pulmonary artery; *SEM,* systolic ejection murmur; *SSN,* suprasternal notch; *S2,* second heart sound; *URSB,* upper right sternal border.

TABLE 2.7 Differential Diagnosis of Systolic Murmurs at the Lower Left Sternal Border

Condition	Important Physical Findings	ECG Findings	Chest Radiography Findings
Ventricular septal defect (VSD)	*Regurgitant systolic, grade 2 to 5 of 6 May not be holosystolic Well localized at LLSB *Thrill often present P2 may be loud	Normal LVH or BVH	*Increased PVM *LAE and LVE (cardiomegaly)
Endocardial cushion defect (ECD), complete	Similar to findings of VSD *Diastolic rumble at LLSB *Gallop rhythm common in infants	*Superior QRS axis, LVH or BVH	Similar to large VSD
Vibratory innocent murmur (Still's)	SEM, grade 2 to 3 of 6 *Musical or vibratory with midsystolic accentuation *Maximum between LLSB and apex	Normal	Normal
Hypertrophic obstructive cardiomyopathy (HOCM)	SEM, medium pitched, grade 2 to 4 of 6 Maximum at LLSB or apex Thrill (±) *Sharp upstroke of brachial pulses May have murmur of MR	LVH Abnormally deep Q waves in leads V5 and V6	Normal or globular LVE
Tricuspid regurgitation (TR)	*Regurgitant systolic, grade 2 to 3 of 6 *Triple or quadruple rhythm (in Ebstein's anomaly) Mild cyanosis (±) Hepatomegaly with pulsatile liver and neck vein distention when severe	RBBB, RAH and first-degree AV block in Ebstein's	Normal PVM RAE if severe
Tetralogy of Fallot (TOF)	Murmurs can be louder at ULSB	(see Table 2.5)	(see Table 2.5)

*Findings characteristic and important in the diagnosis of the condition.
±, May or may not be present; *AV,* atrioventricular; *BVH,* biventricular hypertrophy; *ECG,* electrocardiogram; *LAE,* left atrial enlargement; *LLSB,* lower left sternal border; *LVE,* left ventricular enlargement; *LVH,* left ventricular hypertrophy; *MR,* mitral regurgitation; *P2,* pulmonary closure component of the second heart sound; *PVM,* pulmonary vascular markings; *RAE,* right atrial enlargement; *RAH,* right atrial hypertrophy; *RBBB,* right bundle branch block; *SEM,* systolic ejection murmur; *ULSB,* upper left sternal border.

TABLE 2.8 Differential Diagnosis of Systolic Murmurs at the Apex

Condition	Important Physical Findings	ECG Findings	Chest Radiography Findings
Mitral regurgitation (MR)	*Regurgitant systolic, may not be holosystolic, grade 2 to 3 of 6 Transmits to left axilla (less obvious in children) May be loudest in the mid-precordium	LAH and LVH	LAE and LVE
Mitral valve prolapse (MVP)	*Midsystolic click with or without late systolic murmur *High frequency of thoracic skeletal anomalies (pectus excavatum, straight back) (85%)	Inverted T wave in lead aVF	Normal
Aortic valve stenosis	The murmur and ejection click may be best heard at the apex rather than at 2RICS	Normal or LVH with or without "strain"	Mild LVE (±) Prominent ascending aorta or aortic knob
HOCM	The murmur of HOCM may be maximal at the apex (may represent MR)	LVH Abnormally deep Q waves in leads V5 and V6	Normal or globular LVE
Vibratory innocent murmur	This innocent heart murmur may be loudest at the apex (than at the left lower sternal border)	Normal	Normal

*Findings characteristic and important in the diagnosis of the condition.
2RICS, Second right intercostal space; *ECG*, electrocardiogram; *HOCM*, hypertrophic obstructive cardiomyopathy; *LAE*, left atrial enlargement; *LAH*, left atrial hypertrophy; *LVE*, left ventricular enlargement; *LVH*, left ventricular hypertrophy.

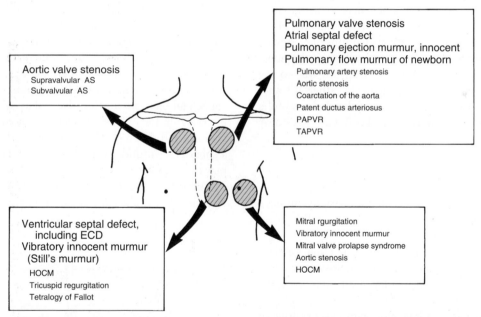

Fig. 2.12 Diagram showing systolic murmurs audible at various locations. Less common conditions are shown in smaller type (see Tables 2.5 to 2.8). *AS*, Aortic stenosis; *ECD*, endocardial cushion defect; *HOCM*, hypertrophic obstructive cardiomyopathy; *PAPVR*, partial anomalous pulmonary venous return; *TAPVR*, total anomalous pulmonary venous return.

innocent murmur in children, which is best audible between the lower left sternal border and apex, has a characteristic "vibratory" or humming quality.

Differential Diagnosis of Systolic Murmurs at Various Locations

Systolic murmurs that are audible at the four locations are presented in Figure 2.12. More common conditions are listed

in larger type and less common conditions in smaller type. For quick reference, characteristic physical, ECG, and radiography findings that are helpful in differential diagnoses are listed in Tables 2.5 through 2.8.

1. **Upper left sternal border (or pulmonary area):** In many conditions, both pathologic and physiologic (i.e., innocent murmur), a systolic murmur is most audible at the upper left sternal border. Audible systolic murmurs at this

location are usually midsystolic murmurs and may be the result of one of the following:

a. PS
b. ASD
c. Innocent (normal) pulmonary flow murmur of newborns
d. Innocent pulmonary flow murmur of older children
e. PA stenosis
f. AS
g. TOF
h. COA
i. PDA with pulmonary hypertension (a continuous murmur of a PDA is usually loudest in the left infraclavicular area)
j. Total anomalous pulmonary venous return (TAPVR)
k. PAPVR

Conditions a through d are more common than the other listed conditions. Table 2.5 summarizes other clinical findings that are useful in the differential diagnosis of systolic murmurs audible at the upper left sternal border.

2. **Upper right sternal border or aortic area:** Systolic murmurs at the upper right sternal border are also midsystolic type. They are all caused by narrowing of the aortic valve or its neighboring vascular structures. The murmur transmits well to the neck. Often it transmits with a thrill over the carotid arteries. The midsystolic murmur of AS may be heard with equal clarity at the upper left sternal border (i.e., "pulmonary area"), as well as at the apex. However, the PS murmur does not transmit well to the upper right sternal border and the neck; rather, it transmits well to the back and the sides of the chest. Systolic murmurs in the upper right sternal border are caused by the following:

a. AS
b. Subvalvular AS (subaortic stenosis)
c. Supravalvular AS

Characteristic physical, ECG, and radiography findings that help in the differential diagnosis of these conditions are presented in Table 2.6.

3. **Lower left sternal border:** Systolic murmurs that are maximally audible at this location may be holosystolic, early systolic, or midsystolic type and may result from one of the following conditions:

a. VSD murmur is either holosystolic or early systolic in timing (a small muscular VSD murmur may be heard best between the lower left sternal border and the apex).
b. Vibratory or musical innocent murmur (e.g., Still's murmur); this murmur may be equally loud or even louder toward the apex, and the maximal intensity may be in the midprecordium.
c. Hypertrophic obstructive cardiomyopathy (HOCM) (formerly known as idiopathic hypertrophic subaortic stenosis)
d. TR
e. TOF

Conditions a and b are more common than the other listed conditions. Characteristic physical, ECG, and radiography

findings that help in the differential diagnosis of these conditions are presented in Table 2.7.

4. **Apical area:** Systolic murmurs that are maximally audible at the apex may be a holosystolic, midsystolic, or late systolic murmur and result from one of the following conditions:

a. MR (holosystolic)
b. MVP (late systolic murmur, usually preceded by a midsystolic click)
c. AS (midsystolic)
d. HOCM (midsystolic)
e. Vibratory innocent murmur (midsystolic)

These are relatively uncommon conditions. Characteristic physical, ECG, and radiography findings are summarized in Table 2.8.

Diastolic Murmurs

Diastolic murmurs occur between the S2 and S1. Based on timing and relation to the heart sounds, they are classified into three types: early diastolic (or protodiastolic), mid-diastolic, and late diastolic (or presystolic) (Fig. 2.13).

1. **Early diastolic decrescendo murmurs** occur early in diastole, immediately after the S2, and are caused by incompetence of the aortic or pulmonary valve (see Fig. 2.13).

Because the aorta is a high-pressure vessel, AR murmurs are high pitched and best heard with the diaphragm of a stethoscope at the third left intercostal space. The AR murmur radiates well to the apex because the regurgitation is directed toward the apex. Bounding peripheral pulses may be present if the AR is significant. AR murmurs are associated with congenital bicuspid aortic valve, subaortic stenosis, after an intervention for AS (i.e., postvalvotomy or after balloon dilatation), and rheumatic heart disease with AR. Occasionally, a subarterial infundibular VSD with prolapsing aortic cusps may cause an AR murmur.

Pulmonary regurgitation murmurs also occur early in diastole. They are usually medium pitched but may be high

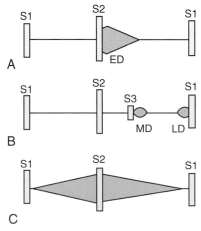

Fig. 2.13 Diagram of diastolic murmurs and the continuous murmur. **A,** Early diastolic (protodiastolic) murmur. **B,** Mid-diastolic and pre-systolic (late diastolic) murmurs. **C,** Continuous murmur. *ED,* Early diastolic or protodiastolic murmur; *LD,* late diastolic or presystolic murmur; *MD,* mid-diastolic murmur.

pitched if pulmonary hypertension is present. They are best heard at the third left intercostal space and radiate along the left sternal border. These murmurs are associated with postoperative TOF (because of surgically induced PR), pulmonary hypertension, postoperative pulmonary valvotomy or after balloon valvuloplasty for PS, and mild deformity of the pulmonary valve.

2. **Mid-diastolic murmurs** start with a loud S3 and are heard in early or mid-diastole but are not temporally midway through diastole (see Fig. 2.13). These murmurs are always low pitched and best heard with the bell of the stethoscope applied lightly to the chest. These murmurs are caused by turbulence caused by the mitral or tricuspid flow secondary to anatomic stenosis or relative stenosis of these valves. Mitral mid-diastolic murmurs are best heard at the apex and are often referred to as an *apical rumble,* although frequently they sound more like a hum than a rumble. These murmurs are associated with MS or a large left-to-right shunt VSD or PDA, which produces relative MS secondary to a large flow across the normal-sized mitral valve.

Tricuspid mid-diastolic murmurs are best heard along the lower left sternal border. These murmurs are associated with ASD, PAPVR, TAPVR, and ECD because they all result in relative tricuspid stenosis (TS). Anatomic stenosis of the tricuspid valve is also associated with these murmurs, but such cases are rare.

3. **Presystolic (or late diastolic) murmurs** are also caused by flow through the AV valves during ventricular diastole. They result from active atrial contraction that ejects blood into the ventricle rather than a passive pressure difference between the atrium and ventricle. These low-frequency murmurs occur late in diastole or just before the onset of systole (see Fig. 2.13) and are found with anatomic stenosis of the mitral or tricuspid valve.

Continuous Murmurs

Continuous murmurs begin in systole and continue without interruption through the S2 into all or part of diastole (see Fig. 2.13). Continuous murmurs are caused by the following:

1. Aortopulmonary or arteriovenous connection (e.g., PDA, arteriovenous fistula, after systemic-to-PA shunt surgery, persistent truncus arteriosus [rarely])
2. Disturbances of flow patterns in veins (e.g., venous hum)
3. Disturbance of flow pattern in arteries (e.g., COA, PA stenosis)

The murmur of PDA in the older child has a machinery-like quality, becoming louder during systole (crescendo), peaking at the S2, and diminishing in diastole (decrescendo). This murmur is maximally heard in the left infraclavicular area or along the upper left sternal border. With pulmonary hypertension, only the systolic portion can be heard, but it is crescendic during systole.

Venous hum is a common innocent murmur that is audible in the upright position, in the infraclavicular region, unilaterally or bilaterally. It is usually heard better on the right side. The murmur's intensity also changes with the position of the neck. When the child lies supine, the murmur usually disappears. Less common continuous murmurs of severe COA may be heard over the intercostal collaterals. The continuous murmurs of PA stenosis may be heard over the right and left anterior chest, the sides of the chest, and in the back.

The combination of a mid-systolic murmur (e.g., VSD, AS, or PS) and a diastolic murmur (e.g., AR or PR) is referred to as a *to-and-fro murmur* to distinguish it from a machinery-like continuous murmur.

Innocent Heart Murmurs

Innocent heart murmurs, also called *functional murmurs,* arise from cardiovascular structures in the absence of anatomic abnormalities. Innocent heart murmurs are common in children. More than 80% of children have innocent murmurs of one type or another sometime during childhood (Table 2.9). All innocent heart murmurs (as well as pathological murmurs) are accentuated or brought out in a high-output state, usually during a febrile illness.

Probably the only way a physician can recognize an innocent heart murmur is to become familiar with the more common forms of these murmurs by auscultating under the supervision of pediatric cardiologists. All innocent heart murmurs are associated with normal ECG and radiography findings. When one or more of the following are present, the murmur is more likely pathologic and requires cardiac consultation:

1. Symptoms
2. Abnormal cardiac size or silhouette or abnormal pulmonary vascularity on chest roentgenograms
3. Abnormal ECG findings
4. Diastolic murmur
5. A systolic murmur that is loud (i.e., grade 3 of 6 or with a thrill), long in duration, and transmits well to other parts of the body
6. Cyanosis
7. Abnormally strong or weak pulses
8. Abnormal heart sounds

Classic Vibratory Murmur

This is the most common innocent murmur in children, first described by Dr. George F. Still of England in 1909. Most vibratory murmurs are detected between 3 and 6 years of age, but the same murmur may be present in neonates, infants, and adolescents. It is maximally audible at the mid-left sternal border or over the midprecordium (between the lower left sternal border and the apex). It is generally of low frequency and best heard with the bell of the stethoscope with the patient in the supine position. The murmur is midsystolic (i.e., not regurgitant) in timing and grade 2 to 3 of 6 in intensity. This murmur is not accompanied by a thrill or ejection click. It has a distinctive quality, described as a "twanging string," groaning, squeaking, buzzing, or vibratory sound, giving a pleasing musical character to the murmur. The murmur is generally loudest in the supine position and often changes in character, pitch, and intensity with upright positioning. The vibratory

TABLE 2.9   Common Innocent Heart Murmurs in Infants and Children

Type (Timing)	Description of Murmur	Age Group
Classic vibratory murmur (Still's murmur) (systolic)	Maximal at MLSB or between LLSB and apex Grade 2 to 3 of 6 *Low-frequency vibratory, "twanging string," groaning, squeaking, or musical	3–6 yr Occasionally in infancy
Pulmonary ejection murmur (systolic)	Maximal at ULSB Grade 1 to 3 of 6 in intensity, early to mid-systolic Blowing in quality	8–14 yr
Pulmonary flow murmur of newborn (systolic)	Maximal at ULSB Transmits well to the left and right chest, axilla, and back Grade 1 to 2 of 6 in intensity	Premature and full-term newborns Usually disappears by 3–6 mo of age
Venous hum (continuous)	*Grade 1 to 3 of 6 continuous murmur, maximal at right (or left) supraclavicular and infraclavicular areas *Inaudible in the supine position (typically heard only in the sitting position) Intensity changes with rotation of the head and compression of the jugular vein	3–6 yr
Carotid bruit (systolic)	Right supraclavicular area and over the carotids Grade 2 to 3 of 6 in intensity Occasional thrill over a carotid	Any age

LLSB, Lower left sternal border; *MLSB,* mid-left sternal border; *ULSB,* upper left sternal border.

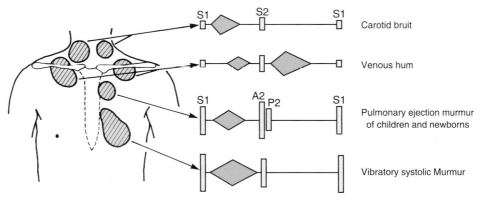

Fig. 2.14 Diagram of innocent heart murmurs in children.

quality may disappear, and the murmur may become softer when the bell is pressed harder, thereby proving its low frequency. The intensity of the murmur increases during febrile illness or excitement, after exercise, and in anemic states. The murmur may disappear briefly at a maximum Valsalva maneuver. The ECG and chest radiography findings are normal (see Table 2.9; Fig. 2.14).

An inexperienced examiner may confuse this murmur with the murmur of a VSD. The murmur of a VSD is usually harsh, grade 2 to 3 of 6 in intensity, holosystolic starting with the S1 rather than midsystolic, and often accompanied by a palpable thrill. The ECG and radiography findings are often abnormal.

The origin of the murmur remains obscure. It is believed to be generated by low-frequency vibrations of normal structures, such as left ventricular "false tendon" or pulmonary valve leaflets, at their attachments during systole or periodic vibrations of a left ventricular false tendon.

Pulmonary Ejection Murmur (Pulmonary Flow Murmur) of Childhood

This is common in children between 8 and 14 years of age but is most frequent in adolescents. The murmur is maximally audible at the upper left sternal border. This murmur represents an exaggeration of normal ejection vibrations within the pulmonary trunk. The murmur is exaggerated by the presence of pectus excavatum, straight back, or kyphoscoliosis. The murmur is midsystolic in timing and slightly grating (rather than vibratory) in quality, with relatively little radiation. The intensity of the murmur is usually a grade 1 to 3 of 6. The S2 is normal, and there is no associated thrill or ejection click (see Table 2.9 and Fig. 2.14). The ECG and chest radiography findings are normal.

This murmur may be confused with the murmur of pulmonary valve stenosis or an ASD. In pulmonary valve stenosis, there may be an ejection click, systolic thrill, widely split S2, right ventricular hypertrophy (RVH) on ECG, and poststenotic dilatation of the main PA segment on chest radiography. Important differential points of ASD include a widely split and fixed S2, a mid-diastolic murmur of relative TS audible at the lower left sternal border if the shunt is large, RBBB or mild RVH on ECG manifested by rsR′ in V1, and chest radiography revealing increased pulmonary vascular markings and enlargement of the right atrium, RV, and main PA.

Pulmonary Flow Murmur of Newborns

This murmur is commonly present in newborns, especially those with low birth weight. The murmur usually disappears by 3 to 6 months of age. If it persists beyond this age, a structural narrowing of the pulmonary arterial tree (i.e., PA stenosis) should be suspected. It is best audible at the upper left sternal border. Although the murmur is only a grade 1 to 2 of 6 in intensity, it transmits impressively to the right and left chest, both axillae, and the back. There is no ejection click. The ECG and chest radiography findings are normal (see Table 2.9 and Fig. 2.14).

In a fetus, the main PA trunk is large, but the branches of the PA are relatively hypoplastic because they receive a small amount of blood flow during fetal life (only 15% of combined ventricular output goes to these vessels). When the ductus closes after birth, the large dome-shaped main PA trunk gives off two small branch pulmonary arteries. The flow through these small vessels produces turbulence with a faster flow velocity, and the turbulence is transmitted along the smaller branches of the PAs. Therefore, this murmur is heard well around the chest wall. The murmur is louder in small preterm babies than in larger full-term neonates.

The murmur resembles the murmur of organic PA stenosis, which may be seen as a component of rubella syndrome, Williams syndrome, or Alagille syndrome. Characteristic noncardiac findings in children with these syndromes lead physicians to suspect that the PA stenosis murmur has an organic cause. Organic PA stenosis is frequently associated with other cardiac defects (e.g., VSD; pulmonary valve stenosis, or TOF), at the site of a previous Blalock-Taussig shunt, or is seen occasionally as an isolated anomaly. The heart murmur of organic PA stenosis persists beyond infancy, and the ECG may show RVH if the stenosis is severe.

Venous Hum

This murmur is commonly audible in children between the ages of 3 and 6 years. At rest, 20% of the cardiac output flows to the brain and the blood returns to the heart via the internal jugular veins. The flow of blood can cause the vein walls to vibrate, creating a humming noise causing venous hums. This is a continuous murmur in which the diastolic component is louder than the systolic component. The murmur is maximally audible at the right, left, or both infraclavicular and supraclavicular areas (see Table 2.9 and Fig. 2.14). The venous hum is heard only in the upright position and disappears in the supine position. It can be obliterated by rotating the head or by gently occluding the neck veins with the fingers.

It is important to differentiate a venous hum from the continuous murmur of a PDA. The murmur of a PDA is loudest at the upper left sternal border or left infraclavicular area and may be associated with bounding peripheral pulses and wide pulse pressure if the shunt is large. The systolic component is louder than the diastolic component. The chest radiographs show increased pulmonary vascular markings and cardiac enlargement. The ECG may be normal (with a small shunt) or show LVH or biventricular hypertrophy (with a large shunt).

Carotid Bruit (or Supraclavicular Systolic Murmur)

This is an early systolic ejection murmur, best heard in the supraclavicular fossa or over the carotid arteries (see Table 2.9 and Fig. 2.14). It is produced by turbulence in the brachiocephalic or carotid arteries. The murmur is a grade 2 to 3 of 6 in intensity. Although it rarely occurs, a faint thrill is palpable over a carotid artery. This bruit may be found in normal children of any age.

The murmur of AS often transmits well to the carotid arteries with a palpable thrill, requiring differentiation from carotid bruits. In AS, the murmur is louder at the upper right sternal border, and a systolic thrill is often present in the upper right sternal border and suprasternal notch, as well as over the carotid artery. An ejection click is often present in aortic valve stenosis. The ECG and radiography findings may appear abnormal.

SOME SPECIAL FEATURES OF THE CARDIAC EXAMINATION OF NEONATES

The following section briefly summarizes some unique aspects of normal and abnormal physical findings in newborns, which are different from those of older infants and children. The difference is caused by the normal RV dominance and elevated pulmonary vascular resistance (PVR) seen in the early neonatal period. Premature infants in general have less RV dominance and a lower PVR than do full-term neonates, adding variability to this generalization.

Normal Physical Findings of Neonates

The following are normal cardiovascular findings in newborn infants:

1. The heart rate generally is faster in newborns than in older children and adults (the newborn rate is usually 100 beats/min, with a normal range of 70 to 180 beats/min).
2. A varying degree of acrocyanosis is the rule rather than the exception.
3. Mild arterial desaturation with arterial Po_2 as low as 60 mm Hg is not unusual in otherwise normal neonates. This may be caused by an intrapulmonary shunt through an as-yet unexpanded portion of the lungs or by a right atrium–to–left atrium shunt through a patent foramen ovale.
4. The RV is relatively hyperactive, with the point of maximal impulse at the lower left sternal border rather than at the apex.
5. The S2 may be single in the first days of life.
6. An ejection click (representing pulmonary hypertension) occasionally is heard in the first hours of life.

7. A newborn may have an innocent heart murmur. Four common innocent murmurs in the newborn period are pulmonary flow murmur of the newborn (see Fig. 2.14), transient systolic murmur of PDA, transient systolic murmur of TR, and vibratory innocent systolic murmur.
   a. Pulmonary flow murmur of the newborn is the most common heart murmur in newborn infants (see previous section).
   b. Transient systolic murmur of PDA is caused by a closing ductus arteriosus and is audible on the first day of life. It is a grade 1 to 2 of 6 only systolic, at the upper left sternal border and in the left infraclavicular area.
   c. Transient systolic murmur of TR is indistinguishable from that of VSD. It is believed that a minimal tricuspid valve abnormality produces regurgitation in the presence of high PVR (and high RV pressure), but the regurgitation disappears as the PVR falls. Therefore, this murmur is more common in infants who had fetal distress or neonatal asphyxia because they tend to maintain high PVR for a longer period.
   d. Vibratory innocent murmur is a counterpart of Still's murmur in older children (see previous section).
8. Peripheral pulses are easily palpable in all extremities, including the feet, in every normal infant. The peripheral pulses normally appear to be bounding in premature babies because of the lack of subcutaneous tissue.

Abnormal Physical Findings in Neonates

The following abnormal physical findings suggest cardiac malformation. Repeated examination is important because physical findings change rapidly in normal infants as well as in infants with cardiac problems.

1. Cyanosis, particularly when it does not improve with the administration of oxygen, suggests a cardiac abnormality.
2. Decreased or absent peripheral pulses in the lower extremities suggest COA. Weak peripheral pulses throughout suggest hypoplastic left heart syndrome (HLHS) or circulatory shock. Bounding peripheral pulses suggest aortic run-off lesions, such as PDA or persistent truncus arteriosus.
3. Tachypnea of greater than 60 breaths/min with or without retraction suggests pulmonary pathology or a cardiac abnormality.
4. Hepatomegaly may suggest a heart defect. A midline liver suggests asplenia or polysplenia syndrome.

5. A heart murmur may be a presenting sign of a congenital heart defect, although innocent murmurs are much more frequent than pathologic murmurs. Most pathologic murmurs should be audible during the first month of life, with the exception of an ASD. However, the time of appearance of a heart murmur depends on the nature of the defect.
   a. Heart murmurs of stenotic lesions (e.g., aortic stenosis, pulmonary stenosis) and those caused by AV valve regurgitation are audible immediately after birth and persist because these murmurs are not affected by the level of PVR.
   b. Heart murmurs of large VSD may not be audible until 1 to 2 weeks of age when the PVR becomes sufficiently low to allow shunt to occur.
   c. The murmur of an ASD appears after 1 or 2 years when the compliance of the RV improves to allow a significant atrial shunt. A newborn or a small infant with a large ASD may not have a heart murmur.
6. Even in the absence of a heart murmur, a newborn infant may have a serious heart defect that requires immediate attention (e.g., severe cyanotic heart defect such as TGA or pulmonary atresia with a closing PDA). Infants who are in severe CHF may not have a loud murmur until the myocardial function is improved through anticongestive measures.
7. An irregular cardiac rhythm and abnormal heart rate suggest a cardiac abnormality.

Role of Pulse Oximetry in Newborn Examination

Although most newborns with CHDs will eventually manifest with abnormal physical findings as shown in this chapter, there are some newborn infants with critical CHD who show no detectable signs of heart defect before discharge from the birth hospital. It is estimated that up to 30% of neonates with critical CHD are discharged after birth without being identified by routine neonatal physical examination. The important role of pulse oximetry screen in detecting some serious CHDs in neonates with mild degrees of hypoxemia (without recognizable cyanosis) was recognized more than a decade ago. Further improvement in the understanding of the beneficial role of the screen has led to making it the standard of care in 2011. At present, the neonatal pulse oximetry screen is the standard of care in nearly all states in the United States. Further discussion of this important topic is presented in Chapter 14.

In the clinical diagnosis and management of congenital or acquired heart disease, the presence or absence of electrocardiographic (ECG) abnormalities is often helpful. Hypertrophies (of ventricles and atria) and ventricular conduction disturbances are the two most common forms of ECG abnormalities. The presence of other ECG abnormalities, such as atrioventricular (AV) conduction disturbances, arrhythmias, and ST segment and T-wave changes, is also helpful in the clinical diagnosis of cardiac problems.

Throughout this chapter, the vectorial approach will be used whenever possible. The vectorial approach is preferred to "pattern reading," which has infinite number of possibilities. The following topics will be discussed in the order listed.
- What is the vectorial approach?
- Comparison of pediatric and adult ECGs
- Basic measurements and their normal values that are necessary for correct interpretation of an ECG. The discussion will include rhythm, heat rate, QRS axis, P and T axes, and so on.
- Atrial and ventricular hypertrophy

- Ventricular conduction disturbances
- ST-segment and T-wave changes, including myocardial infarction (MI)

Cardiac arrhythmias and AV conduction disturbances are discussed separately in Chapters 24 and 25.

For readers who are interested in an in-depth study of the subject, *How to Read Pediatric ECGs*, ed 4, authored by MK Park and WG Guntheroth (Mosby Elsevier, 2016), is recommended.

WHAT IS THE VECTORIAL APPROACH?

The vectorial approach views the standard scalar ECG as three-dimensional vector forces that vary with time. Vector is a quantity that possesses magnitude and direction, but scalar is a quantity that has magnitude only. A scalar ECG, which is routinely obtained in clinical practice, shows only magnitude of the forces against time. However, by combining scalar leads that represent the frontal projection and the horizontal projections of the vectorcardiogram, one can derive the *direction* of the force from scalar ECGs.

The limb leads (leads I, II, III, aVR, aVL, and aVF) provide information about the frontal projection (reflecting superior-inferior and right-to-left forces), and the precordial leads (leads V1–V6, V3R, and V4R) provide information about the horizontal plane, which reflects forces that are right-to-left and anterior-posterior (Fig. 3.1). It is important for readers to become familiar with the orientation of each scalar ECG lead. After they have been learned, the vectorial approach helps readers retain the knowledge gained.

Hexaxial Reference System

It is necessary to memorize the orientation of the hexaxial reference system (see Fig. 3.1A). The hexaxial reference system is made up by the six limb leads (leads I, II, III, aVR, aVL, and aVF) and provides information about the superoinferior and right–left relationships of the electromotive forces. In this system, leads I and aVF cross at a right angle at the electrical center (see Fig. 3.1A). The bipolar limb leads (I, II, and III) are clockwise with the angle between them of 60 degrees. Note that the positive poles of aVR, aVL, and aVF are directed toward the right and left shoulders and the foot, respectively. The positive limb of each lead is shown in a solid line and the negative limb in a broken line. The positive pole of each lead is indicated by the lead labels. The positive pole of lead I is labeled as 0 degree and the negative pole of the same lead as ±180 degrees. The positive pole of aVF is designated as +90 degrees and the negative pole of the same lead as –90 degrees. The positive poles of leads II and III are +60 and +120 degrees, respectively, and so on. The hexaxial reference system is used in plotting the QRS axis, T axis, and P axis.

The lead I axis represents the left–right relationship with the positive pole on the left and the negative pole on the right. The aVF lead represents the superior–inferior relationship with the positive pole directed inferiorly and the negative pole directed superiorly. The R wave in each lead represents the depolarization force directed toward the positive pole; the Q and S waves are the depolarization force directed toward the negative pole. Therefore, the R wave of lead I represents the leftward force, and the S wave of the same lead represents the

rightward force (see Fig. 3.1A). The R wave in aVF represents the inferiorly directed force and the S wave the superiorly directed force. By the same token, the R wave in lead II represents the leftward and inferior force, and the R wave in lead III represents the rightward and inferior force. The R wave in aVR represents the rightward and superior force (pointing to the right shoulder), and the R wave in aVL represents the leftward and superior forces (pointing to the left shoulder).

An easy way to memorize the hexaxial reference system is shown in Fig. 3.2 by a superimposition of a body with stretched arms and legs on the X and Y axes. The hands and feet are the positive poles of electrodes. The left and right hands are the positive poles of leads aVR and aVL, respectively. The left and right feet are the positive poles of leads II and III, respectively. The bipolar limb leads I, II, and III are clockwise in sequence for the positive electrode.

Horizontal Reference System

The horizontal reference system consists of precordial leads (leads V1–V6, V3R, and V4R) (see Fig. 3.1B) and provides information about the anterior–posterior and the left–right relationship. The leads V2 and V6 cross approximately at a right angle at the electrical center of the heart. The V6 axis represents the left–right relationship, and the V2 axis represents the anterior–posterior relationship. The positive limb of each lead is shown in a solid line and the negative limb in a broken line. The positive pole of each lead is indicated by the lead labels (V4R, V1, V2, and so on). The precordial lead V4R is at the mirror image points of V4 in the right chest, and this lead is quite popular in pediatric cardiology because right ventricular forces are more prominent in infants and children.

Therefore, the R wave of V6 represents the leftward force and the R wave of V2 the anterior force. Conversely, the S wave in V6 represents the rightward force and the S wave of V2 the posterior force. The R wave in V1 and V4R represents the rightward and anterior force, and the S wave of these leads represents the leftward and posterior force (see Fig. 3.1B). The R wave of lead V5 in general represents the

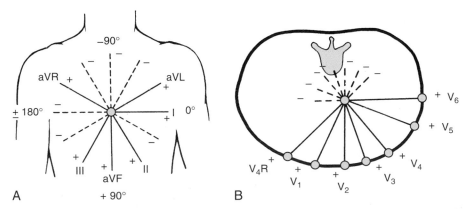

Fig. 3.1 Hexaxial reference system (**A**) shows the frontal projection of a vector loop, and horizontal reference system (**B**) shows the horizontal projection. The combination of (**A**) and (**B**) constitutes the 12- (or 13-) lead electrocardiogram. (From Park MK, Guntheroth WG: *How to Read Pediatric ECGs*, ed 4, Philadelphia, 2006, Mosby Elsevier.)

leftward force, and the R waves of leads V3 and V4 represent a transition between the right and left precordial leads. Ordinarily, the S wave in V2 represents the posterior and thus the left ventricular (LV) force, but in the presence of a marked right axis deviation, the S wave of V2 may represent right ventricular (RV) force that is directed rightward and posteriorly.

Information Available on the 12-Lead Scalar Electrocardiogram

There are three major types of information available in the commonly available form of a 12-lead ECG tracing (Fig. 3.3):

1. The lower part of the tracing is a rhythm strip (of lead II).

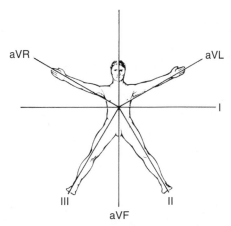

Fig. 3.2 An easy way to memorize the hexaxial reference system. (From Park MK, Guntheroth WG: *How to Read Pediatric ECGs*, ed 4, Philadelphia, 2006, Mosby Elsevier.)

2. The large upper left portion of the recording gives frontal plane information, and the upper right side of the recording presents horizontal plane information. The frontal plane information is provided by the six limb leads (leads I, II, III, aVR, aVL, and aVF) and the horizontal plane information by the precordial leads. In Fig. 3.3, the QRS vector is predominantly directed inferiorly (judged by predominant R waves in leads II, III, and aVF, so-called inferior leads) and is equally anterior and posterior, judged by equiphasic QRS complex in V2.

3. A calibration marker usually appears at the right (or left) margin, which is used to determine the magnitude of the forces. The calibration marker consists of two vertical deflections 2.5 mm in width. The initial deflection shows the calibration factor for the six limb leads, and the latter part of the deflection shows the calibration factor for the six precordial leads. With the full standardization, one millivolt signal introduced into the circuit causes a deflection of 10 mm on the record. With the ½ standardization, the same signal produces 5 mm of deflection. The amplitude of ECG deflections is read in millimeters rather than in millivolts. When the deflections are too big to be recorded, the sensitivity may be reduced to one fourth. With ½ standardization, the measured height in millimeters should be multiplied by 2 to obtain the correct amplitude of the deflection. In Fig. 3.3, the calibration marker indicates that a full standardization was used for the limb leads, and ½ standardization was used for the precordial leads.

Thus, from the scalar ECG tracing, one can gain information of the frontal and horizontal orientations of the QRS (or ventricular) complexes and other electrical activities of the heart as well as the magnitude of such forces.

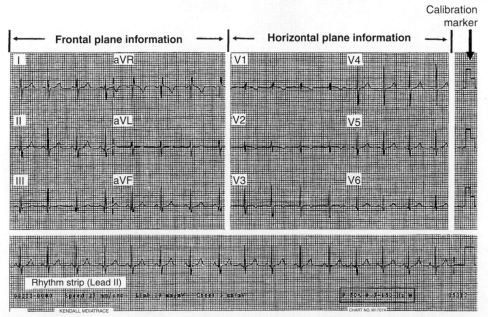

Fig. 3.3 A common form of routine 12-lead scalar electrocardiogram. There are three groups of information available on the recording. Frontal and horizontal plane information is given in the upper part of the tracing. Calibration factors are shown on the *right edge* of the recording. A rhythm strip (lead II) is shown at the *bottom*.

COMPARISON OF PEDIATRIC AND ADULT ELECTROCARDIOGRAMS

Electrocardiograms of normal infants and children are quite different from those of normal adults. The most remarkable difference is RV dominance in infants. RV dominance is most noticeable in newborns, and it gradually changes to LV dominance of adults. By 3 years of age, the child's ECG resembles that of young adults. The age-related difference in the ECG reflects an age-related anatomic difference; the RV is thicker than the LV in newborns and infants, and the LV is much thicker than the RV in adults.

Right ventricular dominance of infants is expressed in the ECG by right axis deviation (RAD) and large rightward or anterior QRS forces (i.e., tall R waves in lead aVR and the right precordial leads [V4R, V1, and V2] and deep S waves in lead I and the left precordial leads [V5 and V6]) compared with an adult ECG.

A normal ECG from a 1-week-old neonate (Fig. 3.4) is compared with that of a young adult (Fig. 3.5). The infant's

ECG demonstrates RAD (+140 degrees) and dominant R waves in the right precordial leads. The T wave in V1 is usually negative. Upright T waves in V1 in this age group suggest right ventricular hypertrophy (RVH). Adult-type R/S progression in the precordial leads (deep S waves in V1 and V2 and tall R waves in V5 and V6, as seen in Fig. 3.5) is rarely seen in the first month of life; instead, there may be *complete reversal* of the adult-type R/S progression, with tall R waves in V1 and V2 and deep S waves in V5 and V6. *Partial reversal* is usually present, with dominant R waves in V1 and V2 as well as in V5 and V6, in children between the ages of 1 month and 3 years.

The normal adult ECG shown in Fig. 3.5 demonstrates the QRS axis near +60 degrees and the QRS forces directed to the left, inferiorly and posteriorly, which are manifested by dominant R waves in I, V5 and V6 (leftward forces), dominant R waves in aVF (inferior forces), and dominant S waves in V1 and V2 (posterior forces). The normal adult ECG shows dominant R waves in the left precordial leads (V5 and V6) and dominant S waves in the right precordial leads, the so-called

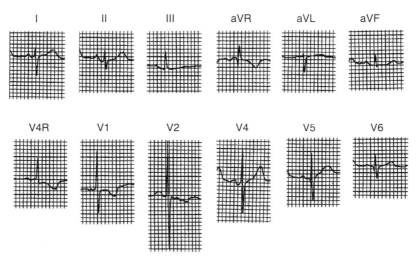

Fig. 3.4 Electrocardiogram from a normal 1-week-old infant.

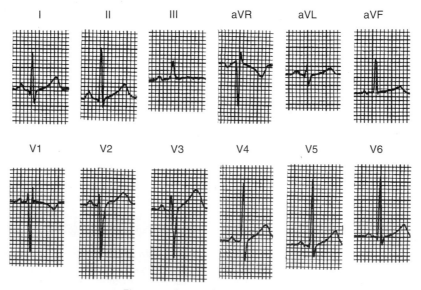

Fig. 3.5 Electrocardiogram from a normal young adult.

adult R/S progression. The T waves are usually anteriorly oriented, resulting in upright T waves in V2 through V6 and sometimes in V1.

BASIC MEASUREMENTS AND THEIR NORMAL AND ABNORMAL VALUES

In this section, basic measurements and their normal values that are necessary for routine interpretation of an ECG are briefly discussed in the order listed. This sequence is one of many approaches that can be used in routine interpretation of an ECG. The methods of their measurements will be followed by their normal and abnormal values and the significance of abnormal values.

1. Rhythm (sinus or nonsinus) by considering the P axis
2. Heart rate (atrial and ventricular rates, if different)
3. The QRS axis, T axis, and QRS-T angle
4. Intervals: PR, QRS, and QT
5. The P-wave amplitude and duration
6. The QRS amplitude and R/S ratio; also abnormal Q waves
7. ST-segment and T-wave abnormalities

Rhythm

Sinus rhythm is the normal rhythm at any age and is characterized by P waves preceding each QRS complex and a normal P axis (0 to +90 degrees); the latter is an often neglected criterion. The requirement of a normal P axis is important in discriminating sinus from nonsinus rhythm. In sinus rhythm, the PR interval is regular but does not have to be of normal interval. (The PR interval may be prolonged as seen in sinus rhythm with first-degree AV block.)

Because the sinoatrial node is located in the right upper part of the atrial mass, the direction of atrial depolarization is from the right upper part toward the left lower part, with the resulting P axis in the lower left quadrant (0 to +90 degrees) (Fig. 3.6A). Some atrial (nonsinus) rhythms may have P waves preceding each QRS complex, but they have an abnormal P axis (Fig. 3.6B). For the P axis to be between 0 and +90 degrees, P waves

must be upright in leads I and aVF or at least not inverted in these leads; simple inspection of these two leads suffices. A normal P axis also results in upright P waves in lead II and inverted P waves in aVR. A method of plotting axes is presented later for the QRS axis, but accurately plotting the P axis is not necessary.

Heart Rate

There are many different ways to calculate the heart rate, but they are all based on the known time scale of ECG papers. At the usual paper speed of 25 mm/sec, 1 mm = 0.04 second, and 5 mm = 0.20 second (Fig. 3.7). The following methods are often used to calculate the heart rate.

1. Count the R-R cycle in six large divisions (1/50 minute) and multiply it by 50 (Fig. 3.8).
2. When the heart rate is slow, count the number of large divisions between two R waves and divide that into 300 (because 1 minute = 300 large divisions) (Fig. 3.9).
3. Measure the R-R interval (in seconds) and divide 60 by the R-R interval. The R-R interval is 0.36 second in Fig. 3.8: 60 ÷ 0.36 = 166.

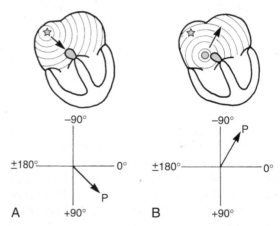

Fig. 3.6 Comparison of P axis in sinus rhythm (**A**) and low atrial rhythm (**B**). In sinus rhythm, the P axis is between 0 and +90 degrees, and P waves are upright in leads I and aVF. In low atrial rhythm, the P wave is superiorly oriented, and P waves are inverted in lead aVF.

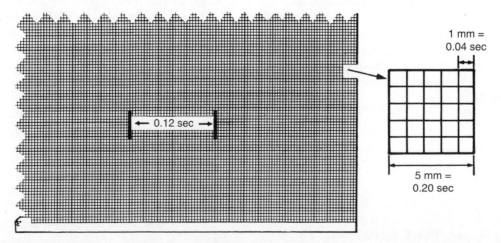

Fig. 3.7 Electrocardiographic paper. Time is measured on the horizontal axis. Each 1 mm equals 0.04 second, and each 5 mm (a large division) equals 0.20 second. Thirty millimeters (or six large divisions) equals 1.2 second or 1/50 minute. (From Park MK, Guntheroth WG: *How to Read Pediatric ECGs*, ed 4, Philadelphia, 2006, Mosby Elsevier.)

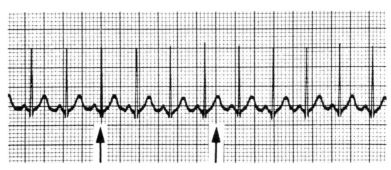

Fig. 3.8 Heart rate of 165 beats/min. There are about 3.3 cardiac cycles (R-R intervals) in six large divisions. Therefore, the heart rate is 3.3 × 50 = 165 (by method 1). By method 3, the RR interval is 0.36 sec. 60 ÷ 0.36 = 166. The rates derived by the two methods are very close.

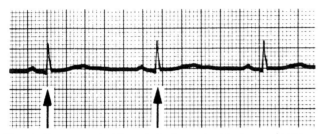

Fig. 3-9 Heart rate of 52 beats/min. By method 2, there are 5.8 large (5 mm) divisions between the two arrows. Therefore, the heart rate is 300 ÷ 5.8 = 52.

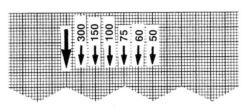

Fig. 3.10 Quick estimation of heart rate. When the R-R interval is 5 mm, the heart rate is 300 beats/min; when the R-R interval is 10 mm, the rate is 150 beats/min, and so on.

4. Use a convenient ECG ruler.
5. An approximate heart rate can be determined by memorizing heart rates for selected R-R intervals (Fig. 3.10). When R-R intervals are 5, 10, 15, 20, and 25 mm, the respective heart rates are 300, 150, 100, 75, and 60 beats/min.

When the ventricular and atrial rates are different, as in complete heart block or atrial flutter, the atrial rate can be calculated using the same methods as described for the ventricular rate; for the atrial rate, the P-P interval rather than the R-R interval is used.

Because of age-related differences in the heart rate, the definitions of bradycardia (<60 beats/min) and tachycardia (>100 beats/min) used for adults do not help distinguish normal from abnormal heart rates in pediatric patients. Operationally, tachycardia is present when the heart rate is faster than the upper range of normal for that age, and bradycardia is present when the heart rate is slower than the lower range of normal. According to age, normal resting heart rates per minute recorded on the ECG are as follows (Davignon et al, 1979/1980).
Newborn: 145 (90–180)
6 months: 145 (105–185)
1 years: 132 (105–170)
2 years: 120 (90–150)
4 years: 108 (72–135)
6 years: 100 (65–135)
10 years: 90 (65–130)
14 years: 85 (60–120)

QRS Axis, T Axis, and QRS-T Angle
QRS Axis

The most convenient way to determine the QRS axis is the successive approximation method using the hexaxial reference system (see Fig. 3.1A). The same approach is also used for the determination of the T axis (see later discussion). For the determination of the QRS axis (as well as T axis), one uses only the hexaxial reference system (or the six limb leads), not the horizontal reference system.

Successive Approximation Method

Step 1: Locate a quadrant using leads I and aVF (Fig. 3.11). In the *top panel* of Fig. 3.11, the net QRS deflection of lead I is positive. This means that the QRS axis is in the left hemicircle (i.e., from -90 degrees through 0 to +90 degrees) from the lead I point of view. The net positive QRS deflection in aVF means that the QRS axis is in the lower hemicircle (i.e., from 0 through +90 degrees to +180 degrees) from the aVF point of view. To satisfy the polarity of both leads I and aVF, the QRS axis must be in the lower left quadrant (i.e., 0 to +90 degrees). Four quadrants can be easily identified based on the QRS complexes in leads I and aVF (see Fig. 3.11).

Step 2: *Among the remaining four limb leads, find a lead with an equiphasic QRS complex* (in which the height of the R wave and the depth of the S wave are equal). The QRS axis is perpendicular to the lead with an equiphasic QRS complex in the predetermined quadrant.

Example: Determine the QRS axis in Fig. 3.12.

Step 1: The axis is in the lower left quadrant (0 to +90 degrees) because the R waves are upright in leads I and aVF.

Step 2: The QRS complex is equiphasic in aVL. Therefore, the QRS axis is +60 degrees, which is perpendicular to aVL.

Normal QRS axis. Normal ranges of QRS axis vary with age. Newborns normally have RAD compared with the adult standard. By 3 years of age, the QRS axis approaches

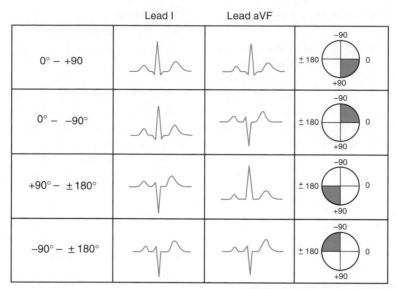

Fig. 3.11 Locating quadrants of mean QRS axis from leads I and aVF. (From Park MK, Guntheroth WG: *How to Read Pediatric ECGs*, ed 4, Philadelphia, 2006, Mosby Elsevier.)

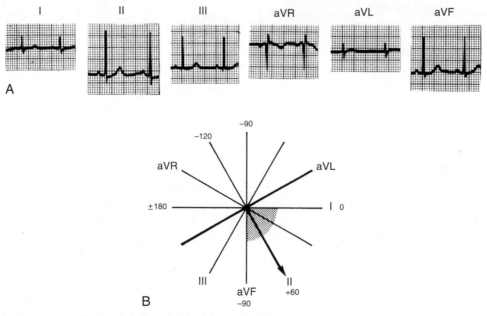

Fig. 3.12 A, Set of six limb leads. B, Plotted QRS axis (+60 degrees).

the adult mean value of +50 degrees. The mean and ranges of a normal QRS axis according to age are shown in Table 3.1.

Abnormal QRS axis. The QRS axis outside normal ranges signifies abnormalities in the ventricular depolarization process.

1. Left axis deviation (LAD) is present when the QRS axis is less than the lower limit of normal for the patient's age. LAD occurs with left ventricular hypertrophy (LVH), left bundle branch block (LBBB), and left anterior hemiblock.
2. RAD is present when the QRS axis is greater than the upper limit of normal for the patient's age. RAD occurs with RVH and right bundle branch block (RBBB).

3. "Superior" QRS axis is present when the S wave is greater than the R wave in aVF. The overlap with LAD and left anterior hemiblock should be noted. Left anterior hemiblock (in the range of −30 to −90 degrees) is seen in congenital heart diseases such as endocardial cushion defect and tricuspid atresia or with RBBB. It is rarely seen in otherwise normal children.

T axis. The T axis is determined by the same methods used to determine the QRS axis. In normal children, including newborns, the mean T axis is +45 degrees, with a range of 0 to +90 degrees, the same as in normal adults. This means that the T waves must be upright in leads I and aVF. The T waves can be flat but must not be einverted in these leads. The T axis outside of the normal quadrant suggests conditions with myocardial dysfunction similar to those listed for abnormal QRS-T angle (see later).

QRS-T angle. The QRS-T angle is formed by the QRS axis and the T axis. A QRS-T angle of greater than 60 degrees is unusual, and one greater than 90 degrees is certainly abnormal. An abnormally wide QRS-T angle with the T axis outside the normal quadrant (0 to +90 degrees) is seen in severe ventricular hypertrophy with "strain," ventricular conduction disturbances, and myocardial dysfunction of a metabolic or ischemic nature.

Intervals

Three important intervals are routinely measured in the interpretation of an ECG: PR interval, QRS duration, and QT interval. The duration of the P wave is also inspected (Fig. 3.13).

TABLE 3.1   Mean and Ranges of Normal QRS Axes by Age

Age	Mean (Range)
1 wk–1 mo	+ 110 degrees (+30 to +180)
1–3 mo	+ 70 degrees (+10 to +125)
3 mo–3 yr	+ 60 degrees (+10 to +110)
Older than 3 yr	+ 60 degrees (+20 to +120)
Adult	+ 50 degrees (–30 to +105)

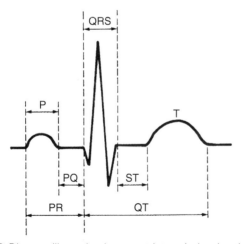

Fig. 3.13 Diagram illustrating important intervals (or durations) and segments of an electrocardiographic cycle.

PR Interval

The normal PR interval varies with age and heart rate (Table 3.2). The PR interval is longer in older individuals and with a slower heart rate.

Prolongation of the PR interval (i.e., first-degree AV block) is seen in myocarditis (rheumatic, viral, or diphtheric), digitalis, amiodarone, or quinidine toxicity, certain congenital heart defects (endocardial cushion defect, atrial septal defect, Ebstein's anomaly), some myocardial dysfunctions, hyperkalemia, and otherwise normal heart with vagal stimulation.

A short PR interval is present in Wolff-Parkinson-White (WPW) preexcitation, Lown-Ganong-Levine syndrome, myocardiopathies of glycogenosis, Duchenne's muscular dystrophy (or relatives of these patients), Friedrich's ataxia, pheochromocytoma, and otherwise normal children. The lower limits of normal PR interval are shown under the topic of WPW preexcitation (see later discussion).

Variable PR intervals are seen in the wandering atrial pacemaker and the Wenckebach phenomena (Mobitz type I second-degree AV block).

QRS Duration

The QRS duration varies with age (Table 3.3). It is short in infants and increases with age.

The QRS duration is prolonged in conditions grouped as ventricular conduction disturbances, which include RBBB, LBBB, preexcitation (e.g., WPW preexcitation), and intraventricular block (as seen in hyperkalemia, toxicity from quinidine or procainamide, myocardial fibrosis, and myocardial dysfunction of a metabolic or ischemic nature). Ventricular arrhythmias (e.g., premature ventricular contractions, ventricular tachycardia, implanted ventricular pacemaker) also produce a wide QRS duration. Because the QRS duration varies with age, the definition of bundle branch block (BBB) or other ventricular conduction disturbances should vary with age (see the section on ventricular conduction disturbances).

QT Interval

The QT interval varies primarily with heart rate. The heart rate-corrected QT (QTc) interval is calculated by the use of Bazett's formula:

$$QTc = QT / \sqrt{RR \ interval}$$

TABLE 3.2   PR Interval According to Age and Rate: Mean (and Upper Limits of Normal)

Rate	0–1 mo	1–6 mo	6 mo–1 yr	1–3 yr	3–8 yr	8–12 yr	12–16 yr	Adults
<60						0.16 (0.18)	0.16 (0.19)	0.17 (0.21)
60–80					0.15 (0.17)	0.15 (0.17)	0.15 (0.18)	0.16 (0.21)
80–100	0.10 (0.12)				0.14 (0.16)	0.15 (0.16)	0.15 (0.17)	0.15 (0.20)
100–120	0.10 (0.12)			(0.15)	0.13 (0.16)	0.14 (0.15)	0.15 (0.16)	0.15 (0.19)
120–140	0.10 (0.11)	0.11 (0.14)	0.11 (0.14)	0.12 (0.14)	0.13 (0.15)	0.14 (0.15)		0.15 (0.18)
140–160	0.09 (0.11)	0.10 (0.13)	0.11 (0.13)	0.11 (0.14)	0.12 (0.14)			(0.17)
160–180	0.10 (0.11)	0.10 (0.12)	0.10 (0.12)	0.10 (0.12)				
>180	0.09	0.09 (0.11)	0.10 (0.11)					

From Park MK, Guntheroth WG: *How to Read Pediatric ECGs*, ed 4, Philadelphia, 2006, Mosby Elsevier.

According to Bazett's formula, the normal QTc interval (mean ± standard deviation [SD]) is 0.40 (±0.014) second with the upper limit of normal 0.44 second in children 6 months and older. The QTc interval is slightly longer in newborn and small infants with the upper limit of normal QTc 0.47 second in the first week of life and 0.45 second in the first 6 months of life.

Long QT intervals may be seen in long QT syndrome (e.g., Jervell and Lange-Nielsen syndrome, Romano-Ward syndrome), hypocalcemia, myocarditis, diffuse myocardial diseases (including hypertrophic and dilated cardiomyopathies), head injury, severe malnutrition, and so on. A number of drugs are also known to prolong the QT interval. Among these are antiarrhythmic agents (especially class IA, IC, and III), antipsychotic phenothiazines (e.g., thioridazine, chlorpromazine), tricyclic antidepressants (e.g., imipramine, amitriptyline), arsenics, organophosphates, antibiotics (e.g., ampicillin, erythromycin, trimethoprim-sulfa, amantadine), and antihistamines (e.g., terfenadine).

A short QT interval is a sign of a digitalis effect or of hypercalcemia. It is also seen with hyperthermia and in short QT syndrome (a familial cause of sudden death with QTc ≤300 msec).

The JT Interval

The JT interval is measured from the J point (the junction between the S wave and the ST segment) to the end of the T wave. A prolonged JT interval has the same significance as a prolonged QT interval. The JT interval is measured only when the QT interval is prolonged or when the QRS duration is prolonged as seen with ventricular conduction disturbances. The JT interval is also expressed as a rate-corrected interval (called *JTc*) using Bazett's formula. Normal JTc (mean ± SD) is 0.32 ± 0.02 second with the upper limit of normal 0.34 second in normal children and adolescents.

P-Wave Duration and Amplitude

The P-wave duration and amplitude are important in the diagnosis of atrial hypertrophy. Normally, the P amplitude is less than 3 mm. The duration of P waves is shorter than 0.09 second in children and shorter than 0.07 second in infants (see the section on criteria for atrial hypertrophy).

QRS Amplitude, R/S Ratio, and Abnormal Q Waves
The QRS Amplitude and R/S Ratio

The amplitudes of the QRS complex and R/S ratio are important in the diagnosis of ventricular hypertrophy. These values also vary with age (Tables 3.4 and 3.5).
1. Because of normal dominance of right ventricular forces in infants and small children, R waves are taller than S waves in the right precordial leads (i.e., V4R, V1, V2), and

S waves are deeper than R waves in the left precordial leads (i.e., V5, V6) in this age group.
2. Accordingly, the R/S ratio (the ratio of the R wave and S wave voltages) is large in the right precordial leads and small in the left precordial leads in infants and small children.

Q Waves

1. Normal mean Q voltages and upper limits are presented in Table 3.6. The average normal Q-wave duration is 0.02 second and does not exceed 0.03 second.
2. Abnormal Q waves may manifest themselves as deep or wide Q waves or as abnormal leads in which they appear.
   a. Deep Q waves may be present in ventricular hypertrophy of the "volume overload" type and in septal hypertrophy.
   b. Deep and wide Q waves are seen in MI.
   c. The presence of Q waves in the right precordial leads (e.g., severe RVH or ventricular inversion) or the absence of Q waves in the left precordial leads (e.g., LBBB or ventricular inversion) is abnormal.

ST Segment and T Waves

1. The normal ST segment is isoelectric. However, in the limb leads, elevation or depression of the ST segment up to 1 mm is not necessarily abnormal in infants and children. An elevation or a depression of the ST segment is judged in relation to the PR segment as the baseline. Some ST-segment changes are normal (nonpathologic), and others are abnormal (pathologic). (See the later section of nonpathologic and pathologic ST-T changes in this chapter.)
2. Tall peaked T waves (taller than half the size of preceding QRS) may be seen in hyperkalemia and LVH (of the "volume overload" type). Flat or low T waves may occur in normal newborns or with hypothyroidism, hypokalemia, pericarditis, myocarditis, and myocardial ischemia.

ATRIAL HYPERTROPHY

Right Atrial Hypertrophy

Tall P waves (>3 mm) indicate right atrial hypertrophy (RAH) or "P pulmonale" (Fig. 3.14).

Left Atrial Hypertrophy

Widened and often notched P wave is seen in left atrial hypertrophy (LAH) or "P mitrale." In V1, the P wave is diphasic with a prolonged negative segment (see Fig. 3.14). A notched P wave in V1 is not diagnostic of LAH; the P wave duration

TABLE 3.3	QRS Duration According to Age: Mean (Upper Limits of Normal[a]) (in Seconds)							
	0–1 mo	1–6 mo	6–12 mo	1–3 yr	3–8 yr	8–12 yr	12–16 yr	Adults
Seconds	0.05 (0.07)	0.055 (0.075)	0.055 (0.075)	0.055 (0.075)	0.06 (0.075)	0.06 (0.085)	0.07 (0.085)	0.08 (0.10)

[a]Upper limit of normal refers to the 98th percentile.
Derived from percentile graphs in Davignon A, Rautaharju P, Boisselle E, Soumis F, Megelas M, Choquette A: Normal ECG standards for infants and children, *Pediatr Cardiol* 1:123–131, 1979/1980.

TABLE 3.4   R Voltages According to Lead and Age: Mean (and Upper Limit[a]) (in mm)

	0–1 mo	1–6 mo	6–12 mo	1–3 yr	3–8 yr	8–12 yr	12–16 yr	Adults
I	4 (8)	7 (13)	8 (16)	8 (16)	7 (15)	7 (15)	6 (13)	6 (13)
II	6 (14)	13 (24)	13 (27)	12 (23)	13 (22)	14 (24)	14 (24)	5 (25)
III	8 (16)	9 (20)	9 (20)	9 (20)	9 (20)	9 (24)	9 (24)	6 (22)
aVR	3 (8)	2 (6)	2 (6)	2 (5)	2 (4)	1 (4)	1 (4)	1 (4)
aVL	2 (7)	4 (8)	5 (10)	5 (10)	3 (10)	3 (10)	3 (12)	3 (9)
aVF	7 (14)	10 (20)	10 (16)	8 (20)	10 (19)	10 (20)	11 (21)	5 (23)
V3R	10(19)	6 (13)	6 (11)	6 (11)	5 (10)	3 (9)	3 (7)	
V4R	6 (12)	5 (10)	4 (8)	4 (8)	3 (8)	3 (7)	3 (7)	
V1	13 (24)	10 (19)	10 (20)	9 (18)	8 (16)	5 (12)	4 (10)	3 (14)
V2	18 (30)	20 (31)	22 (32)	19 (28)	15 (25)	12 (20)	10 (19)	6 (21)
V5	12 (23)	20 (33)	20 (31)	20 (32)	23 (38)	26 (39)	21 (35)	12 (33)
V6	5 (15)	13 (22)	13 (23)	13 (23)	15 (26)	17 (26)	14 (23)	10 (21)

S Voltages According to Lead and Age: Mean (and Upper Limit[a]) (in mm)

	0–1 mo	1–6 mo	6–12 mo	1–3 yr	3–8 yr	8–12 yr	12–16 yr	Adults
I	5 (10)	4 (9)	4 (9)	3 (8)	2 (8)	2 (8)	2 (8)	1 (6)
V3R	3 (12)	3 (10)	4 (10)	5 (12)	7 (15)	8 (18)	7 (16)	
V4R	4 (9)	4 (12)	5 (12)	5 (12)	5 (14)	6 (20)	6 (20)	
V1	7 (18)	5 (15)	7 (18)	8 (21)	11 (23)	12 (25)	11 (22)	10 (23)
V2	18 (33)	15 (26)	16 (29)	18 (30)	20 (33)	21 (36)	18 (33)	14 (36)
V5	9 (17)	7 (16)	6 (15)	5 (12)	4 (10)	3 (8)	3 (8)	
V6	3 (10)	3 (9)	2 (7)	2 (7)	2 (5)	1 (4)	1 (4)	1 (13)

[a]Upper limit of normal refers to the 98th percentile. Voltages measured in millimeters, when 1 mV = 10-mm paper.
From Park MK, Guntheroth WG: *How to Read Pediatric ECGs*, ed 4, Philadelphia, 2006, Mosby Elsevier.

TABLE 3.5   R/S Ratio: Mean and Upper and Lower Limits of Normal According to Age

Lead		0–1 mo	1–6 mo	6 mo–1 yr	1–3 yr	3–8 yr	8–12 yr	12–16 yr	Adults
V1	LLN	0.5	0.3	0.3	0.5	0.1	0.15	0.1	0.0
	Mean	1.5	1.5	1.2	0.8	0.65	0.5	0.3	0.3
	ULN	19	S = 0	6	2	2	1	1	1
V2	LLN	0.3	0.3	0.3	0.3	0.05	0.1	0.1	0.1
	Mean	1	1.2	1	0.8	0.5	0.5	0.5	0.2
	ULN	3	4	4	1.5	1.5	1.2	1.2	2.5
V6	LLN	0.1	1.5	2	3	2.5	4	2.5	2.5
	Mean	2	4	6	20	20	20	10	9
	ULN	S = 0	S = 0	S = 0	S = 0	S = 0	S = 0	S = 0	S = 0

LLN, Lower limits of normal; *ULN,* upper limits of normal.
From Guntheroth WB: *Pediatric Electrocardiography*, Philadelphia, 1965, WB Saunders.

TABLE 3.6   Q Voltages According to Lead and Age: Mean (and Upper Limit[a]) (in mm)

	0–1 mo	1–6 mo	6–12 mo	1–3 yr	3–8 yr	8–12 yr	12–16 yr	Adults
III	1.5 (5.5)	1.5 (6.0)	2.1 (6.0)	1.5 (5.0)	1.0 (3.5)	0.6 (3.0)	1.0 (3.0)	0.5 (4)
aVF	1.0 (3.5)	1.0 (3.5)	1.0 (3.5)	1.0 (3.0)	0.5 (3.0)	0.5 (2.5)	0.5 (2.0)	0.5 (2)
V5	0.1 (3.5)	0.1 (3.0)	0.1 (3.0)	0.5 (4.5)	1.0 (5.5)	1.0 (3.0)	0.5 (3.0)	0.5 (3.5)
V6	0.5 (3.0)	0.5 (3.0)	0.5 (3.0)	0.5 (3.0)	1.0 (3.5)	0.5 (3.0)	0.5 (3.0)	0.5 (3)

[a]Upper limit of normal refers to the 98th percentile. Voltages measured in millimeters, when 1 mV = 10-mm paper.
From percentile graphs in Davignon A, Rautaharju P, Boisselle E, Soumis F, Megelas M, Choquette A: Normal ECG standards for infants and children, *Pediatr Cardiol* 1:123–131, 1979/1980.

has to be abnormally prolonged (with the P duration >0.10 second in children and >0.08 second in infants).

Biatrial Hypertrophy

In biatrial hypertrophy (BAH), a combination of an increased amplitude and duration of the P wave is present (see Fig. 3.14).

VENTRICULAR HYPERTROPHY

General Changes

Ventricular hypertrophy produces abnormalities in one or more of the following: the QRS axis, the QRS voltages, the R/S ratio, the T axis, and miscellaneous areas.

1. Changes in the QRS axis

The QRS axis is usually directed toward the ventricle that is hypertrophied. Although RAD is present with RVH, LAD is seen with volume-overload type but not with pressure-overload type of LVH. Marked LAD (such as that seen with left

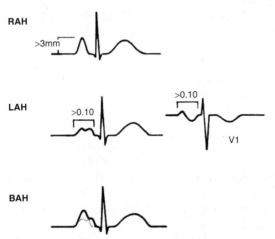

Fig. 3.14 Criteria for atrial hypertrophy. *BAH,* Biatrial hypertrophy; *LAH,* left atrial hypertrophy; *RAH,* right atrial hypertrophy. (From Park MK, Guntheroth WG: *How to Read Pediatric ECGs,* ed 4, Philadelphia, 2006, Mosby Elsevier.)

anterior hemiblock or "superior" QRS axis) usually indicates ventricular conduction disturbances, not hypertrophy.

2. Changes in QRS voltages

Anatomically, the RV occupies the right and anterior aspect, and the LV occupies the left, inferior, and posterior aspect of the ventricular mass. With ventricular hypertrophy, the voltage of the QRS complex increases in the direction of the respective ventricle.

  a. RVH
    1) In the frontal plane: tall R waves in aVR and III and deep S waves in lead I (Fig. 3.15A)
    2) In the horizontal plane: tall R waves in V4R, V1, and V2 and/or deep S waves in V5 and V6 (see Fig. 3.15B)
  b. LVH
    1) In the frontal plane: increased R voltages in leads I, II, aVL, aVF, and sometimes III, especially in small infants (Fig. 3.15A)
    2) In the horizontal plane: tall R waves in V5 and V6 and/or deep S waves in V4R, V1, and V2 (Fig. 3.15B)

3. Changes in R/S ratio

The R/S ratio represents the relative electromotive force of opposing ventricles in a given lead. In ventricular hypertrophy, a change may be seen only in the R/S ratio (see Table 3.5) without an increase in the voltage of the R or S wave.

  a. In RVH, the R/S ratio is increased in the right precordial leads (V4R, V1, V2) and decreased in the left precordial leads (V5, V6).
  b. In LVH, the R/S ratio is increased in the left precordial leads and decreased in the right precordial leads.

4. Changes in the T axis

Changes in the T axis are seen in severe ventricular hypertrophy with relative ischemia of the hypertrophied myocardium.

  a. In the presence of other criteria of ventricular hypertrophy, a wide QRS-T angle (i.e., >90 degrees) with the T axis outside the normal range indicates a "strain" pattern.

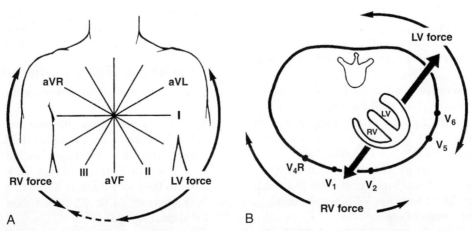

Fig. 3.15 Diagrammatic representation of left and right ventricular forces on the frontal projection (hexaxial reference system) (**A**) and the horizontal plane (**B**). (Park MK, Guntheroth WG: *How to Read Pediatric ECGs,* ed 4, Philadelphia, 2006, Mosby Elsevier.)

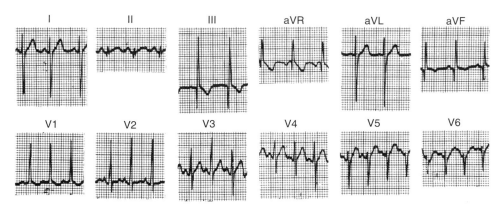

Fig. 3.16 Tracing from a 10-month-old infant with severe tetralogy of Fallot.

b. When the T axis remains in the normal quadrant (0 to + 90 degrees), a wide QRS-T angle indicates a *possible* "strain" pattern.

5. Miscellaneous nonspecific changes
   a. RVH
      1) A q wave in V1 (qR or qRs pattern) suggests RVH, although it may be present in ventricular inversion.
      2) An upright T wave in V1 after 3 days of age is a sign of probable RVH.
   b. LVH. Deep Q waves (>5 mm) and/or tall T waves in V5 and V6 are signs of LVH of "volume overload" type. These may be seen with a large-shunt ventricular septal defect (VSD).

Criteria for Right Ventricular Hypertrophy

In RVH, some or all of the following criteria are present.
1. RAD for the patient's age (see Table 3.1)
2. Increased rightward and anterior QRS voltages (in the absence of prolonged QRS duration) (see Table 3.4); a wide QRS complex with increased QRS voltages suggests ventricular conduction disturbances (e.g., RBBB) rather than ventricular hypertrophy.
   a. R waves in V1, V2, or aVR greater than the upper limits of normal for the patient's age
   b. S waves in I and V6 greater than the upper limits of normal for the patient's age
   In general, the abnormal forces to the right *and* anteriorly is a stronger criteria than abnormal forces to the right or anteriorly only.
3. Abnormal R/S ratio in favor of the RV (in the absence of prolonged QRS duration) (i.e., BBB; see Table 3.5)
   a. R/S ratio in V1 and V2 greater than the upper limits of normal for age
   b. R/S ratio in V6 less than 1 after 1 month of age
4. Upright T waves in V1 in patients more than 3 days of age, provided that the T is upright in the left precordial leads (V5, V6); upright T waves in V1 is not abnormal in patients more than 6 years of age.
5. A q wave in V1 (qR or qRs patterns) suggests RVH. (The physician should ascertain that there is not a small r in an rsR' configuration.)

6. In the presence of RVH, a wide QRS-T angle with T axis outside the normal range (in the 0 to –90 degree quadrant) indicates a "strain" pattern. A wide QRS-T angle with the T axis within the normal range suggests a *possible* "strain" pattern.

Fig. 3.16 is an example of RVH. There is RAD for the patient's age (+150 degrees). The T axis is –10 degrees, and the QRS-T angle is abnormally wide (160 degrees) with the T axis in an abnormal quadrant. The QRS duration is normal. The R-wave voltages in leads III and aVR and the S waves in leads I and V6 are beyond the upper limits of normal, indicating an abnormal rightward force. The R/S ratios in V1 and V2 are larger than the upper limits of normal, and the ratio in V6 is smaller than the lower limits of normal, again indicating RVH. Therefore, this tracing shows RVH with "strain."

The diagnosis of RVH in newborns is particularly difficult because of the normal dominance of the RV during this period of life. Helpful signs in the diagnosis of RVH in newborns are as follows.

1. S waves in lead I that are 12 mm or greater
2. Pure R waves (with no S waves) in V1 that are greater than 10 mm Hg
3. R waves in V1 that are greater than 25 mm or R waves in aVR that are greater than 8 mm
4. A qR pattern seen in V1 (this is also seen in 10% of normal newborns)
5. Upright T waves seen in V1 after 3 days of age
6. RAD with the QRS axis greater than +180 degrees

Criteria for Left Ventricular Hypertrophy

In LVH, some or all of the following abnormalities are present.

1. LAD for the patient's age in some cases (see Table 3.1)
2. QRS voltages in favor of the LV (in the absence of a prolonged QRS duration for age) (see Table 3.4)
   a. R waves in leads I, II, III, aVL, aVF, V5, or V6 greater than the upper limits of normal for age
   b. S waves in V1 or V2 greater than the upper limits of normal for age
   In general, the presence of abnormal forces to more than one direction (e.g., to the left, inferiorly, and posteriorly) is stronger criterion than the abnormality in only one direction

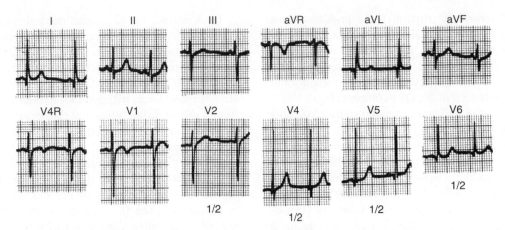

Fig. 3.17 Tracing from a 4-year-old child with a moderate ventricular septal defect. Note that some precordial leads are in ½ normal standardization.

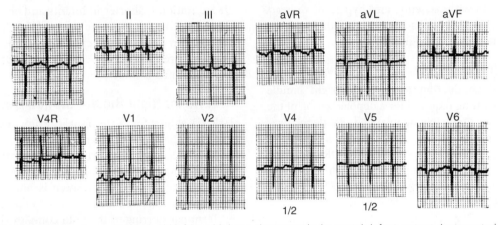

Fig. 3.18 Tracing from a 2-month-old infant with large-shunt ventricular septal defect, patent ductus arteriosus, and severe pulmonary hypertension.

3. Abnormal R/S ratio in favor of the LV: R/S ratio in V1 and V2 less than the lower limits of normal for the patient's age (see Table 3.5)
4. Q waves in V5 and V6, greater than 5 mm, as well as tall symmetrical T waves in the same leads ("LV diastolic overload")
5. In the presence of LVH, a wide QRS-T angle with the T axis outside the normal range indicates a "strain" pattern; this is manifested by inverted T waves in lead I or aVF. A wide QRS-T angle with the T axis within the normal range suggests a possible "strain" pattern.

Fig. 3.17 is an example of LVH. There is LAD for the patient's age (0 degrees). The R waves in leads I, aVL, V5, and V6 are beyond the upper limits of normal, indicating abnormal leftward force. The QRS duration is normal. The T axis (+55 degrees) remains in the normal quadrant. This tracing shows LVH (without "strain").

Criteria for Biventricular Hypertrophy

BVH may be manifested in one of the following ways.
1. Positive voltage criteria for RVH and LVH in the absence of BBB or preexcitation (i.e., with normal QRS duration)
2. Positive voltage criteria for RVH or LVH and relatively large voltages for the other ventricle

3. Large equiphasic QRS complexes in two or more of the limb leads and in the midprecordial leads (i.e., V2 through V5), called the Katz-Wachtel phenomenon (with normal QRS duration)

Fig. 3.18 is an example of BVH. It is difficult to plot the QRS axis because of large diphasic QRS complexes in limb leads. The QRS duration is not prolonged. The R and S voltages are large in some limb leads and in the midprecordial leads (Katz-Wachtel phenomenon). The S waves in leads I and V6 are abnormally deep (i.e., abnormal rightward force), and the R wave in V1 (i.e., rightward and anterior force) is also abnormally large, suggesting RVH. The R waves in leads I and aVL (i.e., leftward force) are also abnormally large, suggesting LVH. Therefore, this tracing shows BVH.

VENTRICULAR CONDUCTION DISTURBANCES

Conditions that are grouped together as ventricular conduction disturbances have abnormal prolongation of the QRS duration in common. Ventricular conduction disturbances include the following:
1. BBB, right and left
2. Preexcitation (e.g., WPW-type preexcitation)
3. Intraventricular block

In BBBs (and ventricular rhythms), the prolongation is in the terminal portion of the QRS complex (i.e., "terminal slurring"). In preexcitation, the prolongation is in the initial portion of the QRS complex (i.e., "initial slurring"), producing "delta" waves. In intraventricular block, the prolongation is throughout the duration of the QRS complex (Fig. 3.19).

Normal QRS duration varies with age; it is shorter in infants than in older children or adults (see Table 3.3). In adults, a QRS duration longer than 0.10 second is considered abnormally prolonged. In infants, a QRS duration of 0.08 second is the upper limit of normal. Depending on the degree of prolongation, complete versus incomplete block may be assigned.

By far the most commonly encountered form of ventricular conduction disturbance is RBBB. WPW preexcitation is uncommon, but it is a well-defined entity that deserves a brief description. LBBB is extremely rare in children, although it is common in adults with ischemic and hypertensive heart disease. Intraventricular block is associated with metabolic disorders and diffuse myocardial diseases.

Right Bundle Branch Block

In RBBB, delayed conduction through the right bundle branch prolongs the time required for a depolarization of the RV. When the LV is completely depolarized, RV depolarization is still in progress. This produces prolongation of the QRS duration, involving the terminal portion of the QRS complex, called "terminal slurring" (see Fig. 3.19B), and the slurring is directed to the *right* and *anteriorly* because the RV is located rightward and anteriorly in relation to the LV.

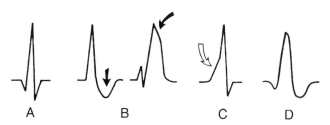

A   B   C   D

Fig. 3.19 Schematic diagram of three types of ventricular conduction disturbances. A, Normal QRS complex. B, QRS complex in right bundle branch block with prolongation of the QRS duration in the terminal portion (*black arrows*, terminal slurring). C, Preexcitation with delta wave (*open arrow*, initial slurring). D, Intraventricular block in which the prolongation of the QRS complex is throughout the duration of the QRS complex.

In a normal heart, synchronous depolarization of the opposing electromotive forces of the RV and LV cancels out the forces to some extent, with the resulting voltages that we call normal. In RBBB (and other ventricular conduction disturbances), asynchronous depolarization of the opposing electromotive forces may produce a lesser degree of cancellation of the opposing forces and thus results in greater manifest potentials for both ventricles. Consequently, abnormally large voltages for both RV and LV may result even in the absence of ventricular hypertrophy. Therefore, the diagnosis of ventricular hypertrophy in the presence of BBB (or WPW preexcitation or intraventricular block) is insecure.

In adults, when the QRS duration is longer than 0.12 second, it is called complete RBBB, and when the QRS duration is between 0.10 and 0.12 second, it is called incomplete right bundle branch block (IRBBB). Normal QRS duration is shorter in infants and children. Therefore, dividing RBBB into complete and incomplete is generally arbitrary and is particularly meaningless in children. Furthermore, in most of pediatric cases of RBBB, the right bundle branch is intact.

Criteria for Right Bundle Branch Block

1. RAD, at least for the terminal portion of the QRS complex (The initial QRS force is normal)
2. The QRS duration clearly longer than the upper limit of normal for the patient's age (see Table 3.3). When the prolongation of the QRS duration is only mild, it could be called incomplete RBBB.
3. Terminal slurring of the QRS complex that is directed to the right and usually, but not always, anteriorly:
   a. Wide and slurred S waves in leads I, V5, and V6
   b. Terminal, slurred R′ in aVR and the right precordial leads (V4R, V1, and V2)
4. ST-segment shift and T-wave inversion are common in adults but not in children.

Fig. 3.20 is an example of RBBB. The QRS duration is increased (0.11 second), indicating a ventricular conduction disturbance. There is slurring of the terminal portion of the QRS complex, indicating a BBB, and the slurring is directed to the right (slurred S waves in leads I and V6 and slurred R waves in aVR) and anteriorly (slurred R waves in V4R and V1), satisfying the criteria for RBBB. Although the S waves in leads I, V5, and

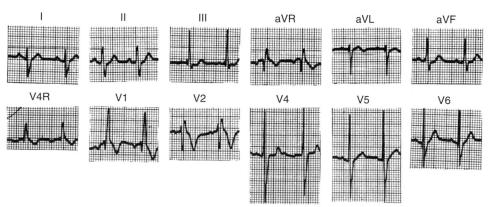

Fig. 3.20 Tracing from a 6-year-old boy who had corrective surgery for tetralogy of Fallot that involved right ventriculotomy for repair of a ventricular septal defect and resection of infundibular narrowing.

V6 are abnormally deep and the R/S ratio in V1 is abnormally large, it cannot be interpreted as RVH in the presence of RBBB.

Two pediatric conditions commonly associated with RBBB are ASD and conduction disturbances after open heart surgery involving right ventriculotomy. Other congenital heart defects often associated with RBBB include Ebstein's anomaly, coarctation of the aorta in infants younger than 6 months of age, endocardial cushion defect, and partial anomalous pulmonary venous return; it is also occasionally seen in normal children. Rarely, RBBB is seen in myocardial diseases (cardiomyopathy, myocarditis), muscle diseases (Duchenne's muscular dystrophy, myotonic dystrophy), and Brugada syndrome.

The significance of RBBB in children is different from that in adults. In several pediatric examples of RBBB, the right bundle is intact. In ASD, the prolonged QRS duration is the result of a longer pathway through a dilated RV rather than an actual block in the right bundle. Right ventriculotomy for repair of VSD or tetralogy of Fallot disrupts the RV subendocardial Purkinje network and causes prolongation of the QRS duration without necessarily injuring the main right bundle, although the latter may occasionally be disrupted.

Incomplete Right Bundle Branch Block

IRBBB is one of the more common ECG abnormalities reported by computer readouts and by physicians alike. Because some physicians are concerned with the rsR′ pattern in V1 or the diagnosis of IBBB, the topic deserves a little more attention.

Although the RSR′ (or rSr′) pattern in V1 is unusual in adults, this pattern is a normal finding in infants, toddlers, and children. From vectorcardiographic points of view, for a newborn ECG pattern to change to the adult pattern, it has to go through a stage in which rSr′ or RsR′ pattern appears. It is almost impossible for a newborn ECG to change to an adult pattern without going through the rSr′ (or rsR′) stage. (For those who are interested in learning about the reason, Park MK, Guntheroth WG: *How to Read Pediatric ECGs*, ed 4, Philadelphia, 2006, Mosby Elsevier, is recommended.)

The following clarifies some issues related to the rSr′ pattern in V1.

1. An rsR′ pattern in V1 is normal if it is associated with normal QRS duration and normal QRS voltage.
2. If the rSr′ pattern is associated with only slightly prolonged QRS duration (not to satisfy the criterion of RBBB), it is then incomplete RBBB. The QRS voltage may be slightly increased in some cases for the same reason as discussed under RBBB.
3. If the rsR′ pattern is associated with slightly prolonged QRS duration and an abnormal QRS voltage, it is still IRBBB, not ventricular hypertrophy.
4. RVH is justified only if an abnormal QRS voltage is present in the presence of normal QRS duration.

The pathophysiology and clinical significance of IRBBB are similar to that of RBBB as discussed earlier. Whether to call it "complete" or "incomplete" is arbitrary in children. When structural and functional cardiac anomalies are ruled out, IRBBB does not have much clinical significance in the pediatric population. Some cardiologists prefer the term "right ventricular conduction delay" rather than a "block" as in IRBBB. The prevalence of IRBBB in the pediatric population is not

known, although a large epidemiologic study from Japan suggests it is around 1% among the normal pediatric population. The prevalence of IRBBB in the adult population is estimated to be 5% to 10%, and it tends to increase with advancing age. A recent report suggests it may be a marker for lone atrial fibrillation in adults (which is defined as atrial fibrillation in the absence of identifiable cardiovascular or pulmonary disease).

Left Bundle Branch Block

Left bundle branch block is extremely rare in children. In LBBB, the duration of the QRS complex is prolonged for age, and the slurred terminal portion of the QRS complex is directed *leftward* and *posteriorly* (to the direction of the LV). A Q wave is absent in V6. A prominent QS pattern is seen in V1, and a tall R wave is seen in V6.

Left bundle branch block in children is associated with cardiac disease or surgery in the LV outflow tract, septal myomectomy, and replacement of the aortic valve. Other conditions rarely associated with LBBB include LVH, myocarditis, cardiomyopathy, MI, aortic valve endocarditis, and premature ventricular contractions (PVCs) or ventricular tachycardia (VT) originating in the RV outflow tract.

Intraventricular Block

In intraventricular block, the prolongation is throughout the duration of the QRS complex (see Fig. 3.19D). This usually suggests serious conditions such as metabolic disorders (e.g., hyperkalemia), diffuse myocardial diseases (e.g., myocardial fibrosis, systemic diseases with myocardial involvement), severe hypoxia, myocardial ischemia, or drug toxicity (quinidine or procainamide).

Wolff-Parkinson-White Preexcitation

Wolff-Parkinson-White preexcitation results from an anomalous conduction pathway (i.e., bundle of Kent) between the atrium and the ventricle, bypassing the normal delay of conduction in the AV node. The premature depolarization of a ventricle produces a delta wave and results in prolongation of the QRS duration (see Fig. 3.19C).

Criteria for Wolff-Parkinson-White Syndrome

1. Short PR interval, less than the lower limit of normal for the patient's age. The lower limits of normal of the PR interval according to age are as follows.

Less than 12 mo: 0.075 second
   1 to 3 years: 0.080 second
   3 to 5 years: 0.085 second
   5 to 12 years: 0.090 second
   12 to 16 years: 0.095 second
   Adults: 0.120 second

2. Delta wave (initial slurring of the QRS complex)
3. Wide QRS duration beyond the upper limit of normal

Patients with WPW preexcitation are prone to attacks of paroxysmal supraventricular tachycardia (SVT) (see Chapter 24). When there is a history of SVT, the diagnosis of WPW syndrome is justified. WPW preexcitation may mimic other ECG abnormalities such as ventricular hypertrophy, RBBB, or myocardial disorders. In the presence of preexcitation, the diagnosis of ventricular hypertrophy cannot be safely made. Large QRS deflections are often seen in this condition because of an asynchronous depolarization of the ventricles rather than ventricular hypertrophy.

Fig. 3.21 is an example of WPW preexcitation. The most striking abnormalities are a short PR interval (0.08 second) and a wide QRS duration (0.11 second). There are delta waves in most of the leads. Some delta waves are negative, as seen in leads III, aVR, V4R, and V1. The ST segments and T waves are shifted in the opposite direction of the QRS vector, resulting in a wide QRS-T angle. The QRS complexes show large leftward voltages, but the diagnosis of LVH cannot safely be made in the presence of WPW preexcitation.

There are two other forms of preexcitation that can also results in extreme tachycardia (SVT).

1. Lown-Ganong-Levine syndrome is characterized by a short PR interval and normal QRS duration. In this condition, James fibers (which connect the atrium and the bundle of His) bypass the upper AV node and produce a short PR interval, but the ventricles are depolarized normally through the His-Purkinje system. When there is no history of SVT, the tracing cannot be read as Lown-Ganong-Levine syndrome; it should read simply as short PR interval.

2. Mahaim-type preexcitation syndrome is characterized by a normal PR interval and long QRS duration with a delta wave. There is an abnormal Mahaim fiber that connects the AV node and one of the ventricles, bypassing the bundle of His and "short circuiting" into the ventricle.

Ventricular Hypertrophy versus Ventricular Conduction Disturbances

Two common ECG abnormalities in children, ventricular hypertrophy and ventricular conduction disturbances, are not always easy to distinguish; both present with increased QRS amplitudes. An accurate measurement of the QRS duration is essential. The following approach may aid in the correct diagnosis of these conditions (Fig. 3.22).

1. When the QRS duration is normal, normal QRS voltages indicate a normal ECG. Increased QRS voltages indicate ventricular hypertrophy.

2. When the QRS duration is clearly prolonged, a ventricular conduction disturbance is present whether the QRS voltages are normal or increased. An additional diagnosis of ventricular hypertrophy should not be made.

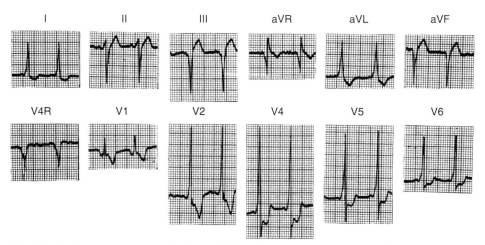

Fig. 3.21 Tracing from an asymptomatic 2-year-old boy whose ventricular septal defect underwent spontaneous closure. The tracing shows the Wolff-Parkinson-White preexcitation (see text for interpretation).

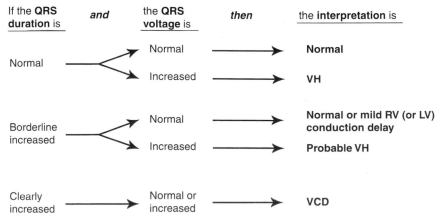

Fig. 3.22 Algorithm for differentiating between ventricular hypertrophy (VH) and ventricular conduction disturbances (VCDs). *LV,* Left ventricle; *RV,* right ventricle.

3. When the QRS duration is borderline prolonged, distinguishing between these two conditions is difficult. Normal QRS voltages favor a normal ECG or a mild (RV or LV) conduction disturbance. An increased QRS voltage favors ventricular hypertrophy.

ST-SEGMENT AND T-WAVE CHANGES

Electrocardiographic changes involving the ST segment and the T wave are common in adults but relatively rare in children. This is because there is a high incidence of ischemic heart disease, BBB, MI, and other myocardial disorders in adults.

ST-Segment Shift

An elevation or a depression of the ST segment is judged in relation to the PR segment as the baseline. Some ST-segment shifts are normal (nonpathologic), but others are abnormal (pathologic).

Nonpathologic ST-Segment Shift

Not all ST-segment shifts are abnormal. A slight shift of the ST segment is common in normal children. Elevation or depression of up to 1 mm in the limb leads and up to 2 mm in the precordial leads is within normal limits. Two common types of nonpathologic ST-segment shifts are J-depression and early repolarization. The T vector remains normal in these conditions.

J-depression

J-depression is a shift of the junction between the QRS complex and the ST segment (J-point) without sustained ST segment depression (Fig. 3.23A). The J-depression is seen more often in the precordial leads than in the limb leads (Fig. 3.24).

Early Repolarization

In early repolarization, all leads with upright T waves have elevated ST segments, and leads with inverted T waves have depressed ST segments (see Fig. 3.24). The T vector remains normal. This condition, seen in healthy adolescents and young adults, resembles the ST-segment shift seen in acute pericarditis; in the former, the ST segment is stable, and in the latter, the ST segment returns to the isoelectric line.

Pathologic ST-Segment Shift

Abnormal shifts of the ST segment often are accompanied by T-wave inversion. A pathologic ST-segment shift assumes one of the following forms:

1. Downward slant followed by a diphasic or inverted T wave (see Fig. 3.23B)
2. Horizontal elevation or depression sustained for longer than 0.08 second (see Fig. 3.23C)

Pathologic ST-segment shifts are seen in LVH or RVH with "strain" (discussed under ventricular hypertrophy); digitalis effect; pericarditis, including postoperative state; myocarditis (see under myocarditis, Chapter 19); MI; and some electrolyte disturbances (hypokalemia and hyperkalemia).

T-Wave Changes

T-wave changes usually are associated with the conditions manifesting with pathologic ST-segment shift. T-wave changes

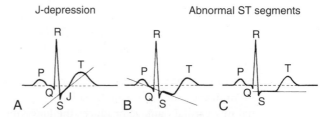

Fig. 3.23 Nonpathologic (nonischemic) and pathologic (ischemic) ST-segment and T-wave changes. A, Characteristic nonischemic ST-segment change called J-depression; note that the ST slope is upward. B and C, Examples of pathologic ST-segment changes; note that the downward slope of the ST segment (B) or the horizontal segment is sustained (C). (From Park MK, Guntheroth WG: *How to Read Pediatric ECGs*, ed 4, Philadelphia, 2006, Mosby Elsevier.)

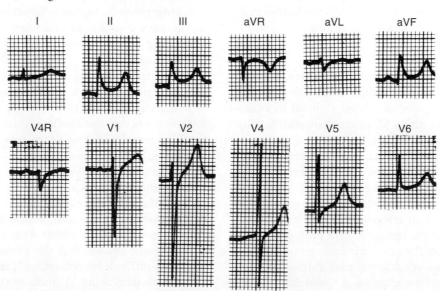

Fig. 3.24 Tracing from a healthy 16-year-old boy that exhibits early repolarization and J-depression. The ST segment is shifted toward the direction of the T wave and is most marked in II, III, and aVF. J-depression is seen in most of the precordial leads.

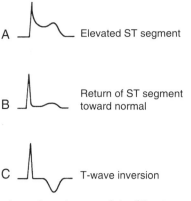

Fig. 3.25 Time-dependent changes of the ST segment and T wave in pericarditis. The initial change is ST-segment elevation (**A**) followed by return of ST segment elevation toward normal (**B**) and T-wave inversion with isoelectric ST segment (**C**). (From Park MK, Guntheroth WG: *How to Read Pediatric ECGs*, ed 4, Philadelphia, 2006, Mosby Elsevier.)

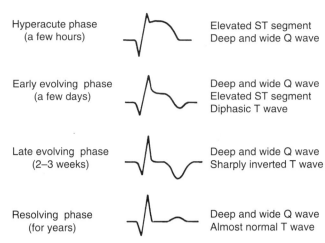

Fig. 3.26 Sequential changes of the ST segment and T wave in myocardial infarction. (From Park MK, Guntheroth WG: *How to Read Pediatric ECGs*, ed 4, Philadelphia, 2006, Mosby Elsevier.)

with or without ST-segment shift are also seen with BBB and ventricular arrhythmias.

Pericarditis

The ECG changes seen in pericarditis are the result of subepicardial myocardial damage or pericardial effusion and consist of the following:

1. Pericardial effusion may produce low QRS voltages (QRS voltages <5 mm in every one of the limb leads).
2. Subepicardial myocardial damage produces the following time-dependent changes in the ST segment and T wave (Fig. 3.25):
   a. ST-segment elevation occurs in the leads representing the LV.
   b. The ST-segment shift returns to normal within 2 to 3 days.
   c. T-wave inversion (with isoelectric ST segment) occurs 2 to 4 weeks after the onset of pericarditis.

Myocardial Infarction

Myocardial infarction is rare in infants and children, but correctly diagnosing the condition is important for proper care. All conditions that have been associated with MI in adults have been described as causing MI in children, such as atherosclerosis, inflammatory disease of the myocardium, lupus erythematosus, polyarteritis nodosa, hypertension, and diabetes mellitus. Uncommon causes of MI in pediatric patients include anomalous origin of the left coronary artery from the pulmonary artery, endocardial fibroelastosis, coronary artery embolization resulting from infective endocarditis or from interventional or diagnostic catheterization procedures performed on the left side of the heart, and inadvertent surgical interruption of the coronary artery during cardiac surgery. In recent years, early and late sequelae of Kawasaki's disease, surgical complications of the arterial switch operation for transposition of the great arteries, and dilated cardiomyopathy have emerged as important causes of MI in the pediatric population.

TABLE 3.7   Leads Showing Abnormal Electrocardiographic Findings in Myocardial Infarction

Location of Infarct	Limb Leads	Precordial Leads
Lateral	I, aVL	V5, V6
Anterior		V1, V2, V3
Anterolateral	I, aVL	V2–V6
Diaphragmatic	II, III, aVF	
Posterior		V1–V3[a]

[a]None of the leads is oriented toward the posterior surface of the heart. Therefore, in posterior infarction, changes that would have been present in the posterior surface leads will be seen in the anterior leads as a mirror image (e.g., tall and slightly wide R waves in V1 and V2, comparable to abnormal Q waves, and tall and wide, symmetric T waves in V1 and V2).

The ECG findings of adult MI are time dependent and are illustrated in Fig. 3.26.

1. Changes seen during the hyperacute phase are short-lived.
2. The more common ECG findings are those of the early evolving phase. These consist of pathologic Q waves (abnormally wide and deep), ST-segment elevation, and T-wave inversion. The duration of the Q wave is 0.04 second or greater in adults, and it should be at least 0.03 second in children.
3. Over the next few weeks (late evolving phase), the elevated ST segment gradually returns toward the baseline, but inverted T waves persist.
4. The pathologic Q waves persist for years after myocardial infarction (see Fig. 3.26).

Leads that show these abnormalities vary with the location of the infarction and are summarized in Table 3.7.

In most pediatric patients with MI, the time of onset is not clearly known, and the evolution of the different phases is difficult to document. Frequent ECG findings in children with acute MI include the following (Towbin et al, 1992):

1. Wide Q waves (>0.035 second) with or without Q-wave notching
2. ST segment elevation (>2 mm)

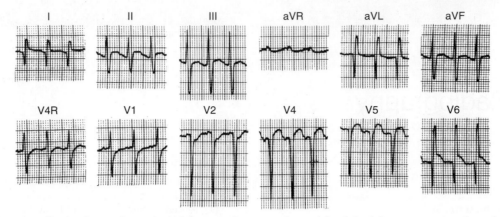

Fig. 3.27 Tracing from a 2-month-old infant who has anomalous origin of the left coronary artery from the pulmonary artery. An abnormally deep and wide Q wave (0.04 second) seen in I, aVL, and V6 and a QS pattern seen in V2 through V6 are characteristic of anterolateral myocardial infarction.

3. Prolongation of QTc interval (>0.44 second) with accompanying abnormal Q waves

The width of the Q wave is more important than the depth; the depth of the Q wave varies widely in normal children (see Table 3.6).

Fig. 3.27 is an ECG of MI in an infant with anomalous origin of the left coronary artery from the pulmonary artery. The most important abnormality is the presence of a deep and wide Q wave (0.04 second) in leads I, aVL, and V6. A QS pattern appears in V2 through V5, indicating anterolateral MI (see Table 3.7).

Electrolyte Disturbances

Two important serum electrolytes that produce ECG changes are calcium and potassium.

Calcium

Calcium ion affects the duration of the ST segment and thus changes the relative position of the T wave. Hyper- or hypocalcemia does not produce ST-segment shift or T-wave changes. Hypocalcemia prolongs the ST segment and, as a result, prolongs the QTc interval (Fig. 3.28). Hypercalcemia shortens the ST segment, resulting in shortening of the QTc interval (see Fig. 3.28).

Potassium

1. Hypokalemia produces one of the least specific ECG changes. When the serum potassium level is below 2.5 mEq/L, ECG changes consist of a prominent U wave with apparent prolongation of the QTc, flat or diphasic T waves, and ST-segment depression (Fig. 3.29). With further lowering of serum potassium levels, the PR interval becomes prolonged, and sinoatrial block may occur.
2. Hyperkalemia. The earliest ECG abnormality seen in hyperkalemia is tall, peaked, symmetrical T waves with a narrow base, so-called tented T wave. In hyperkalemia, sinoatrial block, second-degree AV block (either Mobitz I or II), and accelerated junctional or ventricular escape rhythm may occur. Severe hyperkalemia may result in either ventricular fibrillation or arrest. The following ECG sequence is associated with a progressive increase in the serum potassium level (see Fig. 3.29):

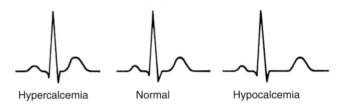

Hypercalcemia   Normal   Hypocalcemia

Fig. 3.28 Electrocardiographic findings of hypercalcemia and hypocalcemia. Hypercalcemia shortens and hypocalcemia lengthens the ST segment. (From Park MK, Guntheroth WG: *How to Read Pediatric ECGs*, ed 4, Philadelphia, 2006, Mosby Elsevier.)

SERUM K

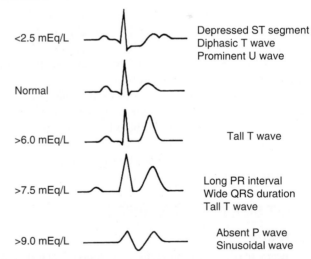

<2.5 mEq/L	Depressed ST segment Diphasic T wave Prominent U wave
Normal	
>6.0 mEq/L	Tall T wave
>7.5 mEq/L	Long PR interval Wide QRS duration Tall T wave
>9.0 mEq/L	Absent P wave Sinusoidal wave

Fig. 3.29 Electrocardiographic findings of hypokalemia and hyperkalemia. (From Park MK, Guntheroth WG: *How to Read Pediatric ECGs*, ed 4, Philadelphia, 2006, Mosby Elsevier.)

a. Tall, tented T waves
b. Prolongation of the QRS duration (intraventricular block)
c. Prolongation of the PR interval (first-degree AV block)
d. Disappearance of the P wave
e. Wide, bizarre diphasic QRS complex ("sine wave")
f. Eventual asystole

These ECG changes are usually seen best in leads I and II and the left precordial leads.

4

Chest Radiography

Chest radiography was an essential part of cardiac evaluation before echocardiography and Doppler studies became widely available to cardiologists. This simple test remains very useful to physicians who do not have access to echocardiography and Doppler studies. Cardiovascular abnormalities may be incidentally suspected by radiographic films that were obtained for other reasons. Chest radiography also supplements information that is not gained by the echocardiography study, such as information on the lung parenchyma, airways, and vascular structures connected to the heart.

Chest radiographic films can provide the following information: heart size and silhouette; enlargement of specific cardiac chambers; pulmonary blood flow or pulmonary vascular markings; and other information regarding lung parenchyma, spine, bony thorax, abdominal situs, and so on. Posteroanterior and lateral views are routinely obtained.

HEART SIZE AND SILHOUETTE

Heart Size

Measurement of the cardiothoracic (CT) ratio is by far the simplest way to estimate the heart size in older children (Fig. 4.1). The CT ratio is obtained by relating the largest transverse diameter of the heart to the widest internal diameter of the chest:

$$\text{CT ratio} = (A + B) - C$$

in which A and B are maximal cardiac dimensions to the right and left of the midline, respectively, and C is the widest internal diameter of the chest. A CT ratio of more than 0.5 indicates cardiomegaly. However, the CT ratio cannot be used with accuracy in newborns and small infants, in whom a good inspiratory chest film is rarely obtained. In this situation, the

degree of inadequate inspiration should be taken into consideration. Also, an estimation of the cardiac volume should be made by inspecting the posteroanterior and lateral views instead of the CT ratio.

To determine the presence or absence of cardiomegaly, the lateral view of the heart should also be inspected. For example, isolated right ventricular enlargement may not be obvious on a posteroanterior film but will be obvious on a lateral film. In a patient with a flat chest (or narrow anteroposterior diameter of the chest), a posteroanterior film may erroneously show cardiomegaly.

An enlarged heart on chest radiographs more reliably reflects a volume overload than a pressure overload. Electrocardiograms (ECGs) better represent a pressure overload than chest radiographic films.

Normal Cardiac Silhouette

The structures that form the cardiac borders in the posteroanterior projection of a chest radiograph are shown in Figure 4.2. The right cardiac silhouette is formed superiorly by the superior vena cava (SVC) and inferiorly by the right atrium (RA). The left cardiac border is formed from the top to the bottom by the aortic knob, the main pulmonary artery (PA), and the left ventricle (LV). The left atrial appendage (LAA) is located between the main PA and the LV and is not prominent in a normal heart. The right ventricle (RV) does not form the cardiac border in the posteroanterior view. The lateral projection of the cardiac silhouette is formed anteriorly by the RV and posteriorly by the left atrium (LA) above and the LV below. In a normal heart, the lower posterior cardiac border (i.e., LV) crosses the inferior vena cava (IVC) line above the diaphragm (see Fig. 4.2).

However, in newborns, a typical normal cardiac silhouette is rarely seen because of the presence of a large thymus and because the films are often exposed during expiration. The thymus is situated in the superoanterior mediastinum. Therefore, the base of the heart may be widened, with resulting alteration in the normal silhouette in the posteroanterior view. In the lateral view, the retrosternal space, which is normally clear in older children, may be obliterated by the large thymus.

Abnormal Cardiac Silhouette

Although discerning individual chamber enlargement often helps diagnose an acyanotic heart defect, the overall shape of the heart sometimes provides important clues to the type of defect, particularly in dealing with cyanotic infants and children. A few examples follow, relating it to the status of pulmonary blood flow or pulmonary vascular markings.

1. A "boot-shaped" heart with decreased pulmonary blood flow is typical in infants with cyanotic tetralogy of Fallot (TOF). This is also seen in some infants with tricuspid atresia. Typical of both conditions is the presence of a hypoplastic main PA segment (Fig. 4.3A).

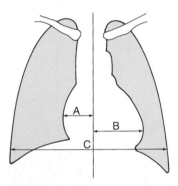

Fig. 4.1 Diagram showing how to measure the cardiothoracic (CT) ratio from the posteroanterior view of a chest radiographic film. The CT ratio is obtained by dividing the largest horizontal diameter of the heart (A + B) by the longest internal diameter of the chest (C).

2. A narrow-waisted and "egg-shaped" heart with increased pulmonary blood flow in a cyanotic infant strongly suggests transposition of the great arteries (TGA). The narrow waist results from the absence of a large thymus and the abnormal relationship of the great arteries (see Fig. 4.3B).

3. The "snowman" sign with increased pulmonary blood flow is seen in infants with the supracardiac type of total anomalous pulmonary venous return (TAPVR). The left vertical vein, left innominate vein, and dilated SVC make up the snowman's head (see Fig. 4.3C).

EVALUATION OF THE CARDIAC CHAMBERS AND GREAT ARTERIES

Individual Chamber Enlargement

Identification of individual chamber enlargement is important in diagnosing a specific lesion, particularly when dealing with acyanotic heart defects. Although enlargement of a single chamber is discussed here, more than one chamber is usually involved.

Left Atrial Enlargement

An enlarged LA causes alterations not only of the cardiac silhouette but also of the various adjacent structures (Fig. 4.4). Mild LA enlargement is best appreciated in the lateral projection by the posterior protrusion of the LA border. Enlargement of the LA may produce "double density" on the posteroanterior view. With further enlargement, the LAA becomes prominent on the left cardiac border. The left mainstem bronchus is elevated.

Left Ventricular Enlargement

In the posteroanterior view, the apex of the heart is not only farther to the left but also downward. In the lateral view of LV enlargement, the lower posterior cardiac border is displaced farther posteriorly and meets the IVC line below the diaphragm level (Fig. 4.5).

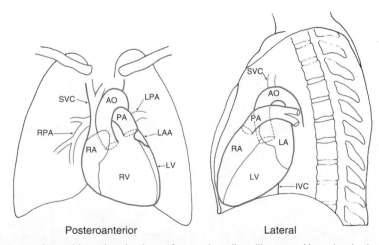

Posteroanterior   Lateral

Fig. 4.2 Posteroanterior and lateral projections of normal cardiac silhouette. Note that in the lateral projection, the right ventricle (RV) is contiguous with the lower third of the sternum and that the left ventricle (LV) normally crosses the posterior margin of the inferior vena cava (IVC) above the diaphragm. *AO,* Aorta; *LA,* left atrium; *LAA,* left atrial appendage; *LPA,* left pulmonary artery; *PA,* pulmonary artery; *RA,* right atrium; *RPA,* right pulmonary artery; *SVC,* superior vena cava.

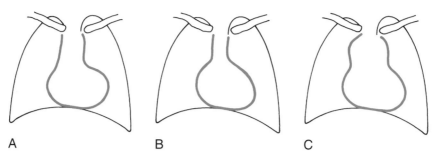

Fig. 4.3 Abnormal cardiac silhouettes. **A,** "Boot-shaped" heart seen in cyanotic tetralogy of Fallot or tricuspid atresia. **B,** "Egg-shaped" heart seen in transposition of the great arteries. **C,** "Snowman" sign seen in total anomalous pulmonary venous return (supracardiac type).

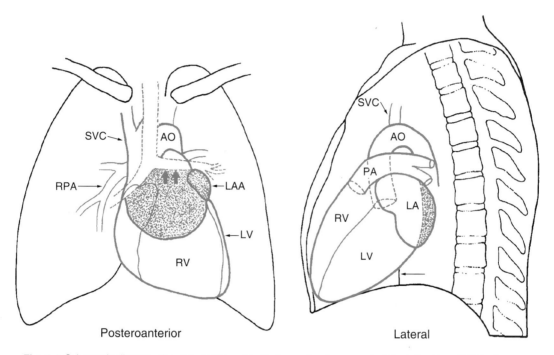

Fig. 4.4 Schematic diagram showing radiographic findings of enlargement of the left atrium (LA) in the posteroanterior and lateral projections. *Arrows* show left mainstem bronchus elevation. In the posteroanterior view, "double density" and prominence of the left atrial appendage (LAA) are also illustrated. In the lateral view, posterior protrusion of the LA border is illustrated. The isolated enlargement of the LA shown here is only hypothetical because it usually accompanies other changes. Other abbreviations are the same as those in Figure 4.2.

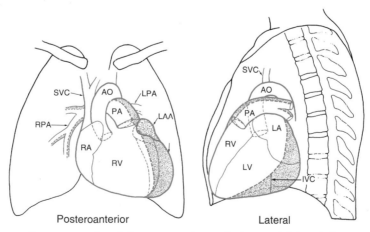

Fig. 4.5 Diagrammatic representation of changes seen in ventricular septal defect. Left ventricle (LV) enlargement in addition to enlargement of the left atrium (LA) and a prominent pulmonary artery (PA) segment. Other abbreviations are the same as those in Figure 4.2.

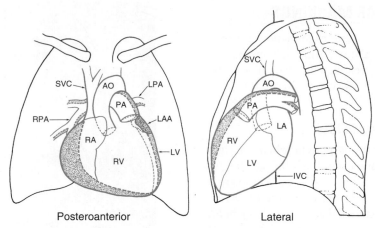

Fig. 4.6 Schematic diagrams of posteroanterior and lateral chest radiographs of atrial septal defect (ASD). There are enlargements of the right atrium (RA) and right ventricle (RV), prominence of the pulmonary artery (PA), and an increased pulmonary vascularity. Other abbreviations are the same as those in Figure 4.2.

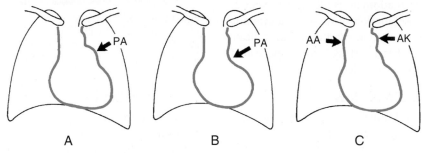

Fig. 4.7 Abnormalities of the great arteries. **A,** Prominent main pulmonary artery (PA) segment. **B,** Concave PA segment resulting from hypoplasia of the main PA. **C,** Dilatation of the aorta may be seen as a bulge on the right upper mediastinum by a dilated ascending aorta (AA) or as a prominence of the aortic knob (AK) on the left upper cardiac border.

Right Atrial Enlargement

Right atrial enlargement is most obvious in the posteroanterior projection as an increased prominence of the lower right cardiac silhouette (Fig. 4.6). However, this is not an absolute finding because both false-positive and false-negative results are possible.

Right Ventricular Enlargement

Isolated right ventricular enlargement may not be obvious in the posteroanterior projection, and the normal CT ratio may be maintained because the RV does not make up the cardiac silhouette in the posteroanterior projection. RV enlargement is best recognized in the lateral view, in which it manifests itself by filling of the retrosternal space (see Fig. 4.6, lateral view).

Size of the Great Arteries

As in the enlargement of specific cardiac chambers, the size of the great arteries often helps make a specific diagnosis.

Prominent Main Pulmonary Artery Segment

The prominence of a normally placed PA in the posteroanterior view (Fig. 4.7A) results from one of the following:
1. Poststenotic dilatation (e.g., pulmonary valve stenosis)

2. Increased blood flow through the PA (e.g., atrial septal defect [ASD], ventricular septal defect [VSD])
3. Increased pressure in the PA (e.g., pulmonary hypertension)
4. Occasional normal finding in adolescents, especially girls

Hypoplasia of the Pulmonary Artery

A concave main PA segment with a resulting "boot-shaped" heart is seen in TOF and tricuspid atresia (see Fig. 4.7B); obviously, malposition of the PA must be ruled out.

Dilatation of the Aorta

An enlarged ascending aorta may be observed in the frontal projection as a rightward bulge of the right upper mediastinum, but a mild degree of enlargement may easily escape detection. Aortic enlargement is seen in TOF and aortic stenosis (as poststenotic dilatation/aortopathy) and less often in patent ductus arteriosus (PDA), coarctation of the aorta (COA), Marfan's syndrome, or systemic hypertension. When the ascending aorta and aortic arch are enlarged, the aortic knob may become prominent on the posteroanterior view (see Fig. 4.7C).

PULMONARY VASCULAR MARKINGS

One of the major goals of radiologic examination is assessment of the pulmonary vasculature. Although many textbooks explain how to detect increased pulmonary blood flow, this is one of the more difficult aspects of interpreting chest radiographs of cardiac patients.

Increased Pulmonary Blood Flow

Increased pulmonary vascularity is present when the right and left PAs appear enlarged and extend into the lateral third of the lung field, where they are not usually present; there is increased vascularity to the lung apices where the vessels are normally collapsed; and the external diameter of the right PA visible in the right hilus is wider than the internal diameter of the trachea.

Increased pulmonary blood flow in an acyanotic child represents ASD, VSD, PDA, endocardial cushion defect, aortopulmonary window, partial anomalous pulmonary venous return (PAPVR), or any combination of these. In a cyanotic infant, increased pulmonary vascular markings may indicate TGA, TAPVR, hypoplastic left heart syndrome, persistent truncus arteriosus, or a single ventricle.

Decreased Pulmonary Blood Flow

Decreased pulmonary blood flow is suspected when the hilum appears small, the remaining lung fields appear black, and the vessels appear small and thin. Ischemic lung fields are seen in cyanotic heart diseases with decreased pulmonary blood flow such as critical stenosis or atresia of the pulmonary or tricuspid valves, including TOF.

Pulmonary Venous Congestion

Pulmonary venous congestion is characterized by a hazy and indistinct margin of the pulmonary vasculature. This is caused by pulmonary venous hypertension secondary to LV failure or obstruction to pulmonary venous drainage (e.g., mitral stenosis, TAPVR, cor triatriatum). Kerley's B lines are short, transverse strips of increased density best seen in the costophrenic sulci. This is caused by engorged lymphatics and interstitial edema of the interlobular septa secondary to pulmonary venous congestion.

Normal Pulmonary Vasculature

Pulmonary vascularity is normal in patients with obstructive lesions such as pulmonary stenosis or aortic stenosis. Unless the stenosis is extremely severe, pulmonary vascularity remains normal in pulmonary stenosis. Patients with small left-to-right shunt lesions also show normal pulmonary vascular markings.

SYSTEMATIC APPROACH

The interpretation of chest radiographs should include a systematic routine to avoid overlooking important anatomic changes relevant to cardiac diagnosis.

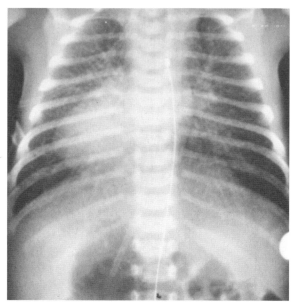

Fig. 4.8 A chest radiographic film of the chest and upper abdomen of a newborn infant with polysplenia syndrome. Note a symmetrical liver ("midline liver"), a stomach bubble in the midline, dextrocardia, and increased pulmonary vascularity.

Location of the Liver and Stomach Gas Bubble

The cardiac apex should be on the same side as the stomach or opposite the hepatic shadow. When there is heterotaxia, with the apex on the right and the stomach on the left (or vice versa), the likelihood of a serious heart defect is great. An even more ominous situation exists with a "midline" liver, associated with asplenia (Ivemark's) syndrome or polysplenia syndrome (Fig. 4.8). These infants usually have complex cyanotic heart defects.

Skeletal Aspect of Chest Radiographic Film

Pectus excavatum may flatten the heart in the anteroposterior dimension and cause a compensatory increase in its transverse diameter, creating the false impression of cardiomegaly. Thoracic scoliosis and vertebral abnormalities are frequent in cardiac patients.

Identification of the Aorta

1. Identification of the descending aorta along the left margin of the spine usually indicates a left aortic arch; identification along the right margin of the spine indicates a right aortic arch. The right aortic arch is frequently associated with TOF or persistent truncus arteriosus. Some of the patients with right aortic arch may have vascular ring (see Chapter 16).
2. In a heavily exposed film, the precoarctation and postcoarctation dilatation of the aorta may be seen as a "figure of 3."

Upper Mediastinum

1. The thymus is prominent in healthy infants and may give a false impression of cardiomegaly. It may give the classic "sail sign" (Fig. 4.9). The thymus often has a wavy border because this structure becomes indented by the ribs. On the lateral view, the thymus occupies the superoanterior mediastinum, obscuring the upper retrosternal space.

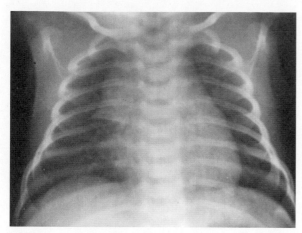

Fig. 4.9 Radiograph showing the typical "sail sign" on the right mediastinal border.

2. The thymus shrinks in cyanotic infants and infants under severe stress from congestive heart failure. In TGA, the mediastinal shadow is narrow ("narrow waist"), partly because of the shrinkage of the thymus gland. Infants with DiGeorge syndrome have an absent thymic shadow and a high incidence of aortic arch anomalies.
3. "Snowman figure" (or figure-of-8 configuration) is seen in infants, who are usually older than 4 months, with anomalous pulmonary venous return draining into the SVC via an ascending vertical vein and the left innominate vein (see Fig. 4.3C).

Pulmonary Parenchyma

1. Pneumonia is a common complication in patients with increased pulmonary blood flow, such as those with a large PDA or VSD.
2. A long-standing density, particularly in the lower left lung field, suggests pulmonary sequestration. In this condition, there is an aberrant, nonfunctioning pulmonary tissue, which does not connect with the bronchial tree and derives its blood supply from the descending aorta. The venous drainage is usually to the pulmonary venous system.
3. A vertical vascular shadow along the lower right cardiac border may suggest PAPVR from the lower lobe and sometimes the middle lobe of the right lung, called *scimitar syndrome*. Its pulmonary venous drainage is usually to the IVC either just above or below the diaphragm. This syndrome is often associated with other anomalies, including hypoplasia of the right lung and right pulmonary artery, sequestration of right lung tissue receiving arterial supply from the aorta, and ASD.

PART 2

Special Tools in Evaluation of Cardiac Patients

A number of special tools are available to cardiologists in the evaluation of pediatric cardiac patients. Some tools are readily available and frequently used, but others are more specialized and are available only at tertiary centers. Echocardiography is the mainstay of noninvasive imaging tools and is available to almost every cardiologist. This tool usually provides the final diagnosis for most pediatric cardiac problems and is discussed in depth. Magnetic resonance imaging and computed tomography are other noninvasive imaging tools that have gained a supplemental role in cardiac evaluation. The discussion of these tools will be limited to the pros and cons of the techniques. Other noninvasive tools frequently used by cardiologists include exercise stress test and ambulatory electrocardiography (e.g., Holter monitor, event monitor). These tests are discussed in depth. Cardiac catheterization and angiocardiography are invasive tests that usually provide conclusive anatomic and physiologic information and the final diagnosis. Although catheter intervention procedures are not diagnostic, Part II discusses it briefly because they are usually performed with cardiac catheterization. Electrophysiologic evaluation is not included in the discussion because they are too specialized and are only performed by specially trained electrophysiologists.

Noninvasive Imaging Tools

OUTLINE

An ideal modality used for noninvasive imaging of congenital heart defects should be able to delineate all aspects of the cardiac anatomy, including extracardiac vessels; evaluate physiological parameters such as measurement of blood flow, pressure gradients across cardiac valves or blood vessels, and ventricular function; be cost effective, portable, and noninvasive with the least risk and discomfort; and include no exposure to ionizing radiation. No single modality satisfies all of these requirements. Chest radiographic films, the original imaging tool, provide only indirect evidence of intracardiac defects that manifest primarily with volume overload. They do not provide images of the defect itself. They are less informative on pressure overload lesions that do not result in chamber enlargement. Echocardiography has become the main noninvasive imaging modality since the 1980s, providing direct images of intracardiac and some extracardiac anatomy. In recent years, noninvasive radiologic techniques such as magnetic resonance imaging (MRI) and computed tomography (CT) have emerged as supplementary modalities in areas for which echocardiography studies are deficient.

In this chapter, two-dimensional (2D) and M-mode echocardiography are presented in some detail. This is followed by a brief discussion of the two radiologic techniques with emphasis on how to choose an optimal radiologic technique for a given patient.

ECHOCARDIOGRAPHY

Echocardiography (echo) uses ultrasound beams reflected by cardiovascular structures to produce characteristic lines or shapes caused by normal or abnormal cardiac anatomy in one, two, or three dimensions, which are called M-mode, 2D, and three-dimensional (3D) echocardiography, respectively.

An echocardiographic study currently begins with real-time 2D echo, which produces high-resolution tomographic images of cardiac structure, their movement, and vascular structures leaving and entering the heart. The Doppler and color mapping study has added the ability to easily detect valve regurgitation and cardiac shunts during the echo examination. These tests combined provide reliable quantitative information such as ventricular function, pressure gradients across cardiac valves and blood vessels, and estimation of pressures in the great arteries and ventricles. Echo examination can be applied in calculation of cardiac output and the magnitude of cardiac shunts, although this is rarely used. Reliable noninvasive hemodynamic evaluation and confident delineation of cardiovascular structures by echo have dramatically reduced the necessity for cardiac catheterization. Increasingly, patients undergo valvular or congenital heart surgery on the basis of an echo diagnosis. Transesophageal echocardiography (TEE) has markedly improved resolution of echo images. Real-time 3D echocardiography provides improved accuracy of imaging the global perspective visualization of various cardiac anomalies, but this is not presented here because it is mostly performed by specially trained cardiologists.

Discussion of instruments and techniques is beyond the scope of this book. Normal 2D echo images and M-mode measurements and their role in the diagnosis of common cardiac problems in pediatric patients are the focus of this presentation.

Two-Dimensional Echocardiography

Two-dimensional echo examinations are performed by directing the plane of the transducer beam along a number of cross-sectional planes through the heart and great vessels. A routine 2D echocardiogram is obtained from four transducer locations: parasternal, apical, subcostal, and suprasternal notch (SSN) positions. From each transducer position, images of the long- and short-axis views are obtained by manually rotating and angulating the transducer. The parasternal and apical views usually are obtained with the patient in the left lateral decubitus position and the subcostal and suprasternal notch views with the patient in the supine position. Figs. 5.1 through 5.9 illustrate some standard images of the heart and great vessels. Modified transducer positions and different angulations make many other views possible. Measurement of important cardiac structures can be made on the freeze frame of 2D echo studies. Normal values of the dimension of the cardiac chambers, great arteries, and various valve annuli are shown in several tables in Appendix D (see Tables D.1 to D.5).

The Parasternal Views

For parasternal views, the transducer is applied to the left parasternal border in the second, third, or fourth space with the patient in the left lateral decubitus position.

Parasternal Long-Axis Views

The plane of sound is oriented along the major axis of the heart, usually from the patient's left hip to the right shoulder. Three major views are recorded: standard long axis, long axis of the right ventricular (RV) inflow, and long axis of the RV outflow (see Fig. 5.1).

1. The **standard long-axis view** is the most basic view that shows the left atrium (LA), mitral valve, and left ventricular (LV) inflow and outflow tracts (see Fig. 5.1A). This view is important in evaluating abnormalities in or near the mitral valve, LA, LV, left ventricular outflow tract (LVOT), aortic valve, aortic root, ascending aorta, and ventricular septum. In a normal heart, the anterior leaflet of the mitral valve is continuous with the posterior wall of the aorta (i.e., aortic–mitral continuity). The trabecular septum (apicalward) and infracristal outlet septum (near the aortic valve) constitute the interventricular septum in this view. Therefore, ventricular septal defects (VSDs) of tetralogy of Fallot (TOF) and persistent truncus arteriosus are best shown in this view. Detailed discussion of localizing other types of VSDs is presented in Chapter 12. Pericardial effusion is readily imaged in this view. This is the view to evaluate mitral valve prolapse (MVP). Frequently, the coronary sinus can be seen as a small circle in the atrioventricular (AV) groove (see Fig. 5.1A). An enlarged coronary sinus may be seen with persistence of left superior vena cava (LSVC), TAPVR to coronary sinus, coronary AV fistula, and rarely with elevated right atrial (RA) pressure.

2. In the **RV inflow view**, a long-axis view of the RV and RA is obtained. In this view, abnormalities in the tricuspid valve (tricuspid regurgitation [TR], prolapse) and inflow portion of the RV are evaluated (Fig. 5.1B). The ventricular septum in this view consists of the inlet muscular septum (near the AV valve) and trabecular septum (apicalward). The right atrial appendage (RAA) can also be seen in this view. This view is good for recording the velocity of TR (to estimated right ventricular systolic pressure [RVSP]).

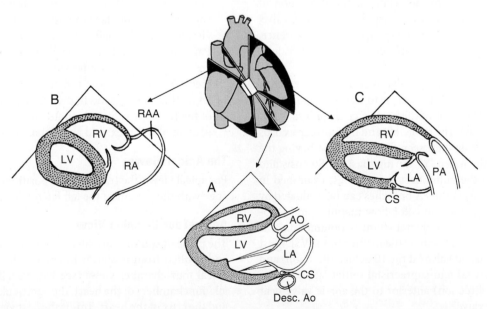

Fig. 5.1 Diagram of important two-dimensional echo views obtained from the parasternal long-axis transducer position. Standard long-axis view (**A**), right ventricular (RV) inflow view (**B**), and RV outflow view (**C**). *AO*, Aorta; *CS*, coronary sinus; *Desc. Ao*, descending aorta; *LA*, left atrium; *LV*, left ventricle; *PA*, pulmonary artery; *RA*, right atrium; *RAA*, right atrial appendage.

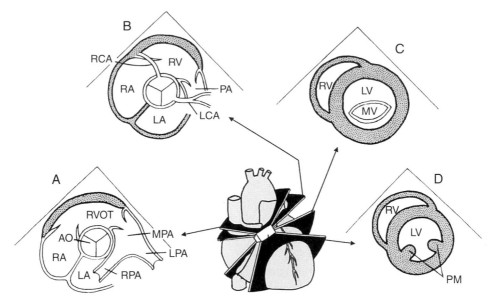

Fig. 5.2 Diagram of a family of the parasternal short-axis views. Semilunar valves and great artery level (**A**), coronary arteries (**B**), mitral valve level (**C**), and papillary muscle level (**D**). *AO,* Aorta; *LA,* left atrium; *LCA,* left coronary artery; *LPA,* left pulmonary artery; *LV,* left ventricle; *MPA,* main pulmonary artery; *MV,* mitral valve; *PM,* papillary muscle; *RA,* right atrium; *RCA,* right coronary artery; *RPA,* right pulmonary artery; *RV,* right ventricle; *RVOT,* right ventricular outflow tract.

3. In the **RV outflow view,** the RV outflow tract (RVOT), pulmonary valve, and proximal main pulmonary artery (PA) are visualized (Fig. 5.1C). The supracristal infundibular (outlet) septum is seen in this view.

Parasternal Short-Axis Views

By rotating the transducer used for the long-axis views clockwise, one obtains a family of important short-axis views (see Fig. 5.2). This projection provides cross-sectional images of the heart and the great arteries at different levels. The parasternal short-axis views are important in the evaluation of the aortic valve (i.e., bicuspid or tricuspid), pulmonary valve, PA and its branches, RVOT, coronary arteries (e.g., absence, aneurysm, stenosis), LA, LV, ventricular septum, AV valves, LV, and right side of the heart.

1. The **aortic valve.** The aortic valve is seen in the center of the image with the RVOT anterior to the aortic valve and the main PA to the right of the aorta ("circle and sausage" view) (see Fig. 5.2A). The right, left, and noncoronary cusps of the aortic valve are best seen from this view, having the appearance of the letter "Y" during diastole. Stenosis and regurgitation of the pulmonary valve is best examined in this plane. Stenosis of the PA branches can be evaluated by Doppler interrogation and color-flow mapping and Doppler interrogation of the ductal shunt is obtained in this plane. Color-flow studies show the membranous VSDs just distal to the tricuspid valve (at the 10 o'clock direction) and both the infracristal and supracristal outlet VSDs (at the 12 to 2 o'clock direction) anterior to the aortic valve near the pulmonary valve.

2. **Coronary arteries.** With a slight manipulation of the transducer from the above plane, the ostia and the proximal portions of the coronary arteries are visualized. The

right coronary artery (RCA) arises from the anterior coronary cusp near the tricuspid valve, which should be confirmed to connect to the aorta; there are some venous structures that run in front of the aorta (cardiac vein) but do not connect to the aorta. The left main coronary artery arises in the left coronary cusp near the main PA. Its bifurcation into the left anterior descending and circumflex coronary artery can usually be seen clearly. The proximal coronary arteries can also be seen in other long-axis views.

3. **Mitral valve.** The mitral valve is seen as a "fish mouth" during diastole. This view is good for measuring the mitral valve area in patients with mitral stenosis, and it is the best view to identify a cleft mitral valve (see Fig. 5.2C).

4. **Papillary muscles.** Two papillary muscles are normally seen at the 4 o'clock (anterolateral) and 8 o'clock (posteromedial) directions. The trabecular septum is seen at this level. This view is good in the assessment of apical portion of the LV such as hypertrophic cardiomyopathy, noncompaction of the apex, and apical mass (see Fig. 5.2D).

The Apical Views

For apical views, the transducer is positioned over the cardiac apex with the patient in the left lateral decubitus position.

Apical Four-Chamber View

The plane of sound is oriented in a nearly coronal body plane and is tilted from posterior to anterior to obtain a family of apical four-chamber views (see Fig. 5.3). This view displays all four chambers of the heart, the ventricular and atrial septa, and the crux of the heart. This is the best view to image the LV apex, where an apical VSD is commonly seen.

1. **Coronary sinus.** In the most posterior plane, the coronary sinus is seen to drain into the right atrium (see Fig. 5.3A).

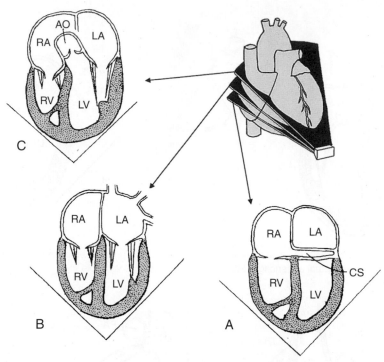

Fig. 5.3 Diagram of two-dimensional echo views obtained with the transducer at the apical position. **A,** The posterior plane view showing the coronary sinus. **B,** The standard apical four-chamber view. **C,** The apical "five-chamber" view is obtained with further anterior angulation of the transducer. *AO,* Aorta; *CS,* coronary sinus; *LA, l*eft atrium; *LV,* left ventricle; *RA,* right atrium; *RV,* right ventricle.

The ventricular septum seen in this view is the posterior trabecular septum.

2. The **apical four-chamber view** (see Fig. 5.3B) evaluates the atrial and ventricular septa and size and contractility of atrial and ventricular chambers, AV valves, and some pulmonary veins and identifies the anatomic RV and LV and detecting pericardial effusion. Normally, the tricuspid valve insertion to the septum is more apicalward than the mitral valve (5–10 mm in older children and adults), with a small portion of the septum (called the AV septum) separating the two AV valves. A defect in this portion of the septum may result in an LV–RA shunt (Gerbode defect). In Ebstein's anomaly, the insertion of the septal tricuspid valve is displaced more apically. The inlet ventricular septum (where an endocardial cushion defect occurs) is well imaged in this view just under the AV valves. VSDs in the entire length of the trabecular septum are well imaged, including apical VSD. The membranous septum is not imaged in this view. The anatomic characteristics of each ventricle are also noted, with the heavily trabeculated RV showing the moderator band. Abnormal chordal attachment of the AV valve (straddling) and overriding of the valve are also noted in this view. The relative size of the ventricles is examined in this view.

3. **Apical "five-chamber" view.** Further anterior angulation of the transducer demonstrates the so-called apical five-chamber view. This view shows the LVOT, aortic valve, subaortic area, and proximal ascending aorta. In this view, color-flow imaging allows qualitative assessment of aortic regurgitation. The membranous VSD is visualized

just under the aortic valve, and the infracristal outlet VSD is also imaged in this plane.

Apical Long-Axis Views

The apical long-axis view (or apical three-chamber view) shows structures similar to those shown in the parasternal long-axis view (see Fig. 5.4A). In the apical two-chamber view, the LA, mitral valve, and LV are imaged. The left atrial appendage can also be imaged (see Fig. 5.4B). The view of the LV apex provides diagnostic clues for cardiomyopathy, apical thrombus, and aneurysm.

The Subcostal Views

Subcostal long-axis (coronal) and short-axis (sagittal) views are obtained from the subxiphoid transducer position, with the patient in the supine position.

Subcostal long-axis (coronal) views are obtained by tilting the coronal plane of sound from posterior to anterior (see Fig. 5.5). The coronary sinus is seen posteriorly draining into the RA, similar to that shown for the apical view (see Fig. 5.5A). Anterior angulation of the transducer shows the atrial and ventricular septa. This is the best view for evaluating the atrial septum, including atrial septal defect (see Fig. 5.5B). Further anterior angulation of the transducer shows the LVOT, aortic valve, and ascending aorta (see Fig. 5.5C). The parts of the ventricular septum visualized in this view (apicalward) are membranous, subaortic outlet, and trabecular septa. The junction of the superior vena cava (SVC) and the RA is seen to the right of the ascending aorta (see Fig. 5.5C). Further anterior angulation shows the entire RV, including the inlet,

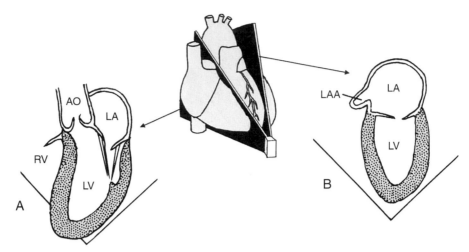

Fig. 5.4 Apical long-axis view. **A,** Apical "three-chamber" view. **B,** Apical "two-chamber" view. *AO,* Aorta; *LA,* left atrium; *LAA,* left atrial appendage; *LV,* left ventricle; *RV,* right ventricle.

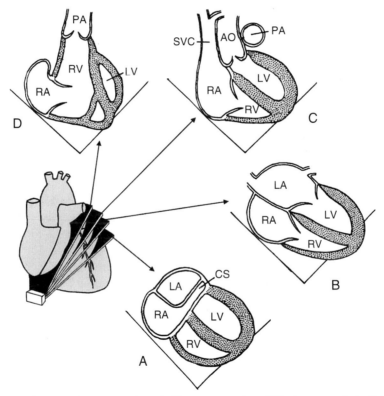

Fig. 5.5 Diagram of subcostal long-axis view. **A,** The coronary sinus (CS) view posteriorly. **B,** Standard subcostal four-chamber view. **C,** View showing the left ventricular outflow tract and the proximal aorta. **D,** View showing the right ventricular outflow tract (RVOT) and the proximal main pulmonary artery. *AO,* Aorta; *LA,* left atrium; *LV,* left ventricle; *PA,* pulmonary artery; *RA,* right atrium; *RV,* right ventricle; *SVS,* superior vena cava.

trabecular and infundibular portions, pulmonary valve, and main PA (see Fig. 5.5D). The ventricular septum seen in this view includes the (apicalward) supracristal outlet, infracristal outlet, and anterior trabecular and posterior trabecular septa.

Subcostal short-axis (or sagittal) views (see Fig. 5.6) are obtained by rotating the long-axis transducer 90 degrees to the sagittal plane.

1. To the right of the patient, both the superior and inferior venae cavae are seen to enter the right atrium (see Fig. 5.6A). A small azygous vein can be seen to enter the SVC,

and the right PA can also be seen on end beneath this vein (see Fig. 5.6A).

2. A leftward angulation of the transducer shows the RVOT, pulmonary valve, PA, and tricuspid valve on end (see Fig. 5.6B). This view is orthogonal to the standard subcostal four-chamber view, and both views combined are good for evaluation of the size of a VSD.

3. Additional leftward angulation of the transducer will show the mitral valve (not shown) and papillary muscle (see Fig. 5.6C), similar to those seen in the parasternal short-axis views.

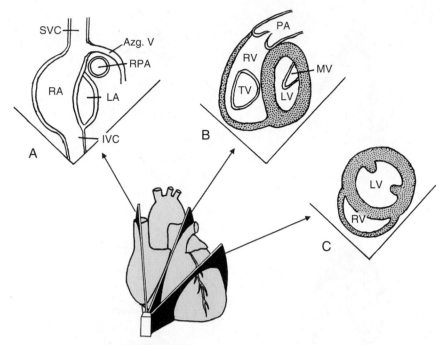

Fig. 5.6 Subcostal short-axis (sagittal) view. **A,** Entry of venae cavae with drainage of the azygous vein (Azg. V). **B,** View showing the right ventricle (RV), right ventricular outflow tract (RVOT), and pulmonary artery (PA). **C,** Short-axis view of the ventricles. *LA,* Left atrium; *LV,* left ventricle; *MV,* mitral valve; *PA,* pulmonary artery; *RA,* right atrium; *RPA,* right pulmonary vein; *SVC,* superior vena cava; *TV,* tricuspid valve.

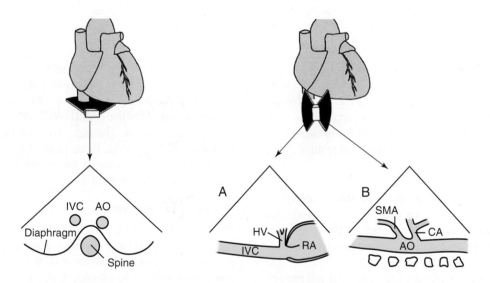

Fig. 5.7 Abdominal views. *Left,* abdominal short-axis view. *Right,* abdominal long-axis view. **A,** Inferior vena cava (IVC) view; **B,** Abdominal descending aorta (AO) view. *CA,* Celiac axis; *HV,* hepatic vein; *RA,* right atrium; *SMA,* superior mesenteric artery.

Subcostal Views of the Abdomen

Abdominal short- and long-axis views (see Fig. 5.7) are obtained from the subxiphoid transducer position, with the patients in supine position.

1. **Abdominal short-axis view** is obtained by placing the transducer in a transverse body plane (see Fig. 5.7, *left*). It demonstrates the descending aorta on the left and the inferior vena cava (IVC) on the right of the spine as two round structures. The aorta should pulsate. Both hemidiaphragms, which move symmetrically with respiration,

are imaged. Asymmetric or paradoxical movement of the diaphragm is seen with paralysis of the hemidiaphragm.

2. **Abdominal long-axis view** is obtained by placing the transducer in a sagittal body plane. The IVC is imaged to the right (see Fig. 5.7A, *right*), and the descending aorta is imaged to the left of the spine (Fig. 5.7B, *right*). The IVC collects the hepatic vein before draining into the right atrium. The eustachian valve may be seen at the junction of the IVC and the RA. The failure of the IVC to join the RA indicates interruption of the IVC (with azygous continuation, which

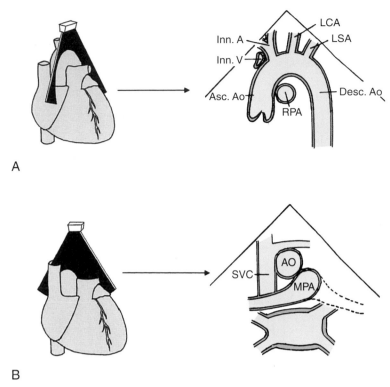

Fig. 5.8 Diagram of suprasternal notch two-dimensional echo views. **A,** Long-axis view. **B,** Short-axis view. *AO,* Aorta; *Asc. Ao,* ascending aorta; *Desc. Ao,* descending aorta; *Inn. A,* innominate artery; *Inn. V,* innominate vein; *LA,* left atrium; *LCA,* left carotid artery; *LSA,* left subclavian artery; *MPA,* main pulmonary artery; *PA,* pulmonary artery; *RPA,* right pulmonary artery; *SVC,* superior vena cava.

is frequently seen with polysplenia syndrome). Major branches of the descending aorta, celiac artery, and superior mesenteric artery are easily visualized. A pulsed-wave Doppler examination of the abdominal aorta in this view is important to identify coarctation by demonstrating persistent diastolic flow and delayed upstroke of systolic flow.

The Suprasternal Views

The transducer is positioned in the suprasternal notch to obtain suprasternal long-axis (see Fig. 5.8A) and short-axis (see Fig. 5.8B) views, which are important in the evaluation of anomalies in the ascending and descending aortas (e.g., coarctation of the aorta), aortic arch (e.g., interruption), size of the PAs, and anomalies of systemic veins and pulmonary veins. In infants, the transducer can be sometimes placed in a high right subclavicular position.

The suprasternal long-axis view (see Fig. 5.8A) is obtained by 45-degree clockwise rotation from the sagittal plane in the suprasternal notch to visualize the entire (left) aortic arch. Failure to visualize the aortic arch in this manner may suggest the presence of a right aortic arch. Three arteries arising from the aortic arch (the innominate, left carotid, and left subclavian arteries in that order) are seen. The innominate vein is seen in cross-section in front of the ascending aorta and the right PA behind the ascending aorta. Manipulation of the transducer farther posteriorly and leftward will image the isthmus and upper descending aorta, a very important segment to study for the coarctation of the aorta.

The suprasternal short-axis view (Fig. 5.8B) is obtained by rotating the ultrasound plane parallel to the sternum. Superior to the circular transverse aorta, the innominate vein is seen to connect to the (right) SVC, which runs vertically to the right of the aorta. The right PA is visualized in its length under the circular aorta. Beneath the RPA is the LA. With a slight posterior angulation of the transducer, four pulmonary veins are seen to enter the LA.

The Subclavicular Views

The right subclavicular view (see Fig. 5.9A) is obtained in the right second intercostal space in a sagittal projection. This view is useful in the assessment of the SVC and right atrial junction as well as the ascending aorta. The right upper pulmonary vein and the azygous vein can also be examined in this view.

The left subclavicular view (see Fig. 5.9B) is useful for examination of the branch PAs. The transducer is positioned in a transverse plane in the second left intercostal space and a little tilted inferiorly. The main PA is seen left of the ascending aorta (*circle*), and it bifurcates into the right and left PA branches.

Quantitative Values Derived from Two-Dimensional Echocardiography

1. **Dimensions of cardiovascular structures.** Several tables of normal values of cardiovascular structures that were measured from still frames of 2D echocardiography are

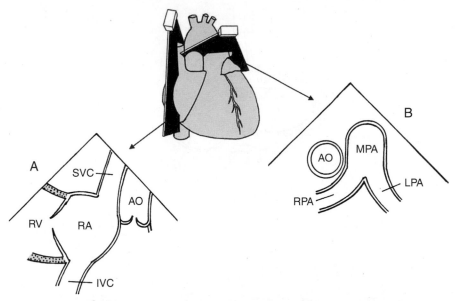

Fig. 5.9 Diagram of subclavicular views. **A,** Right subclavicular view. **B,** Left subclavicular view. *AO,* Aorta; *IVC,* inferior vena cava; *LPA,* left pulmonary artery; *MPA,* main pulmonary artery; *RA,* right atrium; *RPA,* right pulmonary artery; *RV,* right ventricle; *SVC,* superior vena cava.

shown in Appendix D. These tables are frequently useful in the practice of pediatric cardiology. They include M-mode measurements of the LV (Table D.1); stand-alone M-mode measurements of the RV, aorta, and LA (Table D.2); aortic root and aorta (Table D.3); pulmonary valve and PAs (Table D.4); and AV valves (Table D.5). The normal dimension of the coronary arteries is shown in Table D.6.

2. **Left ventricular mass.** LV mass is an indication of left ventricular hypertrophy (LVH). Although the thickness of LV walls (interventricular septum and LV posterior wall) identifies people with increased LV mass, LV mass has become a valuable marker of end-organ damage in patients with systemic hypertension. LV mass can be estimated from M-mode echocardiography or 2D echocardiography measurements.

a. *M-mode echo method.* LV mass is usually derived from 2D-guided M-mode echo measurement, with assumptions that the LV is spherical in shape and the thickness of the wall measured at the basal area of the LV is representative of the entire LV. It is assumed that a smaller sphere formed by the endocardium is inside a larger sphere formed by the pericardium, and therefore, the difference in the volume of the two spheres would be the volume of LV muscle. Although less accurate than the 2D echo method, the M-mode method is simpler to obtain and thus more popular than the 2D method. There is controversy as to indexing the LV mass for body size, having been variably indexed by body weight, height, body surface area, or 2.7 power of height. M-mode–derived LV mass indexed to 2.7 power of height is popular and normal data by that method are presented in Appendix D (Table D.7).

b. *2D echo method.* In the 2D-measured echo technique for calculating LV mass, the LV is assumed to be a bullet shape rather than a sphere, and this technique has been shown to be more accurate than the M-mode method. The LV volume can be estimated from the short- and long-axis views in systole or diastole. The LV area in the short-axis view is calculated by the biplane Simpson's method. The formula for such a volume would be 5/6 the LV area of the short axis multiplied by the length of the ventricle (obtained from the long axis):

$$\text{Volume} = 5/6 \text{ Area} \times \text{Length}$$

The LV volume so calculated is then converted to mass by multiplying it by the specific gravity of muscle (usually taken as 1.05). This cumbersome method is less popular and not routinely performed in most laboratories. Normal values of 2D echo-derived LV mass indexed to the body surface area are presented in Appendix D (Table D.8).

M-MODE ECHOCARDIOGRAPHY

M-mode echocardiography, which graphically displays a one-dimensional slice of cardiac structure varying over time, was one of the earliest tools of echocardiography. Currently, an M-mode echo is obtained as part of 2D tomographic images. M-mode echo is used primarily for the measurement of the dimension (wall thickness and chamber size) and LV function (fractional shortening, wall thickening). It is also useful for assessing the motion of cardiac valves (mitral valve prolapse, mitral stenosis, pulmonary hypertension) and movement of cardiac wall and septa (in RV volume overload).

Fig. 5.10 shows examples of M-mode measurements of the dimension of the RV, LV, LA, and aorta and LV wall thickness during systole and diastole. Line 1 passes through the aorta and LA, where the dimensions of these structures are measured. Line 2 traverses the mitral valve. Line 3 goes through the main body of the RV and LV. Along line 3, the dimensions of the RV and LV and the thickness of the

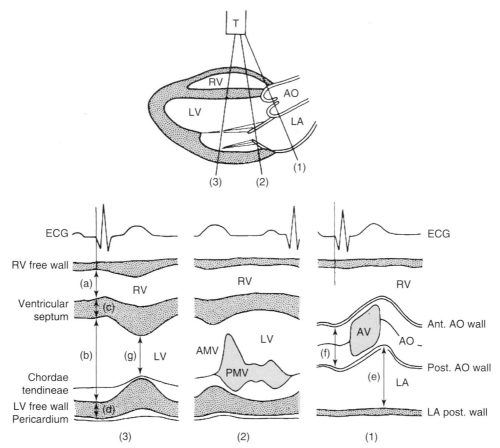

Fig. 5.10 Examples of M-mode measurement of cardiac dimensions. The dimension of the aorta (AO) and left atrium (LA) is measured along line 1. Line 2 passes through the mitral valve. Measurement of chamber dimensions and wall thickness of right ventricle (RV) and left ventricle (LV) is made along line 3. The following measurements are shown in this figure: (a), RV dimension; (b), LV diastolic dimension; (c), interventricular septal thickness; (d), LV posterior wall thickness; (e), LA dimension; (f), aortic dimension; (g), LV systolic dimension. *AMV*, Anterior mitral valve; *ECG*, electrocardiogram; *PMV*, posterior mitral valve; *T*, transducer.

interventricular septum and posterior LV wall are measured during systole and diastole. Pericardial effusion is best detected at this level.

Normal M-Mode Echo Values

Two frequent applications of M-mode echo in clinical practice are measurements of dimension of cardiac structures and LV systolic function.

Cardiac Chamber Dimensions

Most dimensions are measured during diastole, coincident with the onset of the QRS complex; the LA dimension and LV systolic dimension are exceptions (see Fig. 5.10). The dimensions of the cardiac chambers and the aorta increase with increasing age, so normal values are expressed as function of growth (see Appendix D).

Left Ventricular Systolic Function

Left ventricular systolic function is evaluated by the fractional shortening (or shortening fraction) or ejection fraction. The ejection fraction is a derivative of the fractional shortening and offers no advantages over the fractional shortening. Serial determinations of these measurements are important in the

management of conditions in which LV function may change (e.g., in patients with chronic or acute myocardial disease).

Fractional Shortening

Fractional shortening (or shortening fraction) is derived by the following:

$$FS\ (\%) = Dd - Ds/Dd \times 100$$

in which FS is fractional shortening, Dd is end-diastolic dimension of the LV, and Ds is end-systolic dimension of the LV. This is a reliable and reproducible index of LV function, provided there is no regional wall-motion abnormality and there is concentric contractility of the LV. If the interventricular septal motion is flat or paradoxical, the shortening fraction will not accurately reflect ventricular ejection.

Mean normal value of FS is 36%, with 95% prediction limits of 28% to 44%. FS is decreased in a poorly compensated LV regardless of cause (e.g., pressure overload, volume overload, primary myocardial disorders, doxorubicin cardiotoxicity). It is increased in volume-overloaded ventricle (e.g., VSD, patent ductus arteriosus, aortic regurgitation, mitral regurgitation [MR]) and pressure overload lesions (e.g., moderately severe aortic valve stenosis, hypertrophic obstructive cardiomyopathy).

Ejection Fraction

Ejection fraction relates to the change in volume of the LV with cardiac contraction. It is obtained by the following formula:

$$EF\,(\%) = (Dd)^3 - (Ds)^3/(Dd)^3 \times 100$$

in which EF is ejection fraction and Dd and Ds are the end-diastolic and end-systolic dimensions, respectively, of the LV. The volume of the LV is derived from a single measurement of the dimension of the minor axis of the LV. In the preceding formula, the minor axis is assumed to be half of the major axis of the LV; this assumption is incorrect in children. Normal mean ejection fraction is 66% with ranges of 56% to 78%.

DOPPLER ECHOCARDIOGRAPHY

Doppler echocardiography combines the study of cardiac structure and blood flow profiles. The Doppler effect is a change in the observed frequency of sound that results from motion of the source or target. When the moving object or column of blood moves toward the ultrasonic transducer, the frequency of the reflected sound wave increases (i.e., a positive Doppler shift). Conversely, when blood moves away from the transducer, the frequency decreases (i.e., a negative Doppler shift). Doppler ultrasound equipment detects a frequency shift and determines the direction and velocity of red blood cell flow with respect to the ultrasound beam. By convention, velocities of red blood cells moving toward the transducer are displayed above a zero baseline; those moving away from the transducer are displayed below the baseline.

The two commonly used Doppler techniques are continuous wave and pulsed wave. The pulsed wave emits a short burst of ultrasound, and the Doppler echo receiver "listens" for returning information. The continuous wave emits a constant ultrasound beam with one crystal, and another crystal continuously receives returning information. Both techniques have their advantages and disadvantages. Pulsed-wave Doppler can control the site at which the Doppler signals are sampled, but the maximal detectable velocity is limited, making it unusable for quantification of severe obstruction. In contrast, continuous-wave Doppler can measure extremely high velocities (e.g., for the estimation of severe stenosis), but it cannot localize the site of the sampling; rather, it picks up the signal anywhere along the Doppler beam. When these two techniques are used in combination, clinical application expands.

The Doppler echo technique is useful in the study of the following: (1) detecting the presence and direction of cardiac shunts; (2) studying stenosis or regurgitation of cardiac valves; (3) assessing stenosis of blood vessels; (4) assessing the hemodynamic severity of a lesion, including pressures in various compartments of the cardiovascular system; (5) estimating the cardiac output or blood flow; and (6) assessing diastolic function of the ventricle (see later discussion). The Doppler echo is usually used with color flow mapping (see below) to enhance the technique's usefulness.

Normal Doppler velocities in children and adults are shown in Table 5.1. Normal Doppler velocity is less than 1 m/

TABLE 5.1 Normal Doppler Velocities in Children and Adults

	Children Mean (ranges) (m/sec)	Adults Mean (ranges) (m/sec)
Mitral flow	1.0 (0.8–1.3)	0.9 (0.6–1.3)
Tricuspid flow	0.6 (0.5–0.8)	0.6 (0.3–0.7)
Pulmonary artery	0.9 (0.7–1.1)	0.75 (0.6–0.9)
Left ventricle	1.0 (0.7–1.2)	0.9 (0.7–1.1)
Aorta	1.5 (1.2–1.8)	1.35 (1.0–1.7)

From Hatle L, Angelsen B: *Doppler Ultrasound in Cardiology*, ed 2, Philadelphia, 1985, Lea & Febiger.

sec for the PA; it may be up to 1.8 m/sec for the ascending and descending aortas. Mitral and tricuspid inflow velocities are usually less than 1 m/sec.

Measurement of Pressure Gradients

The simplified Bernoulli equation can be used to estimate the pressure gradient across a stenotic lesion, regurgitant lesion, or shunt lesion. One may use one of the following equations.

$$P_1 - P_2\,(mm\,Hg) = 4\left(V_2^2 - V_1^2\right)$$
$$P_1 - P_2\,(mm\,Hg) = 4(V\,max)^2$$

in which $(P1–P2)$ is the pressure difference across an obstruction, V1 is the velocity (m/sec) proximal to the obstruction, and V2 is the velocity (m/sec) distal to the obstruction in the first equation. When V_1 is less than 1 m/sec, it can be ignored, as in the second equation. However, when V_1 is greater than 1.5 m/sec, it should be incorporated into the equation to obtain a more accurate estimation of pressure gradients. This is important in the study of the ascending and descending aortas, where flow velocities are often more than 1.5 m/sec. Ignoring V_1 may significantly overestimate the pressure gradient in patients with aortic stenosis or coarctation of the aorta.

To obtain the most accurate prediction of the peak pressure gradient, the Doppler beam should be aligned parallel to the jet flow, the peak velocity of the jet should be recorded from several different transducer positions, and the highest velocity should be taken. An example of a Doppler study in a patient with moderate pulmonary stenosis is shown in Fig. 5.11. The peak instantaneous pressure gradient calculated from the Bernoulli equation is different from the peak-to-peak pressure gradient measured during cardiac catheterization. The peak instantaneous pressure gradient is usually larger than the peak-to-peak pressure gradient. The difference between the two is more noticeable in patients with mild to moderate obstruction and less apparent in patients with severe obstruction.

Prediction of Intracardiac or Intravascular Pressures

The Doppler echo allows estimation of pressures in the RV, PA, and LV using the flow velocity of certain valvular or shunt jets. Estimation of PA pressure is particularly important in pediatric patients.

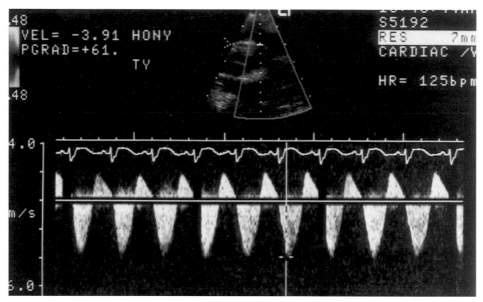

Fig. 5.11 Doppler echocardiographic study in a child with a moderate pulmonary valve stenosis. The Doppler cursor is placed in the main pulmonary artery near the pulmonary valve in the parasternal short-axis view. The maximum forward flow velocity (negative flow) is 3.91 m/sec (with an estimated pressure gradient of 61 mm Hg). There is a small regurgitant (positive) flow seen during diastole.

The following are some examples of such applications:

1. RVSP or pulmonary artery systolic pressure (PASP) can be estimated from the velocity of the TR jet, if present, by the following equation:

$$RVSP \, (or \, PASP) = 4(V)^2 + RA \, pressure$$

in which V is the TR jet velocity.

For example, if the TR velocity is 2.5 m/sec, the instantaneous pressure gradient is $4 \times (2.5)2 = 4 \times 6.25 = 25$ mm Hg. Using an assumed RA pressure of 10 mm Hg, the RVSP (or PASP in the absence of PS) is 35 mm Hg (assuming that the RA pressure of 10 mm Hg is too high for patients who do not have severe TR or RV failure; an RA mean pressure of 5 mm Hg is more reasonable in most children and adolescents).

2. RVSP (or PASP) can also be estimated from the velocity of the VSD jet by the following equation:

$$RVSP \, (or \, PASP) = Systemic \, SP \, (or \, arm \, SP) - 4(V)^2$$

in which V is the VSD jet.

For example, if the VSD jet flow velocity is 3 m/sec, the instantaneous pressure drop between the LV and RV is $4 \times 32 = 36$ mm Hg. That is, the RV SP is 36 mm Hg lower than the left ventricular systolic pressure (LVSP). If LVSP is assumed to be 90 mm Hg, the estimated RV SP is 54 mm Hg (90–36 = 54). In the absence of PS, the PASP will be about 54 mm Hg. Note that the SP obtained in the arm cannot be assumed to be the same as LVSP; the arm pressure is usually 5 to 10 mm Hg higher than the LVSP (see peripheral amplification in Chapter 2).

3. LVSP can be estimated from the velocity of flow through the aortic valve (V) by the following equation:

$$LVSP = 4(V)^2 + Systemic \, SP \, (or \, arm \, SP)$$

in which V is the aortic flow velocity. The same precaution applies as above in that the arm SP is slightly higher than the LVSP.

Measurement of Cardiac Output or Blood Flow

Both systemic blood flow and pulmonary blood flow can be calculated by multiplying the mean velocity of flow and the cross-sectional area as shown in the following equation:

$$Cardiac \, output \, (L/min) = V \times CSA \times 60 \, (sec/min) \div 1000 \, cc/L$$

in which V is the mean velocity (cm/sec) obtained either by using a computer program or by manually integrating the area under the curve. CSA is the cross-sectional area of flow (cm2) measured or computed from the 2D echo. Usually, the PA flow velocity and diameter are used to calculate pulmonary blood flow; the mean velocity and diameter of the ascending aorta are used to calculate systemic blood flow, or cardiac output.

Diastolic Function

Signs of diastolic dysfunction may precede those of systolic dysfunction. Mitral inflow velocities obtained in the apical four-chamber view can evaluate LV diastolic function. There are two flow waves in the AV valves, the E wave and the A wave (Fig. 5.12). The E wave occurs during the early diastolic filling phase, and the A wave occurs during atrial contraction. The E wave is taller than the A wave in normal children and adults. However, the A wave may be normally taller than the E wave in the first 3 weeks of life.

The following simple measurements are useful in evaluating diastolic function of the ventricle (see Fig. 5.12).

1. The E and A wave peak velocities and the ratio of the two (E/A ratio)
2. Deceleration time (DT): the interval from the early peak velocity to the zero intercept of the extrapolated deceleration slope

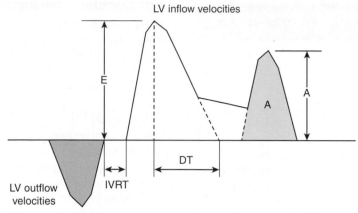

Fig. 5.12 Selected parameters of diastolic function. (See text for discussion.) *A*, Second peak velocity; *DT*, deceleration time; *E*, early peak velocity; *IVRT*, isovolumic relaxation time; *LV*, left ventricle.

3. Atrial filling fraction: the integral of the A velocity divided by the integral of the total mitral inflow velocities
4. Isovolumic relaxation time (IVRT): the interval between the end of the LV outflow velocity and the onset of mitral inflow; this is easily obtained by pulsed-wave Doppler with the cursor placed in the LV outflow near the anterior leaflet of the mitral valve and is measured from the end of the LV ejection to the onset of the mitral inflow

In normal children, the mitral Doppler indexes are as follows. The average peak E velocity is 0.6 m/sec, the average peak A velocity is 0.3 m/sec, and the average E:A velocity ratio is 2.0. Detailed normal values for other measurements are shown in Figure 18.6.

Abnormalities in the diastolic function are easy to find, but they are usually nonspecific and do not provide independent diagnostic information. In addition, they can be affected by loading conditions (i.e., increase or decrease in preload), heart rate, and the presence of atrial arrhythmias. Two well-known patterns of abnormal diastolic function are a decreased relaxation pattern and a "restrictive" pattern (see Fig. 18.6). The decreased relaxation pattern is seen with hypertrophic and dilated cardiomyopathies, LVH of various causes, ischemic heart disease, other forms of myocardial disease, reduced preload (e.g., dehydration), and increased afterload (e.g., during infusion of arterial vasoconstrictors). The "restrictive" pattern is usually seen in restrictive cardiomyopathy but is also seen with increased preload (e.g., seen with MR) and a variety of heart diseases with heart failure.

COLOR-FLOW MAPPING

A color-coded Doppler study provides images of the direction and disturbances of blood flow superimposed on the echo structural image. Although systematic Doppler interrogation can obtain similar information, this technique is more accurate and time saving. In general, red is used to indicate flow toward the transducer, and blue is used to indicate flow away from the transducer. Color may not appear when the direction of flow is perpendicular to the ultrasound beam. The turbulent flow is color coded as either green or yellow.

CONTRAST ECHOCARDIOGRAPHY

Injection of indocyanine green, dextrose in water, saline, or the patient's blood into a peripheral or central vein produces microcavitations and creates a cloud of echoes on the echocardiogram. Structures of interest are visualized or recorded by 2D echo at the time of the injection. This technique has successfully detected an intracardiac shunt, validated structures, and identified flow patterns within the heart. For example, an injection of any liquid into an intravenous line may confirm the presence of a right-to-left shunt at the atrial or ventricular level. To a large extent, this technique has been replaced by color-flow mapping and Doppler studies.

OTHER ECHOCARDIOGRAPHIC TECHNIQUES

Fetal Echocardiography

Improvement in image resolution makes visualization of the fetal cardiovascular structure possible, thereby permitting in utero diagnosis of cardiovascular anomalies. To obtain a complete examination, the transducer is placed at various positions on the maternal abdominal wall. Doppler examination and color mapping are performed at the same time. The optimal timing for performance of a comprehensive transabdominal fetal echo is 18 to 22 weeks of gestation. Images can be more difficult to obtain after 30 weeks of gestation because the ratio of fetal body mass to amniotic fluid increases (Rychik et al, 2004).

Accurate diagnosis of congenital heart defect (CHD) via fetal echo provides many benefits, including improved surgical outcome for infants with CHDs. In addition, fetal echo continues to teach physicians more about human fetal cardiac physiology. It also enables physicians to study the effects of cardiovascular abnormalities and abnormal cardiac rhythms in utero and then assess the need for therapeutic intervention.

Indications for fetal echo are expanding and examples are shown in Box 5.1. Increased nuchal translucency (the amount of fluid at the back of the head and neck of a fetus, which is often associated with chromosomal abnormalities, e.g., trisomies 13, 18, and 21) present on obstetric ultrasound at 10 to

---

BOX 5.1 Examples of Indications for Fetal Echocardiography

Maternal Indications
Family history of CHD
Metabolic disorders (e.g., diabetes, PKU)
Exposure to teratogens
Exposure to prostaglandin synthetase inhibitors (e.g., ibuprofen, salicylates, indomethacin)
Rubella infection
Autoimmune disease (e.g., SLE, Sjögren syndrome)
Familial inherited disorders (Ellis van Creveld syndrome, Marfan syndrome, Noonan disease)
In vitro fertilization

Fetal Indications
Abnormal obstetrical ultrasound screen
Extracardiac abnormality
Chromosomal abnormality
Arrhythmia
Hydrops
Increased first trimester nuchal translucency
Multiple gestation and suspicion of twin-twin transfusion syndrome

---

CHD, Congenital heart disease; *PKU,* phenylketonuria; *SLE,* systemic lupus erythematosus.
From Rychik J, Ayers N, Cuneo B, et al: American Society of Echocardiography guidelines and standards for performance of the fetal echocardiogram, *J Am Soc Echocardiogr* 17:803–810, 2004.

13 weeks gestation has been associated with an increased risk of CHD, even in the absence of chromosomal anomaly. Infants conceived via intracytoplasmic sperm injection and in vitro fertilization have up to a threefold increased prevalence of CHDs.

Transesophageal Echocardiography

By placing a 2D or multiplane transducer at the end of a flexible endoscope, it is possible to obtain high-quality 2D images by way of the esophagus. Color-flow mapping and Doppler examination are usually incorporated in this approach.

If satisfactory images of the heart or blood vessels are not possible from the usual transducer position on the surface of the patient's chest (e.g., in patients with obesity or chronic obstructive pulmonary disease), physicians may use TEE. This approach is especially helpful in assessing thrombus in native or prosthetic valves, endocarditis vegetations, thrombi in the left atrial chamber and appendage, and aortic dissections. TEE is often used for patients who are undergoing cardiac surgery. TEE can monitor LV function throughout the surgical procedure, as well as assess cardiac morphology and function before and after surgical repair of valvular or congenital heart defects. TEE requires general anesthesia or sedation and the presence of an anesthesiologist because a lack of patient cooperation can result in serious complications. Use of this technique in pediatric patients is somewhat limited to intraoperative use and in some obese adolescents and adolescents with complicated heart defects for whom the risk of general anesthesia or sedation is worth taking for the expected benefit. Schematic drawings of biplane images of TEE are shown in Appendix D (see Fig. D.1).

Intravascular Echocardiography

To provide an intravascular echo, the ultrasonic transducer is placed in a small catheter so that vessels can be imaged by means of the lumen. These devices can evaluate atherosclerotic arteries in adults and coronary artery stenosis or aneurysm in children with Kawasaki's disease.

Tissue Doppler Echocardiography

Whereas conventional Doppler echo assesses the direction and the velocity of blood flow, tissue Doppler echo (also known as tissue Doppler imaging) assesses the velocity of myocardial tissue movement at any arbitrary point. When the tissue point is set at the annulus of the AV valve, movement velocities of the annulus summarize the longitudinal shortening of the ventricle during systole and elongation during diastole.

The LV function is assessed from the velocity curves taken from the septal and lateral insertion points of the mitral valve in the four-chamber view. Additional velocity curves taken from the anterior and inferior points of the mitral valve insertion in the two-chamber view may provide a more reproducible measure of the LV function. Peak systolic annular velocity (S′) (Fig. 5.13) of the mitral valve is a reliable measure of the LV function; it decreases in LV systolic dysfunction. For RV function, the lateral point of the tricuspid annulus is used. Likewise, peak tricuspid annular systolic velocity is a measure of the RV systolic function.

The peak mitral annular velocity during early filling phase of diastole (e′) is a measure of LV diastolic function. If there is impaired relaxation (diastolic dysfunction), the (e′) velocity decreases. The late velocity peak (a′) is a function of atrial contraction.

RADIOLOGIC TECHNIQUES: MAGNETIC RESONANCE IMAGING AND COMPUTED TOMOGRAPHY

Although the conventional echo study remains the mainstay of noninvasive evaluation of cardiac patients, it has limitations in complete delineation of cardiac anomalies. In addition to being operator dependent, echocardiography may not provide optimal quality of images of cardiovascular structure because of postoperative scars, chest wall deformities, overlying lung tissue, large body size in adolescents, and obesity. In particular, extracardiac structures such as the PAs, pulmonary veins, and aortic arch cannot always be adequately imaged by echo study because of acoustic window limitations. As to the coronary arteries, only the proximal portion can be adequately imaged by echo studies. Although TEE may improve the quality of images, it is not only a more invasive technique requiring deep sedation or anesthesia, but it does not always provide the needed information for patient care. Cardiac catheterization, with a higher complication rate, may become necessary to make complete anatomic and physiologic evaluation of the patient with complex cardiac pathology. Fortunately, however, some noninvasive radiologic techniques, such as MRI and cardiac

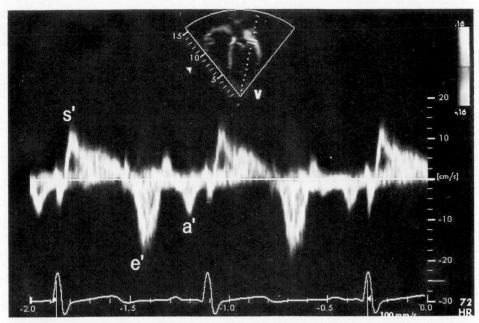

Fig. 5.13 Pulsed-waved tissue Doppler sampling lateral mitral annulus from the apical four-chamber view. The tissue Doppler imaging shows peak velocities in systole (s′), in early diastole (e′), and late diastole (a′) during atrial contraction.

CT, are now available that can obviate the need for cardiac catheterization.

Both MRI and CT can provide images of cardiovascular structures and other intrathoracic structures that are not usually imaged by echo studies. However, one of the radiologic techniques may be better than the other in its capability and its practicality. For example, in young pediatric patients, CT may have a broader appeal because of its short duration of study, but exposure to ionizing radiation and contrast administration requirements are important drawbacks. On the other hand, MRI has capability of offering quantitative ventricular function, myocardial viability, and tissue characterization, which CT lacks. However, MRI requires a longer scanning time and cannot be used in patients with implanted metallic objects, such as pacemakers or intracardiac cardioverter–defibrillators (ICDs).

Physicians and cardiologists often face the situation to make a decision as to which noninvasive technique best serves a patient. This section provides some insights into the advantages and disadvantages of noninvasive radiologic imaging techniques in pediatric patient care. The decision as to which test to order depends on the physician's knowledge, the availability of the technique, and the expertise of cardiovascular radiology consultants in the area. Advantages and disadvantages of MRI and CT are summarized in Box 5.2. Additional discussions on the topic follow.

Magnetic Resonance Imaging

Selected clinical applications and advantages of cardiac MRI in pediatric cardiology include the following.

1. MRI offers excellent images of intracardiac morphology that is better than CT images.
2. Ventricular function. Cardiac MRI has become the gold standard for the quantification of ventricular function for both the LV and RV because it does not rely on geometric assumptions as used in echo study (and cardiac catheterization). It provides accurate information on stroke volume, systolic function, ventricular mass, and regurgitation fraction. A frequent application of RV function study relates to older children who had surgical repair of TOF with resulting pulmonary regurgitation of significant magnitude. MRI studies play a major role in determining the timing of pulmonary valve placement in these patients.
3. Equal quality images of extracardiac structures such as the PAs and their distal branches, the aorta, the pulmonary veins, and the systemic veins as CT does
4. Almost equal quality imaging of trachea and mainstem bronchus
5. Almost equal quality imaging of small vessels such as the coronary artery (in patients who had Kawasaki's disease or the arterial switch operation for transposition of the great arteries)
6. Capability of tissue characterization and myocardial viability, which CT lacks
7. Regional wall motion abnormalities of the LV and RV

The following are considered disadvantages of cardiac MRI:

1. Patients must remain still in the scanner bore for 45 to 60 minutes to minimize motion artifact during image acquisition. Accordingly, many infants and small children require sedation or anesthesia. Most children ages 8 years and older can cooperate sufficiently for a good-quality MRI.
2. Implanted metallic objects are of particular concern in the MRI environment because they could potentially undergo undesirable movement if the magnetic fields are sufficiently strong. MRI can be used to image patients with implanted

BOX 5.2 **Advantages and Disadvantages of Magnetic Resonance Imaging and Computed Tomography**

	Advantages	Disadvantages
MRI	• No radiation • Excellent in assessment of ventricular function (e.g., LV and RV volume, mass, and function, including regurgitation fraction) • Excellent tissue differentiation • Lack of dependence on a rapid bolus of IV contrast	• Long scanning time (45-60 min); needs breath hold (45–60 min) • Need for sedation and anesthesia requiring close monitoring • Metallic artifacts • Contraindicated in patients with pacemakers or ICDs
CT	• Short total scan time (5–10 min) • Fewer requirements of sedation • Excellent quality images of extracardiac vasculatures (e.g., pulmonary arteries and veins, aortic arch, coronary arteries, and aortic collaterals) • Simultaneous evaluation of lungs and airways • High spatial resolution	• Radiation exposure • Risk of iodinated contrast material • Requires breath-hold and a low, regular heart rate • Lack of information on ventricular function (e.g., RV function, pulmonary regurgitation fraction)

CT, Computed tomography; *ICD,* intracardiac cardioverter–defibrillator; *IV,* intravenous; *LV,* left ventricular; *MRI,* magnetic resonance imaging; *RV,* right ventricular.

intravascular coils, stents, and occluding devices when the implants are believed to be immobile. However, the wires and clips may cause localized image artifacts. Surgical clips and sternotomy wires are typically only weakly ferromagnetic.

3. The presence of cardiac pacemaker or ICD is considered a contraindication to MRI.
4. The presence of an intracranial, intraocular, or intracochlear metallic object is also considered a contraindication to MRI.

Computed Tomography

Computed tomography provides excellent quality imaging of extracardiac vasculature and may provide this information much more quickly (5–10 minutes) than MRI. Preferential applications of CT may include the following:

1. Almost equal quality definition of intracardiac anatomy as MRI has
2. Better quality imaging and faster results of coronary artery anomalies than MRI images, a major application of CT angiography
   a. Anomalous origin of left coronary artery
   b. Possible RV-dependent coronary circulation in patients with pulmonary atresia with intact ventricular septum
   c. Postoperative arterial switch operation for D-TGA of the great arteries
   d. Coronary involvement after Kawasaki's disease
3. Comprehensive evaluation of the pulmonary arteries and veins, preoperatively and postoperatively
4. Evaluation of the patency of vascular shunts and conduits, including patients after such operations as Blalock-Taussig shunt, bidirectional Glenn shunt, or Fontan procedure
5. Evaluating status after balloon dilatation with or without stent placement; for example, in the aorta (for coarctation) and pulmonary arteries. CT has a clear advantage over MRI in metallic stent evaluation.

6. Imaging vascular rings and pulmonary artery sling (as an alternative to MRI or cardiac catheterization)
7. Evaluating aortic collaterals prevalent in certain cyanotic CHD, such as TOF
8. Clear imaging of the airways is a unique advantage of CT over other imaging modalities, including vascular or nonvascular narrowing, anomalies, and dynamic obstruction (airway malacia, air trapping)
9. Capability of studying patients with pacemakers and ICD in whom cardiac MRI is prohibited and in patients with metallic implants that create unmanageable artifacts on cardiac MRI (e.g., steel coils)

The following are considered disadvantages of cardiac CT:

1. There is significant radiation exposure associated with CT. Radiation exposure during cardiac CT is estimated to be slightly greater than exposure during a pediatric cardiac catheterization. In children with complex CHDs, the risk may be compounded by their previous or subsequent exposure to ionizing radiation during cardiac catheterization or with serial CT studies.
2. Iodinated contrast materials are more toxic to the kidneys. Adverse reactions with nonionic, iodine-based contrast agents (e.g., hypotension, bradycardia, tachycardia, and even angina) occur at three times the rate of reactions to MRI gadolinium-based compounds.

Choice of Imaging Modalities

The age of the patient may be an important factor in choosing an imaging modality in studying pediatric cardiac patients. Prakash and colleagues (2010) have made the following suggestions.

For infants and children younger than 8 years of age, echo studies can provide accurate diagnosis of even complex CHDs in most cases. Sedation may be required in some infants and children. Therefore, the need for using MRI or CT study arises only rarely. MRI can be used to answer most of the questions regarding ventricular size and function and extracardiac vasculature. However, when the question is primarily the extracardiac vasculature, CT can also be used. Its use should be balanced against the risk of ionizing radiation exposure.

For adolescents and adults, echo remains the primary diagnostic modality. However, MRI plays an increasing role, especially for the evaluation of the extracardiac thoracic vasculature, ventricular volume and function, and flow measurement. MRI is usually preferred over CT or cardiac catheterization in this age group because it avoids exposure to ionizing radiation and can provide a wealth of functional information. CT is used in patients with contraindications to MRI, such as those with cardiac pacemaker or ICD and those in whom concomitant evaluation for coronary disease is necessary.

Other Noninvasive Investigation Tools

Besides imaging, there are other noninvasive investigative tools that are frequently used in the evaluation of cardiac patients. In this chapter, the following are discussed.
- Stress testing
- Long-term electrocardiography (ECG) recording
- Ambulatory blood pressure (BP) monitoring

STRESS TESTING

Stress testing plays an important role in the evaluation of cardiac symptoms by quantifying the severity of the cardiac abnormality, providing important indications of the need for new or further intervention, and assessing the effectiveness of management. The cardiovascular system can be stressed either by exercise or by pharmacologic agents.

The maximum oxygen uptake (Vo_2 max) that can be achieved during exercise is probably the best index of describing fitness or exercise capacity (also called "maximum aerobic power"). Vo_2 max is defined by the plateau of oxygen uptake (Vo_2) that occurs despite continued work. Beyond this level of Vo_2 max, the work can be performed using anaerobic mechanism of energy production, but the amount of work that can be performed using anaerobic means is quite limited. There is a linear relationship between the heart rate and progressive workload or Vo_2 max.

Cardiovascular Response in Normal Subjects

During upright dynamic exercise in normal subjects, the heart rate, cardiac index, and mean arterial pressure increase. In addition, the systemic vascular resistance (SVR) drops, and blood flow to the exercising leg muscles greatly increases. Heart rate increase is the major determinant of increased cardiac output seen during exercise. The heart rate reaches a maximum plateau just before the level of total exhaustion. For subjects between 5 and 20 years of age, the maximal heart rate is about 195 to 215 beats/min. For subjects older than 20 years, the maximal heart rate is 210 to $0.65 \times$ Age.

Blood pressure response varies depending on the type of exercise. During *dynamic exercise*, systolic blood pressure (SBP) increases, but diastolic blood pressure (DBP) and mean arterial pressure remain nearly identical, varying within a few mm Hg from their levels at rest. BP response to *isometric exercise* is quite different from the response to dynamic exercise. With isometric exercise, both SBP and DBP increase.

Although similar changes occur in pulmonary circulation as those seen in the systemic circulation, the increase in the mean pulmonary artery (PA) pressure is more than twice that of systemic mean arterial pressure (e.g., 100% increase), and the drop in pulmonary vascular resistance (PVR) is much less than that in SVR (e.g., 17% decrease in PVR vs 49% decrease in SVR). Because of this, children with pulmonary hypertension or those with RV dysfunction (after Fontan operation or surgery for tetralogy of Fallot [TOF]) may respond abnormally to exercise and demonstrate a decreased exercise capacity.

Cardiovascular Response in Cardiac Patients

1. Congenital heart defects
   a. Patients with minor congenital heart defects (CHDs) (e.g., small left-to-right shunt lesions or mild obstructive lesions) have little or no effect on exercise capacity.

b. Large left-to-right shunt lesions decrease exercise capacity because a ventricle that has a much increased stroke volume at rest has a limited ability to increase the stroke volume further.

c. In patients with severe obstructive lesions, the ventricle may not be able to maintain an adequate cardiac output, so that during exercise, the systemic BP may not increase appropriately, and decreased blood flow to exercising muscles may lead to premature fatigue.

d. In cyanotic lesions, the arterial hypoxemia tends to increased cardiac output and decreased mixed venous oxygen saturation, thereby limiting the usual increment in stroke volume and oxygen extraction that occurs with exercise. Furthermore, these patients have an increased minute ventilation at rest and during exercise. In this way, ventilatory as well as cardiac mechanisms may limit exercise capacity.

2. Postsurgical patients

a. For many patients with CHDs, normal or near-normal exercise tolerance is expected after surgery unless there are significant residual lesions or myocardial damage.

b. After a successful Fontan operation for functional single ventricle, exercise capacity improves, but it remains significantly less compared with normal. This results from both subnormal heart rate response to exercise and abnormal stroke volume (resulting from reduced systemic ventricular function). Cardiac arrhythmias also are common in patients both before and after the Fontan operation and may contribute to the decreased exercise capacity.

c. After arterial switch operation for D-TGA of the great arteries, more than 95% of the children have normal exercise capacity. However, up to 30% of patients have chronotropic impairment with a peak heart rate of less than 180 beats/min. Up to 10% of the patients develop significant ST-segment depression with exercise.

Exercise Stress Testing

Some exercise laboratories have developed bicycle ergometer protocols, but the equipment is not widely used. The treadmill protocols are well standardized and widely used because most hospitals have treadmills. In this chapter, exercise tests, in particular those using the Bruce protocol, will be presented. In the Bruce protocol, the level of exercise increases by increasing the speed and grade of the treadmill for each 3-minute stage.

During exercise stress testing, the patient is continually monitored for symptoms such as chest pain or faintness, ischemic changes or arrhythmias on the ECG, oxygen saturation, and responses in heart rate and BP. In the Bruce protocol, children are not allowed to hold onto the guardrails except to maintain their balance at change of stage because this can decrease the metabolic cost of work and therefore increase the exercise time.

Monitoring During Exercise Stress Testing

1. **Endurance time.** Oxygen uptake is difficult to measure in children. However, there is a high correlation between maximal Vo2 and endurance time, and thus endurance time is the best predictor of exercise capacity in children. The endurance data reported by Cumming et al in 1978 have served as the reference for several decades. In 2001 and 2002, however, two reports from the United States (Ahmed et al, 2001; Chatrath et al, 2002) indicate that the endurance time has been reduced significantly since the 1970s. It is concerning that endurance times reported from two other countries (Italy in 1994; Turkey in 1998) are similar to those published by Cumming et al and are significantly longer than those reported in the two US reports. This may be an indication that US youth are less physically fit than the youth from other countries, possibly secondary to increased obesity prevalence, which may lead to increased risk of coronary artery disease and stroke in the US population. A new set of endurance data from a recent US study is presented in Table 6.1. The endurance times for boys and girls are close until early adolescence, at which time the endurance time of girls diminishes and that of boys increases.

2. **Heart rate.** Heart rate is measured from the ECG signal. A heart rate of 180 to 200 beats/min correlates with maximal oxygen consumption in both boys and girls. Therefore, an effort is made to encourage all children to exercise to attain this heart rate. The mean maximal heart rates for all subjects were virtually identical, 198 ± 11 beats/min for boys and 200 ± 9 beats/min for girls. Heart rate declined abruptly during the first minute of recovery to 146 ± 19 beats/min for boys and 157 ± 19 beats/min for girls.

Inadequate increments in heart rate may be seen with sinus node dysfunction, in congenital heart block, and after cardiac surgery. Sinus node dysfunction is common after surgery involving extensive atrial suture lines, such as the Senning operation or Fontan operation. It is also common after repair of TOF. Marked chronotropic impairment significantly decreases aerobic capacity. Trained athletes tend to have lower heart rates at each exercise level. An extremely high heart rate at low levels of work may indicate physical deconditioning or marginal circulatory compensation.

3. **BP.** BP can be measured with a cuff, a sphygmomanometer, and a stethoscope. Numerous commercially available electronic units are also available to measure BP during exercise. However, one must be concerned with the accuracy of these devices. Accurate measurement of BP, especially DBP, is probably not possible during exercise.

Systolic BP increases linearly with progressive exercise. SBP usually rises to as high as 180 mm Hg (Table 6.2) with little change in DBP. Maximal SBP in children rarely exceeds 200 mm Hg. During recovery, it returns to baseline in about 10 minutes. The DBP ranges between 51 and 76 mm Hg at maximum SBP. DBP also returns to the resting level by 8 to 10 minutes of recovery.

High SBP in the arm, to the level of what is considered hypertensive emergency, probably does not reflect the central aortic pressure, and the usefulness of arm BP in assessing cardiovascular function during upright exercise is questionable except in the case of failure to rise. The major portion of the rise in arm SBP during treadmill exercise probably

TABLE 6.1   Percentiles of Endurance Time (min) by Bruce Treadmill Protocol

| Age Group | PERCENTILES | | | | | Mean ± SD |
	10	25	50	75	90	
BOYS						
4–5	6.8	7.0	8.2	10.0	12.7	8.9 ± 2.4
6–7	6.6	7.7	9.6	10.4	13.1	9.6 ± 2.3
8–9	7.0	9.1	9.9	11.1	15.0	10.2 ± 2.5
10–12	8.1	9.2	10.7	12.3	13.2	10.7 ± 2.1
13–15	9.6	10.3	12.0	13.5	15.0	12.0 ± 2.0
16–18	9.6	11.1	12.5	13.5	14.6	12.2 ± 2.2
GIRLS						
4–5	6.8	7.2	7.4	9.1	10.0	8.0 ± 1.1
6–7	6.5	7.3	9.0	9.2	12.4	8.7 ± 2.0
8–9	8.0	9.2	9.8	10.6	10.8	9.8 ± 1.6
10–12	7.3	9.3	10.4	10.8	12.7	10.2 ± 1.9
13–15	6.9	8.1	9.6	10.6	12.4	9.6 ± 2.1
16–18	7.4	8.5	9.5	10.1	12.0	9.5 ± 2.0

SD, Standard deviation.
From Chatrath R, Shenoy R, Serratto M, Thoele DG: Physical fitness of urban American children, *Pediatric Cardiol* 23:608–612, 2002.

TABLE 6.2   Systolic Blood Pressure Response to Bruce Treadmill Protocol

| Age Group | Rest | Maximal | RECOVERY (MIN) | | |
			6	8	10
BOYS					
5–7	105 ± 10	141 ± 13	111 ± 14	108 ± 9	106 ± 12
8–9	107 ± 10	149 ± 15	111 ± 10	107 ± 9	105 ± 6
10–11	108 ± 7	153 ± 13	112 ± 8	107 ± 9	106 ± 8
12–13	111 ± 12	165 ± 19	118 ± 12	113 ± 15	110 ± 9
14–15	120 ± 12	179 ± 23	124 ± 15	118 ± 16	115 ± 12
16–18	122 ± 14	182 ± 17	136 ± 16	125 ± 13	125 ± 14
GIRLS					
5–7	106 ± 9	143 ± 15	103 ± 4	104 ± 8	98 ± 6
8–9	108 ± 9	149 ± 11	114 ± 14	108 ± 11	108 ± 11
10–11	106 ± 11	145 ± 12	106 ± 10	104 ± 8	102 ± 7
12–13	112 ± 12	163 ± 16	120 ± 14	113 ± 10	108 ± 6
14–15	111 ± 10	166 ± 16	117 ± 13	112 ± 12	111 ± 10
16–18	118 ± 14	170 ± 17	125 ± 14	119 ± 13	117 ± 14

From Ahmad F, Kavey R-E, Kveselis DA, Gaum WE: Response of non-obese white children to treadmill exercise, *J Pediatr* 139:284–290, 2001.

reflects peripheral amplification caused by vasoconstriction in the nonexercising arms (associated with increased blood flow to vasodilated exercising legs); central aortic pressure would probably be much lower than the SBP in the arm in most cases. Figure 6.1 is a dramatic illustration of a relationship between the central and peripheral arterial pressures measured directly with arterial cannulas inserted in to the ascending aorta and radial artery during upright exercise in young adults. Note that when the radial artery SBP is over 230 mm Hg, the aortic pressure is only 160 mm Hg and that there is a very little increase in DBP.

An excessive rise in the peripheral BP has been reported in patients who have had surgical repair of coarctation of the aorta, patients with hypertension and those with the potential to develop hypertension, hypercholesterolemic patients, and patients with aortic regurgitation, but information on the central aortic pressure is lacking in these reports.

Failure of BP to rise to the expected level may be much more significant than the level of the rise in arm BP. The failure reflects an inadequate increase in cardiac output. This is commonly seen with cardiomyopathy, left ventricular outflow tract obstruction, coronary artery diseases, or the onset of ventricular or atrial arrhythmias.

4. **ECG monitoring.** The major reasons for monitoring ECG during exercise testing are to detect exercise-induced arrhythmias and ischemic changes. A complete ECG should be recorded at rest, at least once during each workload, and for several intervals after exercise.

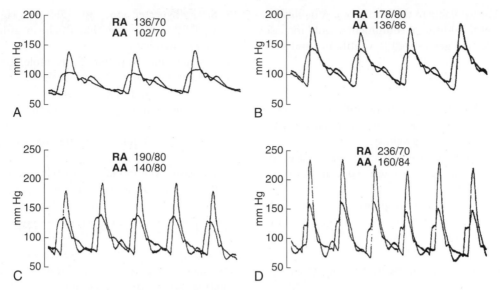

Fig. 6.1 Simultaneous recording of aortic and radial arterial pressure waves in a young adult during rest (**A**) and 28.2% (**B**), 47.2% (**C**), and 70.2% (**D**) of maximal oxygen uptake during treadmill exercise. *AA*, Ascending aorta; *RA*, radial artery. (From Rowell LB, Brengelmann GL, Blackmon JR, Bruce RA, Murray JA: Disparities between aortic and peripheral pulse pressure induced by upright exercise and vasomotor changes in man, *Circulation* 37:954–964, 1968.)

a. **Exercise-induced arrhythmias.** Arrhythmias that increase in frequency or begin with exercise are usually significant and require thorough evaluation. The type and frequency before and after the exercise and occurrence of new or more advanced arrhythmias should be noted. The occurrence of serious ventricular arrhythmias may be an indication to terminate the test. Changes in the QTc duration, including the recovery period, should be evaluated.

b. **Changes suggestive of myocardial ischemia.** ST-segment depression is the most common manifestation of exercise-induced myocardial ischemia. For children, downsloping of the ST segment or sustained horizontal depression of the ST segment of 2 mm or greater when measured at 80 msec after the J point is considered abnormal (see Fig. 3.23). Most guidelines for adult exercise testing, however, recommend the ST-segment depression of 1 mm or greater as an abnormal response. With progressive exercise, the depth of ST-segment depression may increase, involving more ECG leads, and the patient may develop anginal pain. Five to 10 minutes after the termination of the exercise, the ST changes (and T-wave inversion) may return to the baseline. Occasionally, the ischemic ST-segment response may appear only in the recovery phase.

The following lists some points in the evaluation of ST-segment shift in certain situations.

1) Specificity of the exercise ECG is poor in the presence of ST-T abnormalities on a resting ECG or with digoxin use.

2) If the ST segment is depressed at rest (which occurs occasionally), the J point and ST segment measured at 60 to 80 msec should be depressed an additional 1 mm or greater to be considered abnormal.

3) When there is an abnormal depolarization, such as bundle branch block, ventricular pacemaker, or Wolff-Parkinson-White preexcitation, interpretation of ST-segment displacement is impossible.

4) In patients with early repolarization and resting ST-segment elevation, return to the PQ junction is normal. In such cases, ST depression should be determined from the PQ point, not from the elevated J point.

5) There is a poor correlation between ST-segment changes and nuclear perfusion imaging in such conditions as anomalous origin of the coronary artery from the PA, Kawasaki's disease, and postoperative arterial switch operation.

5. **Oximetry.** Pulse oximetry measurement of blood oxygen saturation is useful during exercise testing of children who have CHD. Normal children maintain oxygen saturation greater than 90% during maximal exercise when monitored by pulse oximetry. Desaturation (<90%) during exercise is considered an abnormal response and may reflect pulmonary, cardiac, or circulatory compromise. Children who received lateral tunnel Fontan operation with fenestration may desaturate during exercise because of right-to-left shunt through the fenestration.

Safety of Exercise Testing

A properly supervised exercise study is safe. Exercise testing should be performed under the supervision of a physician who has been trained to conduct the test, with patient safety in mind. The examiner should pay close attention to the subject during the treadmill exercise testing and be alert to stopping the treadmill when the patient can no longer exercise or appears to be in jeopardy. At these times, an observer should be positioned to assist the subject. A well-stocked crash cart should be available in the laboratory. A defibrillator should be present. Additional equipment should include a delivery system for oxygen as well as ventilation and suction apparatus.

Indications

Indications of stress testing vary with institutions and cardiologists. However, some of the more common indications for exercise testing in children are as follows:

1. Evaluate specific signs or symptoms that are induced or aggravated by exercise, such as chest pain, dizziness, or syncope with exertion.
2. Assess or identify abnormal responses to exercise in children with cardiac, pulmonary, or other organ disorders, including the presence of myocardial ischemia and arrhythmias.
3. Assess the efficacy of specific medical or surgical treatments.
4. Assess the functional capacity for recreational, athletic, and vocational activities.
5. Evaluate a prognosis, including both baseline and serial testing measurements.
6. Establish baseline data for institution of cardiac, pulmonary, or musculoskeletal rehabilitation.

Contraindications

Good clinical judgment should be foremost in deciding contraindications for exercise testing. Absolute contraindications include patients with acute myocardial or pericardial inflammatory diseases or patients with severe obstructive lesions in whom surgical intervention is clearly indicated (American Heart Association [AHA], 2006, Clinical Stress Testing in Pediatric Age Group).

The patients with following diagnoses are considered a high-risk group.

1. Acute myocarditis or pericarditis
2. Severe aortic or pulmonary stenosis
3. Pulmonary hypertension
4. Documented long QT syndrome
5. Uncontrolled resting hypertension
6. Unstable arrhythmias
7. Routine testing on Marfan's syndrome
8. Routine testing after heart transplantation

Termination of Exercise Testing

Three general indications to terminate an exercise test are (1) when diagnostic findings have been established and further testing would not yield any additional information, (2) when monitoring equipment fails, and (3) when signs or symptoms indicate that further testing may compromise the patient's well-being. The following indications for termination of exercise testing have been recommended by the AHA 2006 Clinical Stress Testing in Pediatric Age Group.

1. Failure of heart rate to increase or a decrease in ventricular rate with increasing workload associated with symptoms (e.g., extreme fatigue, dizziness)
2. Progressive fall in SBP with increasing workload

3. Severe hypertension, above 250 mm Hg SBP or 125 mm Hg DBP, or BP higher than can be measured by the laboratory equipment
4. Dyspnea that the patient finds intolerable
5. Symptomatic tachycardia that the patient finds intolerable
6. Progressive fall in oxygen saturation to less than 90% or a 10-point drop from resting saturation in a patient who is symptomatic
7. Presence of 3 mm or greater flat or downward-sloping ST-segment depression
8. Increasing ventricular ectopy with increasing workload
9. Patient requests termination of the study

ALTERNATIVE STRESS TESTING PROTOCOLS

Besides treadmill exercise, there are other types of stress testing that can be performed, including the 6-minute walk test, pharmacologic stress tests, and exercise-induced bronchospasm (EIB) provocation tests.

Six-Minute Walk Test

This simple test has been used to quantify functional exercise capacity in individuals with various cardiopulmonary diseases. Therefore, this test may be more appropriate for assessing exercise tolerance in children with moderate to severe exercise limitation for traditional exercise testing. The patient is instructed to walk as fast as possible (without running) at a steady pace for 6 minutes, to cover as much distance or as many laps possible, around two flagpoles positioned 30 meters apart on a flat ground. Reference values for healthy children from Switzerland (Ulrich et al, 2013) are shown in Appendix A for interested readers (see Fig. A.2).

The usefulness of the test may be found in following disease progression and measuring the response to medical interventions on a given patient rather than the need to relate the patient's exercise tolerance against healthy population. Patients using supplemental oxygen should perform the test with oxygen. Portable oximeters may be used if available to the patient. If monitoring equipment is not available, oxygen saturation and heart rate are monitored before and after the test. The total distance walked is the primary outcome. At least two practice tests performed on a separate day are advisable.

Pharmacologic Stress Protocols

This protocol is used when conventional exercise testing is unsuitable or impractical, such as for patients who are too young and those who are unable to perform exercise tests. After pharmacologic stimulations, either echocardiography or nuclear imaging is performed. Two types of pharmacologic agents are used:

- Agents that increase myocardial oxygen consumption (dobutamine, isoproterenol), which simulate the effects of exercise.
- Agents that cause coronary dilatation (adenosine, dipyridamole). Adenosine causes dilatation of normal coronary artery segments, resulting in a shunting of myocardial

blood flow away from diseased segments. Dipyridamole inhibits adenosine reuptake, resulting in the same physiology.

The following are the dosages of the pharmacologic agents recommended in a statement from the AHA (Paridon et al, 2006). Dobutamine is administered in gradually increasing doses from a starting dose of 10 mcg/kg/min to a maximal dose of 50 mcg/kg/min in 3- to 5-minute stages to achieve the target heart rate. Atropine (0.01 mg/kg up to 0.25 mg aliquots every 1–2 minutes up to a maximum of 1 mg) can be administered to augment the heart rate, usually given at 50 mcg/kg/min of dobutamine. Esmolol (10 mg/mL dilution at a dose of 0.5 mg/kg) should be available to rapidly reverse the effects of dobutamine in the event of adverse reaction or development of ischemia. If echocardiography is used, the imaging should be performed at rest and at each dosing stage. Radioisotope for nuclear myocardial perfusion scan should be injected 1 minute before the infusion of dobutamine at maximal dosage is stopped.

Adenosine is infused at 140 mcg/kg/min for 6 minutes. If echocardiography imaging is used, it should be continuous throughout the infusion. Nuclear isotope is given at 3 minutes into the infusion. Dipyridamole is infused over the same time period at a dose of 0.6 mg/kg/min. Radioisotope delivery and echocardiography imaging should be performed at the peak physiologic effect of the dipyridamole, usually 3 to 4 minutes after completion of the infusion. Administration of aminophylline is routinely used in many centers after termination of the dipyridamole infusion.

Adenosine stress magnetic resonance imaging (MRI) with myocardial perfusion imaging is known to be a safe modality and is a useful tool in the evaluation of adequacy of blood supply to the myocardium to guide treatment options. The most common pediatric indications of the procedure are congenital heart disease, Kawasaki's disease, anomalous coronary artery, or myocardial mass (Biko et al. 2018).

Exercise-Induced Bronchospasm Provocation

Bronchial reactivity is measured while the subject exercises for 5 to 8 minutes on a treadmill at an intensity of 80% of maximum capacity. The exercise room should be as cool (temperature, 20°–25°C) and dry as possible.

The exercise protocol should be to quickly increase the intensity to 80% maximum capacity within 2 minutes (using predicted heart rate maximum as a surrogate). If the intensity is not reached quickly, the patient may develop refractoriness to bronchospasm. An incremental work used in many exercise tests, such as the Bruce protocol, is less likely to be effective in evaluating EIB because of too short a duration of high ventilation; therefore, it should not be used in the evaluation of EIB.

Exercise is preceded by baseline spirometry. Spirometry is repeated immediately after exercise and again at minutes 5, 10, and 15 of recovery. Most pulmonary function test nadirs occur within 5 to 10 minutes after exercise. Accepted criteria for a significant decline in forced expiratory volume in 1 second (FEV1) after exercise are variable. Declines of 12% to 15% in FEV1 are typically diagnostic.

LONG-TERM ECG RECORDING

Long-term ECG recording is the most useful method to document and quantitate the frequency of arrhythmias, correlate the arrhythmia with the patient's symptoms, and evaluate the effect of antiarrhythmic therapy. There are several different types of long-term ECG recorders, which detect arrhythmias for varying lengths of time. The Holter monitor is used to record events occurring in 24 hours (or up to 7 days), event recorders record arrhythmic episodes for up to 30 days, and implantable loop recorders and insertable cardiac monitors record rhythm up to 3 years. For ease and enhanced compliance, lightweight water-resistant Holter patches for extended continuous monitoring (up to 7 days) have been developed and introduced to the market. Furthermore, Food and Drug Administration–approved smartphone compatible personal ECG monitoring devices are now available, with which heart rhythms could be recorded, stored, and e-mailed to the health care provider.

Holter Recording

The Holter monitor, invented by Dr. Norman Holter, is a device that records the heart rhythm continuously for 24 hours (or up to 7 days) using ECG electrodes attached on the chest. The heart rhythm is recorded onto a memory flash card or wirelessly and then processed at a heart center. Three simultaneous channels are usually recorded. This helps distinguish artifacts from arrhythmias. This recorder is useful when a child has symptoms almost daily. This type of monitoring is not helpful in the detection of episodes that occur infrequently (e.g., once a week or once a month). Patients are given a diary so they can record symptoms and activities. The monitor has a built-in timer that is used with the patient's diary to allow subsequent correlation of symptoms and activities with arrhythmias. The importance of keeping an accurate and complete diary must be impressed on patients and parents. Events of interest can be picked out and printed for review. A wide variety of information can be obtained from the recording, including heart rates, abnormal heartbeats, and recording of rhythm during any symptoms.

The Holter recordings should reveal the frequency, duration, and types of arrhythmias, as well as their precipitating or terminating events. Significant arrhythmias rarely cause symptoms such as palpitation, chest pain, and syncope (<10% of cases). Marked bradycardia (<50 beats/min in infants, <40 beats/min in older children), supraventricular tachycardia with a rate faster than 200 beats/min, and ventricular tachycardia are potentially life threatening. These arrhythmias do occur and may worsen during sleep.

Indications

Ambulatory ECG monitoring is obtained for the following reasons:

1. To determine whether symptoms such as chest pain, palpitations, and syncope are caused by cardiac arrhythmias
2. To evaluate the adequacy of medical therapy for an arrhythmia
3. To screen high-risk cardiac patients such as those with hypertrophic cardiomyopathy or those who have had operations known to predispose to arrhythmias (e.g., Mustard, Senning, Fontan-type operation)
4. To evaluate possible intermittent pacemaker failure in patients who have an implanted pacemaker
5. To determine the effect of sleep on potentially life-threatening arrhythmias

Interpretations

Interpretation of the results usually includes the following:
1. A description of the basic rhythm and the range of the heart rate
2. For bradycardia, a description of its rate, rhythm, duration (or number of beats) and the presence of escape beats
3. For extreme tachycardia, a description of the rhythm, mode of initiation and termination, and its duration
4. Description of any abnormalities in atrioventricular (AV) conduction
5. Description of any arrhythmias, including their characteristics, duration, and frequency
6. Correlation of the arrhythmias with the patient's activities and symptoms
7. Description of correlation of ST-segment changes with activities if the patient complained of anginal pain

Holter Findings in Normal Children

Meaningful interpretation of the Holter recordings performed in patients with organic heart disease or significant systemic illness requires knowledge of the range of heart rate and rhythm variations in normal subjects of comparable age. Holter ECG recordings of healthy pediatric populations have demonstrated that variations in rate and rhythm, which were previously thought to be abnormal, occur quite frequently.

Premature or Low-Birth-Weight Infants

The minimum heart rate of premature or low-birth-weight infants can be as low as 73 beats/min; the maximum heart rate can be as high as 211 beats/min. Junctional rhythm may be observed in 18% to 70%, premature atrial contractions (PACs) in 2% to 33%, and premature ventricular contractions (PVCs) in 6% to 17%. First-degree AV block or Wenckebach's second-degree AV block occurs in 4% to 6%. Sudden sinus bradycardia and sinus pause occur especially frequently.

Full-Term Neonates

In full-term neonates, the heart rate can be as low as 75 beats/min and as high as 230 beats/min. Junctional rhythm may be present in 28%, PACs in 10% to 35%, and PVCs in 1% to 13%. First-degree AV block or Wenckebach's (Mobitz type 1) second-degree AV block may be recorded in 25% of neonates. Sinus pause is quite frequent.

Children

Southall et al (1981) reported the following findings in healthy 7- to 11-year-old children.
- The mean highest heart rate was 164 ± 17 beats/min.
- The mean lowest heart rate was 49 ± 6 over 3 beats' and 56 ± 6 over 9 beats' duration.
- At their lowest rate, 45% had junction escape rhythm, lasting up to 25 minutes.
- AV conduction:
  - PR interval of 0.20 sec or greater in 9%
  - Mobitz type I second degree AV block in 3%
- Isolated supraventricular or ventricular premature beats in 19% (<1 per hour)
- Sinus pause seen in 65%. The maximum duration of sinus pause on each child was 1.36 ± 0.23 seconds.

Adolescent Boys

Dickinson and Scott (1984) reported the following in healthy 14- to 16-year-old boys.
- Sinus arrhythmia in all cases with heart rate ranging from 45 to 200 beats/min during the day
- During sleep, the heart rate can become as low as 23 beats/min.
- At their lowest rate, escape rhythm was present in 26%.
- AV conduction:
  - Sudden variation in PR interval was noted in 41%.
  - Sinus arrest or sinoatrial block (15%)
  - First-degree AV block (12%)
  - Wenckebach's (Mobitz type 1) second-degree AV block (11%)
- PVCs (occurring in 26%–57%), which include multiform PVCs; PACs (occurring in 13%–20%) were also observed.
- Short episodes of ventricular tachycardia were present in 3%.

Event Recorders

Event monitors are devices that are used by patients over a longer period (weeks to months, typically 1 month). The monitor is used when symptoms suggestive of an arrhythmia occur infrequently. Nowadays, the information collected by the event monitor is monitored continuously and can be communicated to the cardiologist through website or faxed to the health care provider. Two general types of cardiac event monitors are available.
1. Looping memory (presymptom) event monitor
The term "looping" refers to the memory of the monitor, which means that when activated, the monitor can save a preceding or ongoing rhythm for a period of up to 5 minutes in the memory loop. Three to five electrodes are attached on the chest. The monitor is always on but only stores and transmits the patient's rhythm when the patient or caregiver pushes the button or, automatically, when the monitor detects a heart rate that fulfills preset criteria. The stored ECGs are wirelessly transmitted to the event monitoring center directly. This feature is especially useful for people who pass out when their heart problems occur and can press the button only after they wake up.

2. Nonlooping memory (postsymptom) event monitor

This monitor is capable of real-time recording of the cardiac rhythm without having electrodes attached to the chest. This device is used to record symptoms that last longer than 45 to 60 seconds. It is a small device that has small metal discs that function as the electrodes. When symptoms occur, the device is pressed against the chest to start the recording. The device records and stores the events in solid-state memory. It can store up to four to six such events before it is necessary to transmit the information by phone.

Implantable Loop Recorder and Insertable Cardiac Monitor

For patients with very infrequent symptoms, such as once every 6 months, neither Holter recorders nor 30-day event recorders may yield diagnostic information. In such patients, MRI-compatible, insertable cardiac monitors, about the size of a 1¾-inch paper clip, are implanted beneath the skin in the upper left chest. A reader, part of a nearby patient-care-link portal, is activated by the patient and the information is then transmitted via the portal to the health care provider. This device was shown to be instrumental in establishing the diagnosis in patients with infrequent syncope on whom other recording devices failed to document the cause of syncope.

Patch Electrocardiogram Recording Devices

The major shortcomings of the standard 24-hour Holter monitors include poor detection rates of transient arrhythmic events. The advancements in electronic and adhesive technologies have enabled the development of the wearable patch ECG Monitors (Holter patches) capable of continuously recording ECG signals for 7 to 14 days or an even longer period (Lobodzinski et al, 2012). These monitors attach directly to the skin and record ECG signals without visible electrodes and lead wires. They are waterproof, offer good adhesion to the skin, and can operate as either recorders or wireless streaming devices. They enable very long-term monitoring of patients while they are carrying out daily activities.

AMBULATORY BLOOD PRESSURE MONITORING

Blood pressure is not a static variable; rather, it changes not only from daytime to nighttime but also from minute to minute. Casual BP measurement provides only a snapshot of the daytime BP pattern, which is higher than nighttime readings. In some patients, there is a transient elevation of SBP, DBP, or mean BP when BP is measured in a health care facility (i.e., "white-coat hypertension"). This could lead to an overdiagnosis of hypertension and to unnecessarily aggressive and costly diagnostic studies and treatment. Ambulatory BP monitoring (ABPM) has emerged as a technology that addresses some of the limitations of casual BP measurements because it permits the observation of BP throughout day and night in a nonmedical environment. Many antihypertensive organizations recommend BP measurement outside the clinic setting, including self-measurement of BP at home or any other place. Although self-measurement of BP was better than clinic BP measurement, ABPM was even better than self-measured BP in the diagnosis of hypertension. Some researchers advocate the use of ABPM in all patients with casual BP elevation.

Indications

Indications for routine performance of ABPM include the following.

1. ABPM is critical in distinguishing "white-coat hypertension" from true hypertension and confirming the presence of sustained hypertension.
2. To evaluate for the presence of "masked hypertension" when there is a clinical suspicion of it. Masked hypertension is defined as a normal clinic BP but elevated ambulatory BP levels.
3. To assess BP patterns in high risk patients
   a. To assess for abnormal circadian variation in BP such as blunted dipping or isolated sleep hypertension (in patients with diabetes mellitus, chronic kidney disease, solid organ transplant, and severe obesity with or without sleep-disordered breathing)
   b. To assess the severity and persistence of BP elevation in patients at high risk for hypertensive target-organ damage
4. To evaluate effectiveness of drug therapy for hypertension
   a. Confirm BP control in treated patients, especially those with secondary forms of hypertension
   b. Evaluate for apparent drug-resistant hypertension
   c. Determine whether symptoms can be attributed to drug-related hypotension

Procedure

Multiple BP measurements are obtained with a preapplied BP cuff using either the oscillometric or the auscultatory method (with or without the ECG's R-wave gating) for a 24-hour period while children participate in their normal daily activities.

1. Most centers use oscillometric devices. One should use only the device that has been validated according to Association of the Advancement of Medical Instrumentation or British Hypertension Society standards.
2. Monitors should be applied to the nondominant arm with appropriate size of BP cuff.
3. The device should record BP every 15 to 20 minutes during waking hours and every 20 to 30 minutes during sleep.
4. Patient diaries are critical tools in the proper use of ABPM and should at minimum record the sleep times, nap times, and periods of physical activities.
5. A sufficient number of valid BP recordings are needed for a study to be considered interpretable:
   a. Minimum of 1 reading per hour, including during sleep
   b. At least 40 to 50 readings for a full 24-hour report
   c. 65% to 75% of all possible BP readings for a partial day report (depends on frequency of recording programmed into the monitor)

TABLE 6.3	Suggested Revised Schema of Ambulatory Blood Pressure Levels in Children		
Classification	Office BP[a]	Mean Ambulatory SBP or DBP[b,c]	SBP or DBP Load[c,d]
Normal BP	<90th percentile	<95th %tile	<25%
White-coat hypertension	≥95th percentile	<95th %tile	<25%
Prehypertension (now called elevated BP)	≥90th percentile or >120/80 mm Hg	<95th %tile	≥25%
Masked hypertension	<95th %tile	>95th %tile	≥25%
Ambulatory (or sustained) hypertension	>95th %tile	>95th %tile	25-50%
Severe ambulatory hypertension (at risk for end-organ damage)	>95th %tile	>95th %tile	>50%

[a]Based on National High Blood Pressure Education Program Task Forces normative data.
[b]Based on normative ABEATS/MIN value in Appendix B (Tables B.8 and B.9).
[c]For either the wake or sleep period of the study or both.
[d]For patients with elevated load but normal mean ambulatory blood pressure (BP) and office BP that is either normal (<90th percentile) or hypertensive (≥95th percentile), no specific ambulatory BP classification can be assigned based on current evidence and expert consensus. These "unclassified" patients should be evaluated on a case-by-case basis, taking into account the presence of secondary hypertension or multiple cardiovascular risk factors.
%tile, Percentile; *DBP*, diastolic blood pressure; *SBP*, systolic blood pressure.
Adapted from Flynn JT, Daniels SR, Hayman LL, et al: Update: ambulatory blood pressure monitoring in children and adolescents. A scientific statement from the American Heart Association, *Hypertension* 63:1116–1135, 2014.

6. The use of ABPM is usually limited to children 5 to 6 years of age or older. Successful recording has been reported in more than 70% of children younger than 6 years of age.
7. According to the updated recommendation of 2014, outlier data are first filtered out before making calculations of ABPM. Values that fall outside of the following range should be discarded.
- SBP of 60 to 220 mm Hg
- DBP of 35 to 120 mm Hg
- Heart rate of 40 to 180 beats/min
- Pulse pressure of 40 to 120 beats/min

Standard Calculations

In the 2014 updated recommendations, the following basic calculations of ABPM are recommended. Unlike the 2008 recommendation, which used only SBP, the new recommendations include additional calculations using DBP.
1. Mean ambulatory SBP and DBP during the entire 24-hour period, awake, and during sleep periods
2. BP load, which is defined as the percentage of valid BP measures above the 95th percentile for age, gender, and height
3. Nocturnal dipping is calculated by [Mean awake BP minus – Sleep BP ÷ Mean awake BP × 100] for both SBP and DBP. Normal nocturnal dipping was generally defined as a 10% or greater decline in mean SBP and mean DBP from daytime BP levels. Nondipping was defined as a decline of less than 10%.

Ambulatory Blood Pressure Monitoring Standards

The 2014 update on ABPM (Flynn et al, 2014) has recommended two sets of normative standards for ABPM: one by height and the other by age. Normative data based on age are presented in Appendix B (Table B.8 for boys and Table B.9 for girls).

Staging of Ambulatory Blood Pressure Monitoring Levels

Table 6.3 is a suggested schema for staging ABPM by the 2014 update on ABPM (Flynn, 2014).

Invasive Procedures

Two kinds of invasive procedures are used in the practice of pediatric cardiology. The first is cardiac catheterization and angiocardiography, which together are used for diagnosis (diagnostic catheterization). The second treats certain structural heart defects nonsurgically using specially designed catheters and implantable devices that are delivered through cardiac catheters (therapeutic cardiac catheterization).

CARDIAC CATHETERIZATION AND ANGIOCARDIOGRAPHY

Cardiac catheterization and angiocardiography usually constitute the final definitive diagnostic tests for most cardiac patients. They are carried out under general sedation using various sedatives (discussed later). For newborns, cyanotic infants, and hemodynamically unstable children, general anesthesia with intubation may be used.

Under local anesthesia and with strict aseptic preparation of the skin, catheters are placed in peripheral (most commonly the femoral) vessels and advanced to the heart and central vessels under fluoroscopy with image intensification to reduce radiation exposure. At each position in the heart and blood vessels, values of pressure and oxygen saturation of blood are obtained. The oxygen saturation data provide information on the site and magnitude of the left-to-right or right-to-left shunt, if any. The pressure data provide information on the site and severity of obstruction. Cardiac output may be obtained from oxygen saturation data (e.g., the Fick principle) or by indicator dilution (e.g., indocyanine green dye) or thermodilution (e.g., cold saline injection) technique. Selective angiocardiography is usually performed as part of the catheterization procedure (described later).

Normal Hemodynamic Values

Normal oxygen saturation on the right side of the heart is usually 70%, but it may vary between 65% and 80%, depending on cardiac output. Left-sided saturations are usually 95% to 98% in room air. In newborns and heavily sedated children, the oxygen saturation may be lower. Pressures are lower in the right side than in the left side of the heart, with systolic pressures in the right ventricle (RV) and pulmonary artery (PA) about 20% to 30% of those in the left side of the heart (Fig. 7.1).

Routine Hemodynamic Calculations

The following calculations are routinely obtained: flow and resistance for systemic and pulmonary circuits and left-to-right or right-to-left shunt.

Flows (Cardiac Output) and Shunts. Flow is calculated by use of the Fick formula:

$$\text{Pulmonary flow}(Q_p) = {}^{V_{O_2}}\!/C_{PV} - C_{PA}$$

$$\text{Left-to-right shunt} = Q_P - Q_S$$

in which flows are in L/minute, V_{O_2} is oxygen consumption (mL/mine), C is oxygen content (mL/L) at various positions, PV is pulmonary vein, PA is pulmonary artery, AO is aorta, and MV is mixed systemic venous blood (superior vena cava or right atrium). Normal systemic flow or pulmonary flow in the absence of a shunt is 3.1 ± 0.4 L/min/m^2 (i.e., cardiac index).

Oxygen consumption is either directly measured during the procedure or estimated from a table for children 3 years and older (see Appendix A, Table A.6). Assumed oxygen consumption of 150 to 160 mL/min/m^2 is used in older infants and children. In infants younger than 2 to 3 weeks of age, 120 to 130 mL/min/m^2 may be used. *Oxygen capacity* is the maximum quantity of oxygen that can be bound to each gram of hemoglobin (i.e., 1.36 mL × Hemoglobin level; each gram of hemoglobin combines maximally with 1.36 mL of oxygen). *Oxygen saturation* is the amount of oxygen bound to hemoglobin compared with the oxygen capacity, and it is expressed as a percentage.

When there is a pure left-to-right or right-to-left shunt, the magnitude of the shunt is calculated as follows:

$$\text{Left-to-right shunt} = Q_P - Q_S$$

$$\text{Right-to-left shunt} = Q_S - Q_p$$

The flow data are subject to much error because of difficulties in measuring accurate oxygen consumption or because of the frequent use of assumed oxygen consumption in pediatric patients. Therefore, the ratio of pulmonary-to-systemic flow $\dot{Q}P - \dot{Q}s$ is frequently used because it does not require an oxygen consumption value. The ratio provides information on the magnitude of the shunt. A Qp/Qs ratio of 1:1 would indicate no shunting in either direction or bidirectional shunting of equal magnitude. A ratio of 2:1 implies that there is a left-to-right shunt equal to systemic blood flow. A ratio of 0.8:1 signifies that the pulmonary blood flow is 20% less than the systemic blood flow (e.g., the flow ratio seen in a cyanotic patient). Patients with a flow ratio greater than 2:1 are usually surgical candidates.

Resistance. Hydraulic resistance (R) is defined by analogy to Ohm's law as the ratio of the mean pressure drop (ΔP) to flow (Q) between two points in a liquid flowing in a tube (R = $\Delta P/Q$). Therefore, pulmonary vascular resistance (PVR) and systemic vascular resistance (SVR) are calculated using the following formulas:

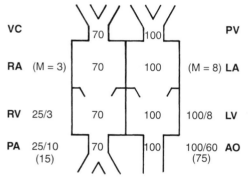

Fig. 7.1 Average values of pressure and oxygen saturation in normal children. Values inside the chambers indicate oxygen saturation (%) and those outside indicate pressure (mm Hg). *AO,* Aorta; *LA,* left atrium; *LV,* left ventricle; *M,* mean pressure; *PA,* pulmonary artery; *PV,* pulmonary vein; *RA,* right atrium; *RV,* right ventricle; *VC,* vena cava.

PVR = Mean PA pressure - Mean left atrium (LA) pressure/Q_p

SVR = Mean aortic pressure - Mean right atrium (RA) pressure/Q_s

The normal SVR is about 20 units/m^2 in children, but it varies markedly between 15 and 30 units/m^2. In newborn infants, the SVR is lower (10–15 units/m^2) and rises gradually to about 20 units/m^2 by 12 to 18 months of age. The normal PVR is high at birth but approaches adult values by about 6 to 8 weeks after birth. Normal values in children and adults are 1 to 3 units/m^2. Accordingly, the ratios of PVR to SVR range from 1:10 to 1:20. High PVR values increase the risk associated with corrective surgery for many congenital cardiac defects.

Selective Angiocardiography

Information derived from echocardiography and oxygen saturation and pressure data from catheterization help determine the number and sites of selective angiocardiograms required to delineate cardiovascular structures. A radiopaque dye is rapidly injected into a certain site, and angiograms are recorded, often on biplane views. Depending on the cardiovascular anomaly under study, special views are obtained by moving the fluoroscopic camera (or by positioning the patient at desired angles). Multiple injection sites are often necessary to obtain a complete anatomic diagnosis (Fig. 7.2A).

Contrast agents used in angiocardiography are opaque because of the iodine content and are classified either as ionic (high osmolality) or nonionic (low osmolality) compounds. Old contrast agents (e.g., Renografin 76, Renovist, Hypaque M-75, Vascoray) are ionic agents with high osmolality (i.e., osmolality of 1690–2150 mOsm/kg; much [five to eight times] higher than serum osmolality of 275–300 mOsm/L). Nonionic contrast agents (e.g., Isovue, Omnipaque) are low-osmolality agents (i.e., osmolality of 200–300 mOsm/

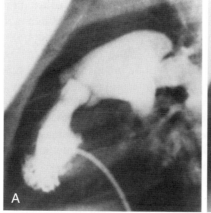 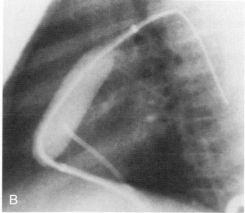

Fig. 7.2 Angiocardiography and balloon valvuloplasty. **A,** Lateral view of a right ventriculogram showing a thick, dome-shaped pulmonary valve and a marked poststenotic dilatation of the pulmonary artery. **B,** A maximally inflated sausage-shaped valvuloplasty balloon is seen, which suggests that the stenotic pulmonary valve has been widened. The balloon catheter was introduced over a guidewire, which was positioned in the left pulmonary artery.

kg), and some are hypotonic to the serum. After the injection of a high-osmolality contrast medium, there is a rapid shift of fluid from the interstitial and intracellular spaces into the intravascular space. This causes volume expansion, a slight drop in hematocrit, and a change in electrolyte concentration. These changes adversely affect newborns and infants with congestive heart failure. Low-osmolality agents cause less volume shift and are safer. Other toxic effects of high-osmolality agents include decreased red cell pliability, increased viscosity, osmolar diuresis, proteinuria, hematuria, and renal failure (occasionally). Therefore, nonionic media are routinely used for the pediatric patients with complex congenital defects. It is important to obtain the important hemodynamic data before the use of a significant amount of contrast agents.

Risk

Cardiac catheterization and angiocardiography can lead to serious complications and occasionally death.

- Complications related to catheter insertion and manipulation include serious arrhythmias; heart block; cardiac perforation; cardiac valve injury; hypoxic spells; vascular injury, perforation, or tears; hemorrhage (that requires transfusion); and infection.
- Complications related to contrast injection include reactions to the contrast material, intramyocardial injection, and renal complications (e.g., hematuria, proteinuria, oliguria, anuria).
- Complications related to exposure, anesthesia, sedation, and medications include hypothermia, acidemia, hypoglycemia, convulsions, hypotension, respiratory depression, diffuse central nervous system injury, stroke, and even death. These complications are more likely to occur in newborns.
- Complications also include exposure to ionized radiation.

The risk of cardiac catheterization and angiocardiography varies with the patient's age and illness, the type of lesion, and the experience of the physician doing the procedure. The reported rate of fatal complications varies from lower than 1% to as high as 5% in the newborn period. In one study, the incidence of significant but nonfatal complications requiring treatment (e.g., arrhythmias and arterial complications) was 12% in infants younger than 4 months old. In comparison, the incidence of such complications was 1.5% in older infants. Major complications (e.g., ventricular arrhythmias, hypotension, arterial complications, perforation of the heart, breakage or knotting of catheters, allergic reactions, hypoxic spells) occurred 1.4% of the time, and minor complications occurred 6.8% of the time. With better preparation and monitoring, as well as the use of prostaglandin infusion in critically ill newborns, the mortality and morbidity rates can be minimized.

Indications

Details of anatomy, including situs, venous and arterial connections, septal integrity, severity of valvular stenosis or regurgitation, size of pulmonary arteries, coronary artery origins, and aortic arch anatomy, are easily established with echocardiography to the degree of certainty required for surgical intervention. When additional information is needed for intervention, it can be obtained by other noninvasive techniques, such as cardiac magnetic resonance imaging or cardiac computed tomography. In centers where these noninvasive imaging techniques are not available and when echocardiography does not provide sufficient detail, cardiac catheterization is indicated (Feltes et al, 2011). In most centers, two thirds of cardiac catheterizations are for interventional purposes, and only one third are for diagnostic purposes.

- Most congenital heart defects, such as ventricular septal defect (VSD), atrial septal defect (ASD), atrioventricular (AV) canal, tetralogy of Fallot (TOF), double outlet right ventricle, coarctation of the aorta (COA), hypoplastic left heart syndrome (HLHS) , and other complex congenital heart disease (CHD) do not need diagnostic catheterization. Most of them can be adequately diagnosed by noninvasive methods. It is indicated when complete diagnosis cannot be made by noninvasive testing or when such testing yields incomplete information.
- The following lists some circumstances that suggest the need for diagnostic catheterization.
  a. To determine accurate pressure gradients in combined aortic stenosis and aortic regurgitation (AR) or pulmonary stenosis (PS) and pulmonary regurgitation or multiple levels of obstruction. Doppler assessment of pressure gradient is different from true peak-to-peak gradient measurement.
  b. Assessment of pulmonary hypertension and its responsiveness to vasodilator therapy
  c. To calculate PVR and pulmonary arterial pressure in the setting of low-flow lesions, such as seen in patients after cavopulmonary anastomosis or after complete Fontan operation or as preoperative assessment of the hemodynamics before these procedures
  d. Patients with pulmonary atresia with intact ventricular septum or pulmonary atresia with complex ventricular anatomy (to determine details of pulmonary vascular supply, the aortopulmonary collateral supply, and the coronary artery anatomy)
  e. To find answers to postoperative problems. Some of these situations may require interventional procedures at the time of catheterization.
    1) Excessive desaturation after a systemic-to-pulmonary shunt (to rule out shunt stenosis or occlusion and branch PA stenosis)
    2) Excessive desaturation after cavopulmonary anastomosis (to rule out venovenous, venoatrial, or pulmonary AV malformation)
    3) When excessive aortopulmonary collateral is suspected
    4) Suspected RV outflow tract obstruction after TOF surgery
  f. Cardiac transplantation (for both CHD and cardiomyopathy), to assess preoperatively and for surveillance of vasculopathy, and to obtain endomyocardial biopsy for rejection identification
  g. Assessment of cardiomyopathy or myocarditis
  h. To assess coronary circulation in some cases of Kawasaki's disease

Sedation

A number of sedatives have been used by different institutions with equal success rates. Smaller doses of sedatives are usually used in cyanotic infants. General anesthesia is usually used, especially when an interventional procedure is planned.

Among the sedatives that have been used are chloral hydrate, diphenhydramine, meperidine (Demerol), promethazine (Phenergan), chlorpromazine (Thorazine), ketamine, and morphine. It should be kept in mind that ketamine has important hemodynamic effects; it increases the SVR and blood pressure.

Preparation and Monitoring

Adequate preparation of the patient before the procedure and careful monitoring during the procedure can minimize complications and fatality from the invasive studies. The following studies should be considered for children undergoing cardiac catheterization.

1. A 12-lead electrocardiogram (ECG), chest radiographs (both posteroanterior and lateral), two-dimensional echocardiography, urinalysis, and a complete blood count within days or weeks in advance of the study
2. Baseline coagulation studies and a platelet count for deeply cyanotic children
3. Blood type and cross-match for infants less than 5 kg of body weight

The following preparation and monitoring are particularly important for the safety of patients:

1. Increasing the temperature in the cardiac catheterization laboratory when an infant is being studied
2. Using a warming blanket and a rectal thermistor to monitor rectal temperature to avoid hypothermia
3. Checking arterial blood gases and pH and correcting acidemia and hypoxemia
4. Correcting hypoglycemia or hypocalcemia before and during the procedure
5. Monitoring oxygen saturation and administering oxygen (if indicated) during the procedure
6. All patients undergoing catheterization should have a reliable intravenous (IV) line (for sedation, resuscitation, or volume replacement).
7. Children with high hemoglobin levels should be given overnight IV fluid to reduce the risk of dehydration, thrombosis, and hypotension.
8. Digitalis should be held beginning the night before catheterization to reduce the risks of catheterization-induced arrhythmias.
9. Angiotensin-converting enzyme inhibitors should be held 24 hours before a planned anesthesia because of an increased risk of significant hypotension on induction.
10. Having emergency medications (e.g., atropine, epinephrine, bicarbonate) drawn up and ready
11. Initiating prostaglandin infusion in cyanotic infants who seem to be ductus dependent
12. Intubating or readiness for intubating infants with respiratory difficulties
13. Whenever possible, having another physician (preferably an anesthesiologist) available to monitor the noncardiac aspects of the patient so that the operator can concentrate on the procedure

CATHETER INTERVENTION PROCEDURES

Recent advances have allowed for the development of a variety of therapeutic procedures using specially modified catheters and catheter-delivered devices. The lives of critically ill neonates may be saved by these procedures. They may also eliminate or delay the need for elective surgical procedures in children with certain CHDs. These procedures can open things that are closed, widen things that are too small, and close things that are open. More specifically, blood vessels and heart valves that are too small can be enlarged using balloon catheters or implantable devices known as stents. Too small an opening in the atrial septum can be enlarged by using balloon or blade catheter. An opening can be created in an intact atrial septum for left-to-right or right-to-left shunt to occur. Abnormal connections within the heart (ASDs and VSDs) can be closed using devices. Abnormal blood vessels (patent ductus arteriosus [PDA] or collaterals) can also be closed using coils or plugging devices. In recent years, to a greater extent, percutaneous valve replacements in the aortic or pulmonary position have been implemented.

Balloon and Blade Atrial Septostomy

In balloon atrial septostomy (Rashkind's procedure), a special balloon-tipped catheter is placed in the left atrium (LA) from the right atrium (RA) through a patent foramen ovale or an existing ASD. The balloon is inflated with diluted contrast material, and the catheter is rapidly pulled back to the RA through the interatrial communication, thereby creating a large opening in the atrial septum. This procedure is mostly effective in infants younger than 1 month of age.

This procedure is indicated in patients with an intact or nearly intact atrial septum in whom a better mixing of systemic and pulmonary venous blood would benefit their oxygenation, cardiac output, or both. Infants who have transposition of the great arteries (TGA), with or without associated ASD, are candidates for the procedure unless an arterial switch operation is to be performed immediately. It is indicated in patients with single ventricle associated with hypoplastic RV or left ventricle (LV) or significantly stenotic tricuspid or mitral valves. It is also indicated in infants with total anomalous pulmonary venous return in rare instances with restrictive ASD if surgery is delayed for some reason. The procedure may be appropriate in selected patients with pulmonary atresia, mitral atresia, and tricuspid atresia.

In infants older than 1 month of age, the atrial septum may be too thick to allow an effective balloon septostomy. In such cases, the atrial septum can be opened with a blade catheter (i.e., Park Blade Septostomy Catheter). The blade catheter uses a small blade that unfolds from the tip of the catheter to actually incise the atrial septum as the catheter tip is withdrawn from the LA to the RA. The opening can be torn further with a balloon catheter. Conditions for which the procedure is necessary are the same as those listed for balloon atrial septostomy.

Balloon Valvuloplasty

The balloons used in these interventional procedures are made of special plastic polymers and retain their predetermined diameters. A long guidewire is advanced far beyond the valve of interest, and the balloon catheter is placed over the wire. The middle of the elongated, sausage-shaped balloon is placed in the valve position. The balloon is then inflated with diluted contrast material to relieve obstruction at the valve.

Pulmonary Valve Stenosis

This technique is the treatment of choice for valvular PS in children and, to a large extent, has replaced the surgical pulmonary valvotomy (see Fig. 7.2B). The results of this technique are excellent, and it does not have significant complications.

The technique of balloon valvuloplasty is straightforward. An exchange wire is introduced through an end-hole catheter and positioned in the distal right or left PA. A balloon is chosen to be 120% to 130% of the pulmonary valve annulus, and it is positioned over a guidewire with the valve at its midpoint. As the balloon is inflated, a waist from the stenotic valve initially appears and later disappears at full inflation. When using a double-balloon technique, a combined diameter of 150% to 160% of the pulmonary valve annulus may be used.

Balloon valvuloplasty may be indicated in patients with maximum instantaneous systolic Doppler gradient of as little as 35 mm Hg, when combined with evidence of RV hypertrophy. This technique can be used in neonates with critical PS, although the complication rate is higher. The effectiveness of balloon valvuloplasty for a severe dysplastic pulmonary valve is questionable, but it may be attempted. The procedure is not useful for the treatment of infundibular PS that is not associated with valvular PS.

Aortic Valve Stenosis

This procedure is more difficult and carries a higher complication rate than does pulmonary valve balloon dilatation, especially for infants. The gradient reduction is less effective than for the pulmonary valve, and creating a significant aortic insufficiency is the major risk of the procedure. In contrast to balloon pulmonary valvuloplasty, the result of aortic valvuloplasty is usually palliative in nature and frequently aimed at delaying an inevitable surgical procedure.

In general, aortic valve dilatation is performed retrograde with a catheter introduced into the femoral artery. An end-hole catheter or wire is passed retrograde across the stenotic valve (which is the most difficult maneuver in the entire procedure) to a stable position in the LV. When the balloon is positioned across the stenotic valve, the balloon is rapidly inflated to the recommended maximal pressure and then rapidly deflated. For a single-balloon technique, the initial balloon is chosen with a diameter about 80% to 90% of the measured aortic annulus. With the double-balloon technique, the combined diameter of the two balloons should be approximately 120% of the aortic annulus.

Indications for balloon valvotomy include peak systolic pressure gradients in excess of 60 mm Hg in asymptomatic children and adolescents. In symptomatic patients (with ischemic or repolarization changes on ECG), a pressure gradient of 50 mm Hg should be used. Newborns or small infants with critical valve obstruction with a dilated LV or poor LV function are also candidates for the procedure, regardless of the measured pressure gradient value. This procedure is not suitable for subaortic membrane or fibromuscular subaortic (or "tunnel") stenosis.

Complications include production or worsening of AR, iliofemoral artery injury and occlusion, ventricular fibrillation, and even death in small infants.

Mitral Stenosis

Balloon dilatation valvuloplasty has been effective for rheumatic mitral stenosis (MS) but less effective for congenital MS. Passage of the balloon catheter across the atrial septum is necessary. Complications include perforation of the LV, transient complete AV block, tearing of the anterior leaflet of the mitral valve, and severe mitral regurgitation.

Stenosis of Prosthetic Conduits and Valves within Conduits

The balloon dilatation procedure may reduce the transconduit gradient across stenotic areas of prosthetic conduits and across valves contained within conduits.

Balloon Angioplasty

Balloon catheters similar to those used in balloon valvuloplasties are used for the relief of stenosis of blood vessels. Appropriate guidewires are placed beyond the point of narrowing, and the balloon catheter is placed over the guidewires. The midportion of the balloon is positioned at the point of narrowing, and the balloon is inflated with diluted contrast material to relieve the narrowing of vascular structures. This procedure has been used for COA and PA branch stenosis and for stenosis of the systemic veins. After the balloon procedure, some blood vessels recoil and do not maintain the dilated caliber of the vessel.

Endovascular stents are sometimes used to maintain vessel patency after balloon angioplasty of any vascular structure. The stent prevents recoil of the vessel, providing better acute results and considerably reduced rate of restenosis than with balloon angioplasty alone. The stent is positioned over an angioplasty balloon, and the balloon is inflated after positioning it at an appropriate site. After stent placement, the vascular endothelium grows over the struts over several months, functionally incorporating the stent into the vessel wall. Occasionally, however, the endothelialization may go awry, resulting in a thick neointimal layer causing a functional stenosis. There is also active work in the development of biodegradable stents, which would eliminate some concerns of repeated dilatation in a growing child.

Recoarctation of the Aorta

Balloon angioplasty is an extremely useful tool in the management of postoperative residual obstruction of coarctation of the aorta. It has become the procedure of choice for patients with this condition because reoperation carries a significant risk of morbidity and mortality. The procedure's success rate is close to 80%, and late development of an aortic aneurysm rarely occurs. Some centers use a stent to prevent restenosis and diminish the late incidence of aneurysm formation (see Chapter 13 for further discussion).

Native (or Unoperated) Coarctation of the Aorta

Balloon angioplasty for native unoperated coarctation is controversial. The rate of recoarctation after the balloon procedure appears higher than that following surgery in infants. The complication rate is 17%, with aortic aneurysm formation (both acute and late) occurring in 6% of the patients. The long-term effects of the procedure on aneurysm formation are unknown. Therefore, surgery may be a better choice than the balloon procedure for native coarctation. Some centers use cutting balloons or low-profile stents in very sick infants, which may reduce aneurysm formation.

Branch Pulmonary Artery Stenosis

The most frequent use of stent in the pediatric patients is to treat peripheral PA stenosis. The peripheral PA stenosis may be seen as an isolated lesion but more commonly as a component of complex cyanotic heart defects. Hypoplastic and stenotic branch PAs are seen with postoperative TOF, pulmonary atresia, and HLHS. Because surgical treatment of peripheral PA stenosis is often not possible, attempting the balloon procedure with stent for this condition is well accepted.

The immediate success rate of the balloon procedure is about 60%, but restenosis occurs in a significant number of patients, and aneurysm formation occurs in approximately 3% of patients. High-pressure balloons appear to improve the effectiveness. Vessels resistant to high-pressure balloon respond to either cutting balloon angioplasty alone or that followed by high-pressure ballooning. Cutting balloons have three or four microsurgical blades with a cutting depth of 0.15 mm, which are activated when the balloons are inflated. Use of an intravascular stent has also improved immediate results and may improve the long-term success rate.

Systemic Venous Stenosis

For obstructed venous baffles after the Mustard or Senning operation for TGA, the balloon procedure is an attractive alternative. The procedure is inappropriate for stenosis of the pulmonary vein because restenosis recurs often.

Closure Techniques

Various devices have been used for nonsurgical closure of ASD, PDA, and muscular VSD in cardiac catheterization laboratories. All closure devices are delivered through a catheter that goes through long, large sheaths. The sheaths are inserted into the femoral vein, the femoral artery, or both. These nonsurgical devices have the advantages of a short hospital stay, rapid recovery, and no residual thoracic scar. In many centers, these devices and techniques are considered the procedures of choice for ASD, PDA, and collateral arteries.

Atrial Septal Defect

In the past, a double-umbrella device was used to close secundum ASD, but because of fractures of its arms, it has been taken off the market in this country. In the United States, the Amplatzer Septal Occluder (AGA Medical, Golden Valley, MN) is the most commonly used device to close the secundum ASD. The Helex Septal Occluder (WL Gore and Associates) is less frequently used and appears to be suitable for smaller ASD or PFO.

The use of the closure device may be indicated to close a secundum ASD measuring 4 mm or more in diameter (but <36 mm for the Amplatzer device and <18 mm for the Helex device), and there must be sufficient rims of atrial septal tissue around the defect. The procedure is performed under general anesthesia under the guide of transesophageal echo. The patient is observed overnight and discharged the next morning. Patients take children's aspirin (3–5 mg) daily for 6 months until endothelialization of the device is complete. Follow-up consists of an echo study at 6 months and 1 year. The closure rate is excellent with residual shunt present in fewer than 5% at 1 year follow-up. Rare possible complications include infection, arrhythmia, stroke, cardiac perforation, and device embolization.

Ventricular Septal Defect

Nonsurgical device closure of selected muscular VSDs is possible by using percutaneous devices, mostly the Amplatzer VSD device, when the defect is not too close to cardiac valves. Device closure, although possible, is not popular for the perimembranous VSD because of the risk of post-procedure heart block.

Patent Ductus Arteriosus

The Amplatzer duct occluder (ADO) (AGA Medical) is the most commonly used device to close medium- to large-sized ductus in the United States. Many small PDAs are still being occluded using a variety of coils.

Closure of small PDAs is performed using Gianturco vascular occlusion coils. They are small, coiled wires coated with thrombogenic Dacron strands that open like a small "pigtail" when placed in the vessel. When delivered to the aortic ampulla, a blood clot is formed around the coil, obstructing blood flow with ultimate endothelialization. Good candidates for the coil occlusion are those children weighing 6 kg or more with the ductus 4 mm and smaller. The incidence of minor complications is low (<5%) and include coil embolization, incomplete closure, mild left PA stenosis, and very rarely hemolysis.

For larger PDAs less than 12 mm in diameter, specialized devices, such as the Amplatzer duct occluder (ADO) are available for catheter-based closure. The devices are implanted antegrade from the femoral vein. There is a 98% or greater closure rate at 6 months with minimal complications and no mortality. Very large ducti in small infants are still probably best treated surgically.

Occlusion of Collaterals and Other Vessels

This technique is used for closing aortopulmonary collaterals mostly in patients with single ventricular anatomy (requiring cavopulmonary anastomosis; i.e., Fontan-type surgery), systemic arteriovenous fistulas, pulmonary arteriovenous fistulas, and venous collateral or surgically placed shunts that are no longer needed. When delivered, the coil occludes the vessel by creating a thrombus around the coil. Alternatively, an Amplatzer Duct Occluder or even an Amplatzer Septal Occluder is placed in a selected spot. Both devices need a discrete area of stenosis within a tubular vessel for fixation. Peripheral embolization of the coil or other devices into the PAs or the aorta is a major risk.

Percutaneous Valve Replacement

Since Bonhoeffer and his colleagues first replaced pulmonary valve by percutaneous techniques in 2000 (Bonhoeffer et al, 2000), this technique has gained increased experience. Candidates for this technique are typically those who received surgery for TOF and late development of severe pulmonary regurgitation. This technique is expected to reduce the need for repeated cardiac surgeries by replacing surgically placed conduits. Most of the reported cases used the Melody transcatheter pulmonary valve (Medtronic, Minneapolis, MN). The Edwards SAPIEN valve (Edwards Lifescience, Irvine, CA) is a newer valve that can be placed in RV outflow tract up to 29 mm in size compared with the Melody valve, with a maximum size of 22 mm. This technique has sparked the development of other valve replacement procedures such as transcatheter aortic valve replacement in selected adult patients.

PART 3

Pathophysiology

In this section, discussion of fetal and perinatal circulation and the circulatory changes that take place after birth is followed by discussion of the pathophysiology of some representative congenital and acquired heart diseases.

Knowledge of fetal and perinatal circulation is extremely helpful in understanding the clinical manifestations and natural history of congenital heart diseases. A few examples of clinical importance in relation to fetal and perinatal circulation will be examined.

In discussing the pathophysiology of congenital and acquired heart diseases, attempts are made to explain why particular electrocardiographic (ECG) changes, abnormalities in chest radiographs (or echocardiographic study), and physical findings are associated with each defect based on hemodynamic abnormalities. Chamber enlargements are well reflected in chest radiographic films, but pressure overload is not. Pressure overload is better reflected on ECG. Although echocardiography and Doppler studies have the capability of demonstrating both pressure and volume overload lesions, an old imaging modality, chest radiographic findings, is used rather than the new techniques because these new techniques are not available to noncardiologists.

Even when the diagnosis of a heart problem is known, correct understanding of pathophysiology plays an essential role in the appropriate management of cardiac patients, including recognition of important complications, use of medications, timing and types of surgical interventions, and following up with postoperative patients.

As an introduction to pathophysiology, a simplistic approach was chosen and controversies avoided. Careful study of the pathophysiology section will enable readers not only to explain but also recall and predict the physical findings and abnormalities of the ECG and chest radiographic films (or of echocardiography findings) of many cardiac anomalies.

8

Fetal and Perinatal Circulation

Knowledge of fetal and perinatal circulation is an integral part of understanding the pathophysiology, clinical manifestations, and natural history of congenital heart disease (CHD), especially anomalies seen in the newborn period. Only a brief discussion of clinically important aspects of fetal and perinatal circulation is presented.

FETAL CIRCULATION

Fetal circulation differs from adult circulation in several ways. Almost all differences are attributable to the fundamental difference in the site of gas exchange. In adults, gas exchange occurs in the lungs. In fetuses, the placenta provides the exchange of gases and nutrients.

Course of Fetal Circulation

There are four shunts in fetal circulation: placenta, ductus venosus, foramen ovale, and ductus arteriosus (Fig. 8.1). The following summarizes some important aspects of fetal circulation:

1. The placenta receives the largest amount of combined (i.e., right and left) ventricular output (55%) and has the lowest vascular resistance in fetuses.
2. The superior vena cava (SVC) drains the upper part of the body, including the brain (15% of combined ventricular output), and the inferior vena cava (IVC) drains the lower part of the body and the placenta (70% of combined ventricular output). Because the blood is oxygenated in the placenta, the oxygen saturation in the IVC (70%) is higher than that in the SVC (40%). The highest PO_2 is found in the umbilical vein (32 mm Hg) (see Fig. 8.1).
3. Most of the SVC blood goes to the right ventricle (RV). About one third of the IVC blood with higher oxygen saturation is directed by the crista dividens to the left atrium (LA) through the foramen ovale, and the remaining two thirds enters the RV and pulmonary artery (PA). The result is that the brain and coronary circulation receive blood

with higher oxygen saturation (Po2 of 28 mm Hg) than the lower half of the body (Po2 of 24 mm Hg) (see Fig. 8.1).
4. Less oxygenated blood in the PA flows through the widely open ductus arteriosus to the descending aorta and then to the placenta for oxygenation.

Dimensions of Cardiac Chambers

The proportions of the combined ventricular output traversing the heart chambers and the major blood vessels are reflected in the relative dimensions of these chambers and vessels (see Fig. 8.1).

1. Because the lungs receive only 15% of combined ventricular output, the branches of the PA are small. This is important in the genesis of the pulmonary flow murmur of newborns (see Chapter 2).
2. The RV is larger and more dominant than the left ventricle (LV). The RV handles 55% of the combined ventricular output, and the LV handles 45% of the combined ventricular output. In addition, the pressure in the RV is identical to that in the LV (unlike in adults). This fact is reflected in electrocardiograms (ECGs) of newborns, which show more RV force than adult ECGs.

Fetal Cardiac Output

Unlike the adult heart, which increases its stroke volume when the heart rate decreases, the fetal heart is unable to increase stroke volume when the heart rate falls because it has a low compliance. Therefore, the fetal cardiac output depends on the heart rate; when the heart rate drops, as in fetal distress, a serious fall in cardiac output results.

CHANGES IN CIRCULATION AFTER BIRTH

The primary change in circulation after birth is a shift of blood flow for gas exchange from the placenta to the lungs. The placental circulation disappears, and the pulmonary circulation is established.

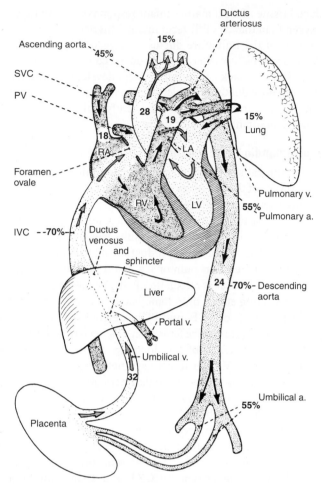

Fig. 8.1 Diagram of the fetal circulation showing the four sites of shunts: placenta, ductus venosus, foramen ovale, and ductus arteriosus. Intravascular shading is in proportion to oxygen saturation, with the lightest shading representing the highest PO_2. The numerical value inside the chamber or vessel is the PO_2 for that site in mm Hg. The percentages outside the vascular structures represent the relative flows in major tributaries and outlets for the two ventricles. The combined output of the two ventricles represents 100%. *a*, Artery; *IVC*, inferior vena cava; *LA*, left atrium; *LV*, left ventricle; *PV*, pulmonary vein; *RA*, right atrium; *RV*, right ventricle; *SVC*, superior vena cava; *v*, vein. (From Guntheroth WG, Kawabori I, Stevenson JG: Physiology of the circulation: fetus, neonate and child. In Kelley VC [ed]: *Practice of Pediatrics*, vol 8, Philadelphia, 1983, Harper & Row.)

1. The removal of the placenta results in the following:
   a. An increase in systemic vascular resistance (SVR) results (because the placenta has the lowest vascular resistance in the fetus)
   b. Cessation of blood flow in the umbilical vein results in closure of the ductus venosus
   c. Fall of prostaglandin (PGE_2), which is produced by placenta and promotes ductus arteriosus patency in utero
2. Lung expansion results in the following:
   a. A reduction of the pulmonary vascular resistance (PVR), an increase in pulmonary blood flow, and a fall in PA pressure (Fig. 8.2)
   b. Functional closure of the foramen ovale as a result of increased pressure in the LA in excess of the pressure in

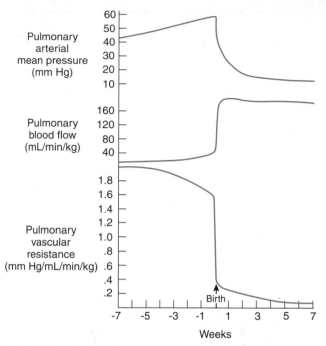

Fig. 8.2 Changes in pulmonary artery pressure, pulmonary blood flow, and pulmonary vascular resistance during the 7 weeks preceding birth, at birth, and in the 7 weeks after birth. The prenatal data were derived from lambs and the postnatal data from other species. (From Rudolph AM: *Congenital Diseases of the Heart*, 1974, Chicago, Mosby.)

the right atrium (RA). The RA pressure falls as a result of closure of the ductus venosus

   c. Closure of patent ductus arteriosus (PDA) as a result of increased arterial oxygen saturation

Changes in the PVR and closure of the PDA are so important in understanding many CHDs that further discussion is necessary.

Pulmonary Vascular Resistance

The PVR is as high as the SVR near or at term. The high PVR is maintained by an increased amount of smooth muscle in the walls of the pulmonary arterioles and alveolar hypoxia resulting from collapsed lungs. (The role of alveolar hypoxia in increasing PVR is further discussed in Chapter 29.)

With expansion of the lungs and the resulting increase in the alveolar oxygen tension, there is an initial, rapid fall in the PVR (Fig. 8.3). This rapid fall is secondary to the vasodilating effect of oxygen on the pulmonary vasculature. Between 6 and 8 weeks after birth, there is a slower fall in the PVR and the PA pressure. This fall is associated with thinning of the medial layer of the pulmonary arterioles. A further decline in the PVR occurs after the first 2 years. This may be related to the increase in the number of alveolar units and their associated vessels.

Several neonatal conditions may interfere with normal maturation (i.e., thinning) of pulmonary arterioles, resulting in the delay in normal decline of PVR and PA pressure: (1) hypoxia (resulting from lung diseases or high altitudes), (2) acidosis, (3) increased pulmonary artery pressure (resulting from large left-to-right shunt lesions), or (4) high pulmonary

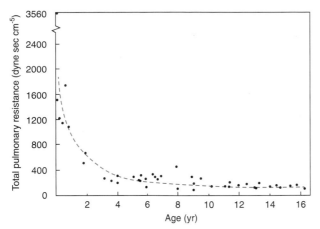

Fig. 8.3 Postnatal changes in pulmonary vascular resistance. (From Moller JH, et al: *Congenital Heart Disease*, Kalamazoo, MI, 1974, Upjohn Company.)

venous pressure (resulting from such condition as mitral stenosis). A few examples of clinical situations follow.

1. Infants with a large ventricular septal defect (VSD) may not develop congestive heart failure (CHF) while living at a high altitude, but they may develop CHF if they move to sea level. This is because of the delayed fall in the PVR associated with high altitudes.
2. Premature infants with VSD or PDA and severe hyaline membrane disease usually do not develop CHF because of their high PVR, which restricts the left-to-right shunt. Acidosis, which is often present in these infants, may contribute to maintaining a high PVR. CHF may develop as their hyaline membrane disease improves because the resulting increase in arterial Po_2 dilates pulmonary arterioles.
3. In infants with large VSDs, a high PA pressure, resulting from a direct transmission of the LV pressure to the PA through the defect, delays the fall in the PVR. As a result, CHF does not develop until 6 to 8 weeks of age or older. In contrast, the PVR falls normally in infants with a small VSD because direct transmission of the LV pressure to the PA does not occur in this situation.

Closure of the Ductus Arteriosus

Functional closure of the ductus arteriosus occurs within 10 to 15 hours after birth by constriction of the medial smooth muscle in the ductus. Anatomic closure is completed by 2 to 3 weeks of age by permanent changes in the endothelium and subintimal layers of the ductus. Oxygen, PGE2 levels, and maturity of the newborn are important factors in closure of the ductus. Acetylcholine and bradykinin also constrict the ductus.

Oxygen and the Ductus

A postnatal increase in oxygen saturation of the systemic circulation (from a Po_2 of 25 mm Hg in utero to 50 mm Hg after lung expansion) is the strongest stimulus for constriction of the ductal smooth muscle, which leads to closure of the ductus. The responsiveness of the ductal smooth muscle to oxygen is related to the gestational age of the newborn; the

ductal tissue of a premature infant responds less intensely to oxygen than that of a full-term infant. This decreased responsiveness of the immature ductus to oxygen is because of its decreased sensitivity to oxygen-induced contraction; it is not the result of a lack of smooth muscle development because the immature ductus constricts well in response to acetylcholine. It may also be caused by persistently high levels of PGE2 in preterm infants (see later section).

Prostaglandin E and the Ductus

A few clinical situations are worth mentioning to show the importance of the PG series in maintaining the patency of the ductus arteriosus in fetuses.

1. A decrease in PGE2 levels after birth results in constriction of the ductus. This decrease results from removal of the placental source of PGE_2 production at birth and from the marked increase in pulmonary blood flow, which allows effective removal of circulating PGE_2 by the lungs.
2. Constricting effects of indomethacin or ibuprofen and the dilator effects of PGE_2 and PGI_2 are greater in the ductal tissues of an immature fetus than of a near-term fetus.
3. Prolonged patency of the ductus can be maintained by intravenous (IV) infusion of a synthetic PGE_2, in newborn infants such as those with pulmonary atresia, whose survival depends on patency of the ductus.
4. Indomethacin or ibuprofen, a cyclooxygenase (COX) inhibitor (or "PG synthetase inhibitor"), can be used to close a significant PDA in premature infants (see Chapter 12).
5. Maternal ingestion of a large amount of aspirin, or any cyclooxygenase enzymes COX1 and COX2 inhibitors, an inhibitor of PG synthetase, may harm fetuses because COX inhibitors may constrict the ductus during fetal life and may result in persistent pulmonary hypertension in the newborn (PPHN). It has been suggested that some cases of PPHN (or persistent fetal circulation syndrome) may be caused by a premature constriction of the ductus arteriosus.

Reopening of a Constricted Ductus

Before true anatomic closure occurs, the functionally closed ductus may be dilated by a reduced arterial $Po2$ or an increased PGE concentration.

1. In some newborn infants, critical congenital heart defects (e.g., hypoplastic left heart syndrome, pulmonary atresia, severe coarctation of the aorta) IV infusion of PGE1 can open a partially or completely constricted ductus.
2. The reopening of the constricted ductus may occur in asphyxia and various pulmonary diseases (as hypoxia and acidosis relax ductal tissues). Ductal closure is delayed at high altitude. There is a much higher incidence of PDA at high altitudes than at sea level.

Responses of Pulmonary Artery and Ductus Arteriosus to Various Stimuli

The PA responds to oxygen and acidosis in the opposite manner from the ductus arteriosus. Hypoxia and acidosis relax the ductus arteriosus but constrict the pulmonary arterioles. Oxygen constricts the ductus but relaxes the pulmonary arterioles. The PAs are also constricted by sympathetic stimulation and α-adrenergic stimulation (e.g., epinephrine, norepinephrine). Vagal stimulation, β-adrenergic stimulation (e.g., isoproterenol), and bradykinin dilate the PAs.

PREMATURE NEWBORNS

Two important problems that premature infants may face are related to the rate at which PVR falls and the responsiveness of the ductus arteriosus to oxygen.

1. The ductus arteriosus is more likely to remain open in preterm infants after birth because the premature infant's ductal smooth muscle does not have a fully developed constrictor response to oxygen. In addition, premature infants have persistently high circulating levels of PGE_2 (caused by decreased degradation in the lungs), and the premature ductal tissue exhibits an increased dilatory response to PGE_2.

2. In premature infants, the pulmonary vascular smooth muscle is not as well developed as in full-term infants. Therefore, the fall in PVR occurs more rapidly than in mature infants. This accounts for the early onset of a large left-to-right shunt and CHF.

9

Pathophysiology of Left-to-Right Shunt Lesions

Before discussing the hemodynamic abnormalities of left-to-right shunt lesions, knowledge of the model that will be used throughout this section is helpful. Figure 9.1 is a block diagram of a normal heart in which one arrow represents a "unit" of normal cardiac output. It is assumed that the cardiac chambers and great arteries and veins indicated by one arrow are normal in size. If a cardiac chamber or great artery has more than one arrow in it, that chamber or blood vessel is going to be dilated. A diagram of a normal cardiac radiograph is presented in Chapter 4 (see Fig. 4.2). Modifications in appearance of chest radiograph secondary to enlargement or reduction of cardiac chambers or great vessels are presented in diagrammatic drawings to aid in the interpretation of chest radiograph films.

ATRIAL SEPTAL DEFECT

In patients with atrial septal defects (ASDs), the direction of the shunt is from left to right, and the magnitude of the left-to-right shunt is determined by the *size* of the defect and the relative *compliance* of the right ventricle (RV) and left ventricle (LV). Because the compliance of the RV is greater than that of the LV, a left-to-right shunt is present. The magnitude of the shunt is reflected in the degree of cardiac enlargement. Let it be assumed that there is a left-to-right shunt of one arrow at the atrial level. As seen in Figure 9.2, the right atrium (RA), RV, and main pulmonary artery (PA) and its branches have two arrows and are therefore dilated. These findings are translated into the chest radiographs (Fig. 9.3), which reveal enlargement of the RA, RV, and PA, as well as an increase in pulmonary vascular markings. Note that the left atrium (LA) is not enlarged (see Figs. 9.2 and 9.3). This is because the increased pulmonary venous return to the LA does not stay in that chamber; rather, it is shunted immediately to the RA. The absence of LA enlargement is one of the helpful radiographic signs for differentiating an ASD from a ventricular septal defect (VSD) in patients with increased pulmonary vascularity.

The dilated RV cavity prolongs the time required for depolarization of the RV because of its longer pathway, producing

either complete or incomplete right bundle branch block (RBBB) pattern (with rsR′ in V1) in the electrocardiogram (ECG). The RBBB pattern in children with ASDs is not the result of actual block in the right bundle.

The heart murmur in ASD is not caused by the shunt at the atrial level. Because the pressure gradient between the atria is so small and the shunt occurs throughout the cardiac cycle, both in systole and diastole, the left-to-right shunt is silent. The heart murmur in ASD originates from the pulmonary valve because of the increased blood flow (denoted by two arrows) passing through this normal-sized valve, producing a relative stenosis of the pulmonary valve. Therefore, the murmur is systolic in timing and is maximal at the pulmonary valve area (i.e., at the upper left sternal border). When the shunt is large, increased blood flow through the tricuspid valve (denoted by two arrows) results in a relative stenosis of this valve, producing a mid-diastolic murmur at the tricuspid valve area (i.e., lower left sternal border). The widely split S2 that is a characteristic finding in ASD results partly from RBBB. The RBBB delays both the electrical depolarization of the RV and the ventricular contraction, resulting in delayed closure of the pulmonary valve. In addition, the large atrial shunt tends to abolish respiration-related variations in systemic venous return to the right side of the heart, resulting in a fixed S2.

It should be noted that infants and small children rarely manifest with the clinical findings described even in the presence of a moderately large ASD (proved by echocardiographic studies) until they are 3 to 4 years of age. It is because the compliance of the RV improves slowly so that any significant shunt does not occur until that age.

Children with ASD rarely experience congestive heart failure (CHF) even in the presence of a large left-to-right shunt. The PAs can handle an increased amount of blood flow for a long time without developing pulmonary hypertension or CHF because there is no direct transmission of the systemic pressure to the PA, and PA pressure remains normal. However, CHF and pulmonary hypertension eventually develop in the third and fourth decades of life if the shunt is large.

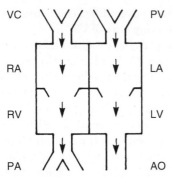

Fig. 9.1 Block diagram of a normal heart. One *arrow* represents a unit of normal cardiac output. *AO,* Aorta; *LA,* left atrium; *LV,* left ventricle; *PA,* pulmonary artery; *PV,* pulmonary vein; *RA,* right atrium; *RV,* right ventricle; *VC,* vena cava.

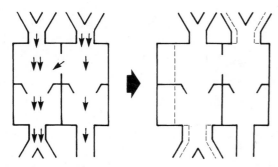

Fig. 9.2 Block diagram of an atrial septal defect. The number of *arrows* in each chamber represents the amount of blood to be handled by that particular chamber. When one redraws the chambers with two *arrows* larger than normal, one can predict which chambers will be enlarged.

VENTRICULAR SEPTAL DEFECT

The direction of the shunt in acyanotic VSD is left to right. The magnitude of the shunt is determined by the size, not the location, of the defect and the level of pulmonary vascular resistance (PVR). With a small defect, a large resistance to the left-to-right shunt occurs at the defect, and the shunt does not depend on the level of PVR. A decrease in the PVR occurs normally in this situation. With a large VSD, the resistance offered by the defect is minimal, and the left-to-right shunt depends largely on the level of PVR. The lower the PVR, the greater the magnitude of the left-to-right shunt. This type of left-to-right shunt is called a *dependent shunt* (in contrast to *obligatory shunt,* to be discussed later in this chapter). Even in the presence of a large VSD in a newborn, the PVR remains elevated, and therefore a large shunt does not occur until the infant reaches 6 to 8 weeks of age, when the shunt increases and CHF may develop.

In a VSD of moderate size, the cardiac chambers or vessels with two arrows enlarge, resulting in enlargement of the main PA, LA, and LV, as well as an increase in pulmonary vascular markings (Fig. 9.4). In VSD, it is the LV that does volume overwork, not the RV. This results in LV enlargement; the RV does not enlarge. Because the shunt of VSD occurs mainly during systole when the RV also contracts, the shunted blood goes directly to the PA rather than remaining in the RV cavity. Therefore, there is no significant volume overload to the RV, and the RV remains relatively normal in size in a VSD with moderate shunt (Fig. 9.4 and 9.5). It should be noted that LA enlargement is present only with VSD but not with ASD. It should also be noted that both VSD and PDA produce an enlargement of the LA and LV.

Figure 9.6 summarizes the hemodynamics of VSDs of varying sizes and helps in the understanding of clinical manifestations. The size of a cardiac chamber directly relates to the amount of blood (or the number of arrows) handled by the chamber. The total number of arrows in the heart diagram

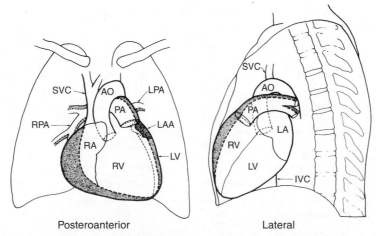

Posteroanterior   Lateral

Fig. 9.3 Diagram of posteroanterior and lateral views of chest radiographs. Enlargement of the right atrium (RA) and pulmonary artery (PA) segment and increased pulmonary vascular markings are present in the posteroanterior view. The right ventricular enlargement is best seen in the lateral view. *AO,* Aorta; *IVC,* inferior vena cava; *LA,* left atrium; *LAA,* left atrial appendage; *LPA,* left pulmonary artery; *LV,* left ventricle; *RPA,* right pulmonary artery; *RV,* right ventricle; *SVC,* superior vena cava.

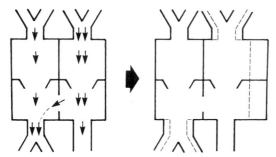

Fig. 9.4 Block diagram of ventricular septal defect that shows the chambers and vessels that will be enlarged. There is an enlargement of the left atrium and left ventricle. The pulmonary artery is prominent, and the pulmonary vascularity is increased. Note the absence of right ventricular enlargement (see text for explanation).

also determines the overall size of the heart. Let us examine Figure 9.6 for varying sizes of VSDs.

With a small VSD, there is only half an arrow coming from the LV to the main PA. In addition, the degree of pulmonary vascular congestion and chamber enlargement is either minimal or too small to result in a significant change in the chest x-ray films (see Fig. 9.6). The degree of volume work imposed on the LV is also too small to produce left ventricular hypertrophy (LVH) on the ECG. The shunt itself produces a heart murmur (regurgitant systolic), and the intensity of the P2 is normal because the PA pressure remains normal.

With a VSD of *moderate* size, one arrow shunts from the LV to the RV, and all the chambers with two arrows enlarge. Therefore, the degree of cardiomegaly on the radiographic

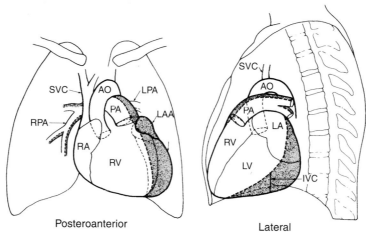

Posteroanterior   Lateral

Fig. 9.5 Diagrams of posteroanterior and lateral views of chest radiographs of a moderate ventricular septal defect. Enlargement of the left atrium (LA), left ventricle (LV), and pulmonary artery (PA) and increased pulmonary vascular markings are present. Note the presence of LA enlargement, which is absent in atrial septal defect. Other abbreviations are the same as those in Figure 9.3.

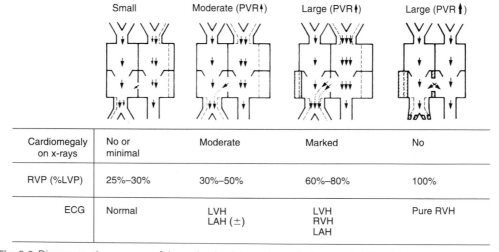

	Small	Moderate (PVR↓)	Large (PVR↓)	Large (PVR↑)
Cardiomegaly on x-rays	No or minimal	Moderate	Marked	No
RVP (%LVP)	25%–30%	30%–50%	60%–80%	100%
ECG	Normal	LVH LAH (±)	LVH RVH LAH	Pure RVH

Fig. 9.6 Diagrammatic summary of the pathophysiology of ventricular septal defect. Most of the radiographic and electrocardiographic findings can be deduced from this diagram (see text for full description). *LAH,* Left atrial hypertrophy; *LVH,* left ventricular hypertrophy; *LVP,* left ventricular pressure; *PVR,* pulmonary vascular resistance; *RVH,* right ventricular hypertrophy; *RVP,* right ventricular pressure.

film is significant. The volume overwork done by the LV is significant, so the ECG shows LVH of the "volume overload" type. Although the shunt is large, the RV is not significantly dilated, and the pressure in this chamber is elevated only slightly (see Fig. 9.6). In other words, in a moderate VSD, the RV is not under significant volume or pressure overload; therefore, ECG signs of right ventricular hypertrophy (RVH) are absent. As in a small VSD, a heart murmur (regurgitant systolic type) is produced by the left-to-right shunt. The normal-sized mitral valve handles two arrows. This relative mitral stenosis produces a mid-diastolic rumble at the apex. The PA pressure is mildly elevated; therefore, the intensity of the P2 may increase slightly.

With *a large* VSD, the overall heart size is larger than that seen with a moderate VSD because there is a much greater shunt. Because there is direct transmission of the LV pressure through the large defect to the RV, in addition to a much greater shunt, the RV becomes enlarged and hypertrophied. Therefore, the chest radiograph shows biventricular enlargement, left atrial enlargement, and greatly increased pulmonary vascularity (see Fig. 9.6). The ECG shows biventricular hypertrophy (BVH) and sometimes left atrial hypertrophy (LAH). A large VSD usually results in CHF in early infancy.

When a large VSD is left untreated, irreversible changes take place in the pulmonary arterioles, producing pulmonary vascular obstructive disease (or Eisenmenger's syndrome). It may take years to develop this condition. When Eisenmenger's syndrome occurs, striking changes take place in the heart size, ECG, and clinical findings. Because the PVR is notably elevated at this stage, approaching the systemic level, the magnitude of the left-to-right shunt decreases. This results in removal of the volume overload placed on the LV as well as the LA. Therefore, the size of the LV and the overall heart size decrease, and the ECG evidence of LVH disappears, leaving only RVH because of the persistence of pulmonary hypertension. Although the heart size becomes small, the PA segment remains enlarged because of persistent pulmonary hypertension. In other words, with the development of pulmonary vascular obstructive disease, the heart size returns to normal except for a prominent PA segment, and a pure RVH on the ECG results. A bidirectional shunt causes cyanosis. Because the shunt is small, the loudness of the murmur decreases, or it may even disappear. The S2 is loud and single owing to pulmonary hypertension.

PATENT DUCTUS ARTERIOSUS

The hemodynamics of PDA are similar to those of VSD. The magnitude of the left-to-right shunt is determined by the *resistance* offered by the ductus (i.e., diameter, length, and tortuosity) when the ductus is small and by the level of PVR when the ductus is large (i.e., dependent shunt). Therefore, the onset of CHF with PDA is similar to that with VSD.

The chambers and vessels that enlarge are the same as those in VSD except for an enlarged aorta to the level of the PDA (i.e., enlarged ascending aorta and transverse arch), which also handles an increased amount of blood flow (Fig. 9.7).

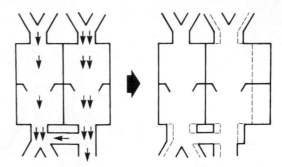

Fig. 9.7 Block diagram of the heart in patent ductus arteriosus (PDA). Note the similarities between PDA and ventricular septal defect as to chamber enlargement. There is enlargement of the aorta to the level of the ductus arteriosus.

Therefore, in PDA, chest radiographic films show enlargement of the LA and LV, a large ascending aorta and PA, and an increase in pulmonary vascular markings (Fig. 9.8). Although the aorta is enlarged, it usually does not produce an abnormal cardiac silhouette because the ascending aorta does not normally form the cardiac silhouette. Therefore, chest radiographic films of PDA are indistinguishable from those of VSD.

Hemodynamic consequences of PDA are similar to those of VSD. In PDA with a small shunt, the LV enlargement is minimal; therefore, the ECG and chest radiographic findings are close to normal. Because there is a significant pressure gradient between the aorta and the PA in both systole and diastole, the left-to-right shunt occurs in both phases of the cardiac cycle, thereby producing the characteristic continuous murmur of this condition. With a small shunt, the intensity of the P2 is normal because the PA pressure is normal.

In PDA with a moderately large shunt, the heart size is moderately enlarged with increased pulmonary blood flow. The chambers enlarged are the LA, LV, and PA segments and the proximal aorta. The ECG shows LVH as in moderate VSD. In addition to the characteristic continuous murmur, there may be an apical diastolic flow rumble as a result of relative stenosis of the mitral valve. The P2 slightly increases in intensity if it can be separated from the loud heart murmur.

In a large PDA, marked cardiomegaly and increased pulmonary vascular markings are present. The volume overload is on the LV and LA, which produces LVH and occasional LAH on the ECG. The free transmission of the aortic pressure to the PA produces pulmonary hypertension and RV hypertension, with resulting RVH on the ECG. Therefore, the ECG shows BVH and LAH, as in a large VSD. The continuous murmur is present, with an apical diastolic rumble owing to relative mitral stenosis. The P2 is accentuated in intensity due to pulmonary hypertension.

An untreated large PDA can also produce pulmonary vascular obstructive disease, with a resulting bidirectional (i.e., right-to-left and left-to-right) shunt at the ductus level. The bidirectional shunt may produce cyanosis only in the lower half of the body (i.e., differential cyanosis). As in VSD with Eisenmenger's syndrome, the heart size returns to normal because of the reduced magnitude of the shunt. The peripheral pulmonary vascularity decreases, but the central hilar vessels

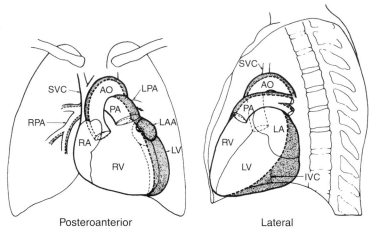

Posteroanterior   Lateral

Fig. 9.8 Diagrams of the posteroanterior and lateral chest radiographs of patent ductus arteriosus (PDA). Note the similarities between PDA and ventricular septal defect. Abbreviations are the same as those in Figure 9.3.

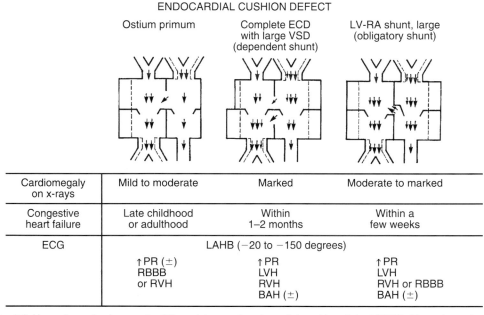

ENDOCARDIAL CUSHION DEFECT

	Ostium primum	Complete ECD with large VSD (dependent shunt)	LV-RA shunt, large (obligatory shunt)
Cardiomegaly on x-rays	Mild to moderate	Marked	Moderate to marked
Congestive heart failure	Late childhood or adulthood	Within 1–2 months	Within a few weeks
ECG	LAHB (−20 to −150 degrees)		
	↑PR (±) RBBB or RVH	↑PR LVH RVH BAH (±)	↑PR LVH RVH or RBBB BAH (±)

Fig. 9.9 Hemodynamic changes in different types of endocardial cushion defect (ECD). Hemodynamics of each type of the defects are described in the text. *BAH*, Biatrial hypertrophy; *LAHB*, left anterior hemiblock; *LVH*, left ventricular hypertrophy; *↑PR*, prolongation of the PR interval on electrocardiogram; *RBBB*, right bundle branch block; *RVH*, right ventricular hypertrophy.

and the main PA segment are greatly dilated owing to severe pulmonary hypertension. The ECG shows pure RVH because the LV is no longer under volume overload. Auscultation no longer reveals the continuous murmur or the apical rumble as a result of the shunt reduction. The S2 is single and loud due to pulmonary hypertension.

ENDOCARDIAL CUSHION DEFECT

During fetal life, the endocardial cushion tissue contributes to the closure of both the lower part of the atrial septum (i.e., ostium primum) and the upper part of the ventricular septum in addition to the formation of the mitral and tricuspid valves. The failure of normal development of this tissue may

be either complete or partial. A simple way of understanding the complete form of endocardial cushion defect (ECD) is that the tissue in the center of the heart is missing, with resulting VSD, the primum type of ASD, and clefts in the mitral and tricuspid valves. In the partial form of the defect, only an ASD is present in the ostium primum septum (primum type of ASD), often associated with a cleft in the mitral valve.

Hemodynamic abnormalities of primum-type ASD are similar to those of secundum-type ASD, in which the RA and RV are dilated with increased pulmonary blood flow (Fig. 9.9). These changes are expressed in the chest radiographs (see Fig. 9.3). The cleft mitral valve is usually insignificant from a hemodynamic point of view because blood regurgitated into the LA is immediately shunted to the RA,

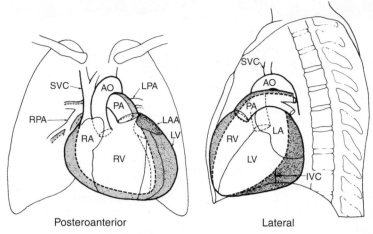

Fig. 9.10 Diagrams of chest radiographs in the complete form of endocardial cushion defect. All four cardiac chambers are enlarged, with increased pulmonary vascular markings. Abbreviations are the same as those in Figure 9.3.

thereby decompressing the LA. The physical findings are also similar to those of secundum ASD: a widely split and fixed S2, a systolic ejection murmur at the upper left sternal border, and a mid-diastolic rumble of relative tricuspid stenosis at the lower left sternal border. In addition, a systolic murmur of mitral regurgitation (MR) is occasionally present. The ECG findings are also similar: RBBB (with rsR′ in V1) or mild RVH. One exception, which is important in differentiating between the two types of ASDs, is the presence of a "superior" QRS axis or left anterior hemiblock (with the QRS axis in the range of −20 to −150 degrees) in the ECG of primum-type ASD. The abnormal QRS axis seen in ECD (both partial and complete forms) is not the result of axis deviation or any of the hemodynamic abnormalities mentioned; rather, the abnormal QRS axis occurs as a result of the primary abnormality in the development of the bundle of His and the bundle branches.

Hemodynamic changes seen with complete ECD are the sum of the changes seen in ASD and VSD. There is volume overload of the LA and LV as in VSD and partially due to MR. In addition, it has volume overload of the RA and RV as in ASD (see Fig. 9.9). The result is biatrial and biventricular enlargement (Fig. 9.10). The magnitude of the left-to-right shunt in complete ECD is determined by the level of PVR (i.e., dependent shunt). The ECG also reflects these

changes as BVH and occasional biatrial hypertrophy (BAH). "Superior" QRS axis is also characteristic of ECD as discussed earlier. Physical examination is characterized by a hyperactive precordium and regurgitant systolic murmurs of VSD and MR, loud and narrowly split S2 (because of pulmonary hypertension), apical or tricuspid diastolic rumble (or both), and signs of CHF. Those who survive infancy may develop pulmonary vascular obstructive disease, as already discussed for large VSD and large PDA.

A direct communication between the LV and RA may occur as part of ECD (or as an isolated defect unrelated to ECD). The direction of the shunt is from the high-pressure LV to the low-pressure RA. The magnitude of the shunt is determined by the *size* of the defect, regardless of the state of PVR; blood shunted to the RA must go forward through the lungs even if the PVR is high. This type of shunt, which is independent of the status of PVR, is called an *obligatory shunt* (see Fig. 9.9). When an LV-RA shunt is present as part of complete ECD, CHF may occur within a few weeks, which is earlier than in the usual VSD. The enlarged chambers are identical to those of the complete form of ECD. Therefore, the chest radiographs and ECG findings are similar to those seen in complete ECD. Physical findings also resemble those of complete ECD, although the holosystolic murmur (resulting from the LV-RA shunt) may be more prominent at the mid-right sternal border.

10

Pathophysiology of Obstructive and Valvular Regurgitant Lesions

This chapter discusses hemodynamic abnormalities of obstructive and valvular regurgitant lesions of congenital and acquired causes. For convenience, they are divided into the following three groups based on their hemodynamic similarities:

1. Ventricular outflow obstructive lesions (e.g., aortic stenosis [AS], pulmonary stenosis [PS], coarctation of the aorta [COA])
2. Stenosis of atrioventricular (AV) valves (e.g., mitral stenosis [MS], tricuspid stenosis [TS])
3. Valvular regurgitant lesions (e.g., mitral regurgitation [MR], tricuspid regurgitation [TR], aortic regurgitation [AR], pulmonary regurgitation [PR])

OBSTRUCTION TO VENTRICULAR OUTPUT

Common congenital obstructive lesions to ventricular output are AS, PS, and COA. All of these obstructive lesions produce the following three pathophysiologic changes (Fig. 10.1):
1. An ejection systolic murmur (as heard on auscultation)
2. Hypertrophy of the respective ventricle (as seen in the electrocardiographic [ECG] or echocardiography study)
3. Poststenotic dilatation (as seen in chest radiographs or echocardiography images; this is not seen with subvalvular stenosis)

Aortic and Pulmonary Valve Stenoses

An ejection type of systolic murmur can best be heard when the stethoscope is placed over the area distal to the obstruction. Therefore, the murmur of AS is usually loudest over the ascending aorta (i.e., aortic valve area or upper right sternal border), and the murmur of PS is loudest over the pulmonary artery (i.e., pulmonary valve area or upper left sternal border). However, the actual location of the aortic valve is under the sternum at the level of the third left intercostal space; therefore, the murmur of AS may be quite loud at the third left intercostal space.

In isolated stenosis of the pulmonary or aortic valve, the intensity and duration of the ejection systolic murmur are directly proportional to the severity of the stenosis. In mild stenosis of a semilunar valve, the murmur is of low intensity (grade 1 to 2 of 6) and occurs early in systole, with the apex of the "diamond" in the first half of systole. With increasing severity of the stenosis, the murmur becomes longer and louder (often with a thrill) with the apex of the murmur moving toward the S2.

With mild pulmonary valve stenosis, the S2 is normal or split widely because of prolonged "hangout time" (see Chapter 2). With severe PS, the murmur is long and may continue beyond the A2 and the S2 splits widely, but the intensity of the P2 decreases (Fig. 10.2A). With severe AS, the S2 becomes single or splits paradoxically because of the delayed closure of the aortic valve (A2) in relation to the P2 (Fig. 10.2B). In semilunar valve stenosis, an ejection click may be audible. The click is produced by a sudden checking of the valve motion or possibly by the sudden distention of the dilated great arteries.

If the obstruction is severe, the ventricle that has to pump blood against the obstruction will hypertrophy. The left ventricle (LV) hypertrophies in AS and the right ventricle (RV) in PS, which results in left ventricular hypertrophy (LVH) and right ventricular hypertrophy (RVH), respectively, on the ECG. Cardiac output is maintained unless myocardial failure occurs in severe cases; therefore, the heart size remains normal (on chest radiographic films or echo study).

The artery distal to the stenotic semilunar valve usually dilates circumferentially (called "poststenotic dilatation"). It occurs only with the semilunar valve stenosis but not with subvalvular stenosis; it is only mild or not seen at all with supravalvular stenosis. In pulmonary valve stenosis, a prominent PA segment is visible on chest radiographic film (see Fig. 4.7A). In aortic valve stenosis, the dilated aorta may look like a bulge on the right upper mediastinum or a prominence of the aortic knob on the left upper mediastinum on chest films (see Fig. 4.7C). Mild dilatation of the ascending aorta secondary to aortic valve stenosis is usually not visible on plain chest radiographic films because the ascending aorta does not form the cardiac border.

In the past, dilated aorta and pulmonary artery associated with stenotic semilunar valves were considered hemodynamic consequences of the stenotic valves, and the term "poststenotic dilatation" was used. The circumferential dilatation seen in the great arteries was thought to have resulted from generalized fatigue of collagen fibers by sustained vibration of the vessel distal to the stenotic valve. In recent years, however, it has become clear that some of the dilated great arteries are primary disorders (aortopathy) genetically determined and not entirely related to hemodynamic abnormalities. Aortopathy is seen in association with bicuspid aortic valve (BAV), coarctation of the aorta (COA), and conotruncal abnormalities (e.g., TOF, pulmonary atresia and VSD, or truncus arteriosus) or seen in genetic syndromes with connective tissue disorders (such as Marfan's, vascular Ehlers-Danlos, and Turner syndromes) (Francois, 2015). Aortopathy is move prominent in BAV than other defects; aortic dilatation in BAV occurs earlier (even in fetuses) and is more prominent than that seen with the stenosis of tricuspid aortic valve in which the pressure gradient is usually greater than in the former. Therefore, dilatation of the aorta

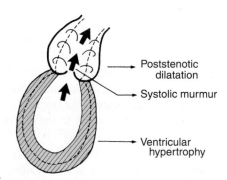

Fig. 10.1 Three secondary changes are seen in aortic valve and pulmonary valve stenosis: an ejection systolic murmur, hypertrophy of the responsible ventricle, and poststenotic dilatation of a great artery. A normal-sized ventricle and a great artery are shown by *broken lines*. The end results of a semilunar valve stenosis are illustrated by *solid lines*.

seen in BAV appears to result from a combination of primary aortopathy (the genetic theory) and hemodynamic changes induced by the bicuspid valve. Histologic abnormalities have been noted in dilated ascending aorta, which include increased amount of collagen and decreased smooth muscle cell content.

Coarctation of the Aorta

In older children with COA, an ejection-type systolic murmur is present over the descending aorta distal to the site of coarctation (i.e., in the left interscapular area). Because many of these patients also have abnormal aortic valves (most commonly bicuspid aortic valves), a soft AS murmur, ejection click, and occasional AR murmur may be heard. Depending on the severity of the obstruction, the femoral pulses are either weak and delayed or absent. The weak pulse results primarily from a slow upstroke of the arterial pulse in the lower extremity sites. On chest radiographs, poststenotic dilatation of the descending aorta (distal to the coarctation) often produces the figure-of-3 sign. The poststenotic dilatation of the descending aorta distal to the coarctation can be easily imaged by echocardiographic study. The ECG shows LVH because of a pressure overload on the LV. In newborns and small infants, RVH or right bundle branch block (RBBB) is commonly seen, but LVH is not (see later section for the reasons).

Clinical presentation of patients with COA occurs in a bimodal distribution: symptomatic newborns and asymptomatic infants and children. The reasons for the bimodality can be explained by the differences in pathology and pathophysiology between the two groups of patients with coarctation of the aorta.

1. Symptomatic newborns with COA

Many patients who become symptomatic early in life have an associated defect such as ventricular septal defect (VSD) or left-sided obstructive lesions. The obstructive lesions may be in the left ventricular outflow tract, the aortic valve, or the proximal aorta (Fig. 10.3A). These associated defects tend to decrease blood flow to the ascending aorta and to the aortic isthmus (i.e., the segment between the left subclavian artery and the ductus arteriosus) during fetal life. As a result, these structures become relatively hypoplastic.

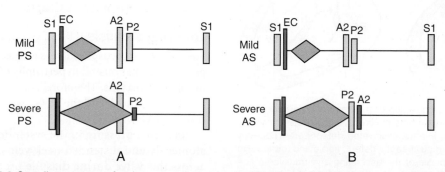

Fig. 10.2 Systolic murmurs of pulmonary valve stenosis (PS) (**A**) and aortic valve stenosis (AS) (**B**). The duration and intensity of the murmur increase with increasing severity of the stenosis. Note the changes in the splitting of S2 (see text). An ejection click (EC) is present in both conditions. Abnormal heart sounds are shown as *black bars*.

These associated anomalies result in more volume work delegated to the RV, which supplies blood to the descending aorta through a large ductus arteriosus. The RV, which is normally dominant, becomes more dilated and hypertrophied, and the LV becomes smaller than normal. This may explain why infants with COA show RVH, rather than LVH, on the ECG. RVH on the ECG is usually replaced with LVH by 2 years of age.

Decreased flow in the proximal aorta does not produce a pressure gradient between the aortic segments proximal and distal to the coarctation (which is supplied by large PDA). The absence of pressure gradient does not stimulate the development of collateral circulation between the ascending and descending aortas. When the ductus closes after birth, the pressure work imposed on the relatively small LV suddenly increases. This results in a noticeable decrease in the perfusion of the descending aorta (with resulting circulatory shock), renal failure, and signs of left heart failure (i.e., dyspnea and pulmonary venous congestion).

2. Asymptomatic coarctation of the aorta

On the contrary, in the absence of the associated defects, the normal amount of blood reaching the isthmus area produces a pressure gradient between the aortic segments above and below the coarctation, and it stimulates the development of collateral circulation between them. Most of these infants, who do not have associated defects, tolerate the postnatal closure of the ductus well and remain asymptomatic (see Fig. 10.3B), although some infants develop LV failure. The ECG will show LVH as expected.

STENOSIS OF ATRIOVENTRICULAR VALVES

Stenosis of the AV valves produces obstruction to pulmonary or systemic venous return. Passive congestion in the pulmonary or systemic venous system causes the clinical manifestations associated with these conditions.

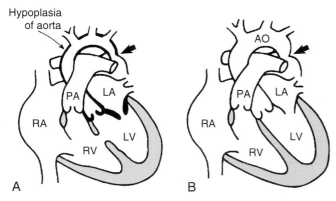

Fig. 10.3 Diagrammatic comparison of the heart and aorta in symptomatic infants and asymptomatic children with coarctation of the aorta. **A,** In symptomatic infants, associated defects are frequently found, which include ventricular septal defect, aortic and mitral valve abnormalities, and hypoplasia of the ascending and transverse aortas. These abnormalities are shown in *heavy lines*. **B,** In asymptomatic children, the coarctation is usually an isolated lesion except for bicuspid aortic valve (not shown). *AO,* Aorta; *LA,* left atrium; *LV,* left ventricle; *PA,* pulmonary artery; *RA,* right atrium; *RV,* right ventricle.

Mitral Stenosis

Stenosis of the mitral valve is more often rheumatic than congenital in origin. It produces a pressure gradient in diastole between the left atrium (LA) and the LV, which in turn produces a series of changes in the structures proximal to the mitral valve (e.g., the LA, pulmonary veins, PAs, and RV). When a significant MS is present, the LA becomes dilated and hypertrophied. The pressure in the LA is raised, which in turn raises pressures in the pulmonary veins and capillaries (Fig. 10.4). Pulmonary edema may result if the hydrostatic pressure in the capillaries exceeds the osmotic pressure of the blood. Therefore, chest radiographs may reveal pulmonary venous congestion or pulmonary edema and enlargement of the LA. Dyspnea with or without exertion and orthopnea may manifest. The high pulmonary capillary pressure results in reflex arteriolar constriction, which in turn causes pulmonary arterial hypertension and eventually hypertrophy of the RV. These changes will be seen as RVH on the ECG and as prominence of the PA segment on chest radiographs. Right heart failure may eventually develop.

The pressure gradient during diastole produces a mid-diastolic rumble that is best heard at the apex on auscultation. When the mitral valve is mobile (not severely stenotic), an opening snap precedes the murmur (mid-diastolic rumble) (see Fig. 21.1). During the last part of diastole, if the pressure gradient still exists between the LA and LV, the LA will contract to push blood forward, producing a presystolic murmur. At the time of the onset of ventricular contraction, the mitral valve leaflets are relatively wide apart because of the prolonged atrial contraction, thereby producing a loud S1. If the cardiac output reduces significantly, thready pulses result. The dilated LA contributes to the frequent occurrence of atrial fibrillation, which may result in the loss of the presystolic murmur.

The following conditions all have in common an elevated pulmonary venous pressure, with similar pathophysiology and must be differentiated from mitral stenosis:
1. Total anomalous pulmonary venous return with obstruction (see Chapter 14)
2. Cor triatriatum (see Chapter 15)
3. Pulmonary vein stenosis (see Chapter 15)
4. Hypoplastic left heart syndrome (see Chapter 14)
5. Left atrial myxoma (see Chapter 22)

Tricuspid Stenosis

Stenosis of the tricuspid valve is rare and usually congenital. It produces dilatation and hypertrophy of the right atrium (RA) for obvious reasons. Therefore, chest radiographs reveal right atrial enlargement, and the ECG may show right atrial hypertrophy (RAH).

Increased pressure in the systemic veins produces hepatomegaly and distended neck veins. A pressure gradient across this valve during diastole produces a mid-diastolic murmur. A prolonged contraction of the RA to push blood through the narrow valve may produce a presystolic murmur.

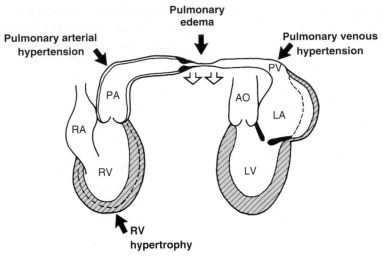

Fig. 10.4 Hemodynamic changes in severe mitral stenosis. Enlargement and hypertrophy of the left atrium (LA), pulmonary venous hypertension, and possible pulmonary edema result. Reflex vasoconstriction of pulmonary arterioles leads to pulmonary arterial hypertension and right ventricular hypertrophy. *AO,* Aorta; *LV,* left ventricle; *PA,* pulmonary artery; *PV,* pulmonary vein; *RA,* right atrium; *RV,* right ventricle.

VALVULAR REGURGITANT LESIONS

Important valvular regurgitant lesions are AR and MR. Severe pulmonary valve regurgitation is relatively rare, except in a postoperative state, such as those seen after surgery for tetralogy of Fallot and other conditions that require conduit placement between the RV and the PA. Significant tricuspid valve regurgitation is also rare except in patients with Ebstein's anomaly.

In general, when regurgitation is severe, the chambers both proximal and distal to a regurgitant valve become dilated, with volume overload of these chambers. Whereas with MR both the LV and LA dilate, with AR the LV enlarges and the aorta enlarges or increases its pulsation. If the regurgitation is minimal, only auscultatory abnormalities indicate its presence.

Mitral Regurgitation

The major problem in MR is volume overload of both the LA and LV, with resulting enlargement of these chambers (Fig. 10.5). Therefore, chest radiographs reveal enlargement of the LA and LV, and the ECG may show LVH and left atrial hypertrophy (LAH).

Regurgitation of blood from the LV to the LA produces a regurgitant systolic murmur that is best heard near the apex. Because of an increased amount of blood flows across the mitral orifice during the rapid filling phase of diastole, the S3 is usually loud. When the regurgitation is severe, a mid-diastolic rumble may be present because of "relative" MS that results from handling an excessive amount of left atrial blood through the normal-sized mitral orifice. The dilated LA chamber tends to dampen the transmission of the pressure from the LV, and the pressure in the LA is usually not notably elevated. Therefore, unlike with mitral stenosis, marked pulmonary hypertension occurs only occasionally with mitral regurgitation.

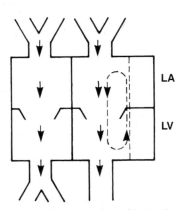

Fig. 10.5 Diagrammatic representation of hemodynamic changes in mitral regurgitation. Note that the chambers with two *arrows* (the left atrium [LA] and left ventricle [LV]) are enlarged.

Tricuspid Regurgitation

In tricuspid regurgitation, hemodynamic changes similar to those described for MR result. The RA and RV enlarge for obvious reasons. The ECG may show RAH and RVH (or RBBB).

A systolic regurgitant murmur, a loud S3, and a diastolic rumble develop, as in MR, but they are audible at the tricuspid area (both sides of the lower sternal border) rather than at the apex. With severe regurgitation, pulsation of the liver and neck veins may occur, reflecting a phasic increase in right atrial pressure by the regurgitation.

Aortic Regurgitation

There is volume overload of the LV because this chamber must handle normal cardiac output in addition to the amount that leaks back to the LV (Fig. 10.6). This is represented as left ventricular enlargement on radiographs and LVH on the ECG. Because of the increase in stroke volume received by the aorta, the aorta pulsates more than normal and becomes

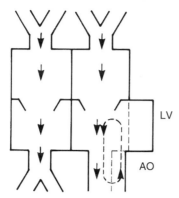

Fig. 10.6 Diagrammatic representation of hemodynamic changes in aortic regurgitation. Note that the left ventricle (LV) and aorta (AO), with two *arrows*, are enlarged.

somewhat dilated, although the aorta does not retain all the increased stroke volume.

An increase in systolic pressure results from an increase in stroke volume. The diastolic pressure is lower because of a continuous leak back to the LV during diastole. This results in a wide pulse pressure and bounding peripheral pulse. The regurgitation during diastole produces a high-pitched, decrescendo diastolic murmur immediately after the S2 (see Fig. 21.4). The regurgitant flow is directed toward the apex; therefore, the diastolic decrescendo murmur is well audible at the apex as well as in the third left intercostal space. The AR flow, which coincides with the forward flow of left atrial blood, produces a flutter motion of the mitral valve, producing an Austin-Flint murmur in diastole. With severe AR, a high left ventricular end-diastolic pressure approximates the mitral valve leaflets at the onset of ventricular systole, resulting in reduced intensity of the S1.

Pulmonary Regurgitation

The pathophysiology of PR is similar to that of AR. The RV dilates, and the PA may enlarge. This is represented in radiographs as right ventricular enlargement and prominence of the PA segment. The ECG may show RVH or RBBB.

Because of the low diastolic pressure of the PA, the murmur of PR is low pitched, and the gap between the S2 and the onset of the decrescendo diastolic murmur is wider than that seen in AR. In the presence of pulmonary hypertension, however, the murmur of PR resembles that of AR. The direction of the regurgitation is to the body of the RV; therefore, the PR murmur is audible along the left sternal border rather than at the apex (where the AR murmur is loud). The different direction of the radiation of the diastolic murmur is helpful in differentiating PR from AR.

11

Pathophysiology of Cyanotic Congenital Heart Defects

CLINICAL CYANOSIS

Detection of Cyanosis

Cyanosis is a bluish discoloration of the skin and mucous membranes resulting from an increased concentration of reduced hemoglobin to about 5 g/100 mL in the cutaneous veins. This level of reduced hemoglobin in the cutaneous vein may result from either desaturation of arterial blood or increased extraction of oxygen by peripheral tissue in the presence of normal arterial saturation (e.g., circulatory shock, hypovolemia, vasoconstriction from cold). Cyanosis associated with desaturation of arterial blood is called *central cyanosis;* cyanosis with normal arterial oxygen saturation is called *peripheral cyanosis.*

Cyanosis is more difficult to detect in children with dark pigmentation. Although cyanosis may be detected on many parts of the body, including the lips, fingernails, oral mucous membranes, and conjunctivae, the tip of the tongue is a good place to look for cyanosis; the color of the tongue is not affected by race or ethnic background, and the circulation is not sluggish in the tongue.

Influence of Hemoglobin Level on Cyanosis

The level of hemoglobin greatly influences the occurrence of cyanosis. This effect is graphically illustrated in Fig. 11.1. As stated earlier, about 5 g/100 mL of reduced hemoglobin in cutaneous veins is required for the appearance of cyanosis. Normally, about 2 g/100 mL of reduced hemoglobin is present in the venules so that an additional 3 g/100 mL of reduced hemoglobin in arterial blood produces clinical cyanosis.

1. For a normal person with hemoglobin of 15 g/100 mL, 3 g of reduced hemoglobin results from 20% desaturation (because 3 is 20% of 15). Thus, cyanosis appears when the oxygen saturation is reduced to about 80%.
2. In a person with polycythemia, cyanosis is recognized at a higher level of oxygen saturation. For example, in a person with hemoglobin of 20 g/100 mL, 3 g of reduced hemoglobin results from only 15% desaturation (or at 85% arterial saturation).
3. In patients with anemia, cyanosis is recognized at a lower level of oxygen saturation. For example, if a patient has a marked anemia (hemoglobin of 6 g/100 mL), 3 g of reduced hemoglobin does not result until the patient's arterial oxygen saturated goes down to 50% desaturation.

Role of Pulse Oximetry in Detection of Hypoxemia

Mild degree of hypoxemia does not manifest with clinical cyanosis. Many neonates with hypoxemia from significant congenital heart diseases (CHDs) may not show cyanosis on routine neonatal examination in the first days of life. About one third of neonates with critical CHDs were estimated to be undetected on routine neonatal examination. In 2011, the pulse oximetry screen was made the standard of care in newborn screen, and it has revolutionized the ability for early detection of critical congenital heart defect (CCHD). In 2017, Abouk et al reported a decline of 33% in critical CHD death rate in eight US states that had implemented CCHD screen. Pulse oximetry can detect mild degree of arterial hypoxemia without recognizable cyanosis in the newborn. Further discussion of the topic is presented in Chapter 14, along with the newborn pulse oximetry algorithm.

First developed in 1972 by Takuo Aoyagi and Michio Kishi of Japan, pulse oximetry monitors a person's arterial oxygen saturation noninvasively. The principle of pulse oximeter is based on the difference in absorption of red light (wavelength of 660 nm) and infrared light (at 940 nm wavelength) by oxygenated hemoglobin and deoxygenated hemoglobin. Oxygenated hemoglobin absorbs more infrared light and allows more red light to pass through. Deoxygenated hemoglobin absorbs more red light and allows more infrared light

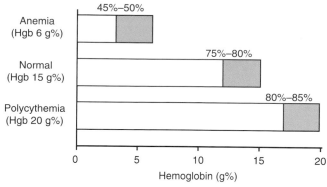

Fig. 11.1 Influence of hemoglobin (Hgb) levels on clinical recognition of cyanosis. Cyanosis is recognizable at a higher arterial oxygen saturation in patients with polycythemia and at a lower arterial oxygen saturation in patients with anemia. See text for explanation.

to pass through. A pair of small light-emitting diodes (LEDs) in the probe emits red and infrared lights, which go through a translucent part of the body (e.g., fingertip or earlobe). Red and infrared lights that passed through are detected by a photodiode on the opposite side of the probe. (Whereas red and infrared light penetrate tissue well, blue, green, yellow, and far-infrared light are significantly absorbed by non-vascular tissues and water.) The pulse oximetry detects oxygen saturation of only arterial blood, not the venous or capillary blood. This ability is based on the principle that the amount of red and infrared light absorbed fluctuate with the cardiac cycle as the arterial blood volume increases during systole and decreases during diastole; in contrast, the blood volume in the veins and capillaries remains relatively constant. The processor of pulse oximeters uses amplitude of the absorbance to calculate the ratio of the red light detected (transmitted light) to the infrared light detected by the photodiode. This ratio represents the ratio of oxygenated hemoglobin to deoxygenated hemoglobin, and the ratio is then converted to peripheral oxygen saturation by the processor.

Causes of Cyanosis

Cyanosis may result from a number of causes (Box 11.1). Central cyanosis (with reduced arterial oxygen saturation) may be caused by cyanotic congenital heart defects (CHDs), lung disease, or central nervous system (CNS) depression. Cyanosis of cardiac origin must be diagnosed early for proper management. Fortunately, detection of a mild hypoxemia is made possible by the neonatal pulse oximetry screen.

Rarely, cyanosis is caused by methemoglobinemia. Methemoglobinemia may occur as a hereditary disorder or be caused by toxic substances. Toxic methemoglobinemia (such as that seen with ingestion of water high in nitrate or exposure to aniline teething gels) is more common than hereditary methemoglobinemia (absence of reductive pathways, or NADH-cytochrome b5 reductase deficiency). When methemoglobin (MHg) levels are greater than 15% of normal hemoglobin, cyanosis is visible, and a level of 70% MHg is lethal. Compensatory polycythemia may occur in this condition. In methemoglobinemia, the color of the blood may

remain brown even after a full oxygenation or a long exposure to room air.

Acrocyanosis, a bluish color of the fingers seen in neonates and infants, is a form of peripheral cyanosis and reflects sluggish blood flow in the fingers. It has no clinical significance unless associated with circulatory shock. *Circumoral cyanosis* refers to a bluish skin color around the mouth. This is a form of peripheral cyanosis seen in healthy children with fair skin because of a sluggish capillary blood flow in association with vasoconstriction. Isolated circumoral cyanosis is of no concern unless it occurs as a result of a low cardiac output.

Cyanosis of Cardiac versus Pulmonary Origin

Differentiation of cardiac cyanosis from cyanosis caused by pulmonary diseases is crucially important for proper management of cyanotic infants. The hyperoxia test helps differentiate cyanosis caused by cardiac disease from that caused by pulmonary disease. In the hyperoxia test, one tests the response of arterial Po_2 to 100% oxygen inhalation. With pulmonary disease, arterial Po_2 usually rises to a level greater than 100 mm Hg. When there is a significant intracardiac right-to-left shunt, the arterial Po_2 does not exceed 100 mm Hg, and the rise is usually not more than 10 to 30 mm Hg, although some exceptions exist. See Chapter 14 for exceptions and further discussion.

Breathing 100% oxygen does not significantly increase Po_2 in the presence of a right-to-left intracardiac shunt. The

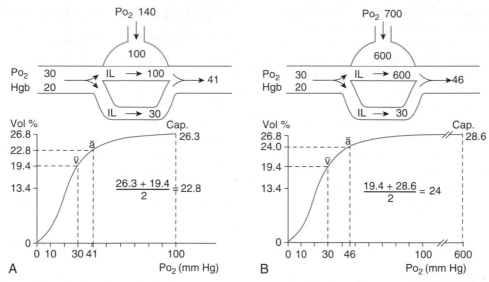

Fig. 11.2 Result of hyperoxitest in cyanotic heart defects. (**A**) Effect of a right-to-left shunt on the arterial Po_2 in room air. (**B**) Effect of a right-to-left shunt on the arterial Po_2 in 100% oxygen. See text for a detailed description. (From Duc G: Assessment of hypoxia in the newborn: Suggestions for a practical approach. Pediatrics 48:469–481, 1971.)

reason for this is explained schematically using Fig. 11.2. Let us assume that this particular patient has a cardiac output of 2 L/min, where 1 L of venous blood is distributed to ventilated alveoli (pulmonary venous return), and 1 L is shunted right-to- left through a cardiac defect.

1. While breathing in *room air* (see Fig. 11.2A)
One liter of venous blood with an oxygen content of 19.4 mL/100 mL (Po_2 of 30 mm Hg) will mix with 1 L of pulmonary venous blood containing 26.3 mL/100 mL (Po_2 of 100 mm Hg) resulting in an oxygen content of 22.8 mL/100 mL). The corresponding Po_2 from the oxygen hemoglobin dissociation curve is 41 mm Hg (shown in the lower panel of Fig. 11.2A). Therefore, mixing 1 L of blood with a Po_2 of 100 mm Hg with 1 L of blood with a Po_2 of 30 mm Hg results in a Po_2 of 41 mm Hg (see Fig. 11.2A), not an arithmetic average of 65 mm Hg. Oxygen content is the amount of oxygen bound to hemoglobin ($1.36 \times$ Hemoglobin concentration $\times$ Arterial O_2 saturation [SaO_2]) plus the amount of oxygen dissolved in arterial blood ($0.0031 \times$ arterial oxygen partial pressure [PaO_2].)

2. While breathing *100% oxygen* (see Fig. 11.2B)
When 1 L of pulmonary venous blood with a Po_2 of 600 mm Hg (oxygen content of 28.6 mg/100 mL) is mixed with 1 L of venous blood with a Po_2 of 30 mm Hg (oxygen content of 19.4 mL/100 mL), the resulting oxygen content is 24 mg/100 mL ([28.6 + 19.4]/2), with a corresponding Po_2 of 46 mm Hg). Thus, breathing 100% oxygen does not significantly alter the Po_2 (an increase from 41 to 46 mm Hg) even though the alveolar Po_2 increases from 100 to 600 mm Hg.

The lower panel of Fig. 11.2 shows the S-shaped oxygen–hemoglobin dissociation curve. The curve describes the relation between the partial pressure of oxygen (Po_2) (x-axis) and the amount of oxygen bound to hemoglobin (y-axis). The

curve demonstrates that more oxygen molecules bind as the Po_2 increases until the Po_2 reaches about 60 mm Hg. At this point, the curve is relatively flat, and the oxygen content of the blood does not increase significantly even with large increases in the Po_2. As can be seen in the figure, there is little difference in oxygen content with Po_2 of 100 or 600 mm Hg.

Consequences and Complications

1. **Polycythemia.** Low arterial oxygen content stimulates bone marrow through erythropoietin release from the kidneys and produces increased number of red blood cells (RBCs). Polycythemia, with a resulting increase in oxygen-carrying capacity, benefits cyanotic children. However, when the hematocrit reaches 65% or higher, a sharp increase in the viscosity of blood occurs, and the polycythemic response becomes disadvantageous, particularly if the patient has congestive heart failure (CHF). Some cyanotic infants have a relative iron deficiency state, with normal or lower than normal hemoglobin and hypochromia on blood smear. A normal hemoglobin in a cyanotic patient represents a relative iron deficiency state. Although less cyanotic, these infants are usually more symptomatic and improve when iron therapy raises the hemoglobin.

2. **Clubbing.** Clubbing is caused by soft tissue growth under the nail bed as a consequence of central cyanosis. The mechanism for soft tissue growth is unclear. One hypothesis is that megakaryocytes present in the systemic venous blood may be responsible for the change. In normal persons, platelets are formed from the cytoplasm of the megakaryocytes by fragmentation during their passage through the pulmonary circulation. The cytoplasm of megakaryocytes contains growth factors (e.g., platelet-derived growth factor and transforming growth factor B). In patients with

right-to-left shunts, megakaryocytes with their cytoplasm may enter the systemic circulation, become trapped in the capillaries of the digits, and release growth factors, which in turn cause clubbing. Clubbing usually does not occur until a child is 6 months of age or older, and it is seen first and is most pronounced in the thumb. In the early stage, it appears as shininess and redness of the fingertips. When fully developed, the fingers and toes become thick and wide and have convex nail beds (see Fig. 2.1). Clubbing is also seen in patients with liver disease or subacute bacterial endocarditis and on a hereditary basis without cyanosis.

3. **CNS complications.** Either very high hematocrit levels or iron-deficient RBCs place individuals with cyanotic CHDs at risk for disorders of the CNS, such as brain abscess and vascular stroke. In the past, cyanotic CHDs accounted for 5% to 10% of all cases of brain abscesses. The predisposition for brain abscesses may partially result from the fact that right-to-left intracardiac shunts may bypass the normally effective phagocytic filtering actions of the pulmonary capillary bed. This predisposition may also result from the fact that polycythemia and the consequent high viscosity of blood lead to tissue hypoxia and microinfarction of the brain, which are later complicated by bacterial colonization. The triad of symptoms of brain abscesses are fever, headache, and focal neurologic deficit.

   Vascular stroke caused by embolization arising from thrombus in the cardiac chamber or in the systemic veins may be associated with surgery or cardiac catheterization. Cerebral venous thrombosis may occur, often in infants younger than 2 years of age who have cyanosis and relative iron-deficiency anemia. A possible explanation for these findings is that microcytosis further aggravates hyperviscosity resulting from polycythemia.

4. **Bleeding disorders.** Disturbances of hemostasis are frequently present in children with severe cyanosis and polycythemia. Most frequently noted are thrombocytopenia and defective platelet aggregation. Other abnormalities include prolonged prothrombin time and partial thromboplastin time and lower levels of fibrinogen and factors V and VIII. Clinical manifestations may include easy bruising, petechiae of the skin and mucous membranes, epistaxis, and gingival bleeding. RBC withdrawal from polycythemic patients and replacement with an equal volume of plasma tend to correct the hemorrhagic tendency and lower blood viscosity.

5. **Hypoxic spells and squatting.** Although most frequently seen in infants with tetralogy of Fallot (TOF), hypoxic spells may occur in infants with other CHDs (see the later section of TOF for further discussion).

6. **Scoliosis.** Children with chronic cyanosis, particularly girls and patients with TOF, often have scoliosis.

7. **Hyperuricemia and gout.** Hyperuricemia and gout tend to occur in older patients with uncorrected or inadequately repaired cyanotic heart defects.

The pathophysiology of individual cyanotic heart defects is discussed in the section to follow.

COMMON CYANOTIC HEART DEFECTS

Complete Transposition of the Great Arteries

Complete transposition of the great arteries (D-TGA) is the most common cyanotic CHD presenting in newborn period and comprises approximately 5% of all CHDs. In this condition, the aorta arises from the right ventricle (RV), and the pulmonary artery (PA) arises from the left ventricle (LV). As the result, the normal anteroposterior relationship of the great arteries is reversed, so that the aorta is anterior to the PA (transposition), but the aorta usually remains to the right of the PA. The prefix D, however, is for d-looping of the cardiac tube during embryogenesis so that the RV ends up on the right (D transposition) and the LV on the left. This is in contrast to L-TGA in which morphologic RV ends up on the left, thus L transposition (see Chapter 14). The atria and ventricles are in normal relationship. The coronary arteries arise from the aorta, as in a normal heart.

Desaturated blood returning from the body to the right atrium (RA) flows out of the aorta without being oxygenated in the lungs and then returns to the RA (Fig. 11.3). Therefore, tissues, including vital organs such as the brain and heart, are perfused by blood with a low oxygen saturation. Conversely, well-oxygenated blood returning to the left atrium (LA) flows out of the PA and returns to the LA. This results in a complete separation of the two circuits. The two circuits are said to be in parallel (Fig. 11.2B) rather than in series, as in normal circulation (see Fig. 11.3A). This defect is incompatible with life unless communication between the two circuits occurs to provide the necessary oxygen to the body. This communication can occur at the atrial, ventricular, or ductal level or at any combination of these levels (see Fig. 11.3B).

In the most frequently encountered form of D-TGA, only a small communication exists between the atria, usually a patent foramen ovale (PFO) (Fig. 11.4A). The newborn is notably cyanotic from birth and has an arterial oxygen saturation of 30% to 50%. The low arterial Po2, which ranges from 20 to 30 mm Hg, causes an anaerobic glycolysis, with resulting metabolic acidosis. Hypoxia and acidosis are detrimental to myocardial function. The normal postnatal decrease in pulmonary vascular resistance (PVR) results in increased pulmonary blood flow

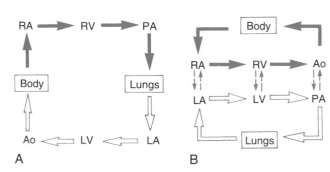

Fig. 11.3 Circulation pathways of normal "in series" circulation (A) and the "in parallel" circulation of transposition of the great arteries (B). *Open arrows* indicate oxygenated blood; *closed arrows* indicate desaturated blood. *AO,* Aorta; *LA,* left atrium; *LV,* left ventricle; *PA,* pulmonary artery; *RA,* right atrium; *RV,* right ventricle.

(PBF) and volume overload to the LA and LV. Severe hypoxia and acidosis (with a resulting decrease in myocardial function) and volume overload to the left side of the heart cause CHF during the first week of life. Unless hypoxia and acidosis are corrected, the condition of these infants deteriorates rapidly. Other metabolic problems encountered are hypoglycemia, which is probably secondary to pancreatic islet hypertrophy and hyperinsulinism, and a tendency toward hypothermia.

Usually no heart murmur is noted in a neonate with D-TGA, although a murmur is commonly found in other forms of cyanotic heart defects. The S2 is single, mainly because the pulmonary valve is farther from the chest wall, causing the P2 to be inaudible. Chest radiographic films show cardiomegaly and increased pulmonary vascularity. The ECG shows right ventricular hypertrophy (RVH), but RVH may be difficult to diagnose in the first days of life because of the normal dominance of the RV at this age. A deeply cyanotic newborn with increased pulmonary vascular markings and cardiomegaly without heart murmur can be considered to have D-TGA until proved otherwise.

The presence of a large atrial septal defect (ASD) is most desirable in infants with TGA. When a large ASD is present, infants have good arterial oxygen saturation (as high as 80% to 90%) because of good mixing (Fig. 11.4B). Therefore, hypoxia

and metabolic acidosis are not the problems in these children. In fact, the idea of the balloon atrial septostomy (Rashkind's procedure) was derived from the natural history of infants with TGA and large ASDs. However, the frequency of a large ASD occurring naturally in TGA is low. Infants who have had successful balloon atrial septostomies behave like those with naturally occurring ASDs. As the PVR falls after birth, PBF increases, with an increase in the size of the LA and LV. Although these infants are not hypoxic or acidotic, CHF develops because of volume overload to the left side of the heart. Because the RV is the systemic ventricle, RVH becomes evident on the ECG.

When associated with a large ventricular septal defect (VSD), only minimal arterial desaturation is present, and cyanosis may be missed (Fig. 11.5A). Therefore, metabolic acidosis does not develop, but left-sided heart failure results within the first few weeks of life as the PBF increases with decreasing PVR. Chest radiographs reflect this, showing cardiomegaly with increased pulmonary vascularity. The ECG may show biventricular hypertrophy (BVH) when the VSD is large: RVH because of the systemic RV and left ventricular hypertrophy (LVH) because of volume overload of the left side of the heart. A heart murmur of VSD is present, and the S2 is single because the P2 is inaudible or pulmonary hypertension is present.

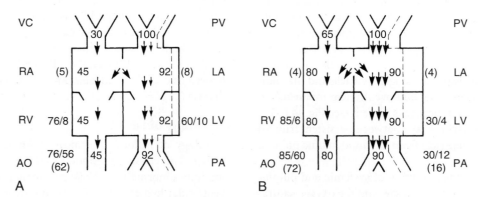

Fig. 11.4 Diagrammatic presentation of the hemodynamics of transposition of the great arteries with inadequate mixing (**A**) and with good mixing at the atrial level (**B**). Numbers within the diagram denote oxygen saturation values, and those outside the diagram denote pressure values. *AO,* Aorta; *LA,* left atrium; *LV,* left ventricle; *PA,* pulmonary artery; *PV,* pulmonary vein; *RA,* right atrium; *RV,* right ventricle; *VC,* vena cava.

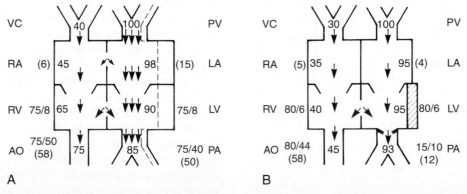

Fig. 11.5 Diagrammatic presentation of the hemodynamic abnormalities in transposition of the great arteries with a large ventricular septal defect (VSD) (**A**) and with VSD and pulmonary stenosis (**B**). Numbers within the diagram denote oxygen saturation values, and those outside the diagram denote pressure values. Abbreviations are the same as those in Fig. 11.4.

When the VSD is associated with pulmonary stenosis (PS) in infants with TGA, although the VSD helps good mixing, the volume of fully saturated blood returning from the lungs is inadequate (see Fig. 11.5B). Likewise, even after a well-performed Rashkind procedure, the arterial oxygen saturation does not increase much because of the decreased PBF. These infants have severe hypoxia and acidosis and may succumb early in life. This is a good illustration of how the magnitude of PBF affects the arterial oxygen saturation in a given cyanotic CHD. Because PBF is not increased, the left cardiac chambers are not under increased volume work; therefore, cardiac enlargement and CHF do not develop. Chest radiographs therefore show normal heart size and normal or decreased pulmonary vascularity. The ECG shows evidence of BVH; LVH is present because of PS, and RVH is present because of the nature of TGA. Physical examination reveals a PS murmur and a single S2 in addition to cyanosis.

Persistent Truncus Arteriosus and Single Ventricle

In persistent truncus arteriosus (Fig. 11.6A), a single arterial blood vessel (truncus arteriosus) arises from the heart. The PA or its branches arise from the truncus arteriosus, and the truncus continues as the aorta. A large VSD is always present in this condition. In single ventricle (also called "double-inlet ventricle") (Fig. 11.6B), two atrioventricular (AV) valves empty into a single ventricular chamber from which a great artery (either the aorta or PA) arises. The other great artery arises from a rudimentary ventricular chamber attached to the main ventricle. The opening between the single ventricle and the rudimentary chamber is called the "bulboventricular foramen." No ventricular septum of significance is present (see Fig. 14.61).

The following similarities exist between persistent truncus arteriosus and single ventricle from a hemodynamic point of view:

1. There is almost complete mixing of systemic and pulmonary venous blood in the ventricle, and the oxygen saturation of blood in the two great arteries is similar.

2. Pressures in both ventricles are identical.
3. The level of oxygen saturation in the systemic circulation is proportional to the magnitude of PBF.

In addition to the level of PVR, the magnitude of PBF is determined by the caliber of the PA in the case of persistent truncus arteriosus and by the presence or absence of PS and the size of the VSD (i.e., the bulboventricular foramen) in the case of single ventricle. When the PBF is large, the patient is minimally cyanotic but may develop CHF because of an excessive volume overload placed on the ventricle. In contrast, when the PBF is small, the patient is severely cyanotic and does not develop CHF because there is no volume overload. This latter group of patients and those with TOF share similar clinical pictures.

Physical examination reveals varying degrees of cyanosis, depending on the magnitude of PBF. A heart murmur of the VSD is rarely audible because of the presence of a huge defect. There may be an ejection systolic murmur caused by the stenosis of the pulmonary valve or of the PA branches. An early diastolic murmur of truncal valve regurgitation may be heard. The ECG usually shows BVH in both conditions. In single ventricle, the QRS complexes of all precordial leads (i.e., V1–V6) are recorded over *one* ventricle; therefore, they are similar (with poor R/S progression), suggestive of BVH. Chest radiographic findings are determined by the magnitude of PBF—if the magnitude of the PBF is large, the heart size is large, and the pulmonary vascularity increases; if the magnitude is small, the heart size is small, and the pulmonary vascularity decreases. With increased PBF and resulting pulmonary hypertension, CHF and later pulmonary vascular obstructive disease (i.e., Eisenmenger's syndrome) may develop.

Tetralogy of Fallot

Tetralogy of Fallot is the most common form of cyanotic CHDs. The classic description of TOF includes the following four abnormalities: VSD, pulmonary stenosis (PS), right ventricular hypertrophy (RVH), and overriding of the aorta. From a physiologic point of view, TOF requires only two abnormalities—a VSD large enough to equalize systolic pressures in both ventricles and a stenosis of the right ventricular outflow tract (RVOT) in the form of infundibular stenosis, valvular stenosis, or both. RVH is secondary to PS, and the degree of overriding of the aorta varies widely and it is not always present. The severity of the RVOT obstruction determines the direction and the magnitude of the shunt through the VSD.

With mild stenosis, the shunt is left to right, and the clinical picture resembles that of a VSD. This is called acyanotic or pink TOF (Fig. 11.7A). With a more severe stenosis, the shunt is right to left, resulting in "cyanotic" TOF (Fig. 11.7B). In the extreme form of TOF, the pulmonary valve is atretic, with right-to-left shunting of the entire systemic venous return through the VSD. In this case, the PBF is provided through a patent ductus arteriosus (PDA) or multiple collateral arteries arising from the aorta. In TOF, regardless of the direction of the ventricular shunt, the systolic pressure in the RV equals that of the LV and the aorta (see Fig. 11.7A and B). The mere

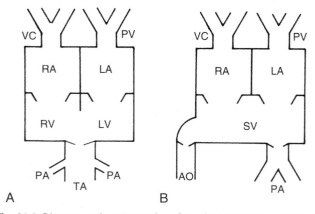

Fig. 11.6 Diagrammatic presentation of persistent truncus arteriosus (A) and a common form of single ventricle (B). *AO,* Aorta; *LA,* left atrium; *LV,* left ventricle; *PA,* pulmonary artery; *PV,* pulmonary vein; *RA,* right atrium; *RV,* right ventricle; *SV,* single ventricle; *TA,* truncus arteriosus; *VC,* vena cava.

combination of a small VSD and a PS is not TOF; the size of the VSD must be nearly as large as the annulus of the aortic valve to equalize the pressure in the RV and LV.

In *acyanotic TOF*, a small to moderate left-to-right ventricular shunt is present, and the systolic pressures are equal in the RV, LV, and aorta (see Fig. 11.7A). There is a mild to moderate pressure gradient between the RV and PA, and the PA pressure may be slightly elevated (because of a less severe stenosis of the RVOT). Because the presence of the PS minimizes the magnitude of the left-to-right shunt, the heart size and the pulmonary vascularity increase only slightly to moderately. These increases are indistinguishable from those of a small to moderate VSD. However, unlike VSDs, the ECG always shows RVH because the RV pressure is always high. Occasionally, LVH is also present. The heart murmurs are caused by the PS and the VSD. Therefore, the murmur is a superimposition of an ejection systolic murmur of PS and a regurgitant systolic murmur of a VSD. The murmur is best audible along the lower left and mid-left sternal borders. Therefore, in a child who has physical and radiographic findings similar to those of a small VSD, the presence of RVH or BVH on the ECG should raise the possibility of acyanotic TOF. (A small VSD is associated with LVH or a normal ECG rather than with RVH or BVH.) Right aortic arch, if present,

confirms the diagnosis. Infants with acyanotic TOF become cyanotic over time, usually by 1 or 2 years of age, and have clinical pictures of cyanotic TOF, including exertional dyspnea and squatting.

In infants with classic *cyanotic TOF*, the presence of severe PS produces a right-to-left shunt at the ventricular level (i.e., cyanosis) with decreased PBF (see Fig. 11.7B). The PAs are small, and the LA and LV may be slightly smaller than normal because of a reduction in the pulmonary venous return to the left side of the heart. Therefore, chest radiograph films show a normal heart size with decreased pulmonary vascularity. The systolic pressures are identical in the RV, LV, and aorta. The ECG demonstrates RVH because of the high pressure in the RV. The right-to-left ventricular shunt is silent, and the heart murmur audible in this condition originates in the PS (ejection-type murmur). The ejection systolic murmur is best audible at the mid-left sternal border (over the infundibular stenosis) or occasionally at the upper left sternal border (in patients with pulmonary valve stenosis). The intensity and the duration of the heart murmur are proportional to the amount of blood flow through the stenotic valve. When the PS is mild, a relatively large amount of blood goes through the stenotic valve (with a relatively small right-to-left ventricular shunt), thereby producing a loud, long systolic murmur (Fig. 11.8A). However,

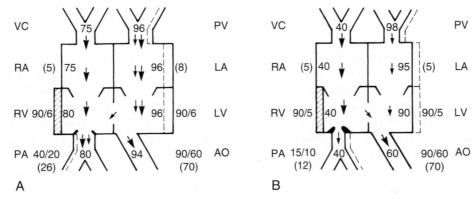

Fig. 11.7 Hemodynamics of acyanotic (**A**) and cyanotic (**B**) tetralogy of Fallot. Numbers within the diagram denote oxygen saturation values, and those outside the diagram denote pressure values. In both conditions, the systolic pressure in the right ventricle (RV) is identical to that in the left ventricle (LV) and the aorta (AO), and there is a significant pressure gradient between the RV and the pulmonary artery (PA). Whereas in the acyanotic form pulmonary blood flow is slightly to moderately increased, in the cyanotic form, pulmonary blood flow is decreased. Other abbreviations are the same as those in Fig. 11.4.

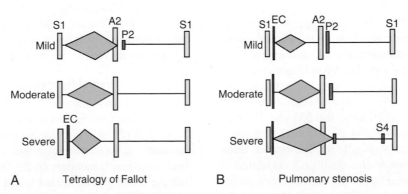

Fig. 11.8 Comparison of ejection systolic murmurs in tetralogy of Fallot (**A**) and isolated pulmonary valve stenosis (**B**) (see text). *EC,* Ejection click.

with severe PS, there is a relatively large right-to-left ventricular shunt that is silent, and only a small amount of blood goes through the PS, thereby producing a short, faint systolic murmur (see Fig. 11.8A). In other words, the intensity and duration of the systolic murmur are inversely related to the severity of the PS. These findings are in contrast to those seen in isolated PS (see Fig. 11.8A and B). Because of low pressure in the PA, the P2 is soft and often inaudible, resulting in a single S2. The heart size on chest radiograph films is normal in TOF because none of the heart chambers handle an increased amount of blood. If a cyanotic infant has a large heart on the chest radiograph films, especially with an increase in pulmonary vascularity, TOF is extremely unlikely unless the child has undergone a large systemic-to-PA shunt operation. Another important point is that an infant with TOF does not develop CHF. This is because no cardiac chamber is under volume overload, and the pressure overload placed on the RV (not higher than the aortic pressure, which is under baroreceptor control) is well tolerated.

The extreme form of TOF is that associated with *pulmonary atresia*, in which the only source of PBF is through a constricting PDA or through multiple collateral arteries (MAPCAs). All systemic venous return is shunted right to left at the ventricular level, resulting in a marked systemic arterial desaturation. Probably the more important reason for such severe cyanosis is the markedly reduced PBF, with resulting reduction of pulmonary venous return to the left side of the heart. Unless the patency of the ductus is maintained, the infant may die. Infusion of prostaglandin E₁ has been successful for a limited time period in keeping the ductus open in this and other forms of cyanotic CHDs that rely on the patency of the ductus arteriosus for PBF. Heart murmur is absent, or a faint murmur of PDA is present. RVH is present on the ECG as in other forms of TOF. Chest radiographs show a small heart and a markedly reduced PBF, as well as absence of main pulmonary trunk (boot-shaped heart).

Hypoxic Spell

Hypoxic spell is an urgent clinical situation that can occur in infants with uncorrected TOF or some other forms of cyanotic CHDs. To handle the situation correctly, physicians should have full understanding of mechanism of the spell, clinical manifestation, and correct management of the situation.

Mechanism of Hypoxic Spell

A sudden increase in right-to-left shunt appears to be the prime event of hypoxic spell, considering the clinical manifestation of the spell. The question is what causes the sudden increase in the right-to-left shunt? Is it a RVOT spasm, as proposed previously by some investigators, or something else?

Because the VSD of TOF is large enough to equalize systolic pressures in both ventricles, the RV and LV may be viewed as a single chamber that ejects blood to the systemic and pulmonary circuits (Fig. 11.9). The ratio of flows to the pulmonary and systemic circuits (Q_p/Q_s) is related to the ratio of resistance offered by the RV outflow obstruction (shown as pulmonary resistance [PR] in Fig. 11.9) and the systemic vascular resistance (SVR). Either an increase in the

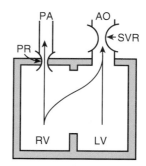

Fig. 11.9 Simplified concept of tetralogy of Fallot that demonstrates how a change in the systemic vascular resistance (SVR) or right ventricular outflow tract obstruction (pulmonary resistance [PR]) affects the direction and the magnitude of the ventricular shunt. *AO,* Aorta; *LV,* left ventricle; *PA,* pulmonary artery; *RV,* right ventricle.

pulmonary resistance or a decrease in the SVR will increase the degree of the right-to-left shunt, producing a more severe arterial desaturation.

Although controversies exist over the role of the spasm of the RVOT as an initiating event for the hypoxic spell, there is no evidence that the spasm actually occurs as a primary event. Pulmonary valve stenosis has a fixed resistance and does not produce spasm. The infundibular stenosis, which consists of disorganized muscle fibers intermingled with fibrous tissue, is almost nonreactive to sympathetic stimulation or catecholamines. Hypoxic spell also occurs in patients with TOF with pulmonary atresia in which the presence or absence of spasm would have no role in the spell. Therefore, the likelihood of the RVOT spasm initiating the right-to-left shunt is remote.

It is more likely that changes in the SVR play a primary role in controlling the degree of the right-to-left shunt and the amount of PBF. A decrease in the SVR increases the right-to-left shunt and decreases the PBF with a resulting increase in cyanosis. In this case, the RVOT dimension may decrease, but it is likely secondary to the decreased amount of blood flowing through it rather than primary spasm. Conversely, an increase in SVR decreases the right-to-left shunt and forces more blood through the stenotic RVOT. In addition to decreased SVR, other causes, such as excessive tachycardia or hypovolemia, can increase the right-to-left shunt through the VSD, resulting in a fall in the systemic arterial oxygen saturation. Tachycardia or hypovolemia may narrow down the RVOT, as a secondary effect. Slowing of the heart rate by β-adrenergic blockers, volume expansion, or interventions that increase the SVR or decrease the PVR (i.e., oxygen) have all been used to terminate the hypoxic spell.

Clinical Features of Hypoxic Spell

The *hypoxic spell,* also called the *cyanotic spell, tet spell,* or *hypercyanotic spell,* occurs in young infants with uncorrected TOF. It is characterized by hyperpnea (i.e., rapid and deep respiration), worsening cyanosis, and disappearance of the heart murmur (secondary to the increased right-to-left ventricular shunt and decreased blood flow through the stenotic RVOT). This occasionally results in complications of the central nervous system and even death. Any event such as crying,

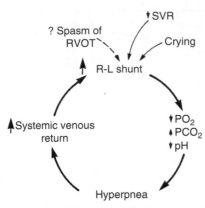

Fig. 11.10 Mechanism of hypoxic spell. A decrease in the arterial Po2 stimulates the respiratory center, and hyperventilation results. Hyperpnea increases systemic venous return. In the presence of a fixed right ventricular outflow tract (RVOT), the increased systemic venous return results in increased right-to-left (R-L) shunt, worsening cyanosis. A vicious circle is established. *SVR*, Systemic vascular resistance.

defecation, or increased physical activity that suddenly lowers the SVR or produces a large right-to-left ventricular shunt may initiate the spell and, if not corrected, establishes a vicious circle of hypoxic spells (as illustrated in Fig. 11.10). The sudden onset of tachycardia or hypovolemia can also cause the spell as discussed earlier. The resulting fall in arterial Po_2, in addition to an increase in Pco_2 and a fall in pH, stimulates the respiratory center and produces hyperpnea. The hyperpnea, in turn, makes the negative thoracic pump more efficient and results in an increase in the systemic venous return to the RV. In the presence of fixed resistance at the RVOT (i.e., pulmonary resistance [PR]) or decreased SVR, the increased systemic venous return to the RV must go out the aorta. This leads to a further decrease in the arterial oxygen saturation, which establishes a vicious circle of hypoxic spells (see Fig. 11.10).

Treatment of Hypoxic Spells

Treatment of the spell is aimed at breaking this cycle by using one or more of the following maneuvers:

1. Picking up the infant in such a way that it assumes the knee–chest position and traps systemic venous blood in the legs, thereby temporarily decreasing systemic venous return and helping to calm the baby. The knee–chest position may also increase SVR by reducing arterial blood flow to the lower extremities.
2. Morphine sulfate suppresses the respiratory center and abolishes hyperpnea.
3. Sodium bicarbonate ($NaHCO_3$) corrects acidosis and eliminates the respiratory center–stimulating effect of acidosis.
4. Administration of oxygen may improve arterial oxygen saturation a little.
5. Vasoconstrictors such as phenylephrine raise SVR and improve arterial oxygen saturation.
6. Ketamine is a good drug to use because it simultaneously increases SVR and sedates the patient. Both effects are known to help terminate the spell.

7. Propranolol has been used successfully in some cases of hypoxic spell, both acute and chronic. Its mechanism of action is not entirely clear. When administered for acute cases, propranolol may slow the heart rate and perhaps reduce the spasm of the RVOT (although not likely as discussed earlier). More important, propranolol may also increase SVR by antagonizing vasodilating effects of β-adrenergic stimulation. The successful use of propranolol in the prevention of hypoxic spell is more likely the result of the drug's peripheral action. The drug may stabilize vascular reactivity of the systemic arteries, thereby preventing a sudden decrease in SVR (see Chapter 14).

Squatting

Infants and toddlers with uncorrected TOF often assume a squatting position after playing hard. During the play, these children become tachypneic and dusky. When they assume a squatting position and rest a little while, these symptoms disappear and then they resume playing. What is the mechanism of recovery from these symptoms during squatting? Squatting position is the same as knee–chest position (which is used to treat hypoxic spells in infants). Squatting or knee chest position increases systemic arterial oxygen saturation as shown in an experimental study (Fig. 11.11). Three mechanisms may be involved. First, reduction of the systemic venous return by trapping venous blood in the lower extremities reduces right-to-left shunt at the ventricular level (evidenced by reduced arterial lactate levels in Fig. 11.11). Second, a reduced arterial blood flow to legs reduces venous washout from leg muscles. Third, squatting might also increase SVR, a known mechanism to reduce right-to-left ventricular shunt.

Tricuspid Atresia

In tricuspid atresia, the tricuspid valve and a portion of the RV do not exist (Fig. 11.12). Because no direct communication exists between the RA and RV, systemic venous return to the RA must be shunted first to the LA through an ASD or PFO. There is usually a VSD (or PDA) for the pulmonary arteries to receive some blood for survival. The great arteries are normally related in about 70% of cases and transposed in about 30% of cases (see Fig. 11.12). In patients with normally related great arteries (see Fig. 11.12A), the VSD is usually small, and the RV and PAs are hypoplastic. In infants with transposed great arteries (see Fig. 11.12B), the VSD and the PAs are usually larger than those seen in patients with normally related great arteries.

For the right-to-left shunt to occur, the RA pressure is elevated in excess of the LA pressure, and enlargement of the RA results (i.e., right atrial hypertrophy [RAH] on the ECG and right atrial enlargement on chest radiographs). The LA and LV receive both systemic and pulmonary venous returns and thereby dilate (i.e., enlargement of the LA and LV on chest radiographs). The volume overload placed on the LV is unopposed by the hypoplastic RV, with resulting LVH on the ECG. Therefore, the ECG shows RAH and LVH, and the chest radiographs show an enlargement of the RA, LA, and LV. In addition, a "superior" QRS axis is a characteristic ECG

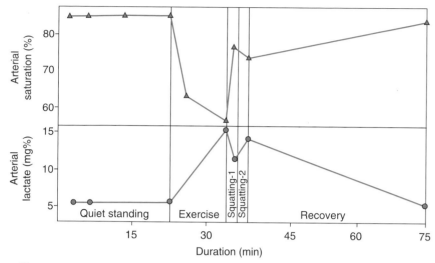

Fig. 11.11 Hemodynamic changes with squatting. An adult patient with tetralogy of Fallot was studied during cardiac catheterization with determinations of arterial oxygen saturation and arterial lactate levels. The latter was used as an indicator of the change in the systemic venous return. With exercise, there is an immediate drop in the arterial saturation and an increase in systemic venous return. With squatting (a knee–chest position), there is an immediate rise in arterial oxygen saturation and a drop in systemic venous return. (From Guntheroth WG, Mortan BC, Mullins GL, Baum D: Venous return with knee-chest position and squatting in tetralogy of Fallot, *Am Heart J* 75:313–318, 1968.)

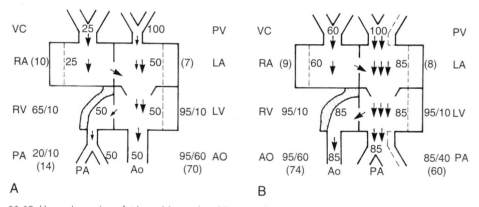

Fig. 11.12 Hemodynamics of tricuspid atresia with normally related (**A**) and transposed (**B**) great arteries. Numbers within the diagram denote oxygen saturations, and those outside the diagram denote pressure values. Abbreviations are the same as those in Fig. 11.4.

finding in tricuspid atresia, as in endocardial cushion defect. Embryologically, there is a similarity between these two defects; tricuspid atresia results from an abnormal development of the endocardial cushion tissue, that is, an incomplete shift of the common AV canal to the right. Developmental abnormalities in the endocardial cushion tissue may explain the similar QRS axis in both conditions.

Oxygen saturation values are equal in the aorta and the PA because there is a complete mixing of systemic and pulmonary venous blood in the LV, from which both the systemic and the pulmonary circulations receive blood. The magnitude of PBF is directly related to the level of arterial oxygen saturation and the overall heart size. In patients with normally related great arteries (see Fig. 11.12A), the PBF is generally reduced (because of a small VSD, hypoplastic RV, or small PAs), and thus, the heart size is small, arterial oxygen saturation is low, and the infant is notably cyanotic. In infants with transposed great arteries (see Fig. 11.12B), the PBF is usually increased. Therefore, these

infants are only mildly cyanotic; their heart size is large, and their pulmonary vascular markings are increased. However, because of an interplay of other factors such as the size of the VSD, the presence or absence of PS or pulmonary atresia, and the patency of the ductus arteriosus, some infants with normally related great arteries may have increased PBF, and some infants with TGA may have decreased PBF.

No physical findings are characteristic of tricuspid atresia. These infants have varying degrees of cyanosis, most have a heart murmur of VSD, and some have a murmur of PS. In patients with increased PBF, an increased amount of blood passing through the mitral valve may produce an apical diastolic rumble. The liver may be enlarged because of increased pressure in the RA, which may result from an inadequate interatrial communication or heart failure.

In summary, tricuspid atresia is the most likely diagnosis if a cyanotic infant has an ECG that shows a "superior" QRS axis, RAH, and LVH and chest radiographic films that show

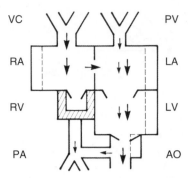

Fig. 11.13 Hemodynamics of pulmonary atresia. The chambers that enlarge are similar to those in tricuspid atresia; therefore, chest radiographic findings are similar in tricuspid atresia and pulmonary atresia. The electrocardiogram also shows left ventricular hypertrophy but without the characteristic "superior" QRS axis of tricuspid atresia. Because of the decreased pulmonary blood flow, the aortic saturation is low, and the infant is notably cyanotic. Abbreviations are the same as those in Fig. 11.4.

enlargement of the RA (with or without left atrial enlargement), a concave PA segment, and decreased pulmonary vascularity.

Pulmonary Atresia

In pulmonary atresia, direct communication between the RV cavity and the PA does not exist; the PDA (or collateral arteries) is the major source of blood flow to the lungs. The RV is usually hypoplastic, and the PAs are also small. The LA and LV are relatively large because they receive both systemic and pulmonary venous returns. The RA dilates and hypertrophies to empty systemic venous return to the LA. The RA enlarges and hypertrophies to maintain a right-to-left atrial shunt (resulting in right atrial enlargement on radiographic films and RAH on the ECG). The RV is usually hypoplastic with a thick ventricular wall, but occasionally, the RV is normal in size; tricuspid regurgitation (TR) is usually present in the latter situation. Systemic and pulmonary venous returns mix in the LA and go to the LV to supply the body and the lungs (Fig. 11.13). The volume load placed on the left side of the heart (i.e., LA and LV) is proportionally related to the magnitude of PBF. Because the PDA is the major source of PBF and it may close after birth, the PBF is usually decreased. When multiple collateral arteries are the only source of pulmonary blood flow, they are usually not adequate and PBF is reduced. Therefore, the infant is severely cyanotic, and the overall heart size is normal or only slightly increased. The hypoplasia of the RV and possible volume overload to the LV produce LVH on the ECG.

The infant is usually notably cyanotic. The S2 is single because there is only one semilunar valve to close. A faint, continuous murmur of PDA may be present. A severely cyanotic newborn with decreased pulmonary vascularity and normal or slightly enlarged heart size on chest radiographic films and RAH or biatrial hypertrophy and LVH on the ECG may have pulmonary atresia. These findings are similar to those seen in infants with tricuspid atresia. However, the QRS axis is usually normal in pulmonary atresia, in contrast to the "superior" QRS axis seen in tricuspid atresia.

Closure of the ductus results in a rapid deterioration of the infant's condition unless there are enough collateral arteries supplying PBF. Reopening or maintaining the patency of the ductus arteriosus with infusion of prostaglandin E_1 increases the PBF, improves cyanosis, and stabilizes the infant's condition.

Total Anomalous Pulmonary Venous Return

In total anomalous pulmonary venous return (TAPVR), the pulmonary veins drain abnormally to the RA, either directly or indirectly through its venous tributaries. An ASD is usually present to send blood from the RA to the LA and LV. Depending on the drainage site, TAPVR may be divided into the following three types (see Fig. 14.30):
1. Supracardiac: The common pulmonary vein drains to the superior vena cava through the vertical vein and the left innominate vein.
2. Cardiac: The pulmonary veins empty into the RA directly or indirectly through the coronary sinus.
3. Infracardiac (or subdiaphragmatic): The common pulmonary vein traverses the diaphragm and drains into the portal or hepatic vein or the inferior vena cava.

Physiologically, however, TAPVR may be divided into two types, obstructive and nonobstructive, depending on the presence or absence of an obstruction to the pulmonary venous return. The infracardiac type is usually obstructive, and the majority of the cardiac and supracardiac types are nonobstructive.

The hemodynamics of the nonobstructive types of TAPVR are similar to those of a large ASD. The amount of blood that goes to the LA through the ASD is determined by the size of the interatrial communication and the relative compliance of the ventricles. Because right ventricular compliance normally increases after birth, with a rapid fall in PVR, and the ASD may be inadequate in size, more blood enters the RV than the LA. Thus, volume overload of the right side of the heart and the pulmonary circulation results, with enlargement of the RA, RV, PA, and pulmonary veins (Fig. 11.14A). Chest radiographs show this as an enlargement of the RA and RV, a prominent PA segment, and increased pulmonary vascular markings. The pressures in the RA, RV, and PA are slightly elevated. The ECG shows right bundle branch block or RVH, as in secundum ASD, and occasional RAH. Because there is complete mixing of systemic and pulmonary venous blood in the RA, oxygen saturation values are almost identical in the aorta and the PA.

Cardiac examination reveals an ejection systolic murmur of PS (at the upper left sternal border) and a diastolic murmur of tricuspid stenosis because the pulmonary and tricuspid valves handle three arrows (see Fig. 11.14A). The S2 splits widely for the same reasons as it does for ASD. This contributes to the characteristic "quadruple" rhythm of TAPVR, which consists of an S1, a widely split S2, and an S3 or S4. Children with large PBF are only minimally desaturated, and cyanosis is often missed because the arterial oxygen saturation ranges from 85% to 90% (see Fig. 11.14A).

If there is an obstruction to the pulmonary venous return, the hemodynamic consequences are notably different from

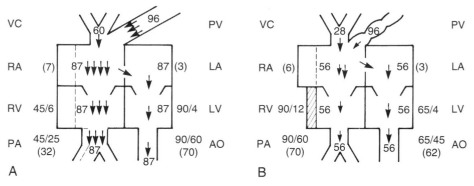

Fig. 11.14 Hemodynamics of total anomalous pulmonary venous return without (**A**) and with (**B**) obstruction to the pulmonary venous return. In the nonobstructive type, the hemodynamics are similar to those of a large atrial septal defect, with the exception of a mild systemic arterial desaturation. In the obstructive type, the hemodynamics are characterized by pulmonary venous hypertension, pulmonary edema, pulmonary arterial hypertension, and marked arterial desaturation. The heart size is not enlarged on chest radiographs. Severe right ventricular hypertrophy is present on the electrocardiogram. Abbreviations are the same as those in Fig. 11.4.

those without pulmonary venous obstruction. The obstruction to the pulmonary venous return causes pulmonary venous hypertension and secondary PA and RV hypertension (see Fig. 11.14B), a situation similar to that seen in mitral stenosis (see Fig. 10.4). Pulmonary edema results when the hydrostatic pressure in the capillaries exceeds the osmotic pressure of the blood. As long as a large ASD permits a right-to-left shunt, the RV cavity remains relatively small (i.e., smaller than one arrow). This is because the RV hypertension prevents the RV compliance from increasing, and the PVR remains elevated. Therefore, chest radiographs show a relatively small heart and characteristic patterns of pulmonary venous congestion or pulmonary edema (i.e., "ground-glass" appearance). The ECG reflects the high pressure in the RV (i.e., RVH). The oxygen saturation values are equal in the aorta and the PA because of the complete mixing of systemic and pulmonary venous return at the RA level, and the arterial saturation is much lower than that found in patients without obstruction. The degree of arterial desaturation or cyanosis inversely relates to the amount of PBF. Infants with obstruction have severe cyanosis and respiratory distress. The latter results from pulmonary edema and may cause pulmonary crackles on auscultation. The pulmonary valve closure sound (P2) is loud because of pulmonary hypertension, which results in a single, loud S2. The heart murmur may be absent or soft because of normal or decreased flow through the pulmonary or tricuspid valve (i.e., smaller than one arrow) (see Fig. 11.14B).

Full comprehension of the relationship between the magnitude of PBF and the systemic arterial oxygen saturation helps in understanding and managing most cyanotic CHDs. The two extreme examples of TAPVR shown in Fig. 11.14 discuss this relationship.

If the PBF is three times as great as the systemic blood flow (i.e., Q_p/Q_s ratio = 3:1), as in most nonobstructive cases (see Fig. 11.14A), the arterial oxygen saturation is close to 90%, and cyanosis does not become obvious. This figure is derived as follows. An assumed pulmonary vein saturation of 96% and a vena caval saturation of 60% result in an average mixed venous saturation of 87%. Of course, the aortic saturation will be 87% in this case (see Fig. 11.14A).

$$[(96 \times 3) + (60 \times 1)] / 4 = 87\ (\%)$$

The difference in the arterial and venous oxygen saturation is kept at 27% to indicate the absence of heart failure (see Fig. 11.14A).

If an obstruction to the pulmonary venous return exists and the PBF is small, a marked arterial desaturation results, based on the following calculation. It assumed that the PBF is 70% of the systemic flow (i.e., Q_p/Q_s ratio = 0.7:1), the pulmonary vein saturation is 96%, and the SVC saturation is 28% (see Fig. 11.14B). The RA saturation (and thus the aortic saturation) will be 56%.

$$[(96 \times 0.7) + (28 \times 1)] / 1.7 = 56\ (\%)$$

It is also assumed that the infant is not experiencing heart failure (i.e., the systemic AV difference is 28%) (see Fig. 11.14B).

This relationship holds true for other forms of cyanotic CHDs. For a given defect, an *increase* in the magnitude of PBF results in a rise in the systemic arterial oxygen saturation; a *decrease* in PBF results in a decrease in the arterial oxygen saturation. An improvement in cyanosis after a systemic-to-PA shunt operation in a cyanotic infant with decreased PBF is an example of this relationship. Conversely, infants with a single ventricle may be in CHF from a large PBF but not be cyanotic. CHF improves after a PA banding operation (which decreases PBF and lowers PA pressure), but the arterial oxygen saturation usually decreases, and cyanosis may appear.

PART 4

Specific Congenital Heart Defects

The next three chapters discuss common left-to-right shunt lesions, obstructive lesions, and cyanotic cardiac defects. Other chapters in this part discuss aortic arch anomalies, primarily "vascular ring" and cardiac malposition. Miscellaneous, rare anomalies that do not belong to these categories are briefly discussed in another chapter. These chapters are intended to be used as a quick reference; therefore, descriptions are brief.

Left-to-Right Shunt Lesions

This chapter discusses common left-to-right shunt lesions such as atrial septal defect (ASD), ventricular septal defect (VSD), patent ductus arteriosus (PDA), endocardial cushion defect (ECD), and partial anomalous pulmonary venous return (PAPVR).

ATRIAL SEPTAL DEFECT

Prevalence

Atrial septal defect (ostium secundum defect) occurs as an isolated anomaly in 3% to 10% of all congenital heart defects (CHDs). It is more common in females than in males (male-to-female ratio of 1:2). About 30% to 50% of children with CHDs have an ASD as part of the cardiac defect.

Pathology

1. Three major types of ASDs exist: secundum defect, primum defect, and sinus venosus defect. Coronary sinus ASD is extremely rare. Patent foramen ovale (PFO) does not ordinarily produce intracardiac shunts (see Chapter 15).

2. Ostium secundum defect is the most common type of ASD, accounting for 50% to 70% of all ASDs. This defect is present at the site of fossa ovalis, allowing left-to-right shunting of blood from the left atrium (LA) to the right atrium (RA) (Fig. 12.1). Anomalous pulmonary venous return is present in about 10% of cases.

3. Ostium primum defects occur in about 30% of all ASDs if those that occur as part of complete ECD are included (see Fig. 12.1). Isolated ostium primum ASD occurs in about 15% of all ASDs. This is discussed in greater detail in the section on partial ECD.

4. Sinus venosus defect occurs in about 10% of all ASDs. The defect is most commonly located at the entry of the superior vena cava (SVC) into the RA (superior vena caval type) and rarely at the entry of the inferior vena cava (IVC) into the RA (inferior vena caval type). The former is commonly associated with anomalous drainage of the right upper pulmonary vein (into the RA), and the latter is often associated with anomalous drainage of the right lung into the IVC ("scimitar syndrome") (see Chapter 15).

5. Coronary sinus ASD is an extremely rare type in which a defect is present in the roof of the coronary sinus. The LA blood shunts through the defect and empties into the RA through the coronary sinus orifice, producing clinical pictures similar to other types of ASD.

6. Mitral valve prolapse (MVP) occurs in 20% of patients with either ostium secundum or sinus venosus defects.

Clinical Manifestations

History

Infants and children with ASDs are usually asymptomatic.

Physical Examination (Fig. 12.2)

1. A relatively slender body build is typical. (The body weight of many is less than the 10th percentile.)

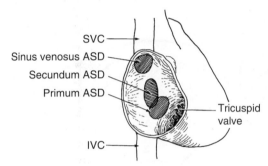

Fig. 12.1 Anatomic types of atrial septal defects (ASDs) viewed with the right atrial wall removed. *IVC,* Inferior vena cava; *SVC,* superior vena cava.

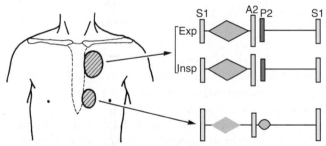

Fig. 12.2 Cardiac findings of atrial septal defect. Throughout this book, heart murmurs with solid borders are the primary murmurs, and those without solid borders are transmitted murmurs or those occurring occasionally. Abnormalities in heart sounds are shown in *black. Exp,* Expiration; *Insp,* inspiration.

2. A widely split and fixed S2 and a grade 2 to 3 of 6 systolic ejection murmur are characteristic findings of ASD in older infants and children. With a large left-to-right shunt, a mid-diastolic rumble resulting from relative tricuspid stenosis may be audible at the lower left sternal border.

3. Classic auscultatory findings (and electrocardiographic [ECG] and radiography findings) of ASD are not present unless the shunt is reasonably large (Q_p/Q_s ratio ≥1.5). The typical auscultatory findings may be absent in infants and toddlers even in those with a large defect because the RV is poorly compliant.

Electrocardiography (Fig. 12.3)

Right axis deviation of +90 to +180 degrees and mild right ventricular hypertrophy (RVH) or right bundle branch block (RBBB) with an rsR′ pattern in V1 are typical ECG findings. In about 50% of patients with sinus venosus ASD, the P axis is less than +30 degrees.

Radiographic Studies (Fig. 12.4)

1. Cardiomegaly with enlargement of the RA and right ventricle (RV) may be present.

2. A prominent pulmonary artery (PA) segment and increased pulmonary vascular markings are seen when the shunt is significant.

Echocardiography

1. A two-dimensional (2D) echocardiographic study is diagnostic. The study shows the position as well as the size of the defect, which can best be seen in the subcostal four-chamber view (Fig. 12.5). In secundum ASD, a dropout can be seen in the midatrial septum. The primum type shows a defect in the lower atrial septum; the SVC type of sinus venosus defect shows a defect in the posterosuperior atrial septum.

2. Indirect signs of a significant left-to-right atrial shunt include RV enlargement and RA enlargement, as well as dilated PA, which often accompanies an increased flow velocity across the pulmonary valve. These findings indicate the functional significance of the defect.

3. Pulsed Doppler examination reveals a characteristic flow pattern with the maximum left-to-right shunt occurring in diastole. Color-flow mapping enhances the evaluation of the hemodynamic status of the ASD.

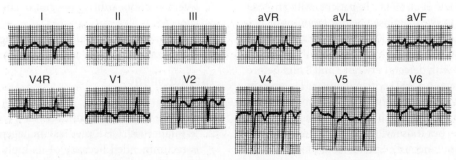

Fig. 12.3 Tracing from a 5-year-old girl with secundum-type atrial septal defect.

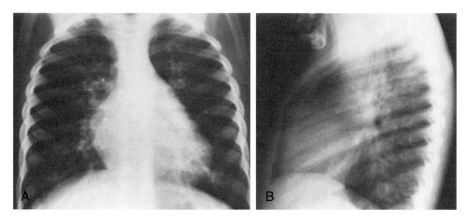

Fig. 12.4 Posteroanterior (**A**) and lateral (**B**) views of chest radiographs from a 10-year-old child with atrial septal defect. The heart is mildly enlarged with involvement of the right atrium (best seen in the posteroanterior view) and the right ventricle (best seen in the lateral view with obliteration of the retrosternal space). Pulmonary vascularity is increased, and the main pulmonary artery segment is slightly prominent.

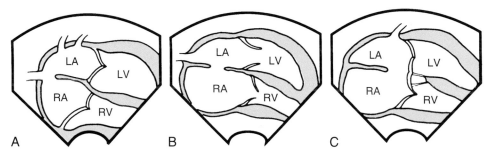

Fig. 12.5 Diagram of two-dimensional echocardiography of the three types of atrial septal defects (ASDs). The subcostal transducer position provides the most diagnostic view. **A,** Sinus venosus defect. The defect is located in the posterosuperior atrial septum, usually just beneath the orifice of the superior vena cava. This defect is often associated with partial anomalous return of the right upper pulmonary vein. **B,** Secundum ASD. The defect is located in the middle portion of the atrial septum. **C,** Primum ASD. The defect is located in the anteroinferior atrial septum, just over the inflow portion of each atrioventricular valve. *LA,* Left atrium; *LV,* left ventricle; *RA,* right atrium; *RV,* right ventricle.

4. M-mode echocardiography may show increased RV dimension and paradoxical motion of the interventricular septum, which are signs of RV volume overload.
5. In older children and adolescents, especially in those who are overweight, adequate imaging of the atrial septum may not be possible with the ordinary transthoracic echocardiographic study. Transesophageal echocardiography (TEE) may be used as an alternative.

Natural History

1. A recent report indicates the overall rate of spontaneous closure to be 87% (Radzic et al, 1993). In patients with an ASD smaller than 3 mm in size diagnosed before 3 months of age, spontaneous closure occurs in 100% of patients at 1 and 1/2 years of age. Spontaneous closure occurs more than 80% of the time in patients with defects between 3 and 8 mm before 1 and 1/2 years of age. An ASD with a diameter larger than 8 mm rarely closes spontaneously. In general, most defects smaller than 5 mm recognized during infancy are likely to spontaneously close, but those with a diameter larger than 8 mm rarely close spontaneously. Spontaneous closure is not likely to occur after 4 years of age.

2. Most children with an ASD remain active and asymptomatic. Rarely, congestive heart failure (CHF) can develop in infancy.
3. If a large defect is untreated, CHF and pulmonary hypertension begin to develop in adults who are in their 20s and 30s, and it becomes common after 40 years of age.
4. With or without surgery, atrial arrhythmias (flutter or fibrillation) may occur in adults. The incidence of atrial arrhythmias increases to as high as 13% in patients older than 40 years of age.
5. Infective endocarditis does not occur in patients with isolated ASDs.
6. Cerebrovascular accident, resulting from paradoxical embolization through an ASD, is a rare complication.

Management
Medical

1. Exercise restriction is unnecessary.
2. In infants with CHF, medical management (with a diuretic) is recommended because of its high success rate and the possibility of spontaneous closure of the defect.

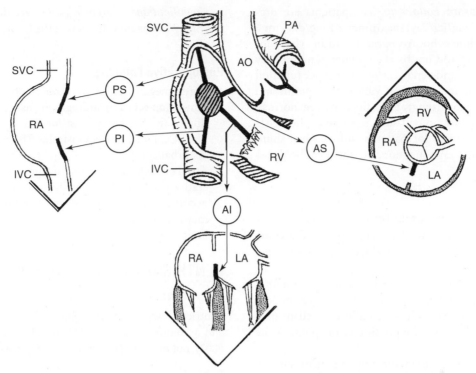

Fig. 12.6 Two-dimensional echocardiographic estimates of the atrial septal defect rim size. The posterosuperior (PS) and posteroinferior (PI) rims are estimated in the bi–vena cava view from the subcostal transducer position, the anteroinferior (AI) rim from the apical four-chamber view, and the anterosuperior (AS) (or retroaortic) rim from the parasternal short-axis view.

Nonsurgical Closure

Nonsurgical closure using a catheter-delivered closure device has become a preferred method, provided the indications are met. Two popular devices used for ASD closure in the United States are the Amplatzer Septal Occluder (AGA Medical) and Gore Cardioform Septal Occluder (WL Gore and Associates). Currently, there are no transcatheter devices designed for closure of sinus venosus, primum, or coronary sinus ASDs.

The use of the closure device may be indicated to close a secundum ASD measuring 5 mm or more in diameter and a hemodynamically significant left-to-right shunt with clinical evidence of RV volume overload (i.e., Q_p/Q_s ratio $\geq 1.5:1$ or greater or RV enlargement). There must be enough rim of septal tissue around the defect for appropriate placement of the device, although some newer devices no longer require a septal rim present along the entire margin of the defect. The size of the rim around the ASD can be estimated by 2D echocardiographic study as diagrammatically shown in Fig. 12.6. The rim size is estimated in four directions: anterosuperior, anteroinferior, posterosuperior, and posteroinferior (Magni et al, 1997).

The timing of the device closure for secundum ASD is not entirely clear. Considering the possibility of spontaneous closure, it is wise not to use the device in infancy unless the patient is symptomatic with heart failure. ASD closure devices can be implanted successfully in children younger than 2 years of age, although common practice suggests that a weight greater than 15 kg may offer some technical advantages and simplify the procedure (Feltes et al, 2011). Closure rates are excellent with small residual shunts seen in fewer than 5% of patients at 1 year of follow-up.

Complications are extremely rare. The overall risk of the procedure is 7.2% with the major complication rate of 1.6%, including device embolism with surgical removal. Other reported complications may include the following.

1. Early ECG abnormalities are common within the first 24 hours after implant, but most of these resolve quickly.
2. Probably the most feared complication with the Amplatzer device (but not with the Helex device) is early or late erosion of the device into the aortic root, with subsequent pericardial tamponade and rare death. It may be related to the oversizing of devices and deficiency of the anterosuperior (or retroaortic) rim (see Fig. 12.6).
3. Rarely, thrombus formation in the right and left atrium occurs (2%–3%), but cerebral embolism is not more frequent than after surgical closure of the defect.
4. Release of nickel from the device (with peak at 1 month after implant) is a rare cause of significant allergic reaction.
5. Transient new onset headache is a rare complaint of the patients.

Advantages of nonsurgical closure include a complete avoidance of cardiopulmonary bypass with its attendant risk, avoidance of pain and residual sternotomy scars, a less than 24-hour hospital stay, and rapid recovery. All of these devices are associated with a higher rate of small residual leak than is operative closure.

Post–Device Closure Follow-up. The patients are prescribed aspirin (3–5 mg/kg/day; maximum, 81 mg/day) for 6 months. Postprocedure echocardiographic studies check for a residual atrial shunt and unobstructed flow of pulmonary veins, coronary sinus, and venae cavae and proper function of the aortic, mitral, and tricuspid valves. If 1-month and 1-year follow-up echocardiographic findings are normal, yearly or biennial follow-up will suffice. Some cardiologists prescribe 81 mg of aspirin for patients with residual shunt to prevent paradoxical embolization, but most cardiologists do not.

Surgical Closure

Indications and Timing. Surgical closure is indicated only when device closure is not considered appropriate. Therefore, most patients with secundum ASD are not candidates for surgical closure of the defect.

1. A left-to-right shunt with a pulmonary-to-systemic blood flow ratio (Q_p/Q_s ratio) of 1.5:1 or greater is a surgical indication. Surgery is usually delayed until 2 to 4 years of age because the possibility of spontaneous closure exists.
2. If CHF does not respond to medical management, surgery is performed during infancy, again if device closure is considered inappropriate.
3. High pulmonary vascular resistance (PVR) (i.e., >10 units/m2, >7 units/m2 with vasodilators) may be a contraindication for surgery (or device closure).

Procedure. For secundum ASD, the defect is traditionally repaired through a midsternal incision under cardiopulmonary bypass by either a simple suture or a pericardial or Teflon patch. Recently, so-called minimally invasive cardiac surgical techniques with smaller skin incisions have become popular, especially for female patients. For ASDs (including simple primum ASDs and sinus venosus defects), one of the following techniques can be used: midline short transxiphoid incision with minimal sternal split (preferred), transverse inframammary incision with vertical or transverse sternotomy, or small lower midline skin incision with either partial or full median sternotomy. The benefit of this technique appears to be an improved cosmetic result; it does not reduce pain, hospital stay, or surgical stress.

For a sinus venosus defect without associated anomalous pulmonary venous return, the defect is closed using an autologous pericardial patch. When it is associated with pulmonary venous anomaly, a tunnel is created between the anomalous pulmonary vein and the ASD by using a Teflon or pericardial patch. A plastic or pericardial gusset is placed in the SVC to prevent obstruction to the SVC. For coronary sinus ASD, the ostium of the coronary sinus is closed with an autologous pericardium with care to avoid conduction tissues, provided it is not associated with persistent left SVC. This will result in drainage of coronary sinus blood into the left atrium.

Mortality. Fewer than 0.5% of patients die; however, there is a greater risk for small infants and those with increased PVR.

Complications. Cerebrovascular accident and postoperative arrhythmias may develop in the immediate postoperative period.

Postoperative Follow-up

1. Cardiomegaly on chest radiographs and enlarged RV dimension on echocardiography as well as the wide splitting of the S2 may persist for 1 or 2 years after surgery. The ECG typically demonstrates RBBB (or RV conduction disturbance).
2. Atrial or nodal arrhythmias occur in 7% to 20% of postoperative patients. Occasionally, sick sinus syndrome, which occurs especially after the repair of a sinus venosus defect, may require antiarrhythmic drugs, pacemaker therapy, or both.

VENTRICULAR SEPTAL DEFECT

Prevalence

Ventricular septal defect is the most common form of CHD and accounts for 17% to 37% of all such defects (Hoffman, 2002), not including those occurring as part of cyanotic CHDs.

Pathology

1. The ventricular septum may be divided into a small membranous portion and a large muscular portion (Fig. 12.7A). The muscular septum has three components: the inlet septum, the trabecular septum, and the outlet (infundibular or conal) septum. The trabecular septum (also simply called the muscular septum) is further divided into anterior, posterior, mid, and apical portions. Therefore, VSD may be classified as a membranous, inlet, outlet (or infundibular), midtrabecular (or midmuscular), anterior trabecular (or anterior muscular), posterior trabecular (or posterior muscular), and apical muscular defect (Fig. 12.7B).
   a. The membranous septum is a relatively small area immediately beneath the aortic valve. The membranous defect involves varying amounts of muscular tissue adjacent to the membranous septum (perimembranous VSD). According to the accompanying defect in the adjacent muscular septum, perimembranous VSDs have been called *perimembranous inlet (atrioventricular [AV] canal type), perimembranous trabecular,* or *perimembranous outlet (tetralogy type) defects.*
   b. Outlet (infundibular or conal) defects account for 5% to 7% of all VSDs in the Western world and about 30% in Far Eastern countries in surgical or autopsy series. The defect is located within the outlet (conal) septum, and part of its rim is formed by the aortic and pulmonary annulus. An aortic leaflet can prolapse through the VSD and cause aortic insufficiency (see later for further discussion). It has been called a *supracristal, conal, subpulmonary,* or *subarterial defect.*
   c. Inlet (or AV canal) defect is located posterior and inferior to the perimembranous defect beneath the septal leaflet of the tricuspid valve (see Fig. 12.7B).

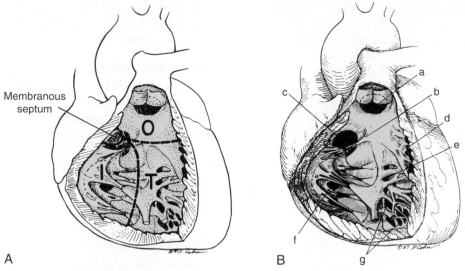

Fig. 12.7 Anatomy of ventricular septum and ventricular septal defect (VSD). **A,** Ventricular septum viewed from the right ventricular (RV) side. The membranous septum is small. The large muscular septum has three components: the inlet septum (I), the trabecular septum (T), and the outlet (or infundibular) septum (O). **B,** Anatomic locations of various VSDs and landmarks viewed with the RV free wall removed. *a,* Outlet (infundibular) defect; *b,* papillary muscle of the conus; *c,* perimembranous defect; *d,* marginal muscular defect; *e,* central muscular defect; *f,* inlet defect; *g,* apical muscular defect. Defects d, e, and g are grouped as muscular VSDs. (From Graham TP Jr, Bender HW, Spach MS et al: *Moss's Heart Disease in Infants, Children, and Adolescents,* Baltimore, 1989, Williams & Wilkins.)

d. Muscular (or trabecular) defect varies in size from tiny defects to large ones. Most small defects close spontaneously. They frequently appear to be multiple when viewed from the right side. A midmuscular defect is posterior to the septal band. An apical muscular defect is near the cardiac apex and is difficult to visualize and repair. The anterior (marginal) defects are usually multiple, small, and tortuous. The "Swiss cheese" type of multiple muscular defect (involving all components of the ventricular septum) is extremely difficult to close surgically.

2. The bundle of His is related to the posteroinferior quadrant of perimembranous defects and the superoanterior quadrant of inlet muscular defects. Defects in other parts of the septum are usually unrelated to the conduction tissue.

3. In an infundibular defect, the right coronary cusp of the aortic valve may herniate through the defect. This may result in an actual reduction of the VSD shunt but may produce aortic regurgitation (AR) and cause an obstruction in the RV outflow tract (RVOT). A similar herniation of the right or noncoronary cusp occasionally occurs through perimembranous defects.

4. Frequency of different subtypes of VSD found may be quite different depending on the diagnostic tools used in the study.
   a. With the use of echocardiography, the incidence of muscular VSD is much higher than perimembranous and other subtypes. Muscular VSD accounted for 59%; perimembranous VSD, 27%; outlet VSD, 1%; and inlet VSD, 1% (Boston Children's Hospital experience). However, many of the muscular (trabecular) VSDs are small in size, and about 85% to 95% of them close spontaneously (Hoffman, 2002).

   b. When studied in surgical and autopsy settings, the prevalence of subtypes of VSD are quite different from the above figures (partly because of small size and spontaneous closure of the muscular VSDs). Perimembranous VSD accounted for 80%; outlet VSD, 5% to 7% (29% in the Far Eastern countries); inlet VSD, 5% to 8%; and muscular VSD, 5% to 20% (McDaniel, 2001).

Clinical Manifestations
History

1. With a small VSD, the patient is asymptomatic with normal growth and development.
2. With a moderate to large VSD, delayed growth and development, decreased level of activity, repeated pulmonary infections, and CHF are relatively common during infancy.
3. With long-standing pulmonary hypertension, a history of cyanosis and a decreased level of activity may be present.

Physical Examination (Figs. 12.8 and 12.9)

1. Infants with small VSDs are well developed and acyanotic. Before 2 or 3 months of age, infants with large VSDs may have poor weight gain or show signs of CHF. Cyanosis and clubbing may be present in patients with pulmonary vascular obstructive disease (Eisenmenger's syndrome).
2. A systolic thrill may be present at the lower left sternal border. Precordial bulge and hyperactivity are present with a large-shunt VSD.
3. The intensity of the P2 is normal with a small shunt and moderately increased with a large shunt. The S2 is loud and single in patients with pulmonary hypertension or pulmonary vascular obstructive disease. A grade 2 to 5 of

6 regurgitant systolic murmur is audible at the lower left sternal border (see Figs. 12.8 and 12.9). It may be holosystolic or early systolic. An apical diastolic rumble is present with a moderate to large shunt (caused by an increased flow through the mitral valve during diastole) (see Fig. 12.9).

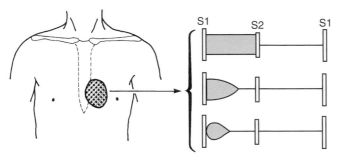

Fig. 12.8 Cardiac findings of a small ventricular septal defect. A regurgitant systolic murmur is best audible at the lower left sternal border; it may be holosystolic or less than holosystolic. Occasionally, the heart murmur is in early systole. A systolic thrill (dots) may be palpable at the lower left sternal border. The S2 splits normally, and the P2 is of normal intensity.

4. With infundibular VSD, a grade 1 to 3 of 6 early diastolic decrescendo murmur of AR may be audible. This murmur may be caused by herniation of an aortic cusp.

Electrocardiography

1. With a small VSD, the ECG is normal.
2. With a moderate VSD, left ventricular hypertrophy (LVH) and occasional left atrial hypertrophy (LAH) may be seen.
3. With a large defect, the ECG shows biventricular hypertrophy (BVH) with or without LAH (Fig. 12.10).
4. If pulmonary vascular obstructive disease develops, the ECG shows RVH only.

Radiography (Fig. 12.11)

1. Cardiomegaly of varying degrees is present and involves the LA, left ventricle (LV), and sometimes RV. Pulmonary vascular markings increase. The degree of cardiomegaly and the increase in pulmonary vascular markings directly relate to the magnitude of the left-to-right shunt.
2. In pulmonary vascular obstructive disease, the main PA and the hilar PAs enlarge noticeably, but the peripheral lung fields are ischemic. The heart size is usually normal.

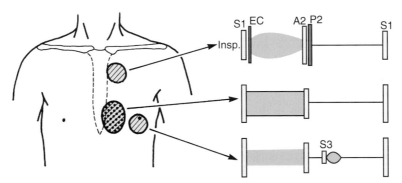

Fig. 12.9 Cardiac findings of a large ventricular septal defect. A classic holosystolic regurgitant murmur is audible at the lower left sternal border. A systolic thrill is also palpable at the same area *(dots)*. There is usually a mid-diastolic rumble, resulting from relative mitral stenosis, at the apex. The S2 is narrowly split, and the P2 is accentuated in intensity. Occasionally, an ejection click (EC) may be audible in the upper left sternal border when associated with pulmonary hypertension. The heart murmurs shown without solid borders are transmitted from other areas and are not characteristic of the defect. Abnormal sounds are shown in black. *Insp,* Inspiration.

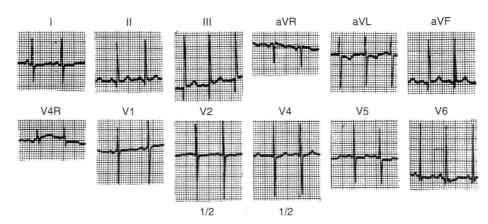

Fig. 12.10 Tracing from a 3-month-old infant with a large ventricular septal defect, patent ductus arteriosus, and pulmonary hypertension. The tracing shows biventricular hypertrophy with left dominance. Note that V2 and V4 are in half standardization.

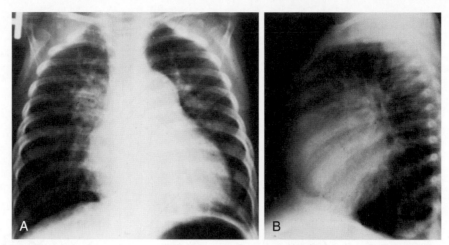

Fig. 12.11 Posteroanterior (**A**) and lateral (**B**) views of chest radiographs of a ventricular septal defect with a large shunt and pulmonary hypertension. The heart size is moderately increased, with enlargement on both right and left sides of the heart. Pulmonary vascular markings are increased, with a prominent main pulmonary artery segment.

Echocardiography

Two-dimensional and Doppler echocardiographic studies can identify the number, size, and exact location of the defect; estimate PA pressure by using the modified Bernoulli equation; identify other associated defects; and estimate the magnitude of the shunt. Because the ventricular septum is a large, complex structure, examination for a VSD should be carried out in a systematic manner to be able to specify the exact location and size of the defect. When possible, more than one view should be obtained, preferably a combination of the long- and short-axis views.

The cardiac valves serve as markers of specific types of VSDs except for the trabecular septum. The membranous VSD is closely related to the aortic valve, the inlet VSD to the tricuspid (or AV) valve, and the infundibular VSD to the semilunar valves. Fig. 12.12 is a collection of selected views of parasternal, apical, and subcostal views, which are useful in locating the site of VSDs.

The *membranous septum* is closely related to the aortic valve. In the apical and subcostal "five-chamber" views, it is seen in the LV outflow tract (LVOT) just under the aortic valve (see Fig. 12.12C3). In the parasternal short-axis view at the level of the aortic valve, it is seen adjacent to the tricuspid valve (see Fig. 12.12B1). These are the best views to confirm the membranous VSD. The membranous VSD is not visible in the standard parasternal long-axis view, but by tilting the transducer slightly to the right, away from the aorta, the membranous VSD becomes visible. Fig. 12.13 shows a membranous VSD imaged in the apical "five-chamber" view.

The inlet septum is best imaged in the apical or subcostal four-chamber view beneath the AV valves (see Fig. 12.12C2 and D1). It can also be seen equally well in the parasternal short-axis view in the posterior interventricular septum at the levels between the mitral valve and the papillary muscle (see Fig. 12.12B2). Simple inlet VSD (not that associated with AV canal defect) is seen beneath the AV valve, but a small amount of tissue remains under the valves. In the AV canal type of

VSD, the AV valves are at the same level. There may be straddling or overriding.

The *infundibular (or outlet) septum* lies inferior to the semilunar valves. The subpulmonary, supracristal infundibular VSD lies under the pulmonary valve (see Fig. 12.12A2 and D3), and the subaortic infracristal VSD (tetralogy of Fallot [TOF] type, also called conoventricular VSD) lies under the aortic valve (see Fig. 12.12A1 and D2). From the RV side, if the outlet septum lies inferior to the pulmonary valve, it is supracristal. The infracristal VSD lies much closer to the aortic valve but away from the pulmonary valve (see Fig. 12.12A1 and C3), and the supracristal is closer to the pulmonary valve (see Fig. 12.12A2, D3, and E1).

The *trabecular septum* is the largest portion of the ventricular septum and extends from the membranous septum to the cardiac apex. The four types of trabecular VSDs are (1) anterior, (2) midmuscular, (3) apical, and (4) posterior. Echocardiographic views that show the locations of different types of trabecular VSDs are shown in Fig. 12.12. The apical VSD occurs near the cardiac apex (see Fig. 12.12A1, A2, C2, C3, D1, and D2). The entire ventricular septum seen at the papillary muscle level is the trabecular septum (see Fig. 12.12B3 and E2). For imaging of an apical muscular VSD, the transducer must be maximally angled toward the cardiac apex.

Natural History

Understanding the natural history of a VSD is important when planning its management.

1. Spontaneous closure of perimembranous and muscular VSDs can occur. It occurs more frequently with small defects and during the first 6 months of life. About 60% of small to moderate muscular VSDs close spontaneously but not after 8 years of age. About 35% of small perimembranous VSDs close spontaneously but not after 5 years of age. These VSDs do not become bigger with age; rather, they decrease in size. However, inlet defects and outlet

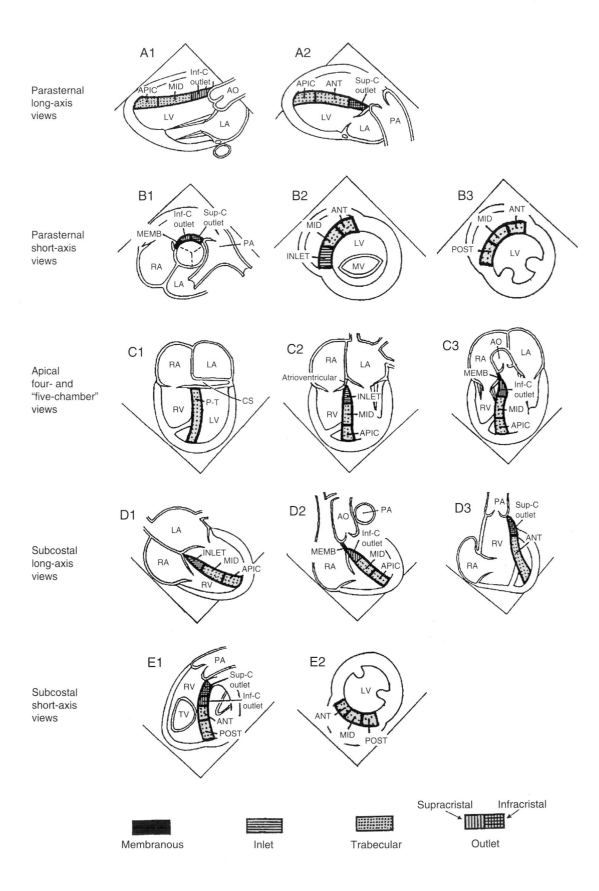

Parasternal long-axis views

Parasternal short-axis views

Apical four- and "five-chamber" views

Subcostal long-axis views

Subcostal short-axis views

Membranous   Inlet   Trabecular   Outlet

Supracristal   Infracristal

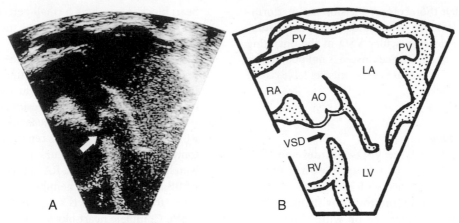

Fig. 12.13 Two-dimensional echocardiogram showing membranous ventricular septal defect (VSD). The membranous VSD is seen underneath the aortic valve in the left ventricular outflow tract (in the apical "five-chamber" view). This view is equivalent to Figure 12.12C3. *AO*, Aorta; *LA*, left atrium; *LV*, left ventricle; *PV*, pulmonary vein; *RA*, right atrium; *RV*, right ventricle.

(infundibular) defects do not become smaller or close spontaneously.

2. CHF develops in infants with large VSDs but usually not until 6 to 8 weeks of age.

3. Pulmonary vascular obstructive disease may begin to develop as early as 6 to 12 months of age in patients with large VSDs, but the resulting right-to-left shunt usually does not develop until the teenage years.

4. Infundibular stenosis may develop in some infants with large defects and result in a decrease in the magnitude of the left-to-right shunt (i.e., acyanotic TOF), with an occasional occurrence of a right-to-left shunt.

Management
Medical

1. Treatment of CHF, if it develops, is indicated with diuretics (with or without digoxin) (see Chapter 27) for 2 to 4 months to see if growth failure can be improved. Some centers do not use digoxin. Addition of spironolactone may be helpful to minimize potassium loss from diuretics. Concomitant use of an afterload reducing agent, such as captopril, has gained popularity. Angiotensin-converting enzyme (ACE) inhibitors may raise the serum potassium level, and spironolactone or potassium supplementation should be discontinued. Frequent feedings of high-calorie formulas, either by nasogastric tube or oral feeding, may help. Anemia, if present, should be corrected by oral iron therapy. These measures often allow delay of surgical treatment and may promote spontaneous reduction or closure of the VSD.

2. No exercise restriction is required in the absence of pulmonary hypertension.

Nonsurgical Device Closure

Nonsurgical percutaneous device closure of selected muscular VSDs is possible in selected patients when the defect is not too close to cardiac valves and when it is difficult to access surgically. Some centers have used so-called hybrid

Fig. 12.12 Selected two-dimensional echo views of the ventricular septum. These schematic drawings are helpful in determining the site of a ventricular septal defect (VSD). Different shading has been used for easy recognition of different parts of the ventricular septum. In the standard parasternal long-axis view (**A1**), the ventricular septum consists of (from the aortic valve toward the apex) the infracristal outlet (Inf-C outlet) septum (the VSD of tetralogy of Fallot is seen here) and the trabecular (mid- and apical) septum. In the parasternal right ventricular outlet tract (RVOT) view (**A2**), the septum consists of the supracristal outlet (Sup-C outlet) septum and the trabecular septum. In the parasternal short-axis view showing the aortic valve (**B1**), the membranous septum is toward the 10 o'clock direction, the infracristal outlet septum at the 12 o'clock direction, and the supracristal outlet septum immediately adjacent to the pulmonary valve. The ventricular septum at the mitral valve (**B2**), the posterior muscular septum is inlet (INLET) septum. The ventricular septum at the papillary muscle (**B3**) is all trabecular septum, so that one can easily classify the defect into anterior (ANT), mid- (MID), and posterior (POST) trabecular defects. In the apical four-chamber view showing the coronary sinus (**C1**), the ventricular septum is the posterior (POST) trabecular septum. In the apical four-chamber view showing both atrioventricular (AV) valves (**C2**), the septum immediately beneath the tricuspid valve is the inlet septum (INLET) and the remainder is the mid- and apical septa. The thin septum between the insertion of the mitral and tricuspid valves is the AV septum (**C2**), a defect which can result in a left ventricle (LV)–to–right atrium (RA) shunt. In the standard apical four-chamber view, the membranous septum is not visible. In the apical "five-chamber" view (**C3**), the membranous (MEMB) septum is seen beneath the aortic valve, and below it is the infracristal outlet (Inf-C outlet) septum. The ventricular septum seen in the subcostal four-chamber view (**D1**) is similar to the apical four-chamber view (**C2**). With anterior angulation of the horizontal transducer, the LV outflow tract (LVOT) is seen (**D2**), and the septum seen here is similar to the apical "five-chamber" view (**C3**). With further anterior angulation, the RVOT is seen (**D3**). The superior part is the supracristal outlet (Sup-C outlet) septum, and the inferior part is the anterior (ANT) trabecular septum (**D3**). The subcostal short-axis view showing the RVOT (**E1**) is orthogonal to the standard subcostal four-chamber view and is an important view for evaluating the site and size of a VSD. In this view, both supracristal outlet (Sup-C outlet) and infracristal outlet (Inf-C outlet) septa (in that order) are seen beneath the pulmonary valve and the trabecular septum (ANT and POST) is seen apical ward. The ventricular septum seen at the papillary muscle (**E2**) is all trabecular septum and is similar to the parasternal short axis view (**B3**).

procedures through left thoracotomy incision and performing "perventricular" device closure without the use of cardiopulmonary bypass to close muscular VSD in the operating room in other selected cases. Device closure is not popular for the perimembranous VSD because of the unacceptable rate of postprocedure heart block.

Surgical

Indications and Timing

1. Small infants who have large VSDs and develop CHF with growth retardation are managed with diuretics and afterload reducing agents, with or without digoxin. If growth failure cannot be improved by medical therapy, the VSD should be operated on within the first 6 months of life, preferably by 3 to 4 months of age. Surgery should be delayed for infants who respond to medical therapy.
2. Infants who have small VSDs and have reached the age of 6 months without CHF or evidence of pulmonary hypertension are usually not candidates for surgery.
3. If the PA pressure is more than 50% of systemic pressure, surgical closure should be done by the end of the first year.
4. After 1 year of age, a significant left-to-right shunt with Q_p/Q_s ratio of at least 2:1 indicates that surgical closure is needed, regardless of PA pressure. Surgery is not indicated for small VSDs with Q_p/Q_s ratio less than 1.5:1.
5. Older infants with large VSDs and evidence of elevated PVR should be operated on as soon as possible.
6. Surgery is contraindicated in patients with a pulmonary to systemic vascular resistance ratio of greater than 0.5 or with pulmonary vascular obstructive disease with a predominant right-to-left shunt.

Procedure

1. PA banding as a palliative procedure is no longer performed unless additional lesions or patient's weight (i.e., preterm infants) make complete repair difficult.
2. Direct closure of the defect is carried out under hypothermic cardiopulmonary bypass, preferably without right ventriculotomy. Patch closure with pericardium or prosthetic material is usually required for large defects. Most perimembranous and inlet VSDs are repaired by a transatrial approach. Outlet (conal) defects are best approached through an incision in the main pulmonary artery. Apical VSD may require apical right ventriculotomy.

As with the closure of ASDs, minimally invasive surgical techniques with smaller skin incisions are becoming popular for the closure of VSDs. The major benefit of this approach appears to be cosmetic.

Mortality. The surgical mortality rate is 0.5%. The mortality rate is higher for small infants younger than 2 months of age, infants with associated defects, or infants with multiple VSDs.

Complications

1. Up to 3% of patients undergoing surgical closure of VSD develop complete heart block. Although the majority of heart block is transient, a small percentage of patients will develop permanent heart block and require pacemaker placement.
2. Residual shunt occurs in fewer than 5%, although some report it in up to 25% of patients undergoing VSD closure. Intraoperative TEE echo has reduced the incidence of the hemodynamically significant residual shunt.
3. Postpericardiotomy syndrome is uncommon.
4. RBBB is frequent in patients repaired via right ventriculotomy (in 50%–90%). It occurs in up to 40% of the patients who had repair through a RA approach.
5. RBBB and left anterior hemiblock, which occurs in fewer than 10% of patients, is a controversial cause of sudden death. Complete heart block requiring pacemaker occurs in 1% to 2% of patients.
6. The incidence of neurologic complications is directly related to the circulatory arrest time.

Surgical Approaches for Special Situations

1. **VSD and PDA.** If the PDA is large, the ductus alone may be closed in the first 6 to 8 weeks in the hope that the VSD is restrictive. If the VSD is large and not restrictive, PDA should be ligated at the time of VSD repair through the median sternotomy.
2. **VSD and coarctation of the aorta (COA).** A VSD is present in 15% to 20% of patients with COA. Several options exist in this controversial situation.
   a. Initial repair of the COA alone if the VSD appears relatively small. The VSD is closed later, if indicated.
   b. Coarctation repair and PA banding when the VSD appears unrestrictive.
   c. Repair of both defects at the same time using one or two incisions.
3. **VSD and AR syndrome.** The prolapsed aortic cusp, with resulting AR, is usually associated with outlet VSD and occasionally with perimembranous VSD. It occurs in about 5% of patients with VSD, but the prevalence is much higher in Far Eastern countries (15%–20%). The adjacent (i.e., right or noncoronary) aortic valve cusps prolapse through the defect into the RVOT, actually reducing the VSD shunt. When AR appears, it gradually worsens. Surgery is usually performed promptly when AR is present even if the Q_p/Q_s ratio is less than 2:1, so that progression of AR (by Venturi effect through the open VSD) is either aborted or abolished. Some centers close the VSD even in the absence of AR if the aortic prolapse is demonstrated. When AR is trivial or mild, the VSD alone is closed. When AR is moderate or severe, the aortic valve is repaired or replaced. Not every case of VSD and AR results from the prolapsed aortic cusps; it may be the result of a VSD and bicuspid aortic valve.

Postoperative Follow-up

1. Office examination should be scheduled every 1 to 2 years.
2. Activity should not be restricted unless complications have resulted from surgery.
3. Although rare these days, patients who had VSD and mild pulmonary hypertension and repair of the VSD after 3

years of age should be checked for possible progressive pulmonary vascular disease.

4. A patient with a postoperative history of transient heart block with or without pacemaker therapy requires long-term follow-up.

PATENT DUCTUS ARTERIOSUS

Prevalence

Patent ductus arteriosus occurs in 5% to 10% of all CHDs, excluding premature infants. It is more common in females than in males (male-to-female ratio of 1:3). PDA is a common problem in premature infants and will be presented under a separate heading in this chapter.

Pathology

1. There is a persistent patency of a normal fetal structure between the PA and the descending aorta, that is, about 5 to 10 mm distal to the origin of the left subclavian artery.
2. The ductus is usually cone shaped with a small orifice to the PA, which is restrictive to blood flow. The ductus may be short or long, straight, or tortuous.

Clinical Manifestations

History

1. Patients are usually asymptomatic when the ductus is small.
2. A large-shunt PDA may cause a lower respiratory tract infection, atelectasis, and CHF (accompanied by tachypnea and poor weight gain).
3. Exertional dyspnea may be present in children with a large-shunt PDA

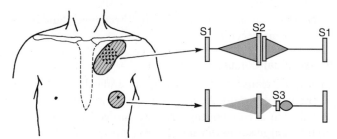

Fig. 12.14 Cardiac findings of patent ductus arteriosus. A systolic thrill may be present in the area shown by *dots*.

Physical Examination (Fig. 12.14)

1. Tachycardia and tachypnea may be present in infants with CHF.
2. Bounding peripheral pulses with wide pulse pressure (with elevated systolic pressure and lower diastolic pressure) are characteristic findings of a large PDA. With a small shunt, these findings do not occur.
3. With a large shunt, the precordium is hyperactive. A systolic thrill may be present at the upper left sternal border. The P2 is usually normal, but its intensity may be accentuated if pulmonary hypertension is present. A grade 1 to 4 of 6 continuous ("machinery") murmur is best audible at the left infraclavicular area or upper left sternal border. An apical diastolic rumble may be heard when the PDA shunt is large. Patients with small ductus may only have a low intensity continuous murmur in the left infraclavicular area.
4. If pulmonary vascular obstructive disease develops, a right-to-left ductal shunt results in cyanosis only in the lower half of the body (i.e., differential cyanosis).

Electrocardiography

The ECG findings in PDA are similar to those in VSD. A normal ECG or LVH is seen with small to moderate PDA. BVH is seen with large PDA. If pulmonary vascular obstructive disease develops, RVH is present.

Radiography

Radiographs are also similar to those of VSD.
1. Chest radiographs may be normal with a small-shunt PDA.
2. Cardiomegaly of varying degrees occurs in moderate to large shunt-PDA with enlargement of the LA, LV, and ascending aorta. Pulmonary vascular markings are increased.
3. With pulmonary vascular obstructive disease, the heart size becomes normal, with a marked prominence of the PA segment and hilar vessels.

Echocardiography

Echocardiography has emerged as the procedure of choice in confirming the diagnosis and assessing functional significance.

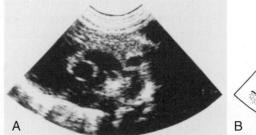
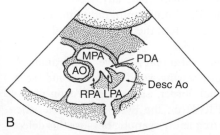

Fig. 12.15 **A** and **B**, Parasternal short-axis view demonstrating patent ductus arteriosus (PDA) that connects the main pulmonary artery (MPA) and the descending aorta (Desc Ao). *AO,* Aorta; *LPA,* left pulmonary artery; *RPA,* right pulmonary artery.

1. The PDA can be imaged in most patients. Its size can be assessed by 2D echo in a high parasternal view or in a suprasternal notch view (Fig. 12.15).
2. Doppler studies that are performed with the sample volume in the PA immediately proximal to the ductal opening provide important functional information (see discussion of PDA in Preterm Neonates).
3. The dimensions of the LA and LV provide an indirect assessment of the magnitude of the left-to-right ductal shunt. The larger the shunt, the greater the dilatation of these chambers.

Natural History

1. Unlike PDA in premature infants, spontaneous closure of a PDA is rare in full-term infants and children. This is because the PDA in term infants results from a structural abnormality of the ductal smooth muscle rather than a decreased responsiveness of the ductal smooth muscle to oxygen.
2. CHF or recurrent pneumonia develops if the shunt is large.
3. Pulmonary vascular obstructive disease may develop if a large PDA with pulmonary hypertension is left untreated.
4. Although rare, an aneurysm of PDA may develop and possibly rupture in adult life.

Differential Diagnosis

The following conditions occur with a heart murmur, which is similar to the continuous murmur of PDA or with bounding pulses, and they require differentiation from PDA:

1. **Coronary arteriovenous fistula.** A continuous murmur is usually maximally audible along the right sternal border, not at the left infraclavicular area or upper left sternal border.
2. **Systemic arteriovenous fistula.** A bounding pulse with a wide pulse pressure and signs of CHF may develop without continuous murmur over the precordium. A continuous murmur is present over the fistula (i.e., head or liver).
3. **Pulmonary arteriovenous fistula.** A continuous murmur is audible over the back. Cyanosis and clubbing are present in the absence of cardiomegaly.
4. **Venous hum.** A venous hum is maximally audible in the right or left infraclavicular and supraclavicular areas when the patient is examined in a sitting position. It usually disappears when the patient lies in a supine position.
5. **Collaterals in COA.** A continuous murmur is audible in the intercostal spaces, usually bilaterally.
6. **VSD with AR.** A to-and-fro murmur, rather than a continuous murmur, is audible at the mid-left sternal border or lower left sternal border.
7. **TOF with absent pulmonary valve syndrome.** A to-and-fro murmur ("sawing wood" sound) is audible at the upper left sternal border. Large hilar PAs on radiographic films and RVH on the ECG are characteristic. These patients are frequently cyanotic because this defect is usually associated with TOF.
8. **Persistent truncus arteriosus.** A continuous murmur is occasionally audible at the second right intercostal space or at the back in a cyanotic infant rather than in the upper left sternal border. The ECG may show BVH, and chest radiographic films show varying degrees of cardiomegaly and increased pulmonary vascularity. A right aortic arch is frequently found.
9. **Aortopulmonary septal defect (aortopulmonary window).** This extremely rare condition produces a bounding pulse, but the murmur resembles that of a VSD. CHF develops in early infancy.
10. **Peripheral PA stenosis.** A continuous murmur is audible all over the thorax. The ECG may show RVH if the stenosis is severe. This often accompanies Williams syndrome or rubella syndrome.
11. **Ruptured sinus of Valsalva aneurysm.** The sudden onset of chest pain and signs of severe heart failure with dyspnea develop. A continuous murmur or a to-and-fro murmur is present at the base. This condition is more commonly seen in patients with Marfan's syndrome.
12. **Total anomalous pulmonary venous return (TAPVR) draining into the RA.** A murmur that sounds similar to a venous hum may be heard along the right sternal border in a child with mild cyanosis. The ECG shows RVH in the presence of cardiomegaly and increased pulmonary vascular markings on chest radiographic films.

Management
Medical

1. Unlike in premature infants with PDAs, indomethacin is ineffective in term infants and should not be used.
2. No exercise restriction is needed in the absence of pulmonary hypertension.
3. Nonsurgical occlusion of PDA has become a standard of care at many centers.

Nonsurgical Closure

Currently, transcatheter closure is standard care beyond the neonatal period. Advances in device and delivery system design are extending this option even to very small infants. Large series of transcatheter closure of PDA in the United States and Europe reported 95% to 100% success rate.

Indications. The following are indications and contraindications for device closure of PDA (Feltes et al. 2011).

1. Closure of PDA is definitely indicated in patients with hemodynamically significant PDA with CHF, failure to thrive, pulmonary overcirculation, or enlargement of the LA and LV.
2. It is reasonable to close a small PDA when the murmur of PDA is audible by standard auscultation techniques.
3. There is controversy related to occlusion of so-called "silent ductus." There are few data on the benefits of occluding the silent ductus because of lack of significant endothelial damage to cause endocarditis.

4. In patients with Eisenmenger syndrome or pulmonary vascular obstructive disease, the response of PVR to balloon occlusion or pulmonary vasodilator (e.g., oxygen or nitric oxide) is tested in cardiac catheterization laboratory. If a good response is obtained, closure is advised. If the response is poor or equivocal, closure may not be recommended. A device closure (without additional surgical insult) may be considered in this setting. The presence of severe pulmonary hypertension with irreversible pulmonary vascular obstructive disease is a contraindication to surgery.

Procedure. Small PDAs smaller than 3 mm in diameter are closed by various kinds of coils and larger ones with the Amplatzer PDA device.

1. Gianturco stainless coils have become the standard device for closure of PDA for all children with ducts less than 3 mm in diameter in the United States. In optimal candidates for the device, the ductus is 2.5 mm in size, but the use of multiple coils can close a ductus up to 5 mm. A retrograde approach is used from the femoral artery. The residual shunt rate is 5% to 15% at 12 months' follow-up. Overall, the procedure is 97% successful (or more) with zero mortality.

2. For larger PDA but smaller than 12 mm in diameter, specialized devices, such as Amplatzer duct occluder, are available for catheter-based closure. The devices are implanted antegrade from the femoral vein. Although original recommendations from the manufacturer exclude patients who weigh less than 6 kg, successful use in infants as small as 2.5 kg has been reported. There is a 98% or greater closure rate at 6 months with minimal complications and no deaths.

The advantages of nonsurgical closure of the ductus include no need for general anesthesia, shorter hospital stay and convalescent period, and elimination of a thoracotomy scar. Disadvantages and potential complications include residual leaks, pulmonary artery coil embolization, hemolysis, left PA stenosis, aortic occlusion with the Amplatzer device, and femoral vessel occlusion.

Surgical Closure

Indications and Timing. Surgical closure is reserved for patients in whom a nonsurgical closure technique is not considered applicable. An interventional device rather than surgery is used to close small ductus with no hemodynamic significance by many centers.

Procedure

1. Ligation and division through left posterolateral thoracotomy without cardiopulmonary bypass is the standard procedure.

2. The technique of video-assisted thoracoscopic surgery (VATS) clip ligation has become the standard of care for surgical management of ductus with adequate length (to allow safe ligation), which is performed through three small ports in the fourth intercostal space.

Mortality. The surgical mortality rate is 0% to 1% for both techniques.

Complications. Complications are rare. Injury to the recurrent laryngeal nerve (hoarseness), the left phrenic nerve (paralysis of the left hemidiaphragm), or the thoracic duct (chylothorax) is possible. Recanalization (reopening) of the ductus is possible, although rare, occurring after ligation alone (without division).

PATENT DUCTUS ARTERIOSUS IN PRETERM NEONATES

Prevalence

Clinical evidence of PDA appears in 45% of infants with a birth weight less than 1750 g and in about 80% of infants with a birth weight less than 1200 g. Significant PDA with CHF occurs in 15% of premature infants with a birth weight less than 1750 g and in 40% to 50% of those with a birth weight less than 1500 g.

Pathophysiology

1. PDA is a special problem in premature infants who are recovering from hyaline membrane disease. With improvement in oxygenation, the PVR falls rapidly, but the ductus remains patent because its responsiveness to oxygen is immature in premature newborns (see Chapter 8). The resulting large left-to-right shunt makes the lung stiff, and weaning the infant from the ventilator and oxygen therapy becomes difficult.

2. If the infant must remain on a ventilator and oxygen therapy for a long time, bronchopulmonary dysplasia develops, with resulting pulmonary hypertension (cor pulmonale) and right-sided heart failure.

3. Premature infants with significant left-to-right shunt may suffer from the consequences of prolonged hypoperfusion to many organs, which may include intracranial hemorrhage, renal dysfunction, myocardial ischemia, and necrotizing enterocolitis. Early recognition and appropriate management of PDA are keys to improving the prognosis of these infants.

Clinical Manifestations

1. The history is important in suspecting a significant PDA in a premature neonate. Typically, a premature infant with hyaline membrane disease shows some improvement during the first few days after birth. This is followed by an inability to wean the infant from the ventilator or a need to increase ventilator settings or oxygen requirements in 4- to 7-day-old premature infants. Episodes of apnea or bradycardia may be the initial sign of PDA in infants who are not on ventilators.

2. The physical examination commonly reveals bounding peripheral pulses, a hyperactive precordium, and tachycardia with or without gallop rhythm. The classic continuous murmur at the left infraclavicular area or upper left sternal border is diagnostic, but the murmur may be only systolic and is difficult to hear in infants who are on ventilators. Premature infants who are fluid overloaded or retaining

fluid may also present with findings of PDA as described earlier (hyperdynamic precordium, systolic ejection murmur, bounding pulses, and wide pulse pressures), requiring differentiation from PDA.

3. The ECG is not diagnostic. It usually is normal but occasionally shows LVH.

4. Chest radiographs show cardiomegaly in larger premature infants who are not intubated. The infant may have evidence of pulmonary edema or increased pulmonary vascular markings, but these may be difficult to assess in the presence of hyaline membrane disease. In infants who are intubated and on high ventilator settings, chest x-ray films may show the heart to be either of normal size or only mildly enlarged.

5. 2D echocardiographic and color-flow Doppler studies provide accurate anatomic and functional information.
   a. 2D echo provides anatomic information about the diameter, length, and shape of the ductus (see Fig. 12.15).
   b. Doppler studies of the ductus (with the sample volume placed at the pulmonary end of the ductus) provide important functional information, such as ductal shunt patterns (pure left-to-right, bidirectional, or predominant right-to-left shunt), pressures in the PA, and magnitude of the ductal shunt or pulmonary perfusion status:

1) Ductal shunt pattern. A continuous positive flow indicates a pure left-to-right shunt with the PA pressure lower than the aortic pressure. In pure right-to-left shunts, flow is continuously negative away from the PA, indicating that the PA pressure is suprasystemic. A bidirectional shunting pattern (with an early negative flow in systole followed by a late positive flow in diastole) is found in infants with PDA and severe pulmonary hypertension.

2) Estimation of PA pressures. A high ductal flow velocity indicates a low PA pressure, and a low flow velocity indicates a high PA pressure. The pressure drop may be underestimated in patients with a small pulmonary end of the ductus, tortuous PDAs, or tunnel-like PDAs with diameters smaller than 3 mm and lengths longer than 10 mm (because of viscous energy loss). However, estimation of the PA systolic pressure could be obtained from the peak velocity of the TR, when it is present.

3) Perfusion status. Increased flow velocity in the left PA suggests a large left-to-right shunt through the ductus. High PA pressure and a lower flow velocity (with a pressure drop of <5 mm Hg) indicate poor perfusion of the lungs, which is a bad prognostic sign during the first 24 to 36 hours.

Management

For symptomatic infants, either pharmacologic or surgical closure of the ductus is indicated. A small PDA that does not cause symptoms should be followed medically for 6 months without surgical ligation because of the possibility of spontaneous closure.

Medical

1. Fluid restriction to 120 mL/kg per day and a diuretic (e.g., chlorothiazide) may be tried for 24 to 48 hours, but these regimens have a low success rate. Use of furosemide is not recommended because it is known to stimulate prostaglandin E_2 synthesis and thus dilate the PDA (Pacifici, 2013). Digoxin is not used because it has little hemodynamic benefit and a high incidence of digitalis toxicity.

2. Pharmacologic closure of the PDA can he achieved with indomethacin (a prostaglandin synthetase inhibitor). Indomethacin inhibits the synthesis and release of prostaglandins, which play a major role in maintaining ductal patency during fetal life.

   Contraindications to the use of indomethacin include high blood urea nitrogen (>25 mg/dL) or creatinine (>1.8 mg/dL) levels, low platelet count (<80,000/mm^3), bleeding tendency (including intracranial hemorrhage), necrotizing enterocolitis, and hyperbilirubinemia.

   Many dosage regimens exist, and dose is dependent on postnatal age of the infant at time of first dose; one example is as follows. The dose is given intravenously every 12 hours a total of 3 doses. For infants less than 48 hours old, 0.2 mg/kg is followed by 0.1 mg/kg times 2. For those who are 2 to 7 days old, 0.2 mg/kg times 3 is given, and for those who are more than 7 days old, 0.2 mg/kg followed by 0.25 mg/kg times 2 is given.

3. Ibuprofen, another inhibitor of prostaglandin synthesis, has also been used in ductal closure in premature infants. A multicenter prospective study from Europe showed that intravenous ibuprofen (10 mg/kg, followed at 24-hour intervals by two doses of 5 mg/kg) starting on the third day of life was equally effective in closing the ductus in preterm newborns as indomethacin. Ibuprofen had a significantly lower incidence of oliguria, and it does not appear to have a deleterious effect on cerebral blood flow. Ibuprofen significantly reduces plasma concentrations of prostaglandin.

4. More recently, acetaminophen is being used for PDA closure in preterm infants. First reported by Hammerman and his colleagues in 2011, acetaminophen, both oral or intravenous, has become another alternative pharmaceutical method for PDA closure with success rates comparable to indomethacin or ibuprofen. Acetaminophen is believed to block the peroxidase segment of prostaglandin synthetase, thus inhibiting prostaglandin production. Because of its different site of action, this drug may not generate vasoconstriction; thus, a non-surgical option for preterm infants with gastrointestinal perforations or reduced renal blood flow. However, its use has been reported to cause elevation of transaminase, so caution is warranted is patient with hepatic injury. A current recommended dosing is 15 mg/kg given every 6 hours.

5. Recent reports from Europe concluded that prophylactic use of ibuprofen in small preterm infants was not useful because, although it reduced the occurrence and the need for surgical ligation of the ductus, it did not reduce the frequency of intraventricular hemorrhage (IVH), mortality, or morbidity. The American Academy of Pediatrics

agrees with this statement. It states further that prophylactic use of indomethacin may be appropriate in settings where rates of IVH are high, but it may not be justified by expected effects on PDA or by an expectation of better long-term outcomes (Benits, 2016).

Surgical

If medical treatment is unsuccessful or if the use of indomethacin is contraindicated, surgical ligation of the ductus may be indicated. The standard operative approach to PDA is through a posterolateral thoracotomy. The PDA is simply ligated or hemoclipped (without division). Many centers now perform PDA ligation in the neonatal intensive care unit at the bedside. The operative mortality rate is 0% to 3%.

Recently, the use of minimally invasive VATS has been reported for the management of PDA in low-birth-weight infants. This technique allows PDA interruption without the muscle cutting or rib spreading of a standard thoracotomy. Reduced compromise of respiratory mechanics and less chest wall deformity associated with a large thoracotomy incision may also be advantages.

COMPLETE ENDOCARDIAL CUSHION DEFECT

Prevalence

Complete ECD (also known as AV canal defect, complete AV canal defect, or AV communis) occurs in about 5% of all CHDs. Of patients with complete ECD, about 70% are children with Down syndrome. Of children with Down syndrome, about 40% have CHDs, and 50% of the defects are ECD. ECD is also a component of heart defects in asplenia and polysplenia syndromes (see Chapter 14).

Pathology

1. Abnormalities seen in complete ECD affect the structures normally derived from the endocardial cushion tissue. Ostium primum ASD, VSD in the inlet ventricular septum, and clefts in the anterior mitral valve and the septal leaflet of the tricuspid valve (forming the common AV valve) are all present in the complete form of ECD (Fig. 12.16). The combination of these defects may result in interatrial and interventricular shunts, LV-to-RA shunt, and AV valve regurgitation. Although rare, the entire atrial septum may be absent (common atrium). When two AV valve orifices are present without an interventricular shunt, the defect is called *partial ECD* or *ostium primum ASD* (which is presented under a separate heading in this chapter).

2. Both complete and partial forms of ECD are characterized by a deficiency of the inlet portion of the ventricular septum, with a "scooped-out" appearance of the muscular septum and an excessively long infundibular septum, as well as by an abnormal position of the aortic valve (i.e., displaced anterosuperiorly rather than being wedged between the right and left AV valves). The latter results in lengthening and narrowing of the LVOT, thereby producing the characteristic "goose-neck deformity" on angiocardiogram (see Fig. 12.21).

3. Whereas in complete ECD, a single valve orifice connects the atrial and ventricular chambers, in the partial form, there are separate mitral and tricuspid orifices. The common AV valve usually has five leaflets (see Fig 12.16). The arrangement of the LV papillary muscles may be abnormal in that either they are closer together or only one papillary muscle is present in the LV, which makes surgical repair difficult.

4. In the majority of complete ECD cases, the AV orifices are equally committed to the RV and LV ("balanced" AV canal). In some patients, however, the orifices are committed primarily to one ventricle, with hypoplasia of the other ventricle (i.e., "unbalanced" AV canal with RV or LV dominance). Hypoplasia of one ventricle may necessitate one ventricular repair (i.e., Fontan operation).

5. A universally accepted classification for complete ECD does not exist. The Rastelli classification was based on the relationships of the anterior bridging leaflets to the crest of the ventricular septum or RV papillary muscles (Fig. 12.17). In type A, the anterior bridging leaflet is

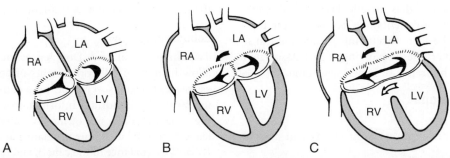

Fig. 12.16 Diagram of the atrioventricular (AV) valve and cardiac septa in partial and complete endocardial cushion defect (ECDs). **A,** Normal AV valve anatomy with no septal defect. **B,** Partial ECD with clefts in the mitral and tricuspid valves and an ostium primum atrial septal defect (ASD) *(solid arrow)*. **C,** Complete ECD. There is a common AV valve with large anterior and posterior bridging leaflets. An ostium primum ASD *(solid arrow)* and an inlet ventricular septal defect *(open arrow)* are present. *LA,* Left atrium; *LV,* left ventricle; *RA,* right atrium; *RV,* right ventricle.

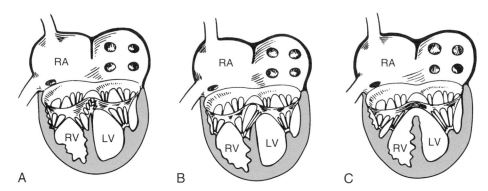

Fig. 12.17 Rastelli's classification of complete endocardial cushion defect. **A,** Type A. **B,** Type B. **C,** Type C. (See text for descriptions.) *LV,* Left ventricle; *RA,* right atrium; *RV,* right ventricle.

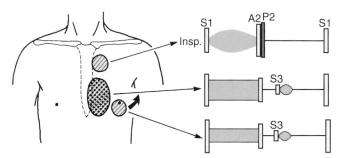

Fig. 12.18 Cardiac findings of complete endocardial cushion defect, which resemble those of a large ventricular septal defect. An apical holosystolic murmur (caused by mitral regurgitation) may transmit toward the left axilla. A systolic thrill may be present at the lower left sternal border *(dotted area),* where the systolic murmur is loudest. *Insp.,* Inspiration.

tightly tethered to the crest of the ventricular septum, occurring in 50% to 70%. This type is commonly associated with Down syndrome. In type B (3%), the anterior bridging leaflet is not attached to the ventricular septum; rather, it is attached to an anomalous RV papillary muscle and is almost always associated with unbalanced AV canal with right dominance. In type C (30%), a free-floating anterior leaflet is attached to the anterior papillary muscle. This type is often seen in visceral heterotaxia and conotruncal malformations.

6. Additional cardiac anomalies include TOF (called "canal tet," occurring in 6% of patients), DORV with more than 50% overriding of the aorta (occurring in 6%), and transposition of the great arteries (occurring in 3%). Associated defects are rare in children with Down syndrome.

Clinical Manifestations

History

Failure to thrive, repeated respiratory infections, and signs of CHF are common.

Physical Examination (Fig. 12.18)

1. Infants with ECD are usually undernourished and have tachycardia and tachypnea (signs of CHF). This defect is common in infants with Down syndrome.

2. Hyperactive precordium with a systolic thrill at the lower left sternal border is common (shown as the area with dots in Fig. 12.18).

3. The S1 is accentuated. The S2 narrowly splits, and the P2 increases in intensity. A grade 3 to 4 of 6 holosystolic murmur is usually audible along the lower left sternal border. The systolic murmur may transmit well to the left axilla and be heard well at the apex when mitral regurgitation (MR) is significant. A mid-diastolic rumble may be present at the lower left sternal border or at the apex as a result of relative stenosis of the tricuspid or mitral valve.

4. Signs of CHF (e.g., hepatomegaly, gallop rhythm) may be present.

Electrocardiography

1. "Superior" QRS axis with the QRS axis between −40 and −150 degrees is characteristic of the defect (Fig. 12.19).

2. Most of the patients have a prolonged PR interval (first-degree AV block).

3. RVH or RBBB is present in all cases, and many patients have LVH, too.

Radiography

Cardiomegaly is always present and involves all four cardiac chambers. Pulmonary vascular markings are increased, and the main PA segment is prominent.

Echocardiography

Two-dimensional and Doppler echocardiographic studies allow imaging of all components of complete ECD and an assessment of the severity of these components. The following surgically important information can be gained: size of the ASD and VSD, size of the AV valve orifices, anatomy of leaflets, chordal attachment, relative and absolute size of the RV and LV (balance of the canal), and papillary muscle architecture (one vs two) in the LV.

1. The apical and subcostal four-chamber views are most useful in evaluating the anatomy and the functional significance of the defect. These views show both an ostium primum ASD and an inlet muscular VSD

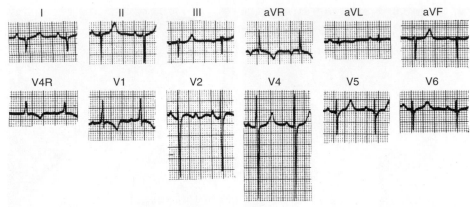

Fig. 12.19 Tracing from a 5-year-old boy with Down syndrome and complete atrioventricular canal. Note the "superior" QRS axis (–110 degrees) and right ventricular hypertrophy.

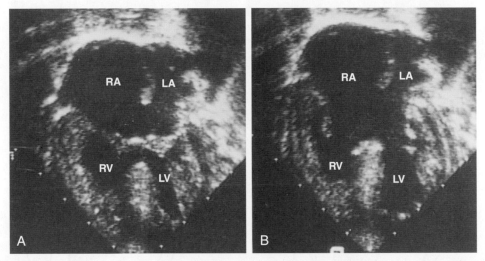

Fig. 12.20 Apical four-chamber views in systole (**A**) and diastole (**B**) from a patient with a complete endocardial cushion defect. In systole, an ostium primum defect and an inlet ventricular septal defect are imaged. The atrioventricular (AV) valve appears to be attached to the crest of the ventricular septum by chordae (type A). When the AV valve opens in diastole, a large deficiency in the center of the heart is visible. Note that there is a common AV valve, instead of two separate AV valves. *LA,* Left atrium; *LV,* left ventricle; *RA,* right atrium; *RV,* right ventricle. (From Snider AR, Serwer GA: *Echocardiography in Pediatric Heart Disease,* St. Louis, 1990, Mosby.)

(Fig. 12.20). Either the anterior bridging leaflet crosses the ventricular septum or the right and left AV valve leaflets can be seen at the same level from the crest of the ventricular septum. The full extent of the ASD and VSD can be imaged during systole when the common anterior leaflet is closed.

2. A combined use of the subcostal transducer position (i.e., ~45 degrees clockwise from a standard four-chamber view) and the parasternal short-axis examination may show a cleft in the mitral valve, the presence of bridging leaflets, the number of AV valve orifices (e.g., double orifice mitral valve), and the AV valve leaflets. These views may also image the abnormal position of the anterolateral papillary muscle, which is displaced posteriorly from its normal position, and the number (i.e., single or triple) of papillary muscles.

3. The subcostal "five-chamber" view may image a gooseneck deformity, which is characteristic of an angiocardiographic finding (Fig. 12.21).

4. In real time, the subcostal and apical four-chamber views can image the chordal attachment of the anterior bridging leaflet to the crest of the ventricular septum (type A), to the right side of the septum (type B), or to a papillary muscle at the apex of the RV or on its free wall (type C).

Natural History

1. Patients with complete ECD develop heart failure 1 to 2 months after birth, and recurrent pneumonia is common. Without surgical intervention, many of these patients die by the age of 2 to 3 years.

2. Survivors begin to develop pulmonary vascular obstructive disease in the latter half of the first year of life. Infants

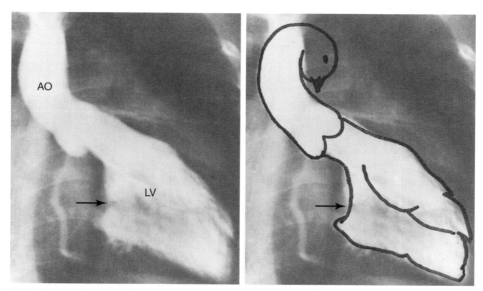

Fig. 12.21 Frontal view of a left ventriculogram of a patient with partial endocardial cushion defect showing a goose-neck deformity. The left ventricular outflow tract is elongated and narrowed. The *arrows* point to the mitral cleft. *AO,* Aorta; *LV,* left ventricle.

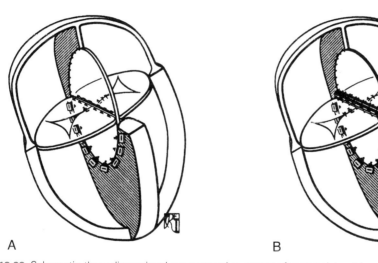

A   B

Fig. 12.22 Schematic three-dimensional reconstructive surgery for complete atrioventricular canal defect. **A,** Single-patch technique. **B,** Two-patch technique. (From Backer CL, Mavroudis C: Atrioventricular canal defect. In Mavroudis C, Backer CL [eds]: *Pediatric Cardiac Surgery,* Philadelphia, 2003, Mosby.)

with Down syndrome are particularly prone to the early development of pulmonary vascular obstructive disease during infancy. Therefore, surgery should be performed during infancy.

Management
Medical

1. In small infants with CHF, anticongestive management with diuretics and ACE inhibitors should be started. Digoxin may also be used (see Chapter 27).
2. Nutrition should be optimized.

Surgical

Indications. The presence of complete ECD indicates the need for surgery because an important hemodynamic derangement is usually present. Most of these infants have

CHF that is unresponsive to medical therapy, and some have elevated pulmonary vascular resistance.

Timing. Although timing varies among institutions and with the hemodynamics of the defect, most centers perform the repair at 2 to 4 months of age. Early surgical repair is especially important for infants with Down syndrome with complete ECD because of their known tendency to develop early pulmonary vascular obstructive disease.

Procedures. **Palliative.** Banding of the PA in early infancy is no longer recommended unless other associated abnormalities make complete repair a high-risk procedure, such as those with "unbalanced" AV canal.

Corrective. Given two ventricles of suitable size and no additional defects, closure of the primum ASD and inlet VSD and construction of two separate and competent AV valves are carried out under cardiopulmonary bypass, deep hypothermia, or both. Some surgeons use a single patch to close the ASD and VSD and reconstruction of the left AV valve as a bileaflet valve; others use a two-patch technique, one patch for the VSD and a second for the ASD (Fig. 12.22). The left AV valve is allowed to persist as a trileaflet structure. A schematic drawing of the surgery is shown in Fig. 12.22. This figure illustrates the complexity of the anatomy of the AV canal. Mitral valve replacement may become necessary in a few patients.

Patients with an unbalanced AV canal (with hypoplasia of RV or LV) may be treated by an earlier PA banding and later by a modified Fontan operation.

Mortality. The mortality rate is about 2.5%. The survival rate is the same for patients with and without Down syndrome. Factors that increase the surgical risk are young age, severe AV valve regurgitation, hypoplasia of the LV, increased and fixed pulmonary vascular resistance, and severe preoperative symptoms. Other defects (e.g., double-orifice mitral valve, single left-sided papillary muscle, additional muscular VSD) increase the surgical risk. The hospital mortality rate for complete ECD and TOF ("canal tet") is around 10%.

Complications
1. MR becomes persistent or worsens 10% of the time.
2. Sinus node dysfunction resulting in bradyarrhythmias may occur.
3. Although complete heart block occurs rarely (in <5% of patients), it occurs more frequently when mitral valve replacement is required (up to 20% of patients).
4. Postoperative arrhythmias occur and are usually supraventricular.

Special Situations
1. Because of the early development of pulmonary vascular obstructive disease in patients with Down syndrome and complete ECD, complete repair should be performed within the first 3 to 6 months of age. Down syndrome itself is not a risk factor.
2. Patients with "unbalanced" AV canal with severe hypoplasia of the LV and low PA pressure may receive a combination of the Damus-Kaye-Stansel operation (similar to Fig. 14.62) and a Fontan-type operation. The proximal PA is anastomosed end to side to the ascending aorta, and systemic venous return is channeled to the right PA, bypassing the RV.
3. In patients with TOF and complete ECD (i.e., "canal tet") who are severely cyanotic, a systemic-to-PA shunt is carried out during infancy. A complete repair is done between 2 and 4 years of age.
4. Parachute deformity of the mitral valve may result in an obstructed mitral orifice. If there is a significant MR, valve replacement may be required.
5. Double-orifice mitral valve (found in 4%) is usually left alone. Incision of the valve may create more problems with MR.

Postoperative Follow-up
1. An office evaluation should be given every 6 months to 1 year.

2. Medications (e.g., diuretics, ACE inhibitors, digoxin) may be required if residual hemodynamic abnormalities are present.
3. Some restriction of activities may be necessary if significant MR or other complications exist.

PARTIAL ENDOCARDIAL CUSHION DEFECT

Prevalence
Partial ECD (partial AV canal defect or ostium primum ASD) occurs in 1% to 2% of all CHDs, which is considerably less than the prevalence of secundum ASD.

Pathology
1. In partial ECD, there is a defect in the lower part of the atrial septum near the AV valves without an interventricular communication (see Fig. 12.1). The anterior and posterior bridging leaflets are fused by a connecting tongue to form separate right and left AV orifices (see Fig. 12.16). There are "clefts" in the septal leaflets of the mitral and tricuspid valves. The conjoined leaflets are displaced into the ventricle and are usually firmly attached to the crest of the ventricular septum. The aortic valve and AV valves are distanced from one another, which accounts for the characteristic "goose-neck" deformity in angiocardiograms (see Fig. 12.21).
2. Less common forms of partial ECD include common atrium, VSD of the inlet septum (i.e., AV canal-type VSD), and isolated cleft of the mitral valve. A common atrium, in which the atrial septum is virtually absent, is either a characteristic lesion in patients with the Ellis-van Creveld syndrome or a component of complex cyanotic heart defects such as those associated with asplenia or polysplenia syndrome.
3. Occasional associated anomalies include secundum ASD and persistent left SVC that drains into the coronary sinus.

Clinical Manifestations

History
1. Patients with ostium primum ASD are usually asymptomatic during childhood.
2. History of symptoms such as dyspnea, easy fatigability, recurrent respiratory infections, and growth retardation may be present early in life if associated with major MR or common atrium.

Physical Examination
1. Cardiac findings are the same as those of secundum ASD (see Fig. 12.2), with the exception of a regurgitant systolic murmur of MR (owing to a cleft mitral valve), which may be present at the apex.
2. Mild cyanosis and clubbing may be present in patients with a common atrium.

Electrocardiography
1. "Superior" QRS axis with the QRS axis ranging from −30 to −150 degrees is characteristic of the condition (see Fig. 12.19).

2. RVH or RBBB (with rsR' pattern in V1) is present, as in secundum ASD.
3. First-degree AV block (i.e., prolonged PR interval) is present in about 50% of cases.

Radiography

The radiography findings are the same as those of a secundum ASD (see Fig. 12.4), except for enlargement of the LA and LV when MR is significant. A characteristic "goose-neck" deformity is seen on a left ventriculogram (see Fig. 12.21).

Echocardiography

1. 2D and Doppler echocardiography allows accurate diagnosis of primum ASD. The defect is in the lower atrial septum (see Fig. 12.5). No visible or Doppler-detectable VSD is present. The septal portions of the AV valves insert at the same level on the crest of the ventricular septum.
2. A cleft in the anterior leaflet of the mitral valve is commonly imaged (which is directed toward the inlet septum or 9 o'clock direction in the parasternal short-axis view). (In case of "isolated mitral cleft," the cleft is directed toward the LVOT or 11 o'clock direction in the short-axis view.)
3. Rare abnormalities of the mitral valve include double-orifice mitral valve and parachute mitral valve.
4. The atrial septum may be completely absent (common atrium) in patients with Ellis-van Creveld syndrome.
5. Color-flow and Doppler studies are useful in the detection of stenosis or regurgitation of the AV valve and in the assessment of the RV and PA pressures.

Natural History

1. Spontaneous closure of the defect does not occur.
2. CHF may develop in childhood earlier than with secundum ASD. CHF is related to major MR or other associated defects.
3. Pulmonary hypertension (i.e., pulmonary vascular obstructive disease) develops in adulthood.

4. Arrhythmias occur in 20% of patients.

Management
Medical

1. No exercise restriction is indicated
2. Anticongestive therapy with diuretics and ACE inhibitors may be indicated for some patients.
3. Device closure of the defect cannot be done.

Surgical

Indications and Timing. The presence of a partial AV canal (or primum ASD) is an indication for surgical repair. Elective surgery can be performed in asymptomatic children between 2 and 4 years of age. Surgery can be performed earlier in infants with CHF, failure to thrive, MR, or a common atrium.

Procedure. Under cardiopulmonary bypass, the primum ASD is closed and the cleft mitral and tricuspid valves are reconstructed. Some surgeons leave the mitral valve as a tri-leaflet valve (without suturing the cleft) by performing various mitral annuloplasty. Recently, minimally invasive cardiac surgical techniques with smaller skin incisions have become popular, especially for female patients (discussed under Atrial Septal Defect).

Mortality. The surgical mortality rate is approximately 2.5%. Risk factors include the presence of CHF or cyanosis, failure to thrive, and moderate to severe MR.

Complications

1. Reoperation is needed in about 15% of the patients who have residual or worsening MR.
2. Atrial or junctional (nodal) arrhythmias occasionally occur.
3. Complete heart block rarely results and requires a permanent cardiac pacemaker.
4. Although rare, subaortic stenosis can develop after surgery. Subaortic stenosis develops more frequently after repair of partial ECD than complete ECD.

Postoperative Follow-up

1. Usually no restriction in activity is indicated.
2. Sinus node dysfunction may require permanent pacemaker therapy.

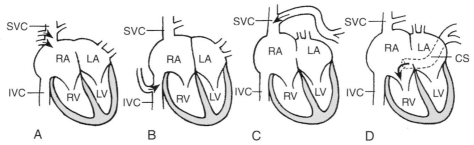

Fig. 12.23 Common types of partial anomalous pulmonary venous return. **A,** The right pulmonary veins drain anomalously to the superior vena cava (SVC). Sinus venosus atrial septal defect (ASD) is usually present. **B,** The right lower pulmonary vein drains anomalously into the inferior vena cava (IVC), usually without an associated ASD. **C,** The left pulmonary veins drain into the left innominate vein. **D,** The left pulmonary veins drain into the coronary sinus (CS). **LA,** Left atrium; **LV,** left ventricle; **RA,** right atrium; **RV,** right ventricle.

3. Periodic echo evaluation for the development of subaortic stenosis and for worsening of MR should be performed.

PARTIAL ANOMALOUS PULMONARY VENOUS RETURN

Prevalence

Partial anomalous pulmonary venous return occurs in fewer than 1% of all CHDs.

Pathology

1. One or more (but not all) pulmonary veins drain into the RA or its venous tributaries such as the SVC, IVC, coronary sinus, and left innominate vein. The right pulmonary veins are involved twice as often as the left pulmonary veins.
2. The right pulmonary veins may drain into the SVC, which is often associated with a sinus venosus defect (Fig. 12.23A), or drain into the IVC (Fig. 12.23B) in association with an intact atrial septum and bronchopulmonary sequestration (see scimitar syndrome in Chapter 15).
3. The left pulmonary veins either drain into the left innominate vein (Fig. 12.23C) or into the coronary sinus (Fig. 12.23D). ASD is usually present with anomalous drainage of the left pulmonary veins.

Pathophysiology

1. Hemodynamic alterations are similar to those in ASD. Pulmonary blood flow increases as a result of recirculation through the lungs.
2. The magnitude of the pulmonary recirculation is determined by the number of anomalous pulmonary veins, the presence and size of the ASD, and the pulmonary vascular resistance.

Clinical Manifestations

History

Children with PAPVR are usually asymptomatic.

Physical Examination

1. Cardiac findings are similar to those of ASD (see Fig. 12.2).
2. When associated with ASD, the S2 is split widely and fixed. When the atrial septum is intact, the S2 is normal. A grade 2 to 3 of 6 midsystolic murmur is present at the upper left sternal border. A mid-diastolic rumble, resulting from relative tricuspid stenosis, may be present.

Electrocardiography

Right ventricular hypertrophy, RBBB, or a normal ECG may be seen.

Radiography

The findings are similar to those of secundum ASD (see Fig. 12.4).

1. Cardiomegaly involving the RA and RV, prominence of the PA segment, and increased pulmonary vascularity are all present.

2. Occasionally, a dilated SVC, a crescent-shaped vertical shadow in the right lower lung (scimitar syndrome) or a distended vertical vein may suggest the site of anomalous drainage.

Echocardiography

The diagnosis of PAPVR requires a high index of suspicion. A systematic attempt to visualize each pulmonary vein should be made during any routine echo studies.

1. The inability to visualize all four pulmonary veins in the presence of mild dilatation of the RA and RV strongly suggests the diagnosis of PAPVR, especially in the presence of a demonstrable ASD.
2. PAPVR is frequently found in patients with ASD of any type and in those with persistent left SVC.
3. In sinus venosus defect, the chance of anomalous drainage of the right upper pulmonary vein is high.

   Cardiac Magnetic Resonance Imaging. Cardiac magnetic resonance imaging can make correct diagnosis of partial anomalous pulmonary venous return, alternative to the invasive cardiac catheterization with exposure to radiation.

Natural History

1. Cyanosis and exertional dyspnea may develop during the third and fourth decades of life. This results from pulmonary hypertension and pulmonary vascular obstructive disease.
2. Pulmonary infections are common in patients with anomalous drainage of the right pulmonary veins to the IVC.

Management

Medical

1. No medical treatment is needed when asymptomatic.
2. Exercise restriction is not required.

Surgical

Indications and Timing. Indications for surgery include a significant left-to-right shunt with a Q_p/Q_s ratio of greater than 2:1 and, if the anatomy is uncomplicated, a ratio of greater than 1.5:1. Surgery is indicated in patients with scimitar syndrome with severe hypoplasia of the right lung even with a Q_p/Q_s ratio less than 2:1. Surgery is carried out between the age of 2 and 5 years. Isolated single-lobe anomaly without an ASD is usually not corrected.

Procedures. Surgical correction is carried out under cardiopulmonary bypass. The procedure to be performed depends on the site of the anomalous drainage.

1. **To the SVC.** A tunnel is created between the anomalous vein and the ASD through the SVC and the RA by using a Teflon or pericardial patch. A plastic or pericardial gusset is placed in the SVC to prevent obstruction to the SVC.
2. **To the IVC.** In scimitar syndrome, the resection of the involved lobe(s) may be indicated without connecting the anomalous vein to the heart. When the anomalous venous drainage is an isolated lesion, the vein is reimplanted to the RA, and an intraatrial tunnel is created to drain into the LA.

3. **To the left innominate vein.** The anomalous left pulmonary vein is anastomosed to the base of the amputated left atrial appendage.

4. **To the coronary sinus.** This defect is repaired in the same manner as for TAPVR to the coronary sinus (see Fig. 14.33C).

Mortality. Surgical mortality occurs less than 1% of the time.

Complications

1. SVC obstruction for those patients with anomalous drainage into the SVC.
2. Postoperative arrhythmias (usually supraventricular) occur.

Postoperative Follow-up

1. An examination should be done every 1 to 2 years or at longer intervals.
2. No restriction in activities is indicated.

Obstructive Lesions

Lesions that produce obstruction to ventricular outflow such as pulmonary stenosis (PS), aortic stenosis (AS), and coarctation of the aorta (COA) are discussed in this chapter.

PULMONARY STENOSIS

Prevalence

Isolated PS occurs in 4% to 8% of all congenital heart defects (CHDs). PS is often associated with other CHDs, such as tetralogy of Fallot (TOF), single ventricle, and others.

Pathology

1. PS may be valvular, subvalvular (infundibular), supravalvular, or within the right ventricular (RV) cavity (i.e., "double-chambered RV").
2. In *valvular PS,* the pulmonary valve is thickened, with fused or absent commissures and a small orifice (Fig. 13.1A). The RV is usually normal in size in children with PS. In neonates with critical PS (with a nearly atretic valve), right-sided structures, including the RV, tricuspid valve, right ventricular outflow tract (RVOT), and pulmonary artery, are commonly underdeveloped. The presence of a hypoplastic TV is an important predictor of

operative mortality. Dysplastic valves (consisting of thickened, irregular, immobile tissue and a variably small pulmonary valve annulus) are frequently seen with Noonan's syndrome.
3. Isolated *infundibular PS* is rare; it is usually associated with a large ventricular septal defect (VSD), as seen in TOF (see Fig. 13.1B).
4. Aberrant hypertrophied muscular bands (running between the ventricular septum and the anterior wall) divide the RV cavity into a proximal high-pressure chamber and a distal low-pressure chamber (double-chambered RV). A "dimple" in the ordinarily smooth RV surface is found during surgery (see Chapter 15).
5. Supravalvular PS (or stenosis of the pulmonary arteries), isolated or in association with other CHDs, occurs in 2% to 3% of all patients with CHD. The stenosis may be single, involving the main pulmonary artery (PA) (see Fig. 13.1) or either of its branches, or multiple, involving both the main and several smaller peripheral PA branches (not shown). Commonly associated defects are pulmonary valve stenosis, VSD, and TOF. Peripheral PA stenosis is often seen in association with congenital syndromes, such as Williams syndrome, Noonan's syndrome, Alagille

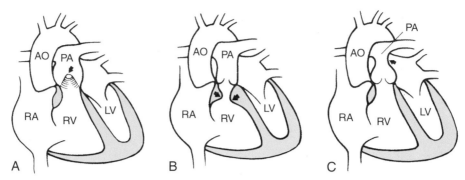

Fig. 13.1 Anatomic types of pulmonary stenoses (PSs). **A,** Valvular stenosis. **B,** Infundibular stenosis. **C,** Supravalvular PS (or stenosis of the main pulmonary artery [PA]). Abnormalities are indicated by *arrows*. *AO,* Aorta; *LV,* left ventricle; *RA,* right atrium; *RV,* right ventricle.

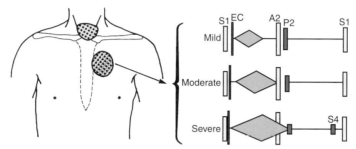

Fig. 13.2 Cardiac findings of pulmonary valve stenosis. Abnormal sounds are shown in *black*. *Dots* represent areas with systolic thrill. *EC,* Ejection click.

syndrome, Ehlers-Danlos syndrome, and Silver-Russell syndrome or congenital rubella syndrome. PA stenosis is discussed further in Chapter 15.

Clinical Manifestations

History

1. Children with mild PS are completely asymptomatic (and restriction of activity is not necessary in children with this condition, except in cases of severe PS).
2. In patients with moderate stenosis, exertional dyspnea and easy fatigability may be present.
3. With severe stenosis (with pressure gradient >70 mm Hg), exertional chest pain or syncope may be present (and even sudden death may occur with strenuous exercise).
4. Newborns with critical PS may present with poor feeding, tachypnea, and cyanosis.

Physical Examination (Fig. 13.2)

1. Most patients are acyanotic and well developed. Newborns with critical PS (who have hypoplastic RV and a right-to-left atrial shunt) are cyanotic and tachypneic.
2. A right ventricular tap and a systolic thrill may be present at the upper left sternal border (and occasionally in the suprasternal notch).
3. A systolic ejection click is present at the upper left sternal border only with valvular stenosis. The S2 may split widely, and the P2 may be diminished in intensity. An ejection-type systolic murmur (grade 2–5 of 6) is best audible at the upper left sternal border, and it transmits

well to the back, too. The louder and longer the murmur, the more severe the stenosis is.
4. Hepatomegaly may be present if congestive heart failure (CHF) develops.
5. In newborns with critical PS, cyanosis may be present (caused by a right-to-left atrial shunt), and signs of CHF with hepatomegaly and peripheral vasoconstriction may be found.
6. In patients with peripheral PA stenosis, a midsystolic murmur in the pulmonary valve area is well transmitted to the axillae and back. Occasionally, a continuous murmur is audible over the involved lung field.

Electrocardiography

1. The electrocardiogram (ECG) findings are normal in mild cases.
2. Right-axis deviation (RAD) and right ventricular hypertrophy (RVH) are present in moderate PS.
3. Right atrial hypertrophy (RAH) and RVH with "strain" may be seen in severe PS.
4. Neonates with critical PS may show left ventricular hypertrophy (LVH) because of a hypoplastic RV and relatively large left ventricle (LV).

Radiography

1. Heart size is usually normal, but the main PA segment may be prominent with valvular stenosis (caused by poststenotic dilatation) (Fig. 13.3). Cardiomegaly is present only if CHF develops.

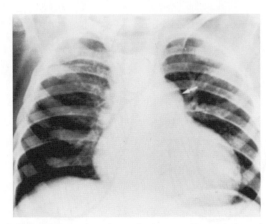

Fig. 13.3 Posteroanterior view of chest radiograph in pulmonary valve stenosis. Note a marked poststenotic dilatation *(arrow)* and normal pulmonary vascularity. (Courtesy Dr. Ewell Clarke, San Antonio, TX.)

2. Pulmonary vascular markings are usually normal but may decrease with severe PS.
3. In neonates with critical PS, lung fields are oligemic with a varying degree of cardiomegaly.

Echocardiography

1. Two-dimensional (2D) echocardiography in the parasternal short-axis view (see Fig. 5.2) shows thick pulmonary valve cusps with restricted systolic motion (doming). The subcostal long-axis view (see Fig. 5.5) may show similar findings. The size of the pulmonary valve annulus can be estimated. The main PA is often dilated (poststenotic dilatation).
2. The Doppler study can estimate the pressure gradient across the stenotic valve by the simplified Bernoulli equation. Multiple echocardiographic views, including parasternal short-axis and subcostal long-axis views, should be used to obtain the maximum flow velocity. The instantaneous pressure gradient estimated by Doppler echo is slightly greater than the peak-to-peak systolic pressure gradient obtained by cardiac catheterization. The severity of PS (by Doppler gradient) may be classified as follows.
   a. Mild: a pressure gradient less than 35 to 40 mm Hg (or RV systolic pressure <50% of the LV pressure)
   b. Moderate: a valve pressure gradient 40 to 70 mm Hg (or RV pressure 50%–75% of the LV pressure)
   c. Severe: a pressure gradient greater than 70 mm Hg (or RV pressure ≥75% LV pressure)
3. Dysplastic valves are characterized by a noticeably thickened and immobile leaflet and hypoplasia of the pulmonary valve annulus.
4. In neonates, Doppler pressure gradient may underestimate the severity of PS because the PA pressure may be higher than normal, especially in those with patent ductus arteriosus (PDA) with a left-to-right shunt.

Natural History

1. The severity of stenosis is usually not progressive in mild PS. For example, more than 95% of patients with an initial Doppler gradient less than 25 mm Hg did not need operation over a 25-year period. The majority of the patients with mild PS (<35 mm Hg) do well without intervention.
2. In moderate or severe PS, the severity tends to progress with age.
3. CHF may develop in patients with severe stenosis. Sudden death is possible in patients with severe stenosis during heavy physical activities.
4. Without appropriate management, most neonates with critical PS die (see Management).

Management
Medical and Balloon Valvuloplasty

1. **Newborns with critical PS.** These cyanotic neonates (with severe pulmonary valve stenosis, hypoplastic RV, and a right-to-left atrial shunt) require emergency treatment to reduce mortality.
   a. These babies may temporarily improve with prostaglandin E_1 (PGE_1) infusion, which reopens the ductus arteriosus, and other supportive measures.
   b. Balloon valvuloplasty is the procedure of choice in critically ill neonates. Immediate reduction in pressure gradient can be achieved in more than 90% of these neonates. Complications of the balloon procedure are more common than in older patients, with a mortality rate of up to 3%, a major complication rate of 3.5%, and a minor complication rate of 15%. About 15% of the patients require reintervention (either repeat valvuloplasty or surgery for infundibular stenosis or dysplastic valve) at a later time.
   c. Even dysplastic valves appear to mature after the balloon procedure.
   d. Some of these infants are not able to maintain effective forward flow through the pulmonary valve because of noncompliant or hypoplastic RV. Some of them may need one of the following: (1) a prolonged PG infusion, (2) ductal stenting, or (3) systemic-to-pulmonary shunt surgery.
2. **Balloon valvuloplasty.** Balloon valvuloplasty is the procedure of choice for the valvular stenosis at all ages.
   a. Indications: Indications for the procedure may include the following.
      1) A resting pressure gradient of greater than 40 mm Hg with the patient sedated in the catheterization laboratory
      2) If the catheterization gradient is 30 to 39 mm Hg, the balloon procedure may be reasonable.
      3) Symptoms attributable to PS with a catheterization gradient greater than 30 mm Hg. The symptoms may include angina, syncope or presyncope, and exertional dyspnea.
      4) The procedure is useful and reasonable in patients with dysplastic pulmonary valve, as commonly seen

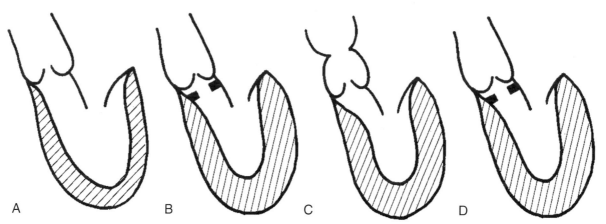

Fig. 13.4 Anatomic types of aortic stenoses. **A,** Normal. **B,** Valvular stenosis. **C,** Supravalvular stenosis. **D,** Subaortic stenosis (discrete type). **E,** Idiopathic hypertrophic subaortic stenosis (this condition is discussed in Chapter 18).

in Noonan's syndrome. It has a lower success rate with the valvuloplasty (65%). If balloon valvuloplasty is unsuccessful, surgery is indicated.

b. Results: The balloon procedure carries an extremely low risk, is painless, is less costly than surgery, and shortens hospital stay (see Chapter 7 for the description of the procedure and Fig. 7.2 for an angiography of the valvuloplasty).

1) A good outcome is achieved in 85% of patients with valvular stenosis. Restenosis after balloon dilatation is extremely rare.

2) Pulmonary regurgitation (PR) after balloon dilatation is common, occurring in 10% to 40% of patients. PR is usually well tolerated, although rarely some of these patients may become candidates for pulmonary valve implantation. Usual balloon sizes used are 120% to 140% of the angiographically measured pulmonary valve annulus.

3) After relief of severe PS (either by balloon or surgery), hypertrophied dynamic infundibulum may cause a persistent pressure gradient, with rare occurrences of fatal outcome ("suicidal right ventricle"). Propranolol may be given to reduce hyperdynamic infundibular obstruction. The reduction of this gradient occurs gradually over weeks.

3. Restriction of activity is not necessary in children with this condition, except in cases of severe PS (Doppler gradient >70 mm Hg).

Surgical

Indications and Timing

1. Surgical valvotomy should be limited to patients with more complex lesions or those in whom balloon procedure is contraindicated or failed.

2. Other types of obstructions (e.g., infundibular stenosis, anomalous RV muscle bundle) with significant pressure gradients require surgery on an elective basis.

3. If balloon valvuloplasty is unsuccessful or unavailable, infants with critical PS and CHF require surgery on an urgent basis.

Procedure

1. Through a midsternal incision, pulmonary valvotomy is performed for pulmonary valve stenosis under cardiopulmonary bypass. The approach is through the PA. Neonates with critical PS may require a transventricular valvotomy or the insertion of a transannular patch (or both) while receiving PGE1 infusion. If severe infundibular hypoplasia is present, a systemic-to-PA shunt is also performed.

2. Dysplastic valves often require complete excision of the valves. Simple valvotomy may be ineffective.

3. Infundibular stenosis requires resection of the infundibular muscle and patch widening of the right ventricular outflow tract.

4. Stenosis at the main PA level requires patch widening of the narrow portion.

5. Anomalous muscle bundles require surgical resection.

Mortality. Surgical mortality occurs in fewer than 1% of older children. The rate is about 10% in critically ill infants.

AORTIC STENOSIS

Prevalence

Left ventricular outflow tract obstruction (LVOTO), which includes stenosis at, below, or above the aortic valve, represents up to 10% of all CHD. Valvular AS is the most frequent (80%–85%) followed by subvalvular stenosis (~15%) and supravalvular stenosis (<5%). Among valvular stenoses, bicuspid aortic valve (BAV) is the most common type (but many of them are undiagnosed until adulthood). Aortic valve stenosis occurs more often in males (male-to-female ratio of 4:1).

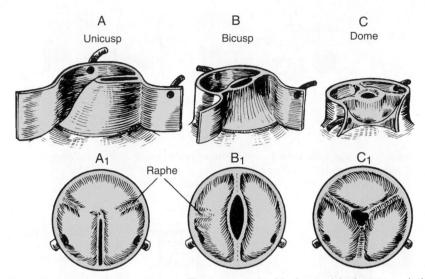

Fig. 13.5 Anatomic types of aortic valve stenoses. The *top row* is the side view, and the *bottom row* is the view as seen in surgery during aortotomy. **A,** Unicuspid aortic valve. **B,** Bicuspid aortic valve. **C,** Stenosis of a tricuspid aortic valve. (From Goor DA, Lillehei CW: *Congenital Malformations of the Heart*, New York, 1975, Grune & Stratton.)

Pathology

1. Stenosis may be at the valvular, subvalvular, or supravalvular level (Fig. 13.4).
2. Valvular AS may be caused by a BAV, a unicuspid aortic valve, or stenosis of the tricuspid (or tricommissural) aortic valve (see Fig. 13.5).
   a. By far the most common type of aortic valve stenosis is BAV, accounting for 75% (see Fig. 13.5B). The diagnosis of this condition has markedly increased since the introduction of echocardiography in clinical practice. More than 50% of patients with BAV have aortic dilatation, which is now considered primary aortopathy (rather than the result of hemodynamic abnormality).
   b. Much less common is the unicuspid valve with one lateral attachment (see Fig. 13.5A).
   c. A valve that has three unseparated cusps with a stenotic central orifice is the least common form (see Fig. 13.5C).
3. Symptomatic neonates with so called "critical neonatal aortic valve stenosis" have primitive, myxomatous valve tissue, with a pinhole opening. The aortic valve ring and ascending aorta are almost always hypoplastic. Hypoplasia of the mitral valve, LV cavity, or LV outflow tract and a VSD are also frequently found, often requiring one ventricular repair (Norwood operation followed by Fontan operation).
4. Supravalvular AS is an annular constriction at the upper margin of the sinus of Valsalva (see Fig. 13.4C). Occasionally, the ascending aorta is diffusely hypoplastic. This is often associated with Williams syndrome (which includes mental retardation, characteristic facies, and multiple pulmonary artery stenosis).
5. Subvalvular (subaortic) stenosis may be in the form of (a) discrete narrowing or (b) long tunnel-like fibromuscular narrowing of the LV outflow tract.
   a. Discrete stenosis occurs more often than tunnel stenosis and it accounts for about 10% of all AS cases. It may be

(a) simple membranous ridge or collar (more common) or (b) fibromuscular ridge with or without membrane.
   1) Two thirds of the patients have associated cardiac lesions, such as VSD, PDA, or COA.
   2) In one third of patients, the stenosis is isolated; familial isolated subaortic membrane has been reported.
   3) In some patients, there is history of surgical intervention, such as membranous VSD closure or PA banding (9 months to 8 years before the development of the membrane).
   b. Tunnel-like subaortic stenosis is often associated with hypoplasia of the ascending aorta and aortic valve ring, as well as thickened aortic valve leaflets. It is usually associated with other LV anomalies, including Shone complex (comprising supramitral ring, parachute mitral valve, subaortic stenosis, and COA).
6. Additional information on BAV
   a. BAV is the most common cardiac malformation with prevalence of 0.4% to 2.25% of the general population (Hoffman, 2002). Most patients with BAV develop stenosis or incompetence after 40 years of age (and thus are not recorded in pediatric population), or they are diagnosed at the postmortem examination.
   b. Concomitant aortic dilatation is an important aspect of BAV. It was initially thought to be a sole consequence of hemodynamic effects, but many studies have pointed out that the dilatation results from a combination of intrinsic aortic wall abnormalities (the genetic theory) and less importantly, hemodynamic changes induced by BAV. Furthermore, aortic dilatation can extend from the aortic annulus to the proximal aortic arch. As a result, some view BAV as a continuum of a disease process affecting the entire aortic root and ascending aorta.

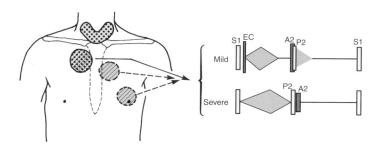

Fig. 13.6 Cardiac findings of aortic valve stenosis. Abnormal sounds are indicated in *black*. Systolic thrill may be present in areas with dots. *EC,* Ejection click.

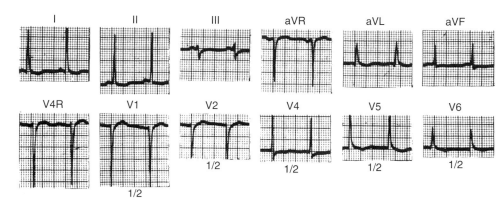

Fig. 13.7 Tracing from a 7-year-old boy with severe aortic stenosis. It shows left ventricular hypertrophy, with a probable "strain" pattern.

c. The prevalence of primary aortic dilatation (aortopathy) is 53% in BAV patients, and 32% of the first-degree relatives have aortic dilatation (Biner, 2009).

d. There is adequate evidence that BAV is an inheritable disorder (i.e., autosomal dominant disease with incomplete penetrance) with a male-to-female ratio of 3:1.

e. Family studies demonstrate the occurrence of a BAV in approximately 9% of first-degree relatives of affected individual. Many patients with BAV have accelerated degradation of the aortic media and a loss of elastic tissue.

Clinical Manifestations

History

1. Neonates with critical or severe stenosis of the aortic valve may develop signs of hypoperfusion or respiratory distress caused by pulmonary edema within days to weeks after birth.

2. Most children with mild to moderate AS are asymptomatic. Occasionally, exercise intolerance may be present. Almost all children with BAV are asymptomatic.

3. Exertional chest pain, easy fatigability, or syncope may occur in children with a severe degree of obstruction.

Physical Examination (Fig. 13.6)

1. Infants and children with AS are acyanotic and are normally developed. Children with BAV may have a completely normal physical examination.

2. Except for neonates with critical AS, blood pressure is normal in most patients, but a narrow pulse pressure is present in severe AS. Patients with supravalvular AS may have a higher systolic pressure in the right arm than in the left (caused by the jet of stenosis directed into the innominate artery, the so-called Coanda effect).

3. A systolic thrill may be palpable at the upper right sternal border, in the suprasternal notch, or over the carotid arteries.

4. An ejection click may be heard with valvular AS. The S2 splits either normally or a bit narrowly. The S2 may split paradoxically in severe AS (see Fig. 13.6). A harsh, grade 2 to 4 of 6, midsystolic murmur is best heard at the second right or left intercostal space, with good transmission to the neck and apex. A high-pitched, early diastolic decrescendo murmur, which results from aortic regurgitation (AR), may be audible in patients with BAV and in those with discrete subvalvular stenosis.

5. Peculiar "elfin facies," mental retardation, and friendly "cocktail party" personalities may be associated with supravalvular AS (e.g., Williams syndrome).

6. Newborns with critical AS may develop signs of reduced peripheral perfusion (with weak and thready pulses; pale, cool skin; and slow capillary refill) triggered by ductal constriction. The clinical picture may mimic overwhelming sepsis with low cardiac output. The heart murmur may be absent or faint but becomes louder when CHF improves.

Electrocardiography

In mild cases, the ECG is normal. LVH with or without strain pattern may be present in severe cases (Fig. 13.7). Correlation of the severity of AS and the ECG abnormalities is relatively poor.

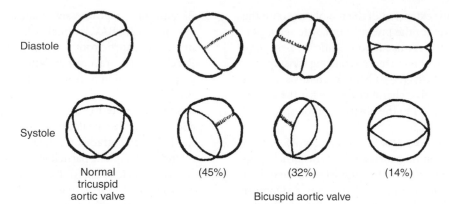

Diastole

Systole

Normal
tricuspid
aortic valve   (45%)   (32%)   (14%)

Bicuspid aortic valve

Fig. 13.8 Diagram of parasternal short-axis scan showing normal tricuspid *(left column)* and bicuspid aortic valves *(three right columns)* during diastole and systole. Three nearly equal-sized aortic cusps are imaged in a normal aortic valve, which opens widely during systole. The systolic opening pattern distinguishes a raphe from a commissure. With a bicuspid aortic valve, various commissural orientations are imaged. The most common pattern demonstrates commissures at the 4 or 5 o'clock and the 9 or 10 o'clock positions, with raphe at the 1 or 2 o'clock position (46%). (Modified from Brandenburg RO Jr, Tajik AJ, Edwards WD, et al: Accuracy of 2-dimensional echocardiographic diagnosis of congenitally bicuspid aortic valve: echocardiographic-anatomic correlation in 115 patients, *Am J Cardiol* 51:1469–1473, 1983.)

Radiography

1. The heart size is usually normal in children, but a dilated ascending aorta or a prominent aortic knob may be seen occasionally in valvular AS, resulting from poststenotic dilatation.
2. Significant cardiomegaly does not develop unless CHF occurs later in life or if AR becomes substantial.
3. Newborns with critical AS show generalized cardiomegaly with pulmonary venous congestion.

Echocardiography

Valvular Aortic Stenosis

1. The parasternal short-axis view of the 2D echocardiography provides optimal assessment of the morphology of the aortic valve. Normal aortic valves are tricuspid, with three cusps of approximately equal size. In diastole the normal aortic cusp margins form a Y pattern (Fig. 13.8), which opens widely during systole. In systole, a BAV appears as a noncircular (i.e., football-shaped) orifice (see Fig. 13.8). Fusion between the right and left coronary cusps is the most common type (occurring up to 70%–85% according to a recent echocardiographic study). Stenosis of the tricuspid aortic valve appears as a heavy Y pattern in diastole and as a small, centrally located orifice in systole, with three thickened commissures distinctly visible. A unicommissural aortic valve, which is seen often in infants with critical AS, is seen as a circular orifice positioned eccentrically within the aortic root and without visible distinct cusps.
2. In the parasternal long-axis view of the 2D echo is the preferred view for measurement of the valve annulus and aortic root dimensions. Doming of the thick aortic valve with restriction to the opening is seen in systole. Reverse doming during diastole commonly occurs in the unicuspid valve, occurs less frequently in the bicuspid valve, and does not occur in the tricuspid aortic valve.

3. Doppler pressure gradient is best obtained from the apical five-chamber view with the cursor placed distal to the stenotic aortic valve in the sinus of Valsalva.
4. Doppler studies can estimate the severity of the stenosis by using the simplified Bernoulli equation (see Chapter 5). The Doppler-derived gradients (i.e., peak instantaneous gradient) are often (~20%) higher than the peak-to-peak systolic pressure gradient obtained during cardiac catheterization. The mean Doppler gradient correlates better with peak-to-peak gradient obtained during cardiac catheterization. However, multiple groups have demonstrated that Doppler-based estimates of disease severity are a reliable means of predicting the need for intervention in pediatric patients, and the 2014 American College of Cardiology (ACC)/American Heart Association (AHA) guidelines used Doppler-derived peak velocities and mean gradient to define disease severity (Nishimura et al, 2014). The severity of the stenosis is defined by a peak velocity across the aortic valve and a mean Doppler gradient across the valve as follows.
   a. Mild: peak velocity of 2.0 to 2.9 msec (or mean Doppler gradient ≤20 mm Hg)
   b. Moderate: peak velocity of 3.0–3.9 msec (or mean Doppler gradient between 20 and 39 mm Hg).
   c. Severe: peak velocity of 4.0 msec or greater (or mean Doppler gradient of ≥40 mm Hg) (or aortic valve area of ≤1.0 cm^2 or indexed valve area ≤0.6 cm^2/m^2)

Subvalvular Aortic Stenosis

1. The type of subaortic stenosis is best imaged in the parasternal long-axis view, apical long-axis view, and apical "five-chamber" view just beneath the aortic valve.
2. One should note whether the stenosis is (a) membrane, (b) fibromuscular ridge, or (c) diffuse tunnel-like fibromuscular narrowing (tunnel stenosis).
3. For the membranous type, one should note (a) the length of the membrane, (b) pressure gradient across the obstruction, (c) the distance of the membrane from the hinge point

of the aortic valve, (d) extension of the membrane onto the aortic or mitral valve, (e) the presence of aortic regurgitation, and (f) associated cardiac lesion. Some of these have been linked to the risk of recurrence requiring for surgery.

4. Pressure gradient across the subaortic stenosis is best obtained in the apical five-chamber view with the cursor placed immediately distal to the obstruction but proximal to the aortic valve.

Supravalvular Aortic Stenosis. Supravalvular AS is seen as a narrowing of the ascending aorta in the parasternal long-axis and apical long-axis views. The suprasternal view best shows diffuse hypoplasia of the ascending aorta. Doppler pressure gradient is obtained with the cursor distal to the stenosis in the ascending aorta.

Magnetic Resonance Imaging

1. Magnetic resonance imaging (MRI) can clarify the level and mechanism of anatomic obstruction if unclear from echocardiographic studies.
2. It may be a reliable tool for serial evaluation of aortic dilatation in patients with BAV.
3. MRI has advantage of simultaneous evaluation of aortic valve pathology, aortic dilatation, and LV dysfunction.

Natural History

1. Chest pain, syncope, and even sudden death (1%–2% of cases) may occur in children with severe AS.
2. Heart failure occurs with severe AS during the newborn period or later in adult life.
3. Progressive aortic dilatation occurs in patients with BAV. Aortic dilatation may lead to aortic aneurysm. Despite the progressive nature of the condition, the incidence of aortic dissection is rare in children and adolescents with BAV.
4. BAVs are nonobstructive during childhood and become stenotic in adult life because of calcification of the valve. Isolated AR tends to occur in younger patients. Signs of calcification occur in the second to third decades of life with worsening of AS and eventual worsening of AR. Valve replacement may be required in many adult patients.
5. Progressive worsening of AR is possible in discrete subaortic stenosis. The jet of the subaortic stenosis damages the aortic valve with resulting AR.

Management
Medical

1. For critically ill newborns with CHF, the patients are stabilized before surgery or balloon valvuloplasty by the use of rapidly acting inotropic agents (usually dopamine) and diuretics to treat CHF and intravenous infusion of PGE_1 to reopen the ductus. Mechanical ventilation may be useful. Neonates and young infants with CHF from critical AS require the balloon valvuloplasty (or surgery) on an urgent basis.
2. For asymptomatic patients with mild to moderate stenosis, a serial echo-Doppler ultrasound evaluation is needed approximately 1- to 2-year intervals. It is needed more often in children with severe stenosis because AS of all severities tends to worsen with time.

3. Because of the progressive nature of aortic dilatation in children with BAV, annual echocardiographic measurement of the aortic root is recommended.
4. Recent AHA recommendations include echocardiographic screening of first-degree relatives of patients with BAV.
5. Exercise stress test (EST) may be indicated in asymptomatic children with peak gradient greater than 50 mm Hg or mean Doppler gradient greater than 30 mm Hg who are interested in athletic participation or in becoming pregnant.
6. Activity restrictions (Graham et al, 2005)
   a. No limitation in activity is required for mild AS.
   b. For patients with moderate AS, varying levels of activity restriction are required:
      1) Those with mild or no LVH by echo, no LV strain on ECG, and normal EST may participate in competitive sports in class IA, IB, and IIA.
      2) Those with supraventricular tachycardia or multiple or complex ventricular tachycardia at rest or with exercise may participate only in low-intensity competitive sports in class IA and IB (see Fig. 35.1).
   c. Patients with severe AS should not participate in any competitive sports.

Balloon Valvuloplasty

Indications for Balloon Valvuloplasty. For valvular AS, percutaneous balloon aortic valvuloplasty has replaced open surgical valvotomy as the treatment of choice for children with moderate to severe congenital aortic valve stenosis in the majority of the centers. For subaortic stenosis, the balloon procedure is not effective, although patients with thin, discrete subaortic membrane may be effectively treated with balloon angioplasty as well. Multiple studies have shown that balloon aortic valvuloplasty has results comparable to surgical repair with very low mortality rate beyond the neonatal period.

The following may be indications for the procedure according to the AHA (Feltes et al, 2011). These recommendations are based on catheter-derived peak systolic ejection gradient as well as clinical symptoms and ECG changes.

- Asymptomatic children and young adults, with a peak systolic ejection gradient of 50 mm Hg or greater
- Symptomatic patients (with angina, syncope), patients with resting or exercise-induced ECG changes, patients planning to become pregnant, or patients who plan to participate in competitive sports if they have a gradient of 40 mm Hg or greater
- Infants with valvular AS with depressed LV systolic function regardless of pressure gradient
- Neonates who require maintenance of a patency of ductus arteriosus for adequate systemic perfusion, regardless of pressure gradient

Results of Valvuloplasty. Although the results of aortic balloon valvuloplasty are promising, they are not as good as those for PS. A technically adequate balloon dilatation will typically reduce the catheter peak-to-peak systolic gradient to 20 to 35 mm Hg. The optimal ratio of balloon-annuls diameter is 0.8 to 0.9. Larger balloon diameter is associated with a greater risk of developing AR after the procedure.

The long-term outcome after a successful valve dilatation is good, but late restenosis and aortic valve regurgitation eventually necessitate reintervention in the majority of patients. The freedom from reintervention was 67% after 5 years in children; it was lower (48%) in newborns (Feltes et al, 2011). Serious complications (e.g., major hemorrhage, loss of the femoral artery pulse, avulsion of part of the aortic valve leaflet, perforation of the mitral valve or left ventricle) can occur.

Surgical

Indications

1. **Valvular AS.** If the balloon valvuloplasty has failed to relieve the pressure gradient or if severe AR results after the balloon procedure

2. **Subaortic membrane.** Patients with the following are considered low risk and are recommended for medical follow-up rather than surgical intervention: those with (a) no or trace AR, (b) Doppler gradient of 30 mm Hg or less, (c) the membrane not in proximity to the aortic valve (>6 mm), and (d) a thin and mobile aortic valve.

   Most commonly accepted indications for surgical intervention are the peak gradient greater than 35 mm Hg and at least mild AR. Occasionally, the presence of one of them may be an indication for intervention. Most centers accept the onset of AR as an indication for surgical removal of the membrane. The risk of recurrence after surgical removal of the membrane has been a concern (see below for further discussion).

3. **Tunnel-type subaortic stenosis.** A gradient of 50 mm Hg or greater is considered an indication for surgery.

4. **Supravalvular AS.** Surgery is advisable for patients with supravalvular AS when there is the peak pressure gradient across the stenosis greater than 50 to 60 mm Hg, severe LVH, or appearance of new AR.

Procedures and Mortality

1. Closed aortic valvotomy, using calibrated dilators or balloon catheters without cardiopulmonary bypass, may be performed in sick infants. This procedure has a low surgical mortality rate.

2. Newborns with "critical AS" (with hypoplasia of the aortic annulus, ascending aorta, and mitral annulus, small LV cavity, and MR from papillary muscle infarction) have a poor prognosis. The Norwood procedure (see Chapter 14) may be preferable (for future Fontan operation) to aortic valvotomy. The mortality rate for sick neonates with critical AS has decreased to around 10%, although it was much higher in the past, up to 40% to 50%.

3. Valvular AS. The following procedures are performed for aortic valve stenosis: aortic valve commissurotomy, aortic valve replacement, or the Ross procedure.

   a. Aortic valve commissurotomy is usually tried if stenosis is the predominant lesion. Fused commissures are divided with a knife to within 1 mm of the aortic wall.

   Only commissures with adequate leaflet attachments to the aortic wall are opened because division of rudimentary commissures produces severe AR.

   b. Aortic valve replacement may be necessary if AR is the predominant lesion. Valve replacement is done by using a mechanical prosthetic valve or homografts. The advantage of the mechanical valve is durability, but it has the tendency of thrombus formation on the valve with a potential embolization. Because of this tendency, patients require warfarin with its attendant risks of bleeding in addition to aspirin. Homografts have the advantage of a lower incidence of thromboembolism but the deterioration of the homograft (caused by degeneration and calcification) is likely to occur within a decade or two.

   Because of accelerated degeneration of homograft or bioprosthesis valves, a mechanical valve is usually used in adolescents. For adolescent girls or women in whom pregnancy is desired, homografts may be a good alternative until the childbearing years are completed because of the known teratogenic effects of warfarin. A recent study in adults suggests that increased serum cholesterol level (>200 mg/dL) may be a risk factor for bioprosthetic valve calcification, and lowering cholesterol levels is recommended.

   c. In the Ross procedure (pulmonary root autografts), the autologous pulmonary valve replaces the aortic valve, and an aortic or a pulmonary allograft replaces the pulmonary valve. The Ross procedure is more complex than simple aortic valve replacement because it requires coronary artery implantation (Fig. 13.9). The pulmonary valve autograft has the advantage of documented long-term durability; it does not require anticoagulation and remains uncompromised by host reactions. There is evidence of the autograft's growth, making it an attractive option for aortic valve replacement in infants and children. Mild regurgitation of the neoaortic valve occurs frequently, which may result from a preexisting pulmonary valve regurgitation. The patient's own aortic valve may be used for pulmonary position after aortic valvotomy ("double" Ross procedure). An early mortality rate for the Ross procedure (and the Ross-Konno procedure) is less than 5%.

4. Subvalvular AS

   a. Excision of the membrane is done for discrete subvalvular AS. There is a tendency for recurrence after surgical excision. The recurrence rate is as high as 25% to 30%. Risk factors for recurrence include (a) younger age (<4 years), (b) high pressure gradient (>50 mm Hg), (c) proximity of the membrane to the aortic valve (<6 mm), and (d) extension of the membrane to the aortic or mitral valves. Some centers delay surgery until after 10 years of age because the recurrence is very rare at this age. More aggressive resection of the membrane and extensive myectomy reduced the recurrence but resulted in higher complication of atrioventricular block (14%). Surgical mortality for subaortic membrane is near zero.

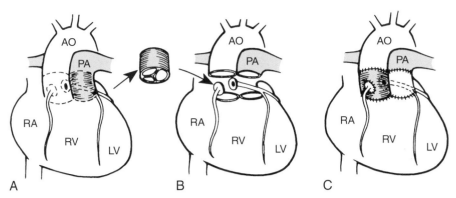

Fig. 13.9 Ross procedure (pulmonary root autograft). **A,** The two *horizontal lines* on the aorta (AO) and pulmonary artery (PA) and two *broken circles* around the coronary artery ostia are lines of proposed incision. The pulmonary valve, with a small rim of right ventricle (RV) muscle, and the adjacent PA are removed. **B,** The aortic valve and the adjacent aorta have been removed, leaving buttons of aortic tissue around the coronary arteries. **C,** The pulmonary autograft is sutured to the aortic annulus and to the distal aorta, and the coronary arteries are sutured to openings made in the PA. The pulmonary valve is replaced with either an aortic or a pulmonary allograft. *LV,* Left ventricle; *RA,* right atrium.

b. For complex LVOT obstruction (e.g., aortic stenosis combined with a diffuse subaortic stenosis or hypoplastic annulus), the Ross procedure can be combined with the Konno operation (the Ross Konno procedure) (Fig. 13.10). The mortality rate for tunnel subaortic stenosis is less than 5%.

5. Supravalvular AS. With the most common hourglass type of supravalvular AS, a reconstructive surgery is done using a Y-shaped patch. For the diffuse form of obstruction, the patch is extended superiorly into the transverse arch to relieve all obstruction. Death occurs for supravalvular stenosis in fewer than 1% of cases, although diffuse narrowing of the ascending aorta and coronary artery ostial stenosis are risk factors.

Postballoon and Postoperative Follow-up

1. Annual follow-up examination is necessary for all patients who had the aortic valve balloon procedure or surgery to detect development of stenosis or regurgitation. In 10% to 30% of patients, significant AR develops after valvotomy or the balloon procedure.

2. Recurrence of discrete subaortic stenosis occurs in 25% to 30% after surgical resection of the membrane and as long as 17 years after the initial procedure, requiring a long, periodic follow-up. Some of these patients require reoperation at a later age.

3. Anticoagulation is needed after a prosthetic mechanical valve replacement. The international normalized ratio (INR) should be maintained between 2.5 and 3.5 for the first 3 months and 2.0 to 3.0 beyond that time. Low-dose aspirin (75–100 mg/day for adolescents) is also indicated in addition to warfarin (ACC/AHA 2006 Guidelines).

4. After aortic valve replacement with bioprosthesis and no risk factors, aspirin (75–100 mg), but not warfarin, is indicated. When there are risk factors (which include atrial fibrillation, previous thromboembolism, LV dysfunction, and hypercoagulable state), warfarin is indicated to achieve an INR of 2.0 to 3.0 (ACC/AHA 2006 Guidelines).

COARCTATION OF THE AORTA

Prevalence

Coarctation of the aorta occurs in 4% to 8% of all cases of CHD. It is more common in males than in females (male-to-female ratio of 2 to 1). Among patients with Turner's syndrome, 30% have COA.

Pathology

1. The usual location of COA is juxtaductal, just distal to the left subclavian artery; less often it is proximal to the origin of the left subclavian artery.

2. The most common associated anomaly is BAV, which occurs in more than 50% and up to 85% of all patients with COA.

3. COA also occurs as part of other CHDs, such as transposition of the great arteries and double-outlet right ventricle (e.g., Taussig-Bing abnormality).

4. Intracerebral aneurysm (berry aneurysm) is present in approximately 10% of patients with COA (Connolly et al, 2003).

5. In symptomatic infants with COA, other associated cardiac defects such as aortic hypoplasia, abnormal aortic valve, VSD, and mitral valve anomalies are often present. In these infants, during fetal life, the descending aorta is supplied mostly via right-to-left ductal flow because the amount of antegrade flow through the relatively small aortic arch and isthmus is reduced (see Fig. 10.3). With ductal closure, a reduced antegrade aortic flow to the descending aorta produces symptoms early in life. Good collateral circulation has not developed in these infants (see Chapter 10). Occasionally, infants without associated defects may become symptomatic because of LV failure, which results from a sudden increase in pressure work in early postnatal life.

6. In *asymptomatic infants and children* with COA, during fetal life, the descending aorta is supplied by both normal amount of antegrade aortic flow through the aortic isthmus and normal ductal flow because associated cardiac

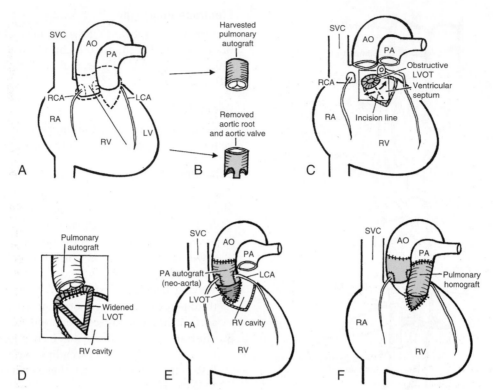

Fig. 13.10 The Ross-Konno procedure. **A,** Intended incision in the ascending aorta and around the aortic annulus and excision boundaries for the pulmonary artery and right ventricle (RV) are shown. Intended incisions to harvest buttons of aortic wall around the coronary artery ostia are also shown. **B,** The pulmonary artery autograft has been harvested (with an extra portion of the RV, not shown) for the Ross procedure. The aortic root and aortic valve are completely excised. **C,** The small obstructed left ventricular outflow tract (LVOT) is shown. The intended incision in the LVOT and the interventricular septum is noted by the *dotted line*, which will result in a V-shaped widening of the LVOT. **D,** The posterior portion of the pulmonary autograft is sutured to the original LVOT. **E,** The LVOT is reconstructed by suturing the extra portion of the RV to the widened V-shaped LVOT. The coronary arteries have been reimplanted. **F,** The right ventricular outflow tract (RVOT) is reconstructed by inserting a pulmonary homograft between the RV body and the distal end of the pulmonary artery. *LCA,* Left coronary artery; *LVOT,* left ventricular outflow tract; *RCA,* right coronary artery; *SVC,* superior vena cava. Other abbreviations used are the same as in Fig. 13.9.

defects are rare in these children except for BAV. Good collateral circulation gradually develops between the proximal aorta and the distal aorta during fetal life.

7. Major collateral circulation between the aortic segments proximal and distal to the coarctation comprises (a) the internal mammary artery anteriorly, (b) arteries arising from the subclavian artery by way of the intercostal arteries, and (c) the anterior spinal artery (Fig. 13.11).

The presentation of patients with COA occurs in a bimodal distribution: newborn infants with circulatory symptoms in the first weeks of life and asymptomatic infants and children (as presented in Chapter 10). Clinical manifestation and management are quite different in these two groups; therefore, they are presented under a separate heading.

Symptomatic Infants-Clinical Manifestations
History

Poor feeding, dyspnea, or signs of acute circulatory shock may develop in the first 6 weeks of life. Figure 13.12 provides an explanation for hemodynamic deterioration in the newborn period. The newborn discharge examination may have been normal as a result of incomplete obliteration of the aortic end of the ductus, which would permit blood flow to the descending aorta. After ductal obliteration, the aortic lumen narrows with loss of the space provided by the aortic end of the ductus.

Physical Examination

1. Infants with COA are pale and experience varying degrees of respiratory distress. Oliguria or anuria, general circulatory shock, and severe acidemia are common. Differential cyanosis may be present; for example, only the lower half of the body is cyanotic because of a right-to-left ductal shunt (particularly after PGE_1 infusion).

2. Peripheral pulses may be weak and thready as a result of CHF. A blood pressure differential may become apparent only after improvement of cardiac function with administration of rapidly acting inotropic agents.

3. The S2 is single and loud; a loud S3 gallop is usually present. No heart murmur is present in 50% of sick infants. A nonspecific ejection systolic murmur is audible over the precordium. The heart murmur may become louder after treatment.

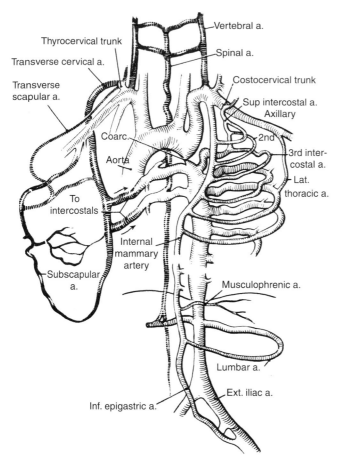

Fig. 13.11 Collateral circulation in coarctation of the aorta. Anteriorly, the internal mammary artery leads to the epigastric arteries for the supply to the lower extremity. The arteries arising from the subclavian artery and supplying the scapula communicate, by way of intercostal arteries, with the descending aorta, thereby supplying blood to the abdominal organs. The anterior spinal artery is also enlarged. *a.,* Artery; *Coarc,* coarctation; *Ext.,* external; *Inf.,* inferior; *Lat.,* lateral; *Sup,* superior. (From Moller JH, Amplatz K, Edwards JE: *Congenital Heart Disease,* Kalamazoo, MI, 1971, Upjohn.)

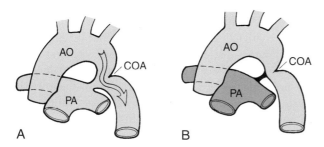

Fig. 13.12 Explanation for hemodynamic deterioration seen in some infants with coarctation of the aorta (COA) in the first days of life. **A,** Coarctation is at the juxtaductal position, so that space is added to the narrowed aorta (AO) by the ductus. **B,** After ductal obliteration, the added lumen is lost, and the aorta becomes severely obstructed, although the severity of the coarctation is unchanged. *PA,* Pulmonary artery.

Electrocardiography

A normal or rightward QRS axis and RVH or right bundle branch block (RBBB) are present in most infants with COA rather than LVH; LVH is seen in older children (see Chapter 10) (Fig. 13.13).

Radiography

Marked cardiomegaly and pulmonary edema or pulmonary venous congestion are usually present.

Echocardiography

Two-dimensional echo and color-flow Doppler studies usually show the site and extent of the coarctation (Fig. 13.14).

1. In the suprasternal notch view, a thin wedge-shaped "posterior shelf" is imaged in the posterolateral aspect of the upper descending aorta, which is distal to the left subclavian artery.
2. Varying degrees of isthmic hypoplasia are present. The third percentile value of normal internal dimension of the aortic isthmus at 40-week gestation is 5.4 mm.
3. The transverse aortic arch may be hypoplastic also. Poststenotic dilatation of the descending aorta is usually imaged. BAV is frequently present. Other associated defects such as VSD can be imaged.
4. Echo diagnosis of neonatal COA in the presence of PDA is difficult. Ramiciotti et al (1993) suggested the following diagnostic criteria for neonatal COA: an aortic isthmus 3 mm or smaller without PDA or an isthmus 4 mm or smaller in the presence of PDA. The ratio of the aortic isthmus to descending aorta at the diaphragm smaller than 0.64 is also a reliable sign of COA in the presence of PDA.
5. Doppler studies above and below the coarctation site should be obtained, as shown in Figure 13.14, in assessing the severity of the coarctation (see Chapter 5 for further discussion).
6. Delayed rate of systolic upstroke and diastolic flow in the abdominal aorta may hint at the presence of coarctation.

Other Imaging

Computed tomography (CT) and MRI have become the imaging modalities of choice after echo diagnosis of the condition. Cardiac catheterization is no longer needed for anatomic assessment. It is performed primarily for interventional treatment.

Natural History

About 20% to 30% of all patients with COA develop CHF by 3 months of age. If a symptomatic infant with COA is undetected and untreated, early death may result from CHF and renal shutdown.

Management
Medical

1. In symptomatic neonates, PGE$_1$ infusion should be started to promote ductal patency and establish flow to the descending aorta and the kidneys.

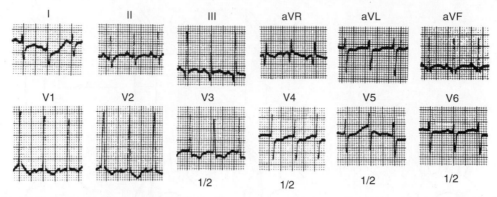

Fig. 13.13 Tracing from a 3-week-old infant with coarctation of the aorta. Note the marked right ventricular hypertrophy.

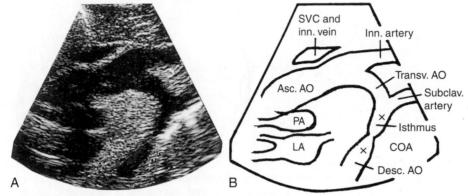

Fig. 13.14 Echocardiogram (**A**) and diagram (**B**) of a suprasternal long-axis view of coarctation of the aorta. A narrowing is present in the upper descending aorta distal to the left subclavian artery. The transverse aortic arch and aortic isthmus are mild to moderately hypoplastic. Doppler estimation of pressure gradients should be obtained at the two *X marks*, proximal and distal to the coarctation for accurate estimation of the pressure gradient.

2. Intensive anticongestive measures with short-acting inotropic agents (e.g., dopamine, dobutamine), diuretics, and oxygen should be started.
3. Metabolic disturbances (e.g., acidosis and hypoglycemia) should be recognized and treated promptly.
4. When the patient is stabilized, either surgical repair or balloon procedure should be performed because the improvement from anticongestive measures is usually temporary.

Nonsurgical

Balloon angioplasty: Although surgical repair has been the primary treatment for COA at most centers, some centers use balloon angioplasty as a palliative strategy in neonates too sick for major surgical procedure. Balloon angioplasty appears to be associated with a higher rate of recoarctation than surgical repair and the rate of complications (including femoral artery injury) is high during infancy. Some centers use low profile endovascular stent in very sick infants, which has the advantage of not producing aneurysm.

Surgical

Indications and Timing

1. If CHF or circulatory shock develops early in life, surgical repair (extended resection with an end-to-end anastomosis) should be performed on an urgent basis. A short period of medical treatment, as described earlier, improves the patient's condition before surgery.
2. If there is a large associated VSD, which occurs in 17% to 33% of patients with COA, one of the following procedures may be performed:
   a. COA and VSD can be repaired in the same operative setting if the VSD is nonrestrictive.
   b. Only coarctation repair is performed if the VSD appear restrictive. Approximately 40% of restrictive VSD close spontaneously.
   c. Pulmonary artery banding is performed if the PA pressure remains high after completing COA surgery. Later the VSD is closed, and the PA band is removed between 6 and 24 months of age.

Procedures. The choice of surgical procedures varies greatly from institution to institution, but the following procedures are popular (Fig. 13.15).

1. Extended resection and end-to-end anastomosis is preferred to other surgical options. It consists of resecting the coarctation segment and anastomosing the proximal and distal aortas (Fig. 13.15, *top*). Because most of symptomatic neonatal COA is associated with hypoplasia of the isthmus and occasionally of the aortic arch, extended

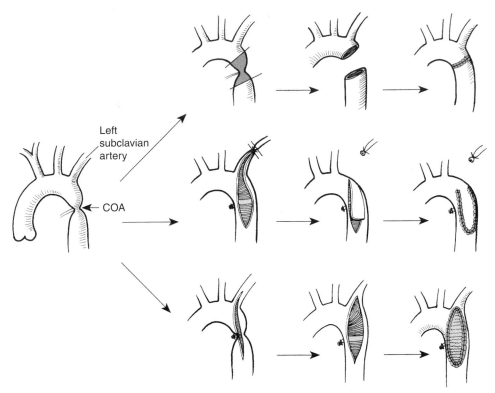

Left
subclavian
artery

← COA

Fig. 13.15 Surgical techniques for repair of coarctation of the aorta (COA). *Top,* End-to-end anastomosis. A segment of coarctation is resected, and the proximal and distal aortas are anastomosed end to end. *Middle,* Subclavian flap procedure. The distal subclavian artery is divided, and the flap of the proximal portion of this vessel is used to widen the coarcted segment. *Bottom,* Patch aortoplasty. An elliptic woven Dacron patch is inserted to expand the diameter of the lumen. Regardless of the type of operative procedure, the ductus arteriosus is always ligated and divided.

resection of hypoplastic parts and an end-to-end anastomosis has resulted in a high success rate with a recurrence rate (4%–11%).

2. Subclavian flap aortoplasty consists of dividing the distal subclavian artery and inserting a flap of the proximal portion of this vessel between the two sides of the longitudinally split aorta throughout the coarctation segment (see Fig. 13.15, *middle*). Need to sacrifice the left subclavicular artery is a concern, which can create subclavian steal. Recurrence rate is lower (10%–40%) than the patch aortoplasty.

3. With patch aortoplasty, the aorta is opened longitudinally through the coarctation segment and extending to the left subclavian artery, and the fibrous shelf and any existing membrane are excised. An elliptic woven Dacron patch is inserted to expand the diameter of the lumen (see Fig. 13.15, *bottom*). Patch aortoplasty has the highest recurrence rate (≤50%).

4. A conduit insertion between the ascending and descending aorta may be performed for severe, long-segment COA (not shown).

Mortality. The mortality rate for COA surgery is less than 1.5%. The mortality rate for repair of COA and VSD at the same time is less than 10%.

Complications

1. Postoperative renal failure is the most common cause of death.

2. Residual obstruction or re-coarctation occurs in 6% to 33% of all patients, but the recurrence rate is lower after surgery than that after balloon angioplasty.

Postoperative Follow-up

1. An examination every 6 to 12 months to check for recurrence of COA is necessary, especially when surgery is performed in the first year of life.

2. Balloon angioplasty (with or without stent) may be performed if a significant recoarctation develops (see Management Algorithm at the end of this chapter).

Asymptomatic Infants and Children-Clinical Manifestations

History. Most children are asymptomatic. Occasionally, a child complains of weakness or pain in the legs after exercise.

Physical Examination (Fig. 13.16)

1. Patients grow and develop normally.

2. Arterial pulses in the leg are either absent or weak and delayed. There is hypertension in the arm, or the leg systolic pressure is equal to or lower than the arm systolic pressure. In normal children, the oscillometric systolic

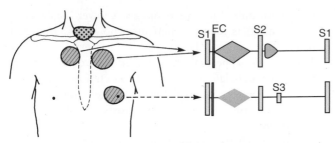

Fig. 13.16 Cardiac findings of coarctation of the aorta. A systolic thrill may be present in the suprasternal notch (area shown by *dots*). *EC,* Ejection click.

pressure in the thigh or calf is 5 to 10 mm Hg higher than that in the arm.

3. A systolic thrill may be present in the suprasternal notch. The S2 splits normally, and the A2 is accentuated. An ejection click is frequently audible at the apex or at the base (or both), which may originate in the associated BAV or from systemic hypertension. An ejection systolic murmur grade 2 to 4 of 6 is heard at the upper right sternal border and mid or lower left sternal border. A well-localized systolic murmur is also audible in the left interscapular area in the back. Occasionally, an early diastolic decrescendo murmur of AR from the BAV may be audible in the third left intercostal space (see Fig. 13.16).

Electrocardiography

Leftward QRS axis and LVH are commonly found. The ECG is normal in approximately 20% of patients.

Radiography

1. The heart size may be normal or slightly enlarged.
2. Dilatation of the ascending aorta may be seen.
3. Overpenetrated films may show an indentation produced by pre- and poststenotic dilations, creating the classic "3 sign."
4. Rib notching between the fourth and eighth ribs may be seen in older children but rarely in children younger than 5 years of age.

Echocardiography

1. The suprasternal notch 2D echo demonstrates a discrete shelf-like membrane in the posterolateral aspect of the descending aorta. Associated findings such as isthmus hypoplasia, poststenotic dilatation, and diminished pulsation in the descending aorta may be present. BAV is frequently present.
2. Doppler examination often demonstrates a pattern of diastolic runoff, especially in patients with robust collaterals or tight stenosis. Continuous-wave Doppler flow profile distal to the coarctation is composed of two superimposed signals representing low-velocity flow in the proximal descending aorta and high-velocity flow across the coarctation. As discussed earlier, a more accurate estimation of the gradient is obtained by the expanded Bernoulli equation, in which the peak velocities obtained from the

segments proximal and distal to the coarctation site are used. This is because the flow velocity proximal to the coarctation is often higher than 1.5 m/sec, and it cannot be ignored in the Bernoulli equation. In severe COA with extensive collaterals, the Doppler-estimated gradient may underestimate the severity of the coarctation because the blood flow through the coarctation site is decreased.

Other Imaging

Magnetic resonance imaging with three-dimensional reconstruction, supplemented by gadolinium contrast, has become the imaging modality of choice. Cardiac catheterization is no longer needed for anatomic assessment.

Natural History

Left ventricular failure, rupture of the aorta, intracranial hemorrhage (i.e., rupture of a berry aneurysm of the arterial circle of Willis), hypertensive encephalopathy, and hypertensive cardiovascular disease are rare complications seen in adulthood.

Management
Medical

Children with mild COA should be watched regularly for hypertension in the arm or for increasing pressure differences between the arm and leg. Reduced blood pressure readings in the lower extremities may be caused by femoral artery injuries resulting from previous surgeries or interventional procedures.

Nonsurgical

1. **Balloon angioplasty.** Balloon angioplasty for native unoperated coarctation is controversial, although most centers perform balloon dilatation for recurrent coarctation. Some centers continue to use the balloon procedure for the native COA, but other centers prefer a surgical approach.

   Indications for balloon intervention include the following according to a recent recommendation by the AHA (Feltes et al, 2011).

   a. Transcatheter systolic gradient across COA of greater than 20 mm Hg and suitable anatomy, irrespective of the patient's age
   b. Transcatheter systolic gradient of less than 20 mm Hg
      1) with evidence of significant anatomic narrowing on imaging with extensive collateral vessels,
      2) in patients with univentricular heart, or
      3) in patients with significant LV dysfunction
   c. It may be reasonable to consider the procedure for native coarctation as a palliative procedure at any age when there is severe LV dysfunction, severe mitral regurgitation, or systemic disease affected by the cardiac condition.

   Common complications of the balloon angioplasty include:

   a. Acute femoral artery injury and thrombosis, especially in small children
   b. Aortic aneurysm formation with serious late complications. Late aneurysm formation was much higher after

balloon angioplasty than surgery (35% vs 0%) (Cowley et al, 2005).

2. **Endovascular stent placement.** A balloon-expandable stainless-steel stent implanted concurrently with balloon angioplasty has gained popularity.

Current recommendations for stent placement in native COA and recoarctation of the aorta are as follows according to the recent recommendations by the AHA (Feltes et al, 2011).

a. For recoarctation, stent placement is indicated in patients who have a transcatheter systolic coarctation gradient greater than 20 mm Hg and are of sufficient size for safe stent placement, which can be expanded to an adult size.

b. For initial treatment of native COA or recurrent coarctation, it is reasonable to consider stent placement if:

1) The transcatheter systolic coarctation gradient is greater than 20 mm Hg

2) A transcatheter systolic gradient is less than 20 mm Hg with systolic hypertension caused by the narrowing of the aorta

3) The long segment coarctation with a transcatheter systolic gradient is greater than 20 mm Hg

c. For patients in whom balloon angioplasty has failed in treatment of native or recurrent COA, it is reasonable to use stent placement.

Advantages of the use of the expandable stent may include the following: (1) it does not require overexpansion of the coarcted segment, thereby reducing the chance of the development of aortic aneurysm; (2) it produces better results with greater reduction of pressure gradient than the balloon procedure alone; and (3) it can be re-expanded to the adult size avoiding repeat surgical procedures.

Successful placement of the stent was reported in 98% of the patients with pressure gradient less than 20 mm Hg. On follow-up, aneurysm was seen in fewer than 1% of the patients and reintervention was needed in 4%.

Surgical

Indications and Timing

1. Significant narrowing of the aorta with pressure gradient greater than 20 to 30 mm Hg is considered an indication for surgery in asymptomatic children.

a. Blood pressure measurement showing hypertension in the arm with a large systolic pressure gradient of 20 to 30 mm Hg or greater by Doppler echo or blood pressure measurement may be a relatively weak indication.

b. Reduction of aortic diameter by 50% at the level of coarctation of the aorta in the presence of pressure gradient of more than 20 to 30 mm Hg is considered an absolute indication for surgery. The dimension of the coarctation segment can be determined by an echo study but an MRI may be a better choice for older children and adolescents.

c. Children with mild COA (<20 mm Hg gradient) may be considered for surgery if a prominent gradient develops with exercise.

2. The preferred age for surgery varies from center to center; some centers prefer ages of 2 and 3 years, and others prefer delaying it until 4 to 5 years of age. A lower incidence of hypertension is found in patients who had COA repair before 1 year of age. However, early surgery (i.e., before 1 year of age) appears to increase the chance of recoarctation. The risk of late recurrence of coarctation is low if the surgery is performed after 2 years of age. Older children are operated on soon after the diagnosis is made.

Procedures

1. Through a left thoracotomy incision, extended resection of the coarctation segment and end-to-end anastomosis is the procedure of choice for discrete COA in children (see Fig. 13.15).

2. Occasionally, subclavian artery aortoplasty or circular or patch grafts may be performed.

Mortality. The mortality rate is less than 1% in older children.

Complications

1. Spinal cord ischemia producing paraplegia may develop after cross-clamping of the aorta during surgery, which is probably related to limited collateral circulation. This develops in 0.4% of cases.

2. Rebound hypertension may occur in the immediate postoperative period as a result of an increased sympathetic activity (with elevated norepinephrine level).

3. Other rare complications may include recurrent laryngeal nerve injury, chylothorax, bleeding, and infection.

Postoperative Follow-up

1. During childhood, annual examinations should pay attention to the possibility of recurrence of coarctation, persistence or resurgence of hypertension, and possible associated anomalies (i.e., BAV or mitral valve disease).

2. Life-long follow-up is indicated because of COA related complications (e.g., aneurysm formation) and frequent association of BAV.

Management Algorithm

Deciding on the optimal treatment for patients with COA can be complicated with many different options available. In general, management is dictated by the age at presentation, complexity of the coarctation, and native versus recurrent coarctation. The following is the management algorithm suggested by Torok et al (2015).

1. For neonates and infants:

a. Surgery (preferably extended resection and end-to-end anastomosis) is recommended by most centers.

b. Surgery is more appropriate especially when the anatomy of the COA is complex, (e.g., transverse arch obstruction) or when repair of associated cardiac defect is required.

c. It is reasonable to choose balloon angioplasty as a palliative strategy in neonates too sick for major surgical procedure.

2. For small children with *native* coarctation:

a. Most centers prefer surgical repair, especially when the COA is associated with complex anatomy (as described earlier).

b. Balloon angioplasty is not a good choice because of its long-term risk of aneurysm.

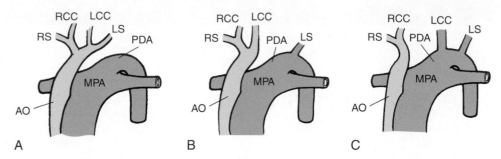

Fig. 13.17 Three types of aortic arch interruptions. **A,** Type A. **B,** Type B. **C,** Type C (see text). *AO,* Aorta; *LCC,* left common carotid; *LS,* left subclavian; *MPA,* main pulmonary artery; *PDA,* patent ductus arteriosus; *RCC,* right common carotid; *RS,* right subclavian.

c. Stent placement is also not a good choice because it requires redilation at a later time, and the arteries are too small to accommodate a stent that can be dilated to adult size.
3. For small children with *recurrent* coarctation:
   a. Balloon angioplasty without stent is a reasonable approach because the child is too small to receive a stent that can be dilated to adult size.
   b. For children with complex anatomy (e.g., tortuous segment of recoarctation), surgery should also be considered.
4. For older children, adolescents and adults:
   a. With a simple, juxtaductal native coarctation, stent placement is a reasonable approach. (Only stents expandable to an adult size should be used.)
   b. Stent placement can also be considered for recurrent coarctation.
   c. Balloon angioplasty (without stent) is not a good choice because it is variably successful, and surgical reintervention may be required.

INTERRUPTED AORTIC ARCH

Prevalence

Interrupted aortic arch accounts for about 1% of critically ill infants who have CHDs.

Pathology

1. This is an extreme form of COA in which the aortic arch is atretic or a segment of the arch is absent.
2. Depending on the location of the interruption, the defect is divided into the following three types (Fig. 13.17):
   a. **Type A:** The interruption is distal to the left subclavian artery (occurring in 30% of cases).
   b. **Type B:** The interruption is between the left carotid and left subclavian arteries (occurs in 43% of cases). An aberrant right subclavian artery is common. DiGeorge syndrome is reported in about 50% of patients with type B.
   c. **Type C:** The interruption is between the innominate and left carotid arteries (occurs in 17% of cases).
3. Interrupted aortic arch is usually associated with PDA and VSD (occurring in >90% of cases). A BAV occurs in 60% of all cases. Often there is mitral valve deformity (10% of

cases), persistent truncus arteriosus (10% of cases), or subaortic stenosis (20% of cases).
4. DiGeorge syndrome occurs in at least 15% of these patients.

Clinical Manifestations

1. Respiratory distress, variable degrees of cyanosis, poor peripheral pulses, and signs of CHF or circulatory shock develop during the first days of life. Differential cyanosis is uncommon because of the frequent association of VSD.
2. Chest radiographs show cardiomegaly, increased pulmonary vascular markings, and pulmonary venous congestion or pulmonary edema. The upper mediastinum may be narrow because of the absence of the thymus, as is commonly found with DiGeorge syndrome. The ECG may show RVH in uncomplicated cases.
3. Echo is useful in the diagnosis of the interruption and associated defects. Cardiac CT or MRI is used more frequently than angiography to clarify the anatomy before surgery.

Management

1. Medical treatment consists of PGE1 infusion (preferably before 4 days of age) with intubation and oxygen administration. Workup for DiGeorge syndrome (i.e., fluorescence in situ hybridization (FISH) for 22q11.2 deletion, serum calcium) should be done. Hyperventilation that causes respiratory alkalosis and tetany should be avoided, and citrated blood (which causes hypocalcemia by chelation) should not be transfused in patients with DiGeorge syndrome. Blood should be irradiated before the transfusion.
2. Primary complete repair of the interruption and the VSD is recommended if the interruption is associated with a simple VSD. If it is associated with complex anomalies, the initial procedures should be banding the PA and repairing the interruption. Debanding and repair of the VSD and other cardiac anomalies should be done at a later date. A primary anastomosis, Dacron vascular graft, or venous homograft may be used to repair the interruption. The surgical mortality rate can be as low as 10% for initial surgery.

14

Cyanotic Congenital Heart Defects

Timely detection and treatment of cyanotic congenital heart defects (CHDs) and other serious heart defects are crucial for survival of the patients. Unfortunately, not all serious CHDs manifest themselves with cyanosis during the neonatal period, especially during the short stay in the nursery. Up to 30% of infants with critical congenital heart disease (CCHD) are discharged after birth without being identified because these infants appear normal on routine examination with no signs of critical CHD in the first days of life. Cyanosis may not be clinically apparent in patients with mild desaturation (>80% saturation). In darkly pigmented infants, cyanosis can be especially difficult to appreciate.

Critical congenital heart disease is a term that refers to a group of serious heart defects that are present from birth for which neonates require early surgical or catheter-based intervention to survive. CCHDs include all cyanotic heart defects and ductal-dependent defects, as well as other rare defects. Ductal-dependent defects are those defects in which survival depends on the patency of the ductus arteriosus, which normally closes after birth, and include such defects as hypoplastic left heart syndrome (HLHS), aortic arch atresia, critical aortic stenosis (AS), critical pulmonary stenosis (PS) or atresia, and tricuspid atresia.

Congenital heart disease is the most common birth defect, and 25% of them are CCHDs. More than 50% of CCHD deaths could be attributed to late or missed diagnosis in the neonatal period (Chang et al, 2008). Therefore, survival of neonates with CCHD depends on early diagnosis and treatment of the defect.

Detection of mild cyanosis has been made much easier in recent years by the use of pulse oximetry in asymptomatic newborns. Newborn screening using pulse oximetry has been strongly supported by recent literature as a valuable tool facilitating the prompt detection of infants CCHDs. In 2011, a group of experts from many medical and scientific societies and governmental agencies developed a screening algorithm for CCHDs in neonates using pulse oximetry. In the same year, universal screening for CCHD was added to the Recommended Uniform Screening Panel by the Secretary of Health and Human Services. Since then, nearly all states in the United States have legislation, regulations, or hospital guidelines in place for newborn screening for CCHD. Neonatal screen with pulse oximetry for CCHD is endorsed by the American Academy of Pediatrics (AAP), American Heart Association, and American College of Cardiology, regardless of whether they live in a state that includes CCHD screening within their newborn screening program. The principle of pulse oximetry is discussed in Chapter 11.

NEONATAL PULSE OXIMETRY SCREEN

The importance of neonatal pulse oximetry screen (POS) is in its ability to detect CCHD or other life-threatening neonatal conditions before the infant is discharged from the birth hospital. Sensitivity of the POS in detecting CCHD has been demonstrated to be high (76.5%) with a specificity up to 99% with a very low false-positive rate, making it a strong test. False-positive cases for heart lesions actually resulted in detection of noncardiac critical conditions that require immediate attention.

Usefulness of Pulse Oximetry

Pulse oximetry screen can detect not only CCHDs but also some noncardiac conditions.

1. All cyanotic CHDs, including ductal-dependent lesions, could be detected by the screen. Timely detection of ductal-dependent lesions is particularly important because interventions to maintain the patency of the ductus are required for survival of the neonate.
2. Some noncardiac conditions that can be detected by POS also require early treatment before deterioration occurs. Examples include hypothermia, infection (including sepsis), lung disease, persistent pulmonary hypertension, hemoglobinopathy, and others.

Neonatal Pulse Oximetry Screen Algorithm

Neonatal POS algorithm varies not only from country to country but also varies on the time of the screen as well as on the site of measurement of oxygen saturation. Presented here is the US pulse oximetry algorithm (Fig. 14.1), which is approved by the AAP.

1. The screen should be done after 24 hours of life or just before early discharge from the hospital. The POS done earlier than 24 hours of age increases false-positive results. Interestingly, however, the false-positive test results detect noncardiac conditions that require prompt attention and treatment.

2. To detect cyanotic CHDs and ductal-dependent lesions, oxygen saturation should be measured in the right hand (for preductal arterial saturation) and either foot (for post-ductal arterial saturation).

Test Results

1. Normal neonates should have oxygen saturation in the right hand and foot higher than 95% and the difference in oxygen saturation between the right hand and the foot should be 3% or less.

2. Positive (abnormal) test results include the following three categories.

   Category 1: oxygen saturation 89% or less in either the right hand or a foot

   Category 2: saturation between 90% and 94% in the right hand and the foot

   Category 3: difference in the saturation 4% or more between the right hand and the foot

   According to the US algorithm, category 1 positive test results require immediate assessment (see Fig. 14.1). Repeat screen is recommended for those with category 2 or 3 positive test results, for up to two times, each separated by 1 hour. Repeat screen may prove negative on some cases. If the positive test results continue to be present on the third screen, action must take place to assess the cases (see Fig. 14.1).

   Cutoff point may require modification in the certain setting such as high altitude, out-of-hospital birth, and infants admitted to neonatal intensive care units. Arterial saturation

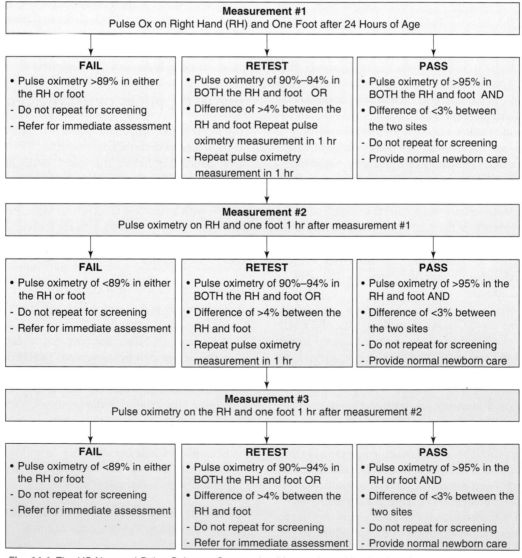

Fig. 14.1 The US Neonatal Pulse Oximetry Screen algorithm endorsed by the American Academy of Pediatrics. *RH*, Right hand.

is expected to be lower in high altitudes (especially above 5000 ft), but the cutoff point has not been established.

What To Do with the Screen Results

Infants who failed the screen:

Infants who failed the screen (or positive test) should not be discharged from the hospital without excluding potentially life-threatening conditions; they should undergo evaluation to identify the cause of hypoxemia.

1. An echocardiography or cardiology consultation is the next step. If a CCHD is identified by echocardiography, urgent consultation with a pediatric cardiologist or transfer to a medical facility with pediatric cardiology expertise is warranted.
2. However, evaluation of the baby using other means (e.g., chest radiograph, blood work) should not be delayed while awaiting an echocardiogram. If a reversible noncardiac cause of hypoxemia is identified and appropriately treated, an echocardiogram may not be necessary. Chest radiography is often helpful in identifying noncardiac causes of hypoxemia.
3. Prostaglandin E_1 (PGE_1) infusion. Infants with ductal-dependent lesions (see earlier for examples) are at increased risk for death and significant morbidity unless interventions are initiated to maintain patency of the ductus arteriosus. Cardiology consultation should be requested on an urgent basis. At the same time, a PGE_1 (Prostin VR Pediatric) intravenous (IV) infusion should be started. The starting dose of Prostin is 0.05 to 0.1 µg/kg/min administered in a continuous IV drip. When the desired effects (increased Po_2, increased systemic blood pressure, improved pH) are achieved, the dose should be reduced step by step to 0.01 µg/kg/min. When the initial starting dose has no effect, it may be increased up to 0.4 µg/kg/min. Three common side effects of IV infusion of PGE_1

are apnea (12%), fever (14%), and flushing (10%). Less common side effects include tachycardia or bradycardia, hypotension, and cardiac arrest.

Infants who passed the screen:

Infants with negative screening results who are clinically well without signs concerning possible CHD (e.g., heart murmur, weak femoral pulses) do not require additional evaluation. However, POS cannot detect all cases of CCHD. If there is clinical suspicion for CCHD, additional evaluation should be pursued even in the setting of a normal POS result.

TRADITIONAL TOOLS IN DIFFERENTIATION OF CENTRAL CYANOSIS

Hypoxemia does not necessarily mean a heart defect is present; it may be caused by pulmonary disease or central nervous system (CNS) depression. Crying may improve the cyanosis caused by lung diseases or CNS depression; however, crying usually worsens cyanosis in patients with cyanotic heart defects. Clinical findings often direct physicians to the correct system that causes cyanosis. Table 14.1 lists some of the differentiating clinical findings of central cyanosis associated with the three common causes of cyanosis.

The following lists some of the traditional tools used in the investigation of cyanotic newborns. When POS is done and echocardiography or cardiology consultation is readily available, some or all of the steps may not be needed, but they are presented here for the sake of completeness.

Initial Evaluation

Although the physical examination, ECG, and chest radiography are not very helpful in diagnosing a specific cyanotic heart defect, these tools are often useful in suspecting cardiac abnormalities.

TABLE 14.1 Causes and Clinical Findings of Central Cyanosis

Systems	Causes	Clinical Findings
CNS depression	Perinatal asphyxia	Shallow irregular respiration
	Heavy maternal sedation	Poor muscle tone
	Intrauterine fetal distress	Cyanosis that disappears when the patient is stimulated or oxygen is given
Pulmonary disease	Parenchymal lung disease (e.g., hyaline membrane disease)	Tachypnea and respiratory distress with retraction and expiratory grunting
		Crackles or decreased breath sounds on auscultation
	Pneumothorax or pleural effusion	Chest radiography may reveal causes (e.g., those listed under causes in this table)
	Diaphragmatic hernia	
	PPHN	Oxygen administration may improve or abolish cyanosis (see Hyperoxia Test)
Cardiac disease	Cyanotic CHD with right-to-left shunt	Tachypnea usually without retraction
		Absence of crackles or abnormal breath sounds unless CHF supervenes
		Heart murmurs may be absent in serious forms of cyanotic CHD
		A continuous murmur (of PDA) may be audible in a cyanotic neonate
		Chest radiography may show cardiomegaly, abnormal cardiac silhouette, increased or decreased pulmonary vascular markings
		Little or no increase in Po_2 with oxygen administration (see Hyperoxia Test)

CHD, Congenital heart defect; *CHF,* congestive heart failure; *CNS,* central nervous system; *PDA,* patent ductus arteriosus; *PPHN,* persistent pulmonary hypertension of newborn.

a. With a cardiac lesion, besides being cyanotic, a neonate may have dyspnea, tachypnea, abnormal heart sounds, heart murmurs, or abnormal peripheral pulses.

b. A midline liver may be palpable (or seen on radiography).

c. Chest radiography may show abnormal lung fields (e.g., increased vascularity, oligemic lung fields, or other abnormalities) and abnormal cardiac shadow (abnormal size or abnormal silhouette).

d. The ECG may show abnormal rhythm and rate, abnormal QRS axis, atrial hypertrophy, or ventricular hypertrophy.

Hyperoxia Test

The test helps differentiate cyanosis caused by cardiac disease from that caused by pulmonary diseases. When central cyanosis has been confirmed by arterial Po_2, one tests the response of arterial Po_2 to 100% oxygen inhalation (hyperoxia test). If not intubated, oxygen should be administered through a plastic hood (e.g., an Oxyhood) for at least 10 minutes to completely fill the alveolar space with oxygen. With pulmonary disease, arterial Po_2 usually rises to greater than 100 mm Hg. When there is a significant intracardiac right-to-left shunt, the arterial Po_2 does not exceed 100 mm Hg, and the rise is usually not more than 10 to 30 mm Hg (see Chapter 11 for details). Exceptions exist in patients with large pulmonary blood flow (PBF) and those with severe lung pathology.

Arterial Po_2 in Preductal and Postductal Arteries

It is important that one obtain arterial blood samples from the right upper body (right radial artery), rather than from the descending aorta, to detect (true) cyanotic CHDs. If a low arterial Po_2 is obtained from an umbilical artery line (or from a lower extremity site), another sample from the right upper body should be obtained, and the Po_2 values from the two sites should be compared to see if there is a right-to-left ductal shunt. Arterial Po_2 from the right radial artery that is 10 to 15 mm Hg higher than that from an umbilical artery catheter is significant. Such a right-to left ductal shunt is caused not only by persistent pulmonary hypertension of the newborn (PPHN) but also by other serious cardiovascular conditions, including severe obstructive lesions of the left ventricle (e.g., severe AS) or aortic obstructive lesions (e.g., interrupted aortic arch, coarctation of the aorta [COA]).

COMPLETE TRANSPOSITION OF THE GREAT ARTERIES

Prevalence

Complete transposition of the great arteries occurs in about 5% to 7% of all CHDs. It is more common in males than in females (male-to-female ratio of 3:1).

Pathophysiology

1. In complete transposition of the great arteries (TGA), the aorta arises anteriorly from the right ventricle (RV) carrying desaturated blood to the body, and the pulmonary artery (PA) arises posteriorly from the left ventricle (LV) carrying oxygenated blood back to the lungs. In the classic complete TGA, the aorta is located anteriorly and to the right (dextro) of the PA. The prefix D, however, is for d-looping of the cardiac tube during embryogenesis so that the RV ends up on the right (D-transposition) and the LV on the left. This is in contrast to L-TGA where morphologic RV ends up on the left, thus L-transposition.

2. The result of D-transposition of the great arteries (D-TGA) is complete separation of the pulmonary and systemic circulations. This results in hypoxemic blood circulating throughout the body and hyperoxemic blood circulating in the pulmonary circuit, which is not compatible with survival (see Fig. 11.4). Defects that permit mixing of the two circulations (e.g., atrial septal defect [ASD], ventricular septal defect [VSD], and patent ductus arteriosus [PDA]) are necessary for survival.

3. About half of these infants do not have associated defects other than a patent foramen ovale (PFO) or a small PDA (i.e., simple TGA).

4. In about 5% of the patients, left ventricular outflow tract (LVOT) obstruction (or subpulmonary stenosis) occurs. The obstruction may be dynamic or fixed. Dynamic obstruction of the LVOT, which occurs in about 20% of such patients, results from bowing of the interventricular septum to the left because of a high RV pressure. Anatomic (or fixed) subpulmonary stenosis or abnormal mitral chordal attachment rarely causes obstruction of the LVOT.

5. VSD is present in 30% to 40% of patients with D-TGA and may be located anywhere in the ventricular septum. A combination of VSD and significant LVOT obstruction (or PS) occurs in about 10% of all patients with D-TGA. Infants with TGA and VSD more commonly have associated defects than those without associated VSD. Such associated defects may include COA, interrupted aortic arch, pulmonary atresia, and an overriding or straddling of the atrioventricular (AV) valve. (Overriding is present when an AV valve annulus commits to both ventricular chambers. It is the result of malalignment of the atria and ventricular septa. Straddling is present when the chordae tendineae insert into the contralateral ventricle through a septal defect. Type A straddling is a mild form in which the chordae insert near the crest of the ventricular septum. In type B, the insertion is along the ventricular septum. In type C straddling, the chordae insert into the free wall of the contralateral ventricle. Overriding and straddling may occur independently or coexist in the same valve.)

Clinical Manifestations
History

1. History of cyanosis from birth is always present.

2. Signs of congestive heart failure (CHF) with dyspnea and feeding difficulties develop during the newborn period.

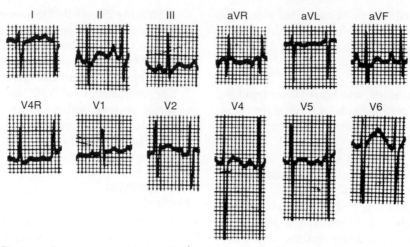

Fig. 14.2 Electrocardiographic tracing from a 6-day-old male infant with complete transposition of the great arteries. The QRS axis is +140 degrees. Note the deep S waves in V5 and V6 and an upright T wave in V1 are consistent with right ventricular hypertrophy.

Physical Examination

1. Moderate to severe cyanosis is present, especially in large male newborns. Such infants are tachypneic but without retraction unless CHF supervenes.
2. The S2 is single and loud. No heart murmur is heard in infants with an intact ventricular septum. An early or holosystolic murmur of VSD may be audible in less cyanotic infants with associated VSD. A soft midsystolic murmur of PS (LVOT obstruction) may be audible.
3. If CHF supervenes, hepatomegaly and dyspnea develop.

Laboratory Studies

1. Severe arterial hypoxemia, usually with acidosis, is present. Hypoxemia does not respond to oxygen inhalation. (See Hyperoxia Test in early section of this chapter.)
2. Hypoglycemia and hypocalcemia are occasionally present.

Electrocardiography (Fig. 14.2)

1. Right ventricular hypertrophy (RVH) is usually present after the first few days of life. The QRS voltages and the QRS axis may be normal in many newborns with the defect. After 3 days of life, an upright T wave in V1 may be the only abnormality suggestive of RVH.
2. Biventricular hypertrophy (BVH) may be present in infants with large VSD, PDA, or pulmonary vascular obstructive disease because all of these conditions produce an additional left ventricular hypertrophy (LVH).
3. Occasionally, right atrial hypertrophy (RAH) is present.

Radiography

1. Cardiomegaly with increased pulmonary vascularity is typically present.
2. An egg-shaped cardiac silhouette with a narrow, superior mediastinum is characteristic (Fig. 14.3).

Echocardiography

Two-dimensional (2D) echo and color-flow Doppler studies usually provide all the anatomic and functional information needed for the management of infants with D-TGA.

1. In the parasternal long-axis view, the great artery arising from the posterior ventricle (LV) has a sharp posterior angulation toward the lungs, which suggests that this artery is the PA (Fig. 14.4A). In contrast to the normal intertwining of the great arteries, the proximal portion of the great arteries runs parallel. Unlike in a normal heart, there is a fibrous continuity between the pulmonary and mitral valves, and subaortic conus is present. (In normal hearts, there is aortic–mitral fibrous continuity with subpulmonary conus.)
2. In the parasternal short-axis view, the "circle and sausage" appearance of the normal great arteries is not visible. Instead, the great arteries appear as "double circles" (Fig. 14.4B). The PA is in the center of the heart, and the coronary arteries do not arise from this great artery. The aorta is usually anterior to and slightly to the right of the PA, and the coronary arteries arise from the aorta.
3. In the apical and subcostal five-chamber views, the PA (i.e., the artery that bifurcates) is seen to arise from the LV, and the aorta arises from the RV.
4. The status of atrial communication, both before and after balloon septostomy, is best evaluated in the subcostal view. Doppler examination and color-flow mapping should aid in the functional evaluation of the atrial shunt.
5. Frequently, associated defects, such as VSD, LVOT obstruction (dynamic or fixed), or pulmonary valve stenosis, are found. Subaortic stenosis or COA rarely occurs.
6. The coronary arteries can be imaged in most patients in the parasternal, subcostal, and apical views (Fig. 14.5).

Other Studies

Cardiac catheterization is performed only for the purpose of balloon atrial septostomy to improve mixing at the atrial level. Rarely, it is performed to look for associated anomalies such as abnormal coronary artery, collateral circulation, or a small aortic isthmus.

Natural History

1. Progressive hypoxia, acidosis, and heart failure result in death in the newborn period. Without surgical intervention, death occurs in 90% of patients before they reach 6 months of age.
2. Infants with an intact ventricular septum are the sickest group but demonstrate the most dramatic improvement after Rashkind balloon atrial septostomy.
3. Infants with large ASD and large VSD are the least cyanotic group but the most likely to develop CHF and pulmonary vascular obstructive disease. Many infants with TGA and a large VSD develop moderate pulmonary vascular

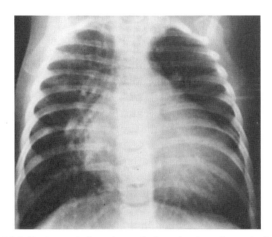

Fig. 14.3 Posteroanterior view of the chest radiograph from a 2-month-old infant with complete transposition of the great arteries. Note the cardiomegaly (cardiothoracic ratio, 0.7), "egg-shaped" heart with a narrow waist, and increased pulmonary vascular markings, which are characteristic of this condition.

obstructive disease by 3 to 4 months of age. Thus, surgical procedures are recommended before that age.

4. Infants with a significant PDA are similar to those with a large VSD in terms of their development of CHF and pulmonary vascular obstructive disease.
5. The combination of VSD and PS allows considerably longer survival without surgery because the pulmonary vascular bed is protected from developing pulmonary hypertension, but this combination carries a high surgical risk for correction.

Management
Medical

1. The following measures should be carried out to stabilize the patient before an emergency cardiac catheterization (if performed) or a surgical procedure is carried out:
   a. Arterial blood gases and pH should be obtained and metabolic acidosis should be corrected. Hypoglycemia and hypocalcemia, if present, should be treated.
   b. PGE$_1$ infusion should be started to improve arterial oxygen saturation by reopening the ductus (see Appendix E for the dosage). This should be continued throughout the cardiac catheterization or until the time of surgery.
   c. Oxygen should be administered for severe hypoxia. Oxygen may help lower pulmonary vascular resistance (PVR) and increase PBF, which in turn increases systemic arterial oxygen saturation.
2. Before surgery, cardiac catheterization and a balloon atrial septostomy (i.e., the Rashkind procedure) are often carried out to have some flexibility in planning surgery. If adequate interatrial communication exists and the anatomic diagnosis of TGA is clear by echo examination, the patient may go to surgery without cardiac catheterization or the balloon atrial septostomy. The need for the balloon septostomy may be determined by inadequate atrial

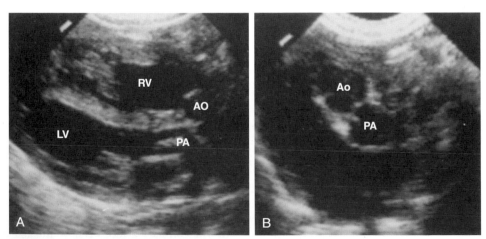

Fig. 14.4 Parasternal echocardiographic views in complete transposition of the great arteries. **A,** In this parasternal long-axis view, the great arteries are seen in parallel alignment. The posterior artery is directed posteriorly, bifurcates into two branches, and is therefore a pulmonary artery (PA). There is a continuity between the pulmonary valve and the mitral valve. **B,** In the parasternal short-axis view, the aorta (AO) and the PA are seen in cross section as *double circles*. The aorta is anterior to and right of the PA. *LV,* Left ventricle; *RV,* right ventricle. (From Snider AR, Serwer GA: *Echocardiography in Pediatric Heart Disease*, St. Louis, 1990, Mosby.)

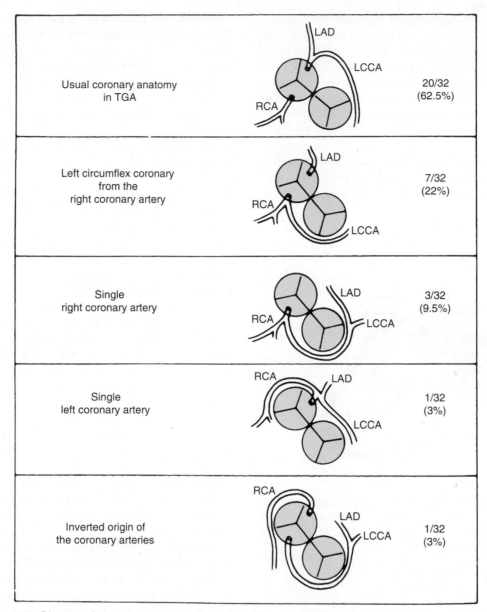

Fig. 14.5 Diagram of the coronary artery anatomy in 32 patients with transposition of the great arteries (TGA). The orientation of the figures is that of a parasternal short-axis echocardiographic view. *LAD,* Left anterior descending artery; *LCCA,* left circumflex coronary artery; *RCA,* right coronary artery. (From Pasquini L, Sanders SP, Parness IA, et al: Diagnosis of coronary artery anatomy by two-dimensional echocardiography in patients with transposition of the great arteries, *Circulation* 75:557–564, 1987.)

mixing through the PFO (evidenced with a high Doppler flow velocity of >1 m/sec, significant hypoxia, or metabolic acidosis) or lack of readiness for surgical intervention.

In the balloon atrial septostomy, a balloon-tipped catheter is advanced into the left atrium (LA) through the PFO. The balloon is inflated with diluted radiopaque dye and abruptly and forcefully withdrawn to the right atrium (RA) under fluoroscopic or echo monitoring. This procedure creates a large defect in the atrial septum through which an improved intracardiac mixing occurs. An increase in the oxygen saturation of 10% or more and a minimal interatrial pressure gradient are considered satisfactory results of the procedure.

3. CHF may be treated with diuretics (and digoxin or angiotensin-converting enzyme [ACE] inhibitors).

4. Cranial magnetic resonance imaging (MRI) is usually performed to rule out associated brain abnormalities preoperatively.

Surgical

No palliative procedure is performed unless arterial switch operation (ASO) cannot be performed early in life. Historically, definitive surgeries performed for TGA were procedures that switched right- and left-sided blood at three levels: the atrial level (intraatrial repair surgeries such as the Senning or Mustard operation), the ventricular level (i.e., Rastelli operation), and the great artery level (ASO). At this time, ASO is clearly the procedure of choice and intraatrial repair surgeries are very rarely performed only under unusual situations. The Damus-Kaye-Stansel operation in conjunction with the Rastelli operation can be performed in patients with VSD and subaortic stenosis. Because of a relatively poor long-term result of the Rastelli operation, other options such as Nikaidoh operation or REV procedure have been entertained on selected patients. For completeness, all of these surgical procedures will be briefly described with schematic illustrations.

Procedures

Atrial Baffle Operations (Mustard and Senning Operations). These procedures reroute pulmonary and systemic venous returns at the atrial level with resulting physiologic

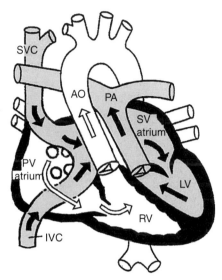

Fig. 14.6 Atrial baffle operation. The hemodynamic results of the Mustard and Senning operations are shown. Systemic venous blood *(shaded)* is redirected at the atrial level to the anatomic left atrium (LA) and left ventricle (LV) and eventually to the pulmonary circulation. Pulmonary venous blood is redirected at the atrial level to the anatomic right atrium (RA) and right ventricle (RV) through the tricuspid valve and to the aorta. *AO,* Aorta; *IVC,* inferior vena cava; *PA,* pulmonary artery; *PV atrium,* pulmonary venous atrium; *SV atrium,* systemic venous atrium; *SVC,* superior vena cava.

correction. The pulmonary venous blood eventually goes to the aorta and the systemic venous blood goes to the PA (see Fig. 14.6 for the hemodynamic results of atrial baffle operation). The Mustard operation uses a pericardial or a prosthetic baffle and the Senning operation uses the patient's own atrial septal flap and the RA free wall to redirect the venous returns.

A number of long-term problems have been reported, including superior vena cava (SVC) obstruction (<5% of all cases), baffle leak (<20%), absence of sinus rhythm (>50%), frequent atrial and ventricular arrhythmias with occasional sudden death, tricuspid valve insufficiency (rare), and RV (i.e., systemic ventricular) dysfunction or failure. The ASO has largely replaced the atrial baffle operation. There are, however, very rare indications for atrial baffle operations, including a situation in which relative contraindications of the ASO exist (e.g., coronary arteries that are difficult to transfer).

Rastelli Operation. In patients with VSD and severe PS, redirection of the pulmonary and systemic venous blood is carried out at the ventricular level. The LV is directed to the aorta by creating an intraventricular tunnel between the VSD and the aortic valve. A valved conduit or a homograft is placed between the RV and the PA (Fig. 14.7). Most surgeons prefer to delay this procedure until after the first year of life.

Complications after the Rastelli operation include conduit obstruction (especially in those containing porcine heterograft valves) and complete heart block (rarely occurs). The conduit needs to be replaced as the child grows. Occasionally, LVOT obstruction occurs at the level of the ventricular septum or at the level of the intraventricular tunnels. More important, the long-term results are not optimal. Two alternative procedures, REV procedure and Nikaidoh procedure (see later discussion of these procedures), could be entertained instead.

Arterial Switch Operation. Arterial switch operation is now firmly established as the procedure of choice. There are almost no situations that would justify the performance of a Senning or Mustard procedure for D-TGA. The coronary arteries are transplanted to the PA, and the proximal great

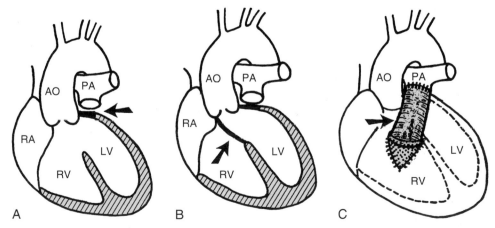

Fig. 14.7 The Rastelli operation. **A,** In patients with D-transposition of the great arteries (D-TGA), ventricular septal defect (VSD) and severe pulmonary stenosis (PS), the pulmonary artery (PA) is divided from the left ventricle (LV), and the cardiac end is oversewn *(arrow).* **B,** An intracardiac tunnel *(arrow)* is placed between the large VSD and the aorta (AO) so that the LV communicates with the aorta. **C,** The right ventricle (RV) is connected to the divided PA by a valved conduit or an aortic homograft. *RA,* Right atrium.

arteries are connected to the distal end of the other great artery, resulting in an anatomic correction (Fig. 14.8). This procedure has advantages over the atrial baffle operations because it is an anatomic (not physiologic) correction, and long-term complications are infrequent. This procedure is indicated not only for simple TGA but also TGA with other associated anomalies (e.g., VSD or PDA) and the Taussig-Bing type of double-outlet right ventricle (DORV) with subpulmonary VSD. The operative mortality rate for neonates with TGA and intact ventricular septum is down to around 2% to 3%.

Complications after the ASO are infrequent. Normal sinus rhythm is usually present, arrhythmias are extremely rare, and LV function is usually normal. The following complications may occur after the ASO:

a. Coronary artery obstruction, which may lead to myocardial ischemia, infarction, and even death, is a serious but rare complication.
b. Supravalvar PS at the anastomosis site (~12%) is the most common cause for reoperation, although the incidence has decreased. Unilateral or bilateral PA branch stenosis is a potential long-term complication in patients undergoing arterial switch with the Lecompte maneuver (see later).
c. Neoaortic valvar regurgitation and supravalvar neoaortic stenosis are rare complications.

The following factors are important for a successful ASO.

a. LV pressure. An LV that can support the systemic circulation after surgery must exist. The LV pressure should be near systemic levels at the time of surgery, so the ASO should be performed shortly after birth. The time limit is 3 weeks of age (although some suggest an upper limit of 8 weeks of age).
b. Coronary artery anatomy. Almost all coronary artery patterns in TGA are amenable to the ASO. However, the risk is slightly higher when either one or both coronary arteries passes between the great arteries or has an intramural course. The single coronary artery is transferable by various surgical techniques.

Currently, other associated anomalies are repaired at the time of the ASO in the neonatal period.

a. For patients with associated VSD, the VSD is repaired through an atrial approach or through the pulmonary valve.
b. For patients with PDA and VSD, PDA is ligated, and the VSD is closed.
c. Mild pulmonary valve stenosis or dynamic subpulmonary stenosis does not preclude a successful ASO.

Two-Stage Switch Operation. In patients whose LV pressure is low (because of missing the chance for an early ASO), it can be raised by PA banding, either with or without a shunt procedure, for 7 to 10 days (in cases of a "rapid two-stage switch operation") or for several months before undertaking the switch operation. LV pressure more than 85% of the RV pressure appears to be satisfactory for the switch operation. The rapid switch is preferable to a longer waiting period, which results in scarring and adhesions of the PA following PA banding. Scarring makes PA reconstruction and anastomosis of the great arteries difficult, and adhesions obscure coronary artery anatomy.

Staged Conversion to Arterial Switch Operation. Some patients who received atrial baffle operation develop RV failure with severe tricuspid valve regurgitation. For these patients, staged conversion to ASO can be done. Initially, a PA band is placed to raise the LV pressure. This is followed by an ASO with a higher mortality rate. Alternatively, after PA band, Damus-Kaye-Stansel operation can be performed, which does not require transfer of coronary arteries. Transfer of coronary arteries is much more difficult in these patients because of dense adhesions.

REV Procedure (Réparation à L'étage Ventriculare). This procedure, first reported by Lecompte, may be performed for patients with D-TGA associated with VSD and severe PS instead of the Rastelli operation. The procedure comprises the following: (1) infundibular resection to en-

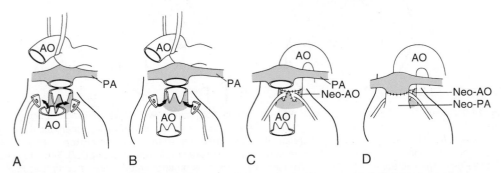

Fig. 14.8 Arterial switch operation. **A,** The aorta (AO; *unshaded*) is transected slightly above the coronary ostia, and the pulmonary artery (PA; *shaded*) is also transected at about the same level. The ascending aorta is lifted, and both coronary arteries are removed from the aorta with triangular buttons. **B,** Triangular buttons of similar size are made at the proper position in the PA trunk. **C,** The coronary arteries are transplanted to the PA trunk. The ascending aorta is brought behind the PA (called the Lecompte maneuver) and is connected to the proximal PA to form a neoaorta (Neo-AO). **D,** The triangular defects in the proximal aorta are repaired, and the proximal aorta is connected to the distal portion of the divided PA. Note that the neo-PA is in front of the neoaorta.

large the VSD, (2) intraventricular baffle to direct LV output to the aorta, (3) aortic transection in order to perform the Lecompte maneuver (by which the RPA is brought anterior to the ascending aorta), and (4) direct RV-to-PA reconstruction by using an anterior patch (Fig. 14.9). This may require fewer reoperations than the Rastelli procedure. Lecompte reported 50 cases (4 months–15 years) with an 18% operative mortality rate.

Nikaidoh Procedure. This procedure is another surgical option for patients with D-TGA, VSD, and severe PS. In this procedure, the aortic root is mobilized and translocated to the pulmonary position. The repair consists of the following: (1) harvesting the aortic root from the RV (with attached coronary arteries in the original procedure), (2) relieving the LVOT obstruction (by enlarging the VSD by means of dividing the outlet septum and excising the pulmonary valve), (3) reconstructing the LVOT (with posteriorly translocated aortic root and the VSD patch), and (4) reconstructing the right ventricular outflow tract (RVOT) (with a pericardial patch or a homograft). In the modified Nikaidoh procedure, one or both coronary arteries are moved to a more favorable position as necessary (not shown), and the Lecompte maneuver

is also performed (Fig. 14.10). The hospital mortality rate is less than 10%.

Damus-Kaye-Stansel Operation. Infants with a large VSD and significant subaortic stenosis may receive the Damus-Kaye-Stansel operation at 1 to 2 years of age. In this procedure, the coronary arteries are not transferred to a neoaorta. Instead, the subaortic stenosis is bypassed by connecting the proximal PA trunk to the ascending aorta. The VSD is closed, and a conduit is placed between the RV and the distal PA (Fig. 14.11).

The Damus-Kaye-Stansel operation is also applicable in patients with single ventricle and TGA with an obstructive bulboventricular foramen (BVF) or DORV with subaortic stenosis (see Fig. 14.62).

Surgical management for patients with TGA and various associated defects is summarized in Fig. 14.12.

Postoperative Follow-up After Arterial Switch Operation. Although the complication rate is much lower for arterial switch than for atrial baffle repair, regular follow-up is needed to detect possible complications, such as stenosis of the PA or aorta in the supravalvular regions, coronary artery obstruction with myocardial ischemia or infarction, ventricular dysfunction,

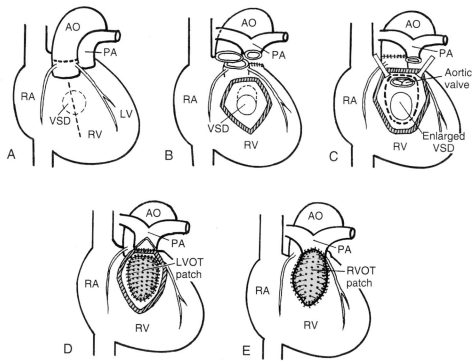

Fig. 14.9 *Réparation à l'étage ventriculare* (REV) procedure for patients with D-transposition of the great arteries (D-TGA), ventricular septal defect (VSD), and severe pulmonary stenosis (PS). A, Schematic drawing of D-TGA with VSD and severe PS (with a relatively small pulmonary artery [PA]). The *broken lines* indicate the planned aortic and right ventricular (RV) incision sites. The *broken circle* indicates a VSD. B, The aorta and PA have been transected, and the right pulmonary artery (RPA) is brought anterior to the aorta (Lecompte maneuver). The proximal PA has been oversewn. The VSD is exposed through the right ventriculotomy. (Note that these figures have expanded ventriculotomy to allow visualization of intracardiac structures.) *Dotted hemi-circular lines* indicate the portion of the infundibular septum to be excised to enlarge the VSD. C, The aortic valve is well shown by retractors. The *broken line* indicates the planned site of a patch placement for the LV–aorta (AO) connection. The transected aorta has been reconnected behind the RPA. D, The completed LV-to-AO tunnel is shown (marked LVOT [left ventricular outflow tract] patch). The superior portion of the right ventriculotomy is sutured directly to the posterior portion of the main PA. E, A pericardial or synthetic patch is used to complete the RV-to-PA reconstruction (marked RVOT [right ventricular outflow tract] patch).

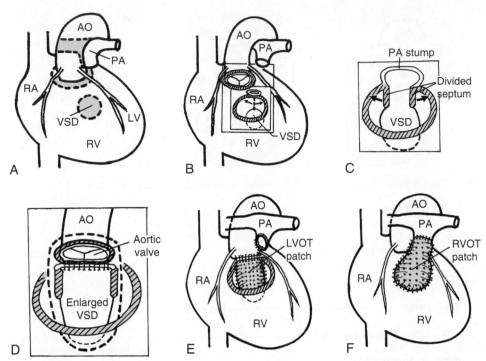

Fig. 14.10 Nikaidoh procedure (for patients with D-transposition of the great arteries [D-TGA], ventricular septal defect [VSD], and severe pulmonary stenosis [PS]). **A,** Schematic drawing of D-TGA with VSD and severe PS (with relatively small pulmonary artery [PA]) is shown. The circular broken line around the aorta is the planned incision site for aortic root mobilization. The *smaller broken circle* indicates a VSD. **B,** The aortic root has been mobilized by a circular incision around the aortic root, which leaves an opening in the right ventricular (RV) free wall. The main PA is also transected. Through the opening, part of the VSD, the ventricular septum, and the hypoplastic PA stump are seen. The *dotted vertical line* in the ventricular septum (in the smaller inset in *B*) is the planned incision through the infundibular septum. **C,** In the inset, the incision in the infundibular septum has created a large opening, which includes the PA annulus and stump and the VSD. **D,** In the *large inset,* the posterior portion of the aorta is directly sutured to the PA stump, which results in a large VSD. This completes translocation of the aorta to the original PA position. The *thick oval-shaped broken line* that goes through the front of the transected aortic root is the planned site for placement of the left ventricular (LV) outflow tract (LVOT) patch, which will direct the LV flow to the aorta. **E,** The completed tunnel is shown (marked LVOT patch, which directs the LV flow to the aorta). The distal segment of the main PA is fixed to the aorta. Some surgeons use the Lecompte maneuver to bring the right pulmonary artery (RPA) in front of the ascending aorta (as shown here). **F,** A pericardial patch is oversewn to complete the RV-to-PA connection (marked RVOT [RV outflow tract] patch).

arrhythmias, and semilunar valve regurgitation. These complications are, for the most part, hemodynamically insignificant or infrequent.

Coronary artery obstruction after the surgery is a concern. In one study, about 5% of postoperative arterial switch patients had coronary arterial abnormalities by coronary angiography; some of them had no signs of ischemia by history, ECG, and echo studies. A periodic follow-up is recommended with ECG, echo, exercise stress test (in older children), MRI or computed tomography (CT), or coronary angiography. MRI can provide a comprehensive anatomic and functional evaluation for coronary ischemia noninvasively, including myocardial perfusion and viability information.

CONGENITALLY CORRECTED TRANSPOSITION OF THE GREAT ARTERIES

Prevalence

Congenitally corrected transposition of the great arteries (or L-TGA) occurs in fewer than 1% of all patients with CHDs.

Pathology

1. In this condition, the visceroatrial relationship is normal, but there is ventricular inversion. The RA is to the right of the LA and receives systemic venous blood. The RA empties into the anatomic LV through the mitral valve, and the LA empties the pulmonary venous blood into the RV through the tricuspid valve. For this to occur, the morphologic RV with tricuspid valve is located to the left of the morphologic LV, which has the mitral valve, which is called *ventricular inversion* (Fig. 14.13). The great arteries are transposed, with the aorta rising from the RV and the PA rising from the LV. The aorta is usually located anterior to and left of the PA. The prefix L is used to indicate *levo* looping of the cardiac tube during embryogenesis; thus, the condition is labeled L-TGA (see Fig. 17.4D). The result is functional correction, in that oxygenated blood coming into the LA goes to the anatomic RV and then flows out to the aorta. This is why the term *corrected* is used to describe this condition.

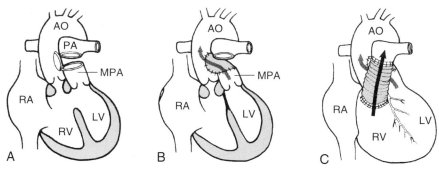

Fig. 14.11 Damus-Kaye-Stansel operation for complete transposition of the great arteries (D-TGA) + ventricular septal defect (VSD) + subaortic stenosis. **A,** D-TGA with VSD and subaortic stenosis is illustrated. The main pulmonary artery (MPA) is transected near its bifurcation. An appropriately positioned and sized incision is made in the ascending aorta (AO). **B,** The proximal MPA is anastomosed end to side to the ascending aorta using either a Dacron tube or Gore-Tex. This channel will direct left ventricular blood to the aorta. The aortic valve is either closed or left unclosed. The VSD is closed (through a right ventriculotomy). **C,** A valved conduit is placed between the right ventricle (RV) and the distal pulmonary artery (PA). This channel will carry RV blood to the PA. *LV,* Left ventricle; *RA,* right atrium.

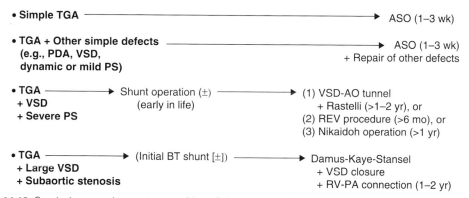

Fig. 14.12 Surgical approaches to transposition of the great arteries with various associated defects. *ASO,* Arterial switch operation; *BT,* Blalock-Taussig; *PDA,* patent ductus arteriosus; *PS,* pulmonary stenosis; *REV,* réparation à l'étage; *TGA,* transposition of the great arteries; *VSD,* ventricular septal defect.

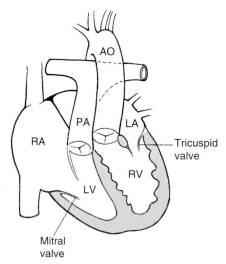

Fig. 14.13 Diagram of congenitally corrected transposition of the great arteries (L-TGA). There is an inversion of ventricular chambers with their corresponding atrioventricular valves. The great arteries are transposed, but functional correction results, with oxygenated blood going to the aorta. Unfortunately, a high percentage of the patients with L-TGA have associated defects, some of which may cause cyanosis. *AO,* Aorta; *LA,* left atrium; *LV,* left ventricle; *PA,* pulmonary artery; *RA,* right atrium; *RV,* right ventricle.

2. Theoretically, no functional abnormalities exist, but unfortunately, most cases are complicated by associated intracardiac defects, AV conduction disturbances, and arrhythmias.
   a. VSD occurs in 80% of all cases.
   b. PS, both valvular and subvalvular, occurs in 50% of patients and is usually associated with VSD.
   c. Systemic AV valve (tricuspid valve) regurgitation occurs in 30% of patients.
   d. Occasionally, complex associated defects are present with hypoplastic ventricle, AV valve abnormalities, or multiple VSDs.
   c. Both varying and progressive degrees of AV block and paroxysmal supraventricular tachycardia (SVT) frequently occur.
3. The cardiac apex is in the right chest (dextrocardia) in about 50% of cases.
4. The coronary arteries show a mirror-image distribution. The right-sided coronary artery supplies the anterior descending branch and gives rise to a circumflex; the left-sided coronary artery resembles a right coronary artery. Essentially, coronary arteries follow the ventricles.

Clinical Manifestations
History

1. During childhood, patients are asymptomatic when L-TGA is not associated with other defects.
2. During the first months of life, most patients with associated defects become symptomatic with cyanosis resulting from VSD and PS or CHF resulting from a large VSD.
3. Exertional dyspnea and easy fatigability may develop with regurgitation of the systemic AV valve (i.e., anatomic tricuspid valve).

Physical Examination

1. The patient is cyanotic if PS and VSD are present.
2. Hyperactive precordium occurs in the presence of a large VSD. Systolic thrill occurs in the presence of PS, with or without VSD.
3. The S2 is loud and single at the upper left or right sternal border. A grade 2 to 4 of 6 harsh holosystolic murmur along the lower left sternal border indicates the presence of VSD or systemic AV valve regurgitation. A grade 2 to 3 of 6 ejection systolic murmur is present at the upper left or right sternal border if PS is present. An apical diastolic rumble may be audible if a large VSD or significant TR is present.
4. Bradycardia, tachycardia, or irregular rhythm requires an investigation for AV conduction disturbances or arrhythmias.

Electrocardiography

1. The absence of Q waves in V5 and V6 or the presence of Q waves in V4R or V1 is characteristic of the condition (Fig. 14.14). This is because the direction of ventricular septal depolarization is from the embryonic LV to RV.
2. The P axis is normal (because of normally related atrial position), but the QRS complexes suggest dominance or hypertrophy of the right-sided ventricle (anatomic LV).
3. Varying degrees of AV block are common. First-degree AV block is present in about 50% of patients. Second-degree AV block may progress to complete heart block. Complete heart block is present in 4% of the patient at birth, and its prevalence increases during follow-up (to 20%–30%).
4. Atrial arrhythmias and Wolff-Parkinson-White (WPW) pre-excitation are occasionally present.
5. Atrial or ventricular hypertrophy (or both) may be present in complicated cases.

Radiography

1. A straight, left upper cardiac border, formed by the ascending aorta, is a characteristic finding (Fig. 14.15).
2. Cardiomegaly and increased pulmonary vascular markings are present when the condition is associated with VSD.
3. Pulmonary venous congestion and left atrial enlargement may be seen with severe left-sided AV valve regurgitation.
4. Positional abnormalities (e.g., dextrocardia, mesocardia) may be present.

Echocardiography

With use of the segmental approach (see Chapter 17), the diagnosis of L-TGA can be made easily, and associated anomalies can be detected and quantitated.

1. The parasternal long-axis view is obtained from a more vertical and leftward scan than with a normal heart. The aorta, which arises from the posterior ventricle, is not in fibrous continuity with the AV valve.
2. In the parasternal short-axis scan, a "double circle" of the semilunar valves is imaged instead of the normal "circle and sausage" pattern. The posterior circle is the PA without demonstrable coronary arteries. The aorta is usually anterior to and left of the PA. The LV, which has two well-defined papillary muscles, is seen anteriorly and on the right and is connected to the characteristic "fish mouth" appearance of the mitral valve.
3. In the apical and subcostal four-chamber views, the LA is connected to the tricuspid valve (which has a more apical attachment to the ventricular septum than the other), and the RA is connected to the mitral valve. The anterior artery (aorta) arises from the left-sided morphologic RV,

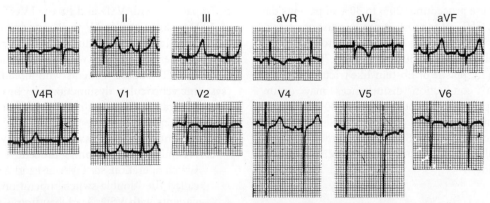

Fig. 14.14 Tracing from an 8-year-old girl with congenitally corrected transposition of the great arteries, ventricular septal defect, and pulmonary stenosis. Note that no Q waves are seen in leads V5 and V6. Instead, the Q waves are seen in V4R and V1. This suggests ventricular inversion. The electrocardiogram also suggests hypertrophy of the right-sided ventricle (anatomic left ventricle).

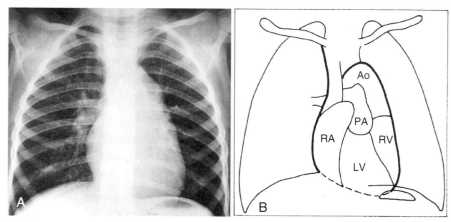

Fig. 14.15 Posteroanterior view of an actual chest radiograph (**A**) and a diagrammatic representation (**B**) from a 10-year-old child with congenitally corrected transposition of the great arteries. Note the straight left cardiac border formed by the ascending aorta (Ao). *LV,* Left ventricle; *PA,* pulmonary artery; *RA,* right atrium; *RV,* right ventricle.

and the posterior artery with bifurcation (PA) arises from the right-sided morphologic LV.

4. The situs solitus of the atria is confirmed by the drainage of systemic veins (i.e., inferior and superior venae cavae) to the right-sided atrium and the drainage of pulmonary veins to the left-sided atrium.

5. The following associated abnormalities should be looked for and their functional significance should be assessed by the Doppler and color-flow studies: type and severity of PS, size and location of VSD, straddling of the AV valve, and so on.

Other Studies

Occasionally, angiography may be necessary to image coronary artery anatomy, although CT or MRI may provide this information noninvasively.

Natural History

The clinical course is determined by the presence or absence of associated defects and complications.

1. Some palliative surgeries are usually needed in infancy when L-TGA is associated with other defects (e.g., PA banding for a large VSD or a systemic-to-PA shunt for severe PS). Without these procedures, 20% to 30% of patients die in the first year. CHF is the most common cause of death.

2. Regurgitation of the systemic AV valve (anatomic tricuspid valve) develops in about 30% of patients. This is often associated with dysplastic or Ebstein-like tricuspid valves.

3. Progressive AV conduction disturbances may occur, including complete heart block in up to 30% of cases. These disturbances occur more often in patients without VSD than in those with VSD. Sudden death rarely occurs.

4. Occasional adult patients without major associated defects are asymptomatic.

Management
Medical

1. Treatment with anticongestive agents is necessary if CHF develops.

2. Antiarrhythmic agents are used for arrhythmias.

Surgical

Palliative Procedures.

1. A modified Blalock-Taussig (BT) shunt is necessary for patients with severe PS (usually associated with VSD).

2. PA banding may be needed for uncontrollable CHF in early infancy.

Definitive Procedures. There are two major approaches to surgical management of L-TGA, classic repair and anatomic repair. Patients with regurgitation of the tricuspid valve (systemic AV valve) or RV dysfunction need the anatomic repair, in which the LV is made the systemic ventricle. Surgical approach for L-TGA is summarized in Fig. 14.16.

Classic Repair. In classic repair, the anatomic RV remains as the systemic ventricle. Competent tricuspid valve (or left AV valve) and good RV function are required. Even after repair, progressive TR and RV failure may develop.

a. In patients with VSD, the VSD is closed through atrial approach. Complete heart block is a complication of the surgery, occurring 15% to 30% of the time. The mortality rate is higher than that for a simple VSD.

b. In patients with VSD and PS (or LVOT obstruction), the VSD is closed and an LV-to-PA conduit is placed.

Anatomic Repair. Anatomic repair makes the anatomic LV the systemic ventricle, which may reduce the likelihood of TR and RV failure. Patients who already have TR or RV (systemic ventricular) dysfunction may be candidates for this type of operation. This repair is technically more difficult than the classic repair and carries a higher risk, but this procedure is a better choice for patients with TR or RV dysfunction.

a. A combination of Senning procedure (which is an atrial switch operation; see Fig. 14.6) and ASO (see Fig. 14.8), called the "double-switch" operation, is performed in patients with VSD. A PA banding is initially placed to delay the procedure until after 1 year of age. Closure of VSD, if present, is performed through the RA. The hospital mortality rate for the "double-switch" operation is

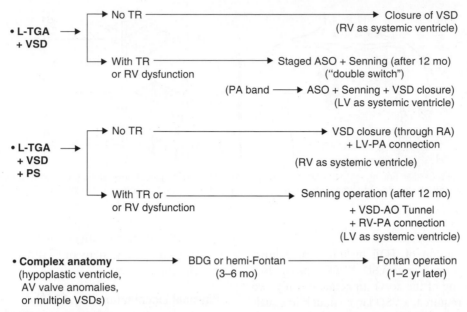

Fig. 14.16 Surgical summary of congenitally corrected transposition of the great arteries (L-TGA). *AO*, aorta; *ASO*, arterial switch operation; *AV*, atrioventricular; *BDG*, bidirectional Glenn; *PA*, pulmonary artery; *RA*, right atrium; *RV*, right ventricle; *PS*, pulmonary stenosis (= LV outflow tract obstruction); *TGA*, transposition of the great arteries; *TR*, tricuspid regurgitation (= left-sided AV valve regurgitation); *VSD*, ventricular septal defect.

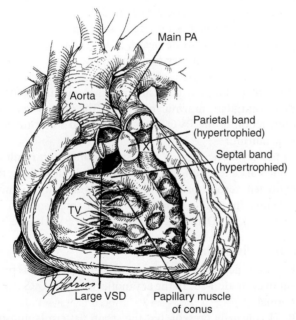

Fig. 14.17 Pathologic anatomy of tetralogy of Fallot viewed with the right ventricular (RV) free wall removed. A large ventricular septal defect (VSD) is present underneath the aortic valve. Hypertrophied parietal and septal bands produce infundibular stenosis (marked *x*). A stenotic and hypoplastic main pulmonary artery (PA) is shown. The RV muscle is hypertrophied. *TV*, Tricuspid valve. (Hirsch JC, Bove EL: *Tetralogy of Fallot*. In Mavroudis C (ed): *Pediatric Cardiac Surgery*, ed 3, Philadelphia, 2003, Mosby. Reproduced with permission.)

approximately 10% with complete heart block occurring from 0% to 23%.

b. In patients with VSD and PS (or LVOT obstruction), a combination of the Senning and Rastelli operations is performed. VSD is closed through a right

ventriculotomy in such a way to connect the VSD to the aorta. Enlargement of the VSD is often necessary. RV-to-PA continuity is established with an extracardiac valved conduit. The hospital mortality rate is around 10%. TR improves after the procedure.

Fontan-Type Operation. In patients with complex intracardiac anatomies, including hypoplasia of one ventricle, straddling AV valves, or multiple VSDs, the bidirectional Glenn operation or full Fontan procedure is indicated.

Other Procedures.

a. **Valve replacement.** For patients with significant TR, valve replacement is required in about 15% of patients, including those without other associated defects.

b. **Pacemaker implantation** is required for either spontaneous or postoperative complete heart block.

c. **Cardiac transplantation.** Some patients with complex L-TGA will eventually become candidates for cardiac transplantation.

Postoperative Follow-up

1. Follow-up every 6 to 12 months is required for a possible progression of AV conduction disturbances, arrhythmias, or worsening of anatomic tricuspid valve regurgitation.

2. Routine pacemaker care, if a pacemaker is implanted, should be conducted.

3. Activity restriction is indicated if significant hemodynamic abnormalities persist.

TETRALOGY OF FALLOT

Prevalence

Tetralogy of Fallot (TOF) occurs in 5% to 10% of all CHDs. This is the most common cyanotic heart defect.

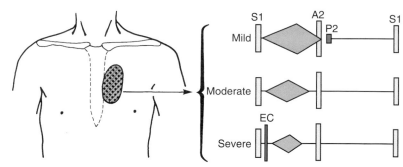

Fig. 14.18 Cardiac findings in cyanotic tetralogy of Fallot (TOF). A long ejection systolic murmur at the upper and mid left sternal border and a loud, single S2 are characteristic auscultatory findings of TOF. *EC,* Ejection click.

Pathology

1. The original description of TOF included the following four abnormalities: a large VSD, RVOT obstruction, RVH, and overriding of the aorta. In actuality, only two abnormalities are required, a VSD large enough to equalize pressures in both ventricles and an RVOT obstruction. The RVH is secondary to the RVOT obstruction, and the overriding of the aorta varies (Fig. 14.17).

2. The VSD in TOF is a large perimembranous defect with extension into the subpulmonary region.

3. The RVOT obstruction is most frequently in the form of infundibular stenosis (45%). The obstruction is rarely at the pulmonary valve level (10%). A combination of the two may also occur (30%). The pulmonary valve is atretic in the most severe form of the anomaly (15%), which is discussed under a separate heading in this chapter.

4. The pulmonary annulus and main PA are variably hypoplastic in most patients. The PA branches are usually small, although marked hypoplasia is uncommon. Stenosis at the origin of the branch PAs, especially the left PA, is common. Occasionally, systemic collateral arteries feed into the lungs, especially in severe cases of TOF.

5. Right aortic arch is present in 25% of cases, with some of them having symptoms of vascular ring.

6. In about 5% of patients with TOF, abnormal coronary arteries are present. The most common abnormality is the anterior descending branch arising from the right coronary artery and passing over the RVOT, which prohibits a surgical incision in the region.

7. Complete AV canal defect occurs in approximately 2% of patients with TOF, more commonly among patients with Down syndrome, called "canal tet." In these patients, the VSD has a large outlet component in addition to the inlet portion associated with the AV canal.

Clinical Manifestations

History

1. A heart murmur is audible at birth.
2. Most patients are symptomatic with cyanosis at birth or shortly thereafter. Dyspnea on exertion, squatting, or hypoxic spells develop later, even in mildly cyanotic infants (see Chapter 11).

3. Occasional infants with *acyanotic* TOF may be asymptomatic or may show signs of CHF from a large left-to-right ventricular shunt.

Physical Examination (Fig. 14.18)

1. Varying degrees of cyanosis, tachypnea, and clubbing (in older infants and children) are present.

2. An RV tap along the left sternal border and a systolic thrill at the upper and mid-left sternal borders are commonly present (50%).

3. An ejection click that originates in the aorta may be audible. The S2 is usually single because the pulmonary component is too soft to be heard. A long, loud (grade 3 to 5 of 6) ejection-type systolic murmur is heard at the mid and upper left sternal borders. This murmur originates from the PS but may be easily confused with the holosystolic regurgitant murmur of a VSD. The more severe the obstruction of the RVOT, the shorter and softer the systolic murmur.

4. In the acyanotic form, a long systolic murmur, resulting from VSD and infundibular stenosis, is audible along the entire left sternal border, and cyanosis is absent. Thus, auscultatory findings resemble those of a small-shunt VSD (but, unlike VSD, the ECG shows RVH or BVH).

Electrocardiography

1. Right axis deviation (RAD) (+120 to +150 degrees) is present in cyanotic TOF. In the acyanotic form, the QRS axis is normal.

2. RVH is usually present, but the strain pattern is unusual (because RV pressure is not suprasystemic). BVH may be seen in the acyanotic form. RAH is occasionally present.

Radiography

Cyanotic Tetralogy of Fallot.

1. The heart size is normal or smaller than normal, and pulmonary vascular markings are decreased. "Black" lung fields are seen in TOF with pulmonary atresia.

2. A concave main PA segment with an upturned apex (i.e., "boot-shaped" heart or coeur en sabot) is characteristic (Fig. 14.19).

3. RA enlargement (25%) and right aortic arch (25%) may be present.

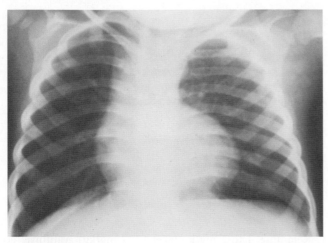

Fig. 14.19 Posteroanterior view of chest roentgenogram in tetralogy of Fallot. The heart size is normal, and pulmonary vascular markings are decreased. A hypoplastic main pulmonary artery segment contributes to the formation of the "boot-shaped" heart.

Acyanotic Tetralogy of Fallot. Radiographic findings of acyanotic TOF are indistinguishable from those of a small to moderate VSD (but patients with TOF have RVH rather than LVH on the ECG).

Echocardiography

Two-dimensional echo and Doppler studies usually make the diagnosis and quantitate the severity of TOF. Careful echo study can delineate anomalous coronary arteries, which has important surgical consequences.

1. A large, perimembranous infundibular VSD and overriding of the aorta are readily imaged in the parasternal long-axis view (Fig. 14.20).
2. Anatomy of the RVOT, the pulmonary valve, the pulmonary annulus, and the main PA and its branches is imaged in the parasternal short-axis and subcostal short-axis views. These views allow systematic evaluation of the severity of obstruction at different levels.
3. Doppler studies estimate the pressure gradient across the RVOT obstruction.
4. Anomalous coronary artery distribution can be imaged in most cases by echo studies (Fig. 14.21), primarily from the parasternal short- and long-axis views. The major concern is to rule out any branch of the coronary artery crossing the RVOT. Thus, preoperative cardiac catheterization solely for the diagnosis of coronary artery anatomy is most of the time no longer necessary; when in doubt, CT or MRI angiography could be used as an alternative, noninvasive imaging modality.
5. Associated anomalies such as ASD and persistence of the left SVC can be imaged.

Other Studies

Two-dimensional echo and Doppler studies are the primary method of evaluation before surgery. CT and MRI angiography may clarify questions on the anomalous coronary arteries. Cardiac catheterization is reserved only for patients with specific unanswered questions after the noninvasive studies.

Natural History

1. Infants with acyanotic TOF gradually become cyanotic. Patients who are already cyanotic become more cyanotic as the infundibular stenosis worsens, and polycythemia develops.
2. Polycythemia develops secondary to cyanosis.[a]
3. Physicians need to watch for the development of relative iron-deficiency state (i.e., hypochromia) (see Chapter 11).[a]
4. Hypoxic spells may develop in infants (see Chapter 11).
5. Growth retardation may be present if cyanosis is severe.[a]
6. Brain abscess and cerebrovascular accident rarely occur (see Chapter 11).[a]
7. Subacute bacterial endocarditis (SBE) is occasionally a complication.[a]
8. Some patients, particularly those with severe TOF, develop aortic regurgitation (AR).
9. Coagulopathy is a late complication of a long-standing cyanosis.[a]

Hypoxic Spell

Hypoxic spell (also called cyanotic spell, hypercyanotic spell, "tet" spell) of TOF is not as common as it used to be because many patients with TOF receive surgery before they develop the spell. However, it is very important for physicians to be able to immediately recognize and treat the spell appropriately because it can lead to serious complications of the CNS.

Hypoxic spells are characterized by a paroxysm of hyperpnea (i.e., *rapid* and *deep* respiration), irritability and prolonged crying, increasing cyanosis, and decreasing intensity of the heart murmur. Hypoxic spells occur in infants, with a peak incidence between 2 and 4 months of age. These spells usually occur in the morning after crying, feeding, or defecation. A severe spell may lead to limpness, convulsion, cerebrovascular accident, or even death. There appears to be no relationship between the degree of cyanosis at rest and the likelihood of having hypoxic spells (see Chapter 11).

Treatment of the hypoxic spell strives to break the vicious circle of the spell (see Fig. 11.10). Physicians may use one or more of the following to treat the spell.

1. The infant should be picked up and held in a knee–chest position.
2. Morphine sulfate, 0.2 mg/kg administered subcutaneously or intramuscularly, suppresses the respiratory center and abolishes hyperpnea (and thus breaks the vicious cycle).
3. Oxygen is usually administered, but it has little demonstrable effect on arterial oxygen saturation.
4. Acidosis should be treated with sodium bicarbonate ($NaHCO_3$), 1 mEq/kg administered intravenously. The same dose can be repeated in 10 to 15 minutes. $NaHCO_3$ reduces the respiratory center–stimulating effect of acidosis.

[a]This occurs in all types of cyanotic CHDs.

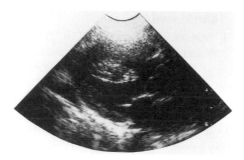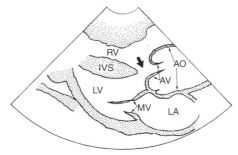

Fig. 14.20 Parasternal long-axis view in a patient with tetralogy of Fallot. Note a large subaortic ventricular septal defect *(arrow)* and a relatively large aorta (AO) overriding the interventricular septum (IVS). *AV,* Aortic valve; *LA,* left atrium; *LV,* left ventricle; *MV,* mitral valve; *RV,* right ventricle.

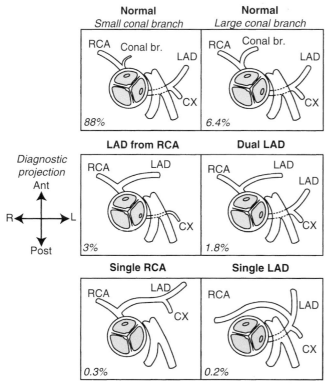

Fig. 14.21 Patterns of coronary artery anatomy in tetralogy of Fallot (TOF) as imaged from the parasternal short-axis view. The percentage of each pattern seen in 598 patients with TOF is indicated in the lower *left corner* of each box. Four types of anomalous coronary arteries shown in the *lower panels* are abnormal, with the left descending artery (LAD) crossing over the right ventricular outflow tract (RVOT), which has important surgical consequences. The LAD branch originating from the right coronary artery (RCA) and from a single coronary artery cross the RVOT in their course toward the left ventricle. *Ant,* Anterior; *br,* branch; *CX,* left circumflex coronary artery; *L,* left; *R,* right; *Post,* posterior. (From Need LR, Powell AJ, del Nide P, Geva T: Coronary echocardiography in tetralogy of Fallot: diagnostic accuracy, resource utilization and surgical implications over 13 years, *J Am Coll Cardiol* 36:1371–1377, 2000.)

With the preceding treatment, the infant usually becomes less cyanotic, and the heart murmur becomes louder, which indicates an increased amount of blood flowing through the stenotic RVOT. If the hypoxic spells do not fully respond to these measures, the following medications can be tried:

1. Ketamine, 1 to 3 mg/kg (average, 2 mg/kg) administered intravenously over 60 seconds, works well. It increases the systemic vascular resistance and sedates the infant.
2. Propranolol, 0.01 to 0.25 mg/kg (average, 0.05 mg/kg) administered by slow IV push, reduces the heart rate and may reverse the spell.

Management
Medical

1. Physicians should recognize and treat hypoxic spells (see the preceding section and Chapter 11). It is important to educate parents to recognize the spell and know what to do.
2. Oral propranolol therapy, 0.5 to 2mg/kg every 6 hours, is occasionally used to prevent hypoxic spells while waiting for an optimal time for corrective surgery in the regions where open-heart surgical procedures are not well established for small infants.
3. Balloon dilatation of the RVOT and pulmonary valve, although not widely practiced, has been attempted to delay repair for several months.
4. Relative iron-deficiency state should be detected and treated. Iron-deficient children are more susceptible to cerebrovascular complications. Normal hemoglobin or hematocrit values or decreased red blood cell indices indicate an iron-deficiency state in cyanotic patients.

Surgical

Palliative Shunt Procedures

Indications. Shunt procedures are performed to increase PBF (Fig. 14.22). Indications for shunt procedures vary from institution to institution. Many institutions, however, prefer primary repair without a shunt operation regardless of the patient's age. However, when the following situations are present, a shunt operation may be chosen usually rather than primary repair.

1. Neonates with TOF and pulmonary atresia
2. Infants with hypoplastic pulmonary annulus, which requires a transannular patch for complete repair
3. Children with hypoplastic PAs
4. Unfavorable coronary artery anatomy
5. Infants younger than 3 to 4 months old who have medically unmanageable hypoxic spells
6. Infants weighing less than 2.5 kg

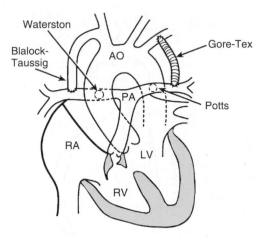

Fig. 14.22 Palliative procedures that can be performed in patients with cyanotic cardiac defect with decreased pulmonary blood flow. The Gore-Tex interposition shunt (or modified Blalock-Taussig shunt) is the most popular systemic–to–pulmonary artery (PA) shunt procedure; others are no longer performed (but are shown for completeness). *AO,* Aorta; *LV,* left ventricle; *RA,* right atrium; *RV,* right ventricle.

Procedures, Complications, and Mortality. Although several other procedures were performed in the past (see Fig. 14.22), a modified BT (Gore-Tex interposition) shunt is the only procedure performed at this time.

1. Classic BT shunt (1945), anastomosed between the subclavian artery and the ipsilateral PA, is usually performed for infants older than 3 months because it is often thrombosed in young infants. A right-sided shunt is performed in patients with left aortic arch; a left-sided shunt is performed for right aortic arch.
2. The Potts operation (1946), anastomosed between the descending aorta and the left PA, is no longer performed either. It may result in heart failure or pulmonary hypertension, as in the Waterston operation. A separate incision (i.e., left thoracotomy) is required to close the shunt during corrective surgery, which is performed through a midsternal incision.
3. The Waterston shunt (1962), anastomosed between the ascending aorta and the right PA, is no longer performed because of a high incidence of surgical complications. Complications resulting from this procedure included too large a shunt, leading to CHF or pulmonary hypertension, and narrowing and kinking of the right PA at the site of the anastomosis. This created difficult problems in closing the shunt and reconstructing the right PA at the time of corrective surgery.
4. Modified BT shunt. A Gore-Tex interposition shunt is placed between the subclavian artery and the ipsilateral PA. This is the most popular procedure for any age, especially for infants younger than 3 months of age. Whereas a right-sided shunt is preferred for patients with left aortic arch, a left-sided shunt is preferred for patients with a right aortic arch. The surgical mortality rate is 1% or less.

Complete Repair Surgery. Timing of this operation varies from institution to institution, but early surgery is generally preferred.

Indications and Timing.

1. Most centers prefer primary elective repair between 3 months and 12 months of age, even if they are asymptomatic, acyanotic (i.e., "pink tet"), or minimally cyanotic. Advantages cited for early primary repair include not only avoiding risks associated with a shunt operation but also diminution of hypertrophy and fibrosis of the RV, normal growth of the PAs and alveolar units, and reduced incidence of postoperative ventricular arrhythmias and possible sudden death.
2. The occurrence of hypoxic spell is generally considered an indication for operation, even in conservative centers.
3. Mildly cyanotic infants who have had previous shunt surgery may have total repair 1 to 2 years after the shunt operation.
4. Patients with coronary artery anomalies may have an early surgery at the same time as those without anomalous coronary arteries. In the past, surgery for these patients was delayed until after 1 year of age because a conduit placement may be required between the RV and the PA.

Procedure. Total repair of the defect is carried out under cardiopulmonary bypass, circulatory arrest, and hypothermia. The procedure includes patch closure of the VSD, preferably through transatrial and transpulmonary artery approach (rather than right ventriculotomy), widening of the RVOT by division or resection of the infundibular tissue, and pulmonary valvotomy, avoiding placement of a transannular fabric patch (Fig. 14.23). At the present time, surgeons aim to avoid right ventriculotomy and placement of transannular patch whenever possible. Widening of the RVOT without placement of patch is more likely to be accomplished if the repair is done in early infancy. However, if the pulmonary annulus and main PA are hypoplastic, transannular patch placement is unavoidable. Some centers advocate placement of a monocusp valve at the time of initial repair, but others advocate pulmonary valve replacement at a later time if indicated.

The surgical approach in patients with TOF is summarized in Fig. 14.24.

Mortality and Complications. For patients with uncomplicated TOF, the mortality rate is 1% to 2% during the first 2 years. Patients at risk are those younger than 3 months and older than 4 years, as well as those with severe hypoplasia of the pulmonary annulus and trunk. Other risk factors may include multiple VSDs, large aortopulmonary collateral arteries, and Down syndrome.

Pulmonary valve regurgitation may occur, but mild regurgitation is well tolerated. Right bundle branch block (RBBB) on the ECG develops after right ventriculotomy (in >90%). Complete heart block (i.e., <1%) and ventricular arrhythmia are both rare.

Anomalous Coronary Artery. Anomalous coronary artery occurs in 2% to 9% of patients with TOF. The left anterior descending artery (LAD) originates from the right coronary

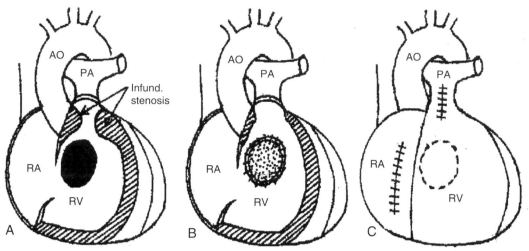

Fig. 14.23 Schematic drawing of surgical correction of tetralogy of Fallot (TOF). **A,** Anatomy of TOF showing a large ventricular septal defect (VSD) and infundibular stenosis seen with the anterior walls of the right atrium and right ventricle removed. **B,** Patch closure of the VSD is done (through a right atrial incision and through the tricuspid annulus), and the resection of the infundibular stenosis is done (through an incision in the pulmonary artery), avoiding right ventriculotomy. **C,** The right atrial incision and the pulmonary artery incision sites are shown. *AO,* Aorta; *Infund.,* infundibular; *PA,* pulmonary artery; *RA,* right atrium; *RV,* right ventricle.

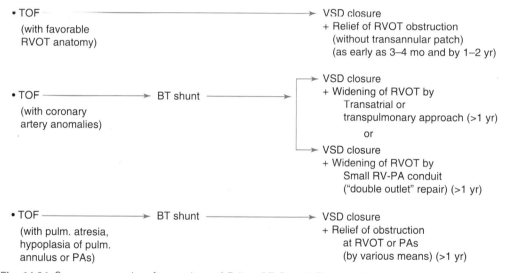

Fig. 14.24 Surgery approaches for tetralogy of Fallot. *BT,* Blalock-Taussig; *PAs,* pulmonary arteries; *pulm.,* pulmonary; *RVOT,* right ventricular outflow tract; *TOF,* tetralogy of Fallot; *RV-PA,* right ventricle-to-pulmonary artery; *VSD,* ventricular septal defect.

artery or from a single coronary artery. The LAD then crosses the RVOT in its course to the LV. The presence of anomalous coronary artery may delay the time of surgery until after 1 year of age because it may require a conduit between the RV and the PA. However, recent reports show that an early repair is possible by using transatrial and trans–pulmonary artery approach without using an extracardiac conduit. Using transatrial and transpulmonary approach, the VSD was closed, and the infundibular stenosis often was relieved by thinning or coring of the infundibular endocardium. Short outflow patch could be placed either above or below the anomalous artery. Some patients received monocusp to a transannular incision. Rarely, a small conduit was necessary between the RV and the PA, in addition to the widened native outflow

tract, so that a "double outlet" (the native outlet and the conduit) resulted from the RV.

Postoperative Follow-up.

1. Long-term follow-up with office examinations every 6 to 12 months is recommended, especially for patients with residual VSD shunt, residual obstruction of the RVOT, residual PA obstruction, arrhythmias, or conduction disturbances.

2. Significant, and usually progressive, pulmonary regurgitation may develop after repair of TOF. Although the PR is well tolerated for a decade or two, moderate to severe PR may eventually lead to significant volume overload to the RV and RV dysfunction. For a period of time, RV dysfunction remains reversible with intervention to abolish PR by

BOX 14.1 Proposed Indications for Pulmonary Valve Replacement in Patients with Repaired Tetralogy of Fallot or Similar Physiology with Right Ventricular Regurgitation Fraction ≥25%

I. Asymptomatic patients with two or more of the following.
  a. RV end-diastolic volume index >150 mL/m² (normal, <108 mL/m²)
  b. RV end-systolic volume index ≥80 mL/m² (normal, <47mL/m²)
  c. RV ejection fraction <47%
  d. LV ejection fraction <55%
  e. Large RVOT aneurysm
  f. QRS duration >160 msec
  g. Sustained tachyarrhythmia related to right-sided heart volume load
  h. Other abnormalities (e.g., RV systolic pressure >70% systemic pressure; severe PA branch stenosis not amenable to transcatheter therapy; moderate or severe TR; residual significant left-to-right shunt at atrial or ventricular level) severe AR

II. Symptomatic patients fulfilling one or more of the quantitative criteria detailed above

Examples of symptoms and signs include (1) exertional intolerance not explained by extracardiac causes, (2) signs and symptoms of heart failure, and (3) syncope attributable to arrhythmia.

III. In the following special situation, with one or more of the quantitative criteria in section
  a. Patients who had surgery at older than 3 yr of age
  b. Women in reproductive age who may get pregnant

AR, Aortic regurgitation *LV*, left ventricular; *PA*, pulmonary artery; *RV*, right ventricular; *RVOT*, right ventricular outflow tract; *TR*, tricuspid regurgitation.
From Geva T: Indications for pulmonary valve replacement in repaired tetralogy of Fallot. The quest continues [editorial], *Circulation* 128:1855–1847, 2013.

insertion of a homograft pulmonary valve by either a transcatheter technique or surgically. Severe PR left untreated may result in irreversible anatomic and functional changes in the RV, but the ideal timing of the valve replacement has been controversial. Although the procedural mortality rate is low, the functional integrity of all available bioprosthesis valves deteriorates within 10 years, posing continuing problems.

Proposed indications for pulmonary valve replacement in patients previously operated for TOF with significant PR are as follows (Geva, 2013). Prerequisite to the use of the proposal is the presence of moderate to severe PR (with RV regurgitation fraction ≥25%) (Box 14.1). RV function is best investigated by MRI; if MRI is complicated or contraindicated because of the presence of metallic objects or cardiac pacemaker, a CT can be used.

3. Some patients, particularly those who had Rastelli operation using valved conduit, develop valvular stenosis or regurgitation. Valvular stenosis may improve after balloon dilatation, but PR may worsen. Nonsurgical percutaneous

pulmonary valve implantation technique developed by Bonhoeffer et al (2000) has been used successfully. Two types of valves are being used: Melody Medtronic, available in diameters 16 mm and 18 mm, and the family of Edwards SAPIEN valves, available in diameters 23 mm, 26 mm, and 29 mm (see further discussion under TOF with Pulmonary Atresia in this chapter).

4. Some children develop late arrhythmias, particularly ventricular tachycardia, which may result in sudden death. Arrhythmias are primarily related to persistent RVH as a result of unsatisfactory repair.

5. Pacemaker therapy is indicated for surgically induced complete heart block or sinus node dysfunction.

6. Varying levels of activity limitation may be necessary.

7. For patients who have residual defects or have prosthetic material for repair, SBE prophylaxis should be observed throughout life.

TETRALOGY OF FALLOT WITH PULMONARY ATRESIA (PULMONARY ATRESIA AND VENTRICULAR SEPTAL DEFECT)

Prevalence

Pulmonary atresia occurs in about 15% to 20% of patients with TOF.

Pathology

1. The intracardiac pathology resembles that of TOF in all respects except for the presence of pulmonary atresia, the extreme form of RVOT obstruction. The atresia may be at the infundibular or valvular level.

2. The PBF is most commonly mediated through a PDA (70%) and less commonly through multiple systemic collaterals (30%), which are referred to as *multiple aortopulmonary collateral arteries (MAPCAs)*. Both PDA and collateral arteries may coexist as the source of PBF.

3. The central PAs are usually confluent in patients with PDA (70%). In patients with MAPCAs, the central PA is frequently nonconfluent, with the right upper lobe frequently supplied by a collateral from the subclavian artery and the left lower lobe by a collateral from the descending aorta. The subgroup of the patients with MAPCAs is designated as pulmonary atresia and ventricular septal defect (PA-VSD).

4. PA anomalies are common in the form of hypoplasia, nonconfluence, and abnormal distribution.
  a. The central PAs are confluent in 85% of patients; they are nonconfluent in 15%.
  b. The central and branch PAs are hypoplastic in most patients, but this occurs more frequently in patients with MAPCAs than in those with PDA (see later for further discussion of hypoplasia of the PAs).
  c. Incomplete arborization (distribution) of one or both PAs is found in 50% of patients with confluent PAs and in 80% of patients with nonconfluent PAs.

5. Collateral arteries arise most commonly from the descending aorta (occurring in two thirds of patients), less commonly

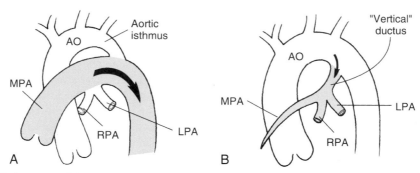

Fig. 14.25 Anatomy of the ductus arteriosus in pulmonary atresia. The size and direction of the ductus arteriosus are different between a normal fetus and a fetus with pulmonary atresia. **A,** In a normal fetus, the ductus is large and joins the aorta (AO) at an obtuse angle. The aortic isthmus (the portion of the aorta between the left subclavian artery and the ductus) is narrower than the descending aorta. **B,** In pulmonary atresia, the ductus is small because flow to the descending aorta does not go through the ductus. Furthermore, because flow is from the aorta to the pulmonary artery, the connection of the ductus with the aorta has an acute inferior angle (sometimes called "vertical" ductus). The aortic isthmus has the same diameter as the descending aorta. This type of ductus arteriosus is also found in some patients with tricuspid atresia. *LPA,* Left pulmonary artery; *MPA,* main pulmonary artery; *RPA,* right pulmonary artery.

from the subclavian arteries, and rarely from the abdominal aorta or its branches.

6. The ductus is small and long and arises from the transverse aortic arch and courses downward ("vertical" ductus) (Fig. 14.25).
7. The McGoon ratio and the Nakata index are used to quantitate the degree of PA hypoplasia. Small values of these measurements may adversely affect the outcome of surgeries in patients with small PAs.
   a. The McGoon ratio is the ratio of the sum of the diameter of the immediately prebranching portion of the right pulmonary artery (RPA) and left pulmonary artery (LPA) divided by the diameter of the descending aorta just above the diaphragm. It is measured by echo, angiography, or MRI. Normal values of McGoon ratio are 2.0 to 2.5. Most survivors of TOF with pulmonary atresia have the ratio greater than 1. Good Fontan candidates should have the ratio greater than 1.8.
   b. The Nakata index is the cross-sectional area of the RPA and LPA (in mm²) divided by the body surface area (BSA). It is measured by angiocardiography or by MRI. The average diameters of both RPA and LPA are measured at the points immediately proximal to the origin of the first lobar branches at maximal and minimal during one cardiac cycle in the anteroposterior view of the pulmonary arteriogram. The cross-sectional area is calculated by using the formula, $\pi \times r^2 \times$ magnification coefficient (in which r is the radius or half of the measured PA diameter). A normal Nakata index is 330 ± 30 mm²/BSA. Patients with TOF with PS should have the index greater than 100 for survival. A good Fontan candidate should have an index greater than 250, and a good Rastelli candidate should have an index greater than 200. (Those with the index less than 200 should have a shunt operation rather than the Rastelli operation.)

Clinical Manifestations

1. These patients are cyanotic at birth. The degree of cyanosis depends on whether the ductus is patent and how extensive the systemic collateral arteries are.
2. Usually a heart murmur cannot be heard. However, a faint, continuous murmur may be audible from the PDA or collaterals. The S2 is loud and single. A systolic click is occasionally present.
3. The ECG shows RAD and RVH.
4. Chest radiography shows a normal heart size. The heart often appears as a boot-shaped silhouette (see Fig. 14.19), and the pulmonary vascularity is usually markedly decreased (i.e., "black" lung field). Rarely, children with MAPCAs have excessive PBF, and CHF may develop.
5. Echo studies show all the anatomic findings of TOF plus the absence of a direct connection between the RV and the PA. In this case, a careful examination of the central PA is necessary with measurements of the size of central and branch PAs. The small branch PAs and "vertical ductus" (see Fig. 14.25) are well imaged from a high parasternal or suprasternal transducer position. Some of the multiple collateral arteries are also imaged by echo and Doppler.
6. Cardiac catheterization and angiograms are sometimes needed for a complete delineation of the collaterals. Alternatively, MRI or CT angiography (CTA) is performed for complete anatomic delineation of the aortic collaterals and PA branches.

Natural History

1. Without immediate attention to the establishment of PBF during the newborn period, most neonates who have this condition die during the first 2 years of life; however, infants with extensive collaterals may survive for a long time, perhaps for more than 15 years.
2. Occasionally, patients with excessive collateral circulation develop hemoptysis during late childhood.

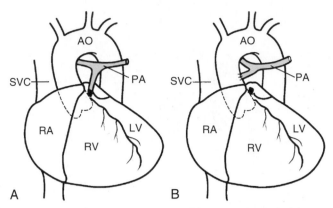

Fig. 14.26 Central end-to-side shunt (Mee procedure). **A,** Diagram of tetralogy of Fallot with pulmonary atresia. **B,** The hypoplastic pulmonary artery (PA) is anastomosed to the ascending aorta (AO) as posteriorly as possible. *LV,* Left ventricle; *RA,* right atrium; *RV,* right ventricle; *SVC,* superior vena cava. (From Watterson KG, Wilkinson JL, Karly TR, Mee RBB: Very small pulmonary arteries: central end-to-side shunt, *Ann Thorac Surg* 52:1131–1137, 1991.)

Management
Medical

1. PGE_1 infusion should be started as soon as the diagnosis is made or suspected to keep the ductus open for additional studies and to prepare for surgery. The starting dose of alprostadil (Prostin VR Pediatric) solution is 0.05 to 0.1 μg/kg/min. When the desired effect is obtained, the dosage should be gradually reduced to 0.01 μg/kg/min.
2. Emergency cardiac catheterization or MRI or CTA is usually needed to delineate the anatomy of the PAs and systemic arterial collaterals.

Surgical

A connection must be established between the RV and true PA as early in life as possible. This may make tiny central PAs to enlarge rapidly during the first year of life with improved arborization (distribution) of the PAs with concurrent development of alveolar units. To achieve this goal, some centers initially use a central shunt procedure, and others proceed with an RV-to-PA connection.

1. **Central shunt operation.** Some centers use a central shunt directly connecting the ascending aorta and the hypoplastic main PA to achieve growth of the peripheral PAs (Mee procedure) (Fig. 14.26). A classic or modified BT shunt is avoided because it is difficult to perform on tiny PAs and may cause stenosis or distortion. This is then followed by unifocalization (see later for explanation), RV-PA connection, and closure of VSD. Other centers skip the shunt procedure and proceed with the connection of the RV and the main PA (see later).
2. **RV to-PA connection**
   a. **Single-stage repair.** Complete, primary surgical repair in patients with TOF and pulmonary atresia is possible only when (1) the true PAs provide most or all PBF (with O_2 saturation of >75%) and (2) the central PA connects without obstruction to sufficient regions of the lungs (i.e., at least equal to one whole lung). If

additional major collaterals are identified, one tests the level of arterial O_2 saturation after occlusion of the collateral in the catheterization laboratory. If the O_2 saturation remains greater than 70% to 75%, coil occlusion of the collaterals is then carried out.

Primary repair of this condition consists of closing the VSD, establishing a continuity between the RV and the unifocalized PA (see later for unifocalization procedure) using either aortic or pulmonary homograft (9–10 mm internal diameter), and interrupting collateral circulation. Good candidates for the repair are those with a Nakata index greater than 200. If the index is less than 200, a shunt procedure is preferable.

   b. **Multiple-stage repair.** When the requirements for single-stage repair are not met, three consequential steps are used to repair this condition. These steps are summarized in Fig. 14.27.
      1) **Stage 1.** RV-to-hypoplastic PA conduit using a relatively small homograft conduit (6–8 mm internal diameter) (see Fig. 14.27B, *top* and *bottom rows*). The major goal of this operation is to make the central PA grow to an adequate size for eventual repair surgery. Interventional catheterization is carried out 3 to 6 months later to identify and coil occlude remaining aortic collaterals, to define PA distribution, and to identify if certain bronchopulmonary segments are receiving duplicate blood supply.
      2) **Stage 2.** Unifocalization procedure is carried out. Unifocalization is a surgical procedure in which aortopulmonary collaterals are divided from their aortic origin and are anastomosed to the true PAs or main PA conduit (see Fig. 14.27C, *top row* and B C, *bottom row*). Post-unifocalization catheterization is carried out 3 to 6 months later to (a) identify multiple peripheral stenosis in both the true as well as the unifocalized collaterals and to do balloon dilatation with or without stenting and (b) assess the need for further unifocalization procedures.
      3) **Stage 3.** Closure of VSD with or without fenestration, usually at 1 to 3 years of age (see Fig. 14.27C). The homograft conduit may need to be replaced at the same time. If the RV pressure is 10% to 20% greater than systemic pressure, a central fenestration of 3 to 4 mm is created. Multiple ballooning and stenting procedures are often necessary to reduce RV pressure to less than 50% systemic if possible.

Surgical steps used in patients with TOF with pulmonary atresia are summarized in Fig. 14.28.

Postoperative Follow-up

1. Frequent follow-up is needed to assess the palliative surgery and decide on appropriate times for further surgeries.
2. Valved conduits or homografts may develop valve degeneration requiring conduit replacement at a later time. Valvular stenosis can be dilated with a balloon to reduce the pressure gradient but often results in a significant valve regurgitation, eventually leading to RV dysfunction.

Confluent PA and collaterals

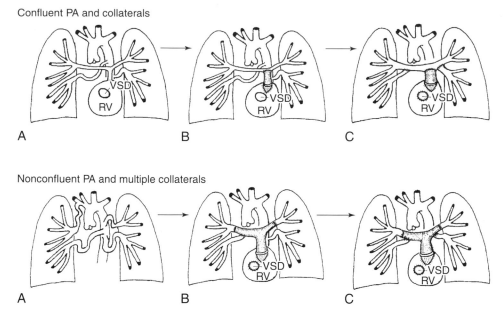

Nonconfluent PA and multiple collaterals

Fig. 14.27 Diagram of multiple-stage repair. *Upper row* (confluent pulmonary artery [PA] and collaterals): **A,** A hypoplastic but confluent central PA and multiple other collateral arteries. **B,** A small right ventricle–to–PA (RV-to-PA) connection is made with pulmonary homograft (shown shaded), with collaterals left alone. **C,** The pulmonary arteries have grown to a larger size, and a larger pulmonary homograft has replaced the earlier small one. Collateral arteries are now anastomosed (unifocalized) to the originally hypoplastic PA branches. The ventricular septal defect (VSD) may be closed at a later time, usually 1 to 3 years of age. The pulmonary homograft is usually replaced with a larger graft at this time. *Bottom row* (nonconfluent PA and multiple collaterals): **A,** Absent central PA and multiple aortic collaterals are shown. **B,** A small pulmonary homograft (6–8 mm internal diameter, shown *shaded*) is used to establish the RV-to-PA connection with some collaterals connected to it (unifocalized) (performed at 3–6 mo). Some collaterals are not unifocalized at this time. **C,** The homograft conduit has been replaced with a larger one. Remaining collateral arteries are anastomosed to the pulmonary homograft to complete unifocalization procedure. The VSD is closed with or without fenestration, usually at 1 to 3 years.

Many of these patients require surgical replacement of the conduit.

3. Bonhoeffer and his colleagues (2000) developed a technique in which a dysfunctional conduit or homograft valve can be replaced by percutaneous replacement of pulmonary valve, and more children and adults have successfully had this procedure done. A bovine jugular venous valve was mounted into the platinum stent and loaded in the delivery system. The assembly was delivered (implanted) in the RVOT according to standard stent-placing technique using an 18-Fr-long sheath through a right femoral approach. This valve is marketed as the Melody transcatheter pulmonary valve (Medtronic, Minneapolis, MN). The other commercially available valve for use in the RVOT is the Edwards SAPIEN valve (Edwards Lifescience, Irvine, CA), a balloon-expandable stainless-steel stent containing a bovine pericardial valve.

4. Survivors of the defect may need antibiotic prophylaxis for SBE for an indefinite period.

5. A certain level of activity restriction is needed because many of these children have exercise intolerance. Most survivors after complete repair are in New York Heart Association (NYHA) class I or II symptomatically.

TETRALOGY OF FALLOT WITH ABSENT PULMONARY VALVE

Prevalence

Tetralogy of Fallot with absent pulmonary valve occurs in approximately 2% of patients with TOF.

Pathology and Pathophysiology

1. The pulmonary valve leaflets are either completely absent or have an uneven rim of rudimentary valve tissue present. The annulus of the valve is stenotic and displaced distally. A massive aneurysmal dilatation of the PAs is present. This anomaly is usually associated with a large VSD, similar to that seen in TOF. It rarely occurs with an intact ventricular septum.

2. The massive PA aneurysm (Fig. 14.29) develops during fetal life resulting from severe pulmonary regurgitation (PR) and an associated increase in RV stroke volume. The aneurysmal PAs compress anteriorly the lower end of the developing trachea and bronchi throughout fetal life, producing hypoplasia of the compressed airways. This produces signs of airway obstruction and respiratory distress during infancy. Pulmonary complications (e.g., atelectasis, pneumonia) are the usual causes of death rather than the intracardiac defect.

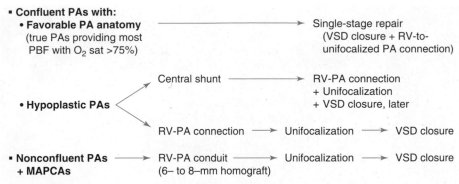

Fig. 14.28 Surgical approaches for tetralogy of Fallot with pulmonary atresia (or pulmonary atresia and ventricular septal defect [VSD]). *MAPCAs,* Multiple aortopulmonary artery collaterals; *PA,* pulmonary artery; *PBF,* pulmonary blood flow; *RV-PA,* right ventricle–to–pulmonary artery, *VSD,* ventricular septal defect.

3. The ductus arteriosus is almost always absent in patients with more severe aneurysmal dilatation of the PAs.
4. A right-sided aortic arch is frequently found (in ~50%), and the condition may be associated with absent or aortic origin of a branch PA.
5. In some infants, tufts of PAs entwine and compress the intrapulmonary bronchi, resulting in reduced numbers of alveolar units, which might be the cause of continuing respiratory problems even after the surgical relief of compression of the main stem bronchus.

Clinical Manifestations

1. Mild cyanosis may be present as a result of a bidirectional shunt during the newborn period when the PVR is relatively high. Cyanosis disappears, and signs of CHF may develop, after the newborn period. Respiratory symptoms vary greatly; ranging from neonates with severe respiratory compromise, those with wheezing or frequent respiratory infection, and those with no respiratory symptoms at all. At times there may be significant hypoxia secondary to airway compression by the dilated main PA, which would respond to prone positioning of the infant.
2. A to-and-fro murmur (with "sawing-wood" sound) at the upper and mid-left sternal borders is a characteristic auscultatory finding of the condition. This murmur occurs because of mild PS and free PR. The S2 is loud and single. The RV hyperactivity is palpable.
3. The ECG shows RAD and RVH.
4. Chest radiography images reveal a noticeably dilated main PA and hilar PAs. The heart size is either normal or mildly enlarged, and pulmonary vascular markings may be slightly increased. The lung fields may show hyperinflated areas, representing partial airway obstruction (see Fig. 14.29A).
5. Echo studies reveal a large, subaortic VSD with overriding of the aorta, distally displaced pulmonary annulus (with thick ridges instead of fully developed pulmonary valve leaflets), and gigantic aneurysm of the PA and its branches. The RV is markedly dilated, often with paradoxical motion of the ventricular septum. Doppler studies reveal evidence of stenosis at the annulus and PR. Cardiac catheterization

and angiocardiography (see Fig. 14.29B) are usually unnecessary for accurate anatomic assessment of the PAs.
6. A CT or MRI scan can define relationship between sites of airway obstruction and dilatation of the central PA. Bronchoscopy provides the degree of airway compression.

Natural History

1. More than 75% of infants with severe pulmonary complications (e.g., atelectasis, pneumonia) die during infancy if treated only medically. The surgical mortality rate of infants with pulmonary complications is 20% to 40%.
2. Infants who survive infancy without serious pulmonary problems do well for 5 to 20 years and have fewer respiratory symptoms during childhood. They become symptomatic later and die from intractable right-sided heart failure.

Management
Medical

In the past, medical management was preferred because of poor surgical results in newborns; however, the mortality rate of medical management is much higher than for surgical management. After the pulmonary symptoms appear, neither surgical nor medical management has good results.

Surgical

Symptomatic neonates should have corrective surgery on an urgent basis. Even asymptomatic child should have elective surgery in the first 3 to 6 months of life.

Primary Repair. Complete primary repair is the procedure of choice. VSD is closed either through right ventriculotomy (across the pulmonary annulus) or a transatrial approach. In symptomatic neonates, a pulmonary homograft is used to replace the dysplastic pulmonary valve and the dilated main and branch PAs. Alternatively, a valved conduit may be used to restore competence of the pulmonary valve, and the aneurysmal PAs are plicated. Some surgeons advocate aortic transection to achieve good exposure of the PAs for an extensive pulmonary arterioplasty into the hila of both lungs. Some surgeons advocate stenting the airway at the time of surgery.

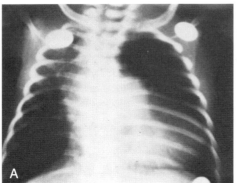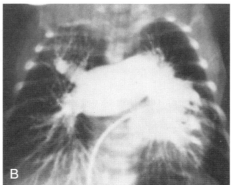

Fig. 14.29 A, Posteroanterior view of plain chest film showing hyperinflated areas in the left upper lobe and right lower portion of the chest in a 1-month-old infant who had tetralogy of Fallot with absence of the pulmonary valve. **B,** Anteroposterior view of pulmonary arteriogram showing massive aneurysmal dilatation of both the right and left pulmonary arteries.

TOTAL ANOMALOUS PULMONARY VENOUS RETURN

Prevalence

Total anomalous pulmonary venous return (TAPVR) accounts for 1% of all CHDs. There is a marked male preponderance for the infracardiac type (male-to-female ratio of 4:1).

Pathology and Pathophysiology

1. No direct communication exists between the pulmonary veins and the LA. Instead, they drain anomalously into the systemic venous tributaries or into the RA. Depending on the drainage site of the pulmonary veins, the defect may be divided into the following four types (Fig. 14.30).
   a. Supracardiac: This type accounts for 50% of TAPVR patients. The common pulmonary venous sinus drains into the right SVC through the left vertical vein and the left innominate vein (see Fig. 14.30A).
   b. Cardiac: This type accounts for 20% of TAPVR patients. The pulmonary veins enter the RA separately through four openings (only two openings are illustrated in Fig. 14.30B), or the common pulmonary venous sinus drains into the coronary sinus (see Fig. 14.30C).
   c. Infracardiac: This type accounts for 20% of TAPVR patients. The common pulmonary venous sinus drains to the portal vein, ductus venosus, hepatic vein, or inferior vena cava (IVC). The common pulmonary vein penetrates the diaphragm through the esophageal hiatus (see Fig. 14.30D).
   d. Mixed type: This type, which is a combination of the other types, accounts for 10% of TAPVR patients.
2. Many patients with supracardiac and cardiac types of TAPVR and most patients with the infracardiac type have pulmonary hypertension secondary to obstruction of the pulmonary venous return. Either the length of the venous channels or the resistance caused by the hepatic sinusoids is the cause of obstruction.
3. In patients with pulmonary venous obstruction, pulmonary arterial hypertension develops. These patients develop progressive pulmonary venous congestion, hypoxemia, and systemic hypoperfusion.
4. An interatrial communication, either an ASD or PFO, is necessary for survival. Most patients do not have restricted flow across the atrial septum.
5. The left side of the heart is relatively small.

Clinical Manifestations

Clinical manifestations differ, depending on whether there is obstruction to the pulmonary venous return.

Without Pulmonary Venous Obstruction
History

1. CHF with growth retardation and frequent pulmonary infection are common in infancy.
2. A history of mild cyanosis from birth is present.

Physical Examination

1. The infant is undernourished and mildly cyanotic. Signs of CHF (e.g., tachypnea, dyspnea, tachycardia, hepatomegaly) are present.
2. Precordial bulge with hyperactive RV impulse is present. Cardiac impulse is maximal at the xyphoid process and the lower left sternal border.
3. Characteristic quadruple or quintuple rhythm is present. The S2 is widely split and fixed, and the P2 may be accentuated. A grade 2 to 3 of 6 ejection systolic murmur is usually audible at the upper left sternal border. A mid-diastolic rumble is always present at the lower left sternal border (caused by increased flow through the tricuspid valve) (Fig. 14.31).

Electrocardiography

Right ventricular hypertrophy of the so-called volume overload type (i.e., rsR′ in V1) and occasional RAH are present.

Radiography

1. Moderate to marked cardiomegaly involving the RA and RV is present with increased pulmonary vascular markings.

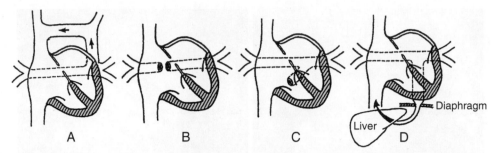

Fig. 14.30 Anatomic classification of total anomalous pulmonary venous return. **A,** Supracardiac. **B** and **C,** Cardiac. **D,** Infracardiac.

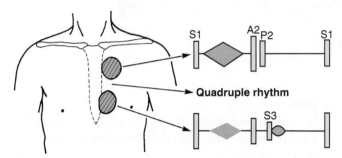

Fig. 14.31 Cardiac findings of total anomalous pulmonary venous return without obstruction to pulmonary venous return.

2. "Snowman" sign or figure-of-8 configuration may be seen in the supracardiac type but rarely before 4 months of age (Fig. 14.32).

With Pulmonary Venous Obstruction

History

1. Marked cyanosis and respiratory distress develop in the neonatal period with failure to thrive.
2. Cyanosis worsens with feeding, especially in infants with the infracardiac type, resulting from compression of the common pulmonary vein by the food-filled esophagus.

Physical Examination

1. Moderate to marked cyanosis and tachypnea with retraction are present in newborns or undernourished infants.
2. Cardiac findings may be minimal. A loud, single S2 and gallop rhythm are present. Heart murmur is usually absent. If present, however, it is usually a faint ejection-type systolic murmur at the upper left sternal border.
3. Pulmonary crackles and hepatomegaly are usually present.

Electrocardiography

Invariably, RVH in the form of tall R waves in the right precordial leads is present. RAH is occasionally present.

Radiography

The heart size is normal or slightly enlarged. The lung fields reveal findings of pulmonary edema (i.e., diffuse reticular pattern and Kerley's B lines). These findings may be confused with pneumonia or hyaline membrane disease.

Echocardiography

Echo and Doppler study is usually diagnostic of the condition and can identify associated anomalies.

1. ***Features common to all types***
   a. A large RV with a compressed LV (i.e., relative hypoplasia of the LV) is the most striking initial finding. A large RA and a small LA, with deviation of the atrial septum to the left and dilated PAs, are also present.
   b. An interatrial communication is usually present. PFO occurs in 70% of patients, and secundum ASD occurs in 30%.
   c. A large, common chamber (i.e., common pulmonary venous sinus) may be imaged posterior to the LA in the parasternal long-axis view.
   d. An M-mode echo may show paradoxical or flat motion of the interventricular septum, as a sign of RV volume overload.
   e. Doppler studies reveal an increased flow velocity in the PA, an increased flow velocity or continuous flow at the site of the pulmonary venous drainage, and findings suggestive of pulmonary hypertension.

2. ***Features of the supracardiac type.*** The most common site of connection is the left SVC (i.e., left vertical vein), with subsequent drainage to the dilated left innominate vein and right SVC. These abnormal pathways can be imaged in the suprasternal notch short-axis view. Color-flow mapping and Doppler ultrasound are helpful in defining the direction of the flow in the left SVC.

3. ***Features of the cardiac type.*** The most common site of entry is to the coronary sinus, occurring in 15% of cases. A dilated coronary sinus, best imaged in the parasternal long-axis view and the apical four-chamber view, may be the first clue to this condition.

4. ***Features of the infracardiac type.*** A dilated vein descending to the abdominal cavity through the diaphragm is imaged using the subcostal sagittal and transverse scans. All four pulmonary veins that connect to the confluence must be imaged. They are best imaged on the subcostal coronal scan or the suprasternal notch short-axis view.

5. ***Possibility of the mixed type.*** Unless it is demonstrated that all four pulmonary veins connect to the confluence, the possibility of the mixed type of TAPVR cannot be eliminated. In the most common mixed type, the left

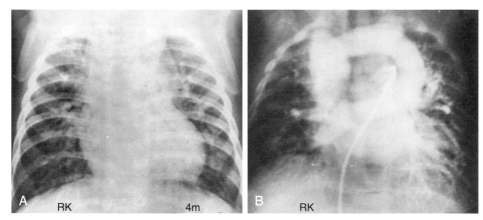

Fig. 14.32 Posteroanterior view of plain chest film demonstrating the "snowman" sign (**A**) and an angio-cardiogram demonstrating anatomic structures that participate in the formation of the "snowman" sign (**B**). The vertical vein (left superior vena cava), the dilated left innominate vein, and the right superior vena cava are opacified.

lung, usually the upper lobe, drains to the left SVC, and the remaining pulmonary veins in both lungs drain to the coronary sinus. When the mixed type is suspected, CTA, MRI, or cardiac catheterization needs to be performed.

Other Studies

Echo is usually diagnostic and can identify the subtypes. Cardiac catheterization is rarely performed for diagnostic purpose; it is occasionally done to perform atrial septostomy to improve atrial shunt or to identify complex mixed type of pulmonary venous return. Alternatively, MRI or cardiac CT can be used for diagnosis in case of complex mixed type; the former is preferable because it does not use ionizing radiation.

Natural History

1. CHF occurs in both types of TAPVR with growth retardation and repeated pneumonias.
2. Without surgical repair, two thirds of the infants without obstruction die before reaching 1 year of age. They usually die from superimposed pneumonia.
3. Patients with the infracardiac type rarely survive for longer than a few weeks without surgery. Most die before 2 months of age.

Management
Medical

1. Intensive anticongestive measures with diuretics should be provided for infants without pulmonary venous obstruction.
2. Metabolic acidosis should be corrected, if present.
3. Infants with severe pulmonary edema (resulting from the infracardiac type and from other types with obstruction) should be intubated, heavily sedated, or even paralyzed if necessary before urgent surgery.
4. If the size of the interatrial communication appears small and immediate surgery is not indicated, balloon atrial septostomy or blade atrial septostomy may be performed to enlarge the communication.

Surgical

Indications and Timing. Corrective surgery is necessary for all patients with this condition. No palliative procedure exists.

1. All infants with pulmonary venous obstruction should be operated on as soon as feasible after diagnosis.
2. Infants who do not have pulmonary venous obstruction but do have heart failure that is difficult to control are usually operated on when stable on a semielective basis.

Procedures. Although procedures vary with the site of the anomalous drainage, all procedures are intended to redirect the pulmonary venous return to the LA (Fig. 14.33). Surgical techniques used vary from surgeon to surgeon; some use the RA approach to reach the LA, and others reach the posterior wall of the LA directly. Some favor use of deep hypothermic (18°–20°C) circulatory arrest.

1. Supracardiac type. A large, side-to-side anastomosis is made between the common pulmonary venous sinus and the LA. The vertical vein is ligated. The ASD is closed with a cloth patch (see Fig. 14.33A).
2. TAPVR to the RA. The atrial septum is excised, and a patch is sewn in such a way that the pulmonary venous return is diverted to the LA (see Fig. 14.33B). The ASD may have to be enlarged.
3. TAPVR to the coronary sinus. An incision is made in the anterior wall of the coronary sinus ("unroofing") to make a communication between the coronary sinus and the LA. A single patch closes the original ASD and the ostium of the coronary sinus. This results in drainage of coronary sinus blood with low oxygen saturation into the LA (see Fig. 14.33C).
4. Infracardiac type. A large vertical anastomosis is made between the common pulmonary venous sinus and the LA. The common pulmonary vein, which descends vertically to the abdominal cavity, is ligated above the diaphragm (see Fig. 14.33D).

Mortality. The surgical mortality rate is between 5% and 10% for infants with the unobstructed type. This rate can be much higher for infants with the obstructed type.

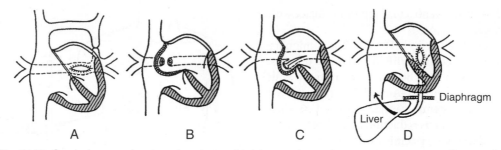

Fig. 14.33 Surgical approaches to various types of total anomalous pulmonary venous returns. See text for description of the procedures.

Two common causes of death are postoperative paroxysms of pulmonary hypertension and the development of pulmonary vein stenosis.

Complications

1. Paroxysms of pulmonary hypertension, which relate to a small and poorly compliant left heart, with resulting cardiac failure and pulmonary edema, may require prolonged respiratory support postoperatively.
2. Postoperative arrhythmias are usually atrial.
3. Obstruction at the site of anastomosis or stenosis of the pulmonary veins rarely occurs.

Postoperative Follow-up

1. An office evaluation every 6 to 12 months is recommended for such late complications as pulmonary vein obstruction and atrial arrhythmias.
2. Pulmonary vein obstruction at the anastomosis site or delayed development of pulmonary vein stenosis may occur in about 10% of patients and requires reoperation. These complications are usually evident within 6 to 12 months after the repair. The possibility of pulmonary vein stenosis requires cardiac catheterization and angiocardiography. If present, it is nearly impossible to correct.
3. Some patients develop atrial arrhythmias, including sick sinus syndrome, that require medical treatment or pacemaker therapy.
4. Activity restriction is usually unnecessary unless pulmonary venous obstruction occurs.

TRICUSPID ATRESIA

Prevalence

Tricuspid atresia accounts for 1% to 3% of CHDs.

Pathology

1. The tricuspid valve is absent, and the RV is hypoplastic, with absence of the inflow portion of the RV. The associated defects such as ASD, VSD, or PDA are necessary for survival.
2. Tricuspid atresia is usually classified according to the presence or absence of TGA and PS (Fig. 14.34). The great arteries are normally related in about 70% of cases and are transposed in 30% of cases. In 3% of cases, the L form of transposition occurs.

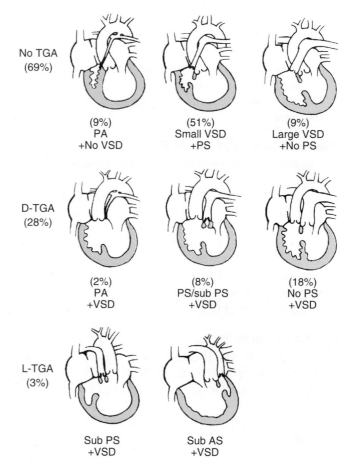

Fig. 14.34 Anatomic classification of tricuspid atresia. In about 70% of cases, the great arteries are normally related, and there is usually a small ventricular septal defect (VSD) with associated hypoplasia of the pulmonary artery (PA). When the great arteries are transposed, the VSD is usually large, and the PAs are large with increased pulmonary blood flow. *AS,* Aortic stenosis; *D-TGA,* complete transposition of the great arteries; *L-TGA,* congenitally corrected TGA; *PA,* pulmonary atresia; *PS,* pulmonary stenosis; *sub AS,* subaortic stenosis; *sub PS,* subpulmonary stenosis; *TGA,* transposition of the great arteries; *VSD,* ventricular septal defect. (Data from Keith JD, Rowe RD, Vlad P: *Heart Disease in Infancy and Childhood,* ed 3, New York, 1978, Macmillan.)

3. In patients with normally related great arteries, the VSD is usually small, and PS is present with resulting hypoplasia of the PAs, and the PBF is reduced. This is the most common type, occurring in about 50% of all patients with tricuspid atresia. Occasionally, the VSD is large with

normal-sized PAs or the ventricular septum is intact with pulmonary atresia.

4. When TGA is present, it is mostly D-TGA. The pulmonary valve is normal with increased PBF in two thirds of cases. In one third of cases, it is either stenotic or atretic with decreased PBF. Patients with TGA need a fairly large VSD to maintain normal systemic cardiac output. Less than adequate size or spontaneous reduction of the VSD creates problems with a decreased systemic cardiac output.

5. COA or interrupted aortic arch is a frequently associated anomaly that is more commonly seen in patients with TGA.

Clinical Manifestations
History

1. Cyanosis is usually severe from birth. Tachypnea and poor feeding usually manifest.
2. History of hypoxic spells may be present in infants with this condition.

Physical Examination (Fig. 14.35)

1. Cyanosis is usually present. Older infants may have clubbing.
2. A systolic thrill is rarely palpable when associated with PS.
3. The S2 is single. A grade 2 to 3 of 6 holosystolic (or early systolic) murmur of VSD is usually present at the lower left sternal border. A continuous murmur of PDA is occasionally present. An apical diastolic rumble is rarely audible in patients with large PBF.
4. Hepatomegaly may indicate an inadequate interatrial communication or CHF.

Electrocardiography

1. "Superior" QRS axis (between 0 and −90 degrees) is characteristic. It appears in most patients without TGA (Fig. 14.36). The "superior" QRS axis is present in only 50% of patients with TGA.
2. LVH is usually present; RAH or biatrial hypertrophy is common.

Radiography

The heart size is normal or slightly increased, with enlargement of the RA and LV. Pulmonary vascularity decreases in most patients (Fig. 14.37), although it may increase in infants with TGA. Occasionally, the concave PA segment may produce a boot-shaped heart, like the x-ray findings of TOF.

Echocardiography

Two-dimensional echo readily establishes the diagnosis of tricuspid atresia.

1. Absence of the tricuspid orifice, a large RA, marked hypoplasia of the RV, and a large LA and LV can be imaged in the apical four-chamber view. The size of the LA is determined by the magnitude of PBF.
2. The bulging of the atrial septum toward the left and the size of the interatrial communication are easily imaged in the subcostal four-chamber view.

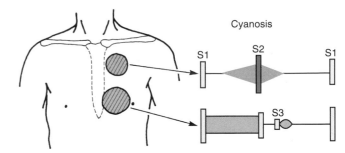

Cyanosis

Fig. 14.35 Cardiac findings of tricuspid atresia associated with patent ductus arteriosus and ventricular septal defect. "Superior" QRS axis on the electrocardiogram and cyanosis are characteristic of the defect.

3. The size of the VSD, the presence and severity of PS, and the presence of TGA should all be investigated.
4. Patients with TGA should be examined for possible subaortic stenosis and aortic arch anomalies, especially the COA.

Other Studies

Echo and color-flow Doppler studies can delineate most anatomic and physiologic issues related to the condition. However, cardiac catheterization with interventional balloon atrial septostomy is indicated when atrial communication is inadequate. Cardiac catheterization is generally recommended before a planned surgical intervention other than the BT shunt or PA banding. Specific information on the PA anatomy, pressure, and LV function is necessary before any Fontan-type operation.

Natural History

1. Few infants with tricuspid atresia and normally related great arteries survive beyond 6 months of age without surgical palliation.
2. Occasionally, patients with increased PBF develop CHF and eventually pulmonary vascular obstructive disease.
3. For patients who survive into their second decade of life without Fontan-type operation, the chronic volume overload of the LV usually results in LV systolic dysfunction, which is a known risk factor for Fontan operation. (The Fontan procedure should be performed before LV dysfunction develops.)

Management
Initial Medical Management

1. PGE_1 should be started in neonates with severe cyanosis to maintain the patency of the ductus before planned cardiac catheterization or cardiac surgery.
2. The Rashkind procedure (balloon atrial septostomy) may be performed as part of the initial catheterization to improve the RA-to-LA shunt, especially when the interatrial communication is considered inadequate by echo studies.
3. Treatment of CHF is rarely needed in infants with TGA and without PS.

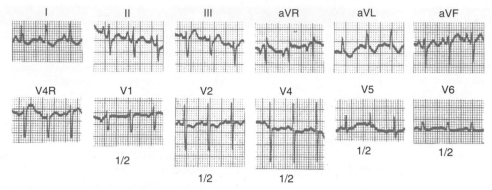

I   II   III   aVR   aVL   aVF

V4R   V1   V2   V4   V5   V6

1/2   1/2   1/2   1/2   1/2

Fig. 14.36 Tracing from a 6-month-old girl with tricuspid atresia showing "superior QRS axis" or left anterior hemiblock (–30 degrees), right atrial hypertrophy, and left ventricular hypertrophy.

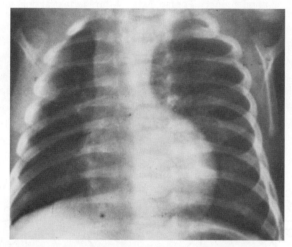

Fig. 14.37 Posteroanterior view of chest roentgenogram in an infant with tricuspid atresia with normally related great arteries. The heart is minimally enlarged. The pulmonary vascular markings are decreased, and the main pulmonary artery segment is somewhat concave.

4. Infants with normally related great arteries and adequate PBF through a VSD do not need any other procedures; rather, they need to be closely watched for decreasing oxygen saturation resulting from spontaneous reduction of the VSD.

Surgical

Most infants with tricuspid atresia require one or more palliative procedures before a Fontan-type operation, the definitive surgery, can be performed. Staged palliative surgical procedures are aimed at producing ideal candidates for future Fontan candidates. Ideal candidates for a Fontan-type operation are those who have normal LV function and low pulmonary resistance.

1. Normal LV function results from prevention of excessive volume or pressure loading of the LV by:
   a. Preventing excessive volume load by using a relatively small systemic-to-pulmonary shunt (e.g., 3.5 mm for neonates)
   b. Avoiding ventricular hypertrophy (e.g., by relieving the LV outflow obstruction)
2. Low pulmonary resistance may results from:

a. Providing adequate PBF which promote the growth of PA branches (with resulting increase in the cross-sectional area of the pulmonary vascular bed)
   b. Preventing distortion of the central PAs. Shunt operation is preferably done on the right PA, which can be incorporated into Fontan operation.
   c. Protecting pulmonary vascular bed from overflow or pressure overload (by PA band when PBF is increased)

Palliative surgical procedures described later, and the Fontan procedure are not just for tricuspid atresia, but they are also performed for other CHDs with functionally single ventricle, such as single ventricle (double-inlet ventricle), some cases of pulmonary atresia with intact ventricular septum, unbalanced AV canal, complicated DORV, HLHS, and heterotaxia (splenic syndromes). Because the Fontan operation is applicable to other defects, staged approach to the Fontan operation is summarized in Box 14.2 for quick reference.

Stage 1. The most frequently done first-stage operation is the BT shunt. Under special circumstances, other procedure (e.g., Damus-Kaye-Stansel operation) may have to be combined with the BT shunt. On rare occasion, a PA banding is indicated for infants with too much PBF.

1. BT shunt. Most patients who have tricuspid atresia with decreased PBF need the BT shunt soon after birth when the PVR is still high (see Fig. 14.22). This procedure results in the volume load on the LV because the LV supplies blood to both the systemic and pulmonary circulations. Thus, the shunt should be relatively small (e.g., 3.5 mm) and should not be left alone too long (before proceeding to stage 2 operation). The BT shunt is done on the right PA.
2. Damus-Kaye-Stansel and shunt operation. For infants with tricuspid atresia with TGA and restrictive VSD, the Damus-Kaye-Stansel procedure may be performed in addition to a systemic-to-PA shunt. In the Damus-Kaye-Stansel operation, the main PA is transected, and the distal PA is sewn over. The proximal PA is connected end to side to the ascending aorta (see Fig. 14.11). A systemic-to-PA shunt is created to supply blood to the lungs. A Fontan-type operation is performed at a later time. This procedure also results in the volume overload to the left

BOX 14.2   **Fontan Pathway**

- **Stage I:** One of the following procedures is done in preparation for a future Fontan operation
  1. The Blalock-Taussig shunt, when PBF is small
  2. PA banding when PBF is excessive
  3. Damus-Kaye-Stansel + shunt operation (for TA + TGA + restrictive VSD)

Medical follow-up after stage I: watch for:
- a. Cyanosis (O_2 saturation <75%): cardiac catheterization or MRI to find the cause of it
- b. Poor weight gain (CHF from too much PBF): tightening of PA band may be necessary
- **Stage II** (at 3 mo or by 6 mo)
  1. Bidirectional Glenn operation or
  2. The hemi-Fontan operation

Medical follow-up after stage II: watch for:
- a. A gradual decrease in O_2 saturation (<75%) may be caused by:
1) Opening of venous collaterals

2) Pulmonary AV fistula (caused by the absence of hepatic inhibitory factor):
  Perform cardiac catheterization (to find and occlude collaterals) or proceed with Fontan operation
- b. Transient hypertension: 1–2 wk postoperatively; may use ACE inhibitors
- a. Cardiac catheterization by 12 mo after stage II
  The following are risk factors. Presence of two or more is a high-risk situation.
  1) Mean PA pressure >18 mm Hg (or PVR >2 U/m²)
  2) LV end diastolic pressure >12 mm Hg (or EF <60%)
  3) AV valve regurgitation
  4) Distorted PAs secondary to previous shunt operation
- **Stage III** (Fontan operation): usually at 2 to 5 yr of age
  1. "Lateral tunnel" Fontan (with 4-mm fenestration): less favorable now
  2. An extracardiac conduit (with or without fenestration)

ACE, Angiotensin-converting enzyme; *AV*, atrioventricular; *CHF*, congestive heart failure; *EF*, ejection fraction; *LV*, left ventricle; *MRI*, magnetic resonance imaging; *PA*, pulmonary artery; *PBF*, pulmonary blood flow; *PVR*, pulmonary vascular resistance; *TA*, tricuspid atresia; *TGA*, transposition of the great arteries; *VSD*, ventricular septal defect.

ventricle, and a stage 2 operation should be performed as early as possible.

3. PA banding. PA banding is rarely necessary for infants with CHF resulting from increased PBF. PA banding protects the pulmonary vasculature from developing pulmonary hypertension, and it may be performed at any age with a mortality rate of less than 5%.

Follow-up Medical Management. After the stage 1 operation, the infant should be watched carefully until the time of the stage 2 palliation with emphasis on the following.
1. Cyanosis (with O_2 saturation <75%) should be investigated by cardiac catheterization or MRI.
2. Poor growth may indicate too large a PBF and tightening of PA band should be considered.

Stage 2. As a stage 2 operation, either a bidirectional Glenn shunt or rarely the hemi-Fontan operation is performed in preparation for the final Fontan operation.
1. Bidirectional Glenn operation. An end-to-side SVC-to-RPA shunt (also called bidirectional superior cavopulmonary shunt) can be performed at 2 to 6 months of age (Fig. 14.38A). By this time, the PVR is sufficiently low to allow venous pressure to be the driving force for the pulmonary circulation. There appears to be no advantage in further delaying the second stage operation beyond 6 months. For this procedure to be successful, the PVR has to be relatively low because the SVC blood flows passively into the PAs. Any previous systemic-to-PA shunt is taken down at the time of the procedure. The azygos vein and, when present, the hemiazygos are divided. The IVC blood still bypasses the lungs.

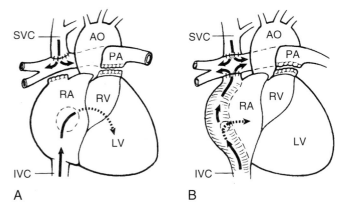

Fig. 14.38 A modified Fontan operation. **A,** Bidirectional Glenn operation or superior vena cava (SVC)–to–right pulmonary artery anastomosis (stage 2 operation). **B,** Completion of the Fontan operation by cavocaval baffle–to–pulmonary artery (PA) connection, with or without fenestration (stage 3 operation). See text for description of these procedures. *AO*, Aorta; *IVC*, inferior vena cava; *LV*, left ventricle; *RA*, right atrium; *RV*, right ventricle.

This procedure satisfactorily increases oxygen saturation, which averages 85%, without adding volume work to the LV. The mortality rate for this procedure is about 2%.
2. The hemi-Fontan operation. An incision is made along the most superior part of the RA appendage and is extended into the SVC (Fig. 14.39). A connection is made between this opening and the lower margin of the central portion of the PA. An intraatrial baffle is placed to direct the SVC blood to the PAs. The BT shunt is taken down, and the native pulmonary valve is oversewn.
  Advantages of hemi-Fontan operation are that (1) it allows supplementation of the central PA area so as to

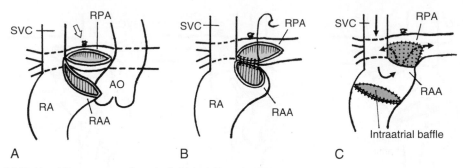

Fig. 14.39 Hemi-Fontan operation. **A,** A Blalock-Taussig (BT) shunt is taken down *(arrow)*. An incision is made in the superior aspect of the right atrial appendage (RAA), extending it into the superior vena cava (SVC), and a horizontal incision is made in the right pulmonary artery (RPA). **B,** The lower margin of the RPA incision and the adjacent margin of the incision in the RAA and SVC are connected. **C,** The connection is completed using pulmonary allograft. An intraatrial patch is placed to direct SVC blood to the pulmonary arteries. *AO,* Aorta; *RA,* right atrium.

optimize flow to the left lung and (2) it simplifies the subsequent Fontan operation. A major disadvantage may be that it involves extensive surgery in the region of the sinus node and sinus node artery, which may result in late sinus node dysfunction.

Follow-up Medical Management. Medical follow-up after the stage 2 operation should focus on the following (see Box 14.2).

1. A remarkable improvement in O_2 saturation (~85%) results after the procedure. However, a gradual deterioration in O2 saturation may occur in the months postoperatively, which may be caused by:
   a. Opening of venous collaterals which decompress the upper body
   b. The development of pulmonary arteriovenous (AV) fistula, which may be related to absence of hepatic inhibitory factor

Pulmonary AV fistulas develop commonly after the SVC-to-PA connection, in which hepatic venous blood does not reach the pulmonary circulation. It has been postulated that the liver may produce vasoconstrictor prostaglandins, which prevent pulmonary vasodilation and development of pulmonary AV fistula. Vasoconstrictor PGs in blood from the liver bypassing the pulmonary circulation may lead to the pulmonary AV fistulas. Song and colleagues (1996) reported that long-term aspirin (a cyclooxygenase inhibitor) therapy has successfully prevented the development of cyanosis, possibly by preventing pulmonary AV fistula formation. A similar pulmonary AV fistula also occurs, with the clinical manifestation of cyanosis, in patients with liver dysfunction (hepatopulmonary syndrome). The diagnosis of pulmonary AV malformation requires pulmonary angiography or, even better, a bubble contrast echo with injection into branch PAs.

2. If a child's O_2 saturation is 75% or less, it is preferable to proceed with Fontan operation. Alternatively, cardiac catheterization may be performed to find a cause of desaturation (systemic veno-venous fistulas, which may be coil occluded).

3. A pre-Fontan cardiac catheterization is performed before the planned procedure.

Stage 3. A modified Fontan operation is the definitive procedure for patients with tricuspid atresia. The whole premise of the Fontan operation is directing the entire systemic venous blood to the PAs without an intervening pumping chamber. The Fontan operation is usually completed when the child is 2 to 5 years of age.

The following are risk factors for the Fontan operation. The presence of two or more of these risk factors constitutes a high-risk situation.

1. High PVR (>2 U/m²) or high mean PA pressure (>18 mm Hg)
2. Distorted PAs secondary to previous shunt operations
3. Poor systolic or diastolic ventricular function, with LV end-diastolic pressure greater than 12 mm Hg or an ejection fraction less than 60%
4. AV valve regurgitation

The surgical technique of completing modified Fontan operation varies according to the type of the second-stage operation performed (bidirectional Glenn operation or hemi-Fontan operation).

After the Bidirectional Glenn Procedure. An intraatrial tubular pathway is created from the orifice of the IVC to the orifice of the SVC (termed *cavocaval baffle* or a *lateral tunnel*). The cardiac end of the SVC is anastomosed to the undersurface of the RPA to complete the operation (see Fig. 14.38B).

Some centers routinely use "fenestration" (4–6 mm) in the baffle, and others use it only in high-risk patients. The fenestration could be considered to be closed later, usually with an ASD closure device in the catheterization laboratory. Cited advantages of fenestration include decompression of the systemic venous circulation and augmentation of cardiac output in the early postoperative period. Disadvantages include systemic arterial desaturation with possible systemic embolization from the systemic veins and the later need to close the fenestration. Alternative to the described procedure, an extracardiac conduit may be used to complete the Fontan operation (see Fig. 14.41H). Fenestration is not necessary for the extracardiac conduit, but some surgeons create the fenestration with this approach.

Early survival rates have improved to greater than 95%. In a large series of 500 Fontan operations, the probabilities of

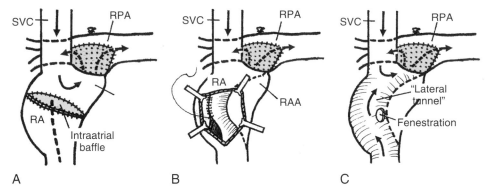

Fig. 14.40 From the hemi-Fontan to Fontan connection. **A,** A vertical incision *(heavy broken line)* is made in the anterior right atrial (RA) wall. **B,** The intraatrial patch is removed, and a lateral tunnel is constructed to direct the inferior vena cava (IVC) blood to the existing conglomerate of RA and right pulmonary artery (RPA). **C,** The direction of blood flow from the superior vena cava (SVC) and IVC is shown.

survival were 85% at 1 month, about 80% at 1 and 5 years, and 70% at 10 years.

After the Hemi-Fontan Operation. The intraatrial patch that was used to direct SVC blood to the PAs is excised, and a lateral atrial tunnel is constructed, directing flow from the IVC to the previously created amalgamation of the SVC with the RPA (Fig. 14.40).

Timing for surgery is the same as for the cavocaval baffle-to-PA anastomosis. The mortality rate of the Fontan procedure for children who have undergone a hemi-Fontan operation is reportedly lower than those who had the bidirectional Glenn operation.

Complications of the Fontan-Type Operation

Early Complications. Early postoperative complications may include the following.

1. Low cardiac output, heart failure, or both are early postoperative complications.
2. Persistent pleural effusion. This is a troublesome complication. Prolonged pleural drainage may lead to protein-losing enteropathy, which carries a poor prognosis. It may be the result of a sudden rise in the systemic venous or RA pressure. It occurs more often on the right side. The presence of aortopulmonary collaterals increases the risk of prolonged pleural effusion. Coil occlusion of these vessels before surgery can ameliorate this problem.

   Extracardiac conduit was associated with increased pleural drainage than intraatrial lateral tunnel, although the former may have a theoretical benefit for lower incidence of late arrhythmias (Rogers et al, 2012). On the other hand, creation of fenestration was associated with a decreased incidence of prolonged effusion.

   The following treatment can be used for this complication: prolonged chest tube drainage, a low-fat diet with a medium-chain triglyceride oil supplement or total parenteral nutrition, chemical or talc pleurodesis, a pleuroperitoneal shunt, and thoracic duct ligation, which is a major surgery.
3. Thrombus formation in the systemic venous pathways may result from a sluggish blood flow, which can be diagnosed by transesophageal echo. Treatment consists of warfarin, thrombolysis with streptokinase, or surgical removal. The risk is highest in the first several weeks to months after the Fontan operation, although the risk is present for the lifetime.
4. Although rare, acute liver dysfunction with alanine transaminase greater than 1000 U/L can occur during the first week after surgery, possibly resulting from hepatic hypoperfusion (caused by low cardiac output).

Late Complications. Regular follow-up is necessary to detect the following late complications:

1. Prolonged hepatomegaly and ascites require treatment with diuretics, afterload-reducing agents, and digitalis.
2. Supraventricular arrhythmia is one of the most troublesome complications. Early-onset arrhythmias occur in 15% of patients. The incidence of late-onset supraventricular arrhythmia continues to increase with longer follow-up after the Fontan procedure (6% at 1 year, 12% at 3 years, and 17% at 5 years). Extra-cardiac conduit (instead of intra-atrial lateral tunnel) may help reduce incidence of late cardiac arrhythmias (see Fig. 14.41H).
3. A progressive decrease in arterial oxygen saturation may result from obstruction of the venous pathways, leakage in the intraatrial baffle, or development of pulmonary AV fistula.
4. Protein-losing enteropathy can result from increased systemic venous pressure that subsequently causes lymphangiectasis. Prolonged pleural drainage is an unfavorable sign to develop this condition. Increased PVR, decreased cardiac index, and increased ventricular end-diastolic pressure were coincidental findings with the condition. The incidence of protein-losing enteropathy among survivors is 4%. The prognosis is poor; although it had previously been reported that about half the patients, regardless of the type of treatment-medical or surgical, die within 5 years, the more recent outcome has improved. Heart transplantation should be considered for these patients.
5. Thromboembolism can occur in up to 10% of the patients after Fontan operation. Some reports suggest stroke occurring in as high as 19% of the patients. Therefore, a long-term thromboprophylaxis is required (see later).

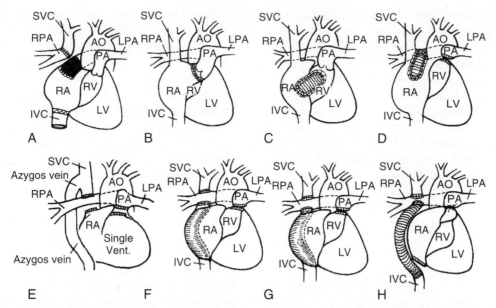

Fig. 14.41 Modifications of the Fontan operation. **A,** The original Fontan operation (Fontan and Baudet, 1971) consisted of an end-to-end anastomosis of the right pulmonary artery (RPA) to the superior vena cava (SVC), an end-to-end anastomosis of the right atrial appendage (RAA) to the proximal end of the RPA by means of an aortic valve homograft, closure of the atrial septal defect (ASD), insertion of a pulmonary valve homograft into the inferior vena cava (IVC), and ligation of the main pulmonary artery (PA). **B,** Modification by Kreutzer et al (1973) consisted of an anastomosis of the RAA and the main PA with its intact pulmonary valve (which was excised from the right ventricle [RV]) after closure of the ASD and ventricular septal defect. A Glenn operation was not performed, and no IVC valve was used. **C,** A later modification by Bjork et al (1979) consisted of a direct anastomosis between the RAA and the right ventricular outflow tract in patients with a normal pulmonary valve using a roof of pericardium to avoid a synthetic tube graft. **D,** Direct anastomosis of the right atrium (RA) to the RPA. **E,** Kawashima et al (1983) first showed that systemic venous returns could be directly connected to the pulmonary circulation without passing through the right heart. **F** and **G,** Separate anastomosis of the two ends of the divided SVC to the RPA and insertion of IVC to SVC intraatrial baffle (total cavopulmonary connection) with (**G**) and without (**F**) fenestration. **H,** Extracardiac conduit between the IVC and the RPA and a bidirectional Glenn operation. *AO,* Aorta; *LPA,* left pulmonary artery; *LV,* left ventricle.

The following are considered an increased risk for thromboembolism: a known hypercoagulable state, presence of intracardiac prosthetic materials, intracardiac shunt (fenestration), dilated atrium, atrial arrhythmias, ventricular dysfunction, low-flow states, stasis in the venous pathways, protein-losing enteropathy, and PA distortion. The use of extracardiac conduit may reduce the risk of thromboembolism.

Results of Fontan Operation. Currently, the operative mortality rate of the Fontan procedure is less than 3%. Mean PA pressure of 15 mm Hg or greater was associated with prolonged hospital stay and unfavorable outcomes (Rogers et al, 2012). The overall survival rate after the Fontan operation is better than 95% at follow-up of 50 months (Hirsch et al, 2008).

Postoperative Medical Follow-up.

1. Patients should maintain a low-salt diet.
2. Medications
   a. Some patients need continued digoxin and diuretic therapy.
   b. An ACE inhibitor is generally recommended. Although not proved, it may augment LV output with consequent improvement in PBF.
   c. Aspirin or even warfarin is used to prevent thrombus formation. Controversy exists as to whether aspirin is adequate for thrombus prophylaxis as compared with warfarin. A recent international report suggests that aspirin (5 mg/kg/day) is as good as properly controlled warfarin therapy (with target international normalized ratio at 2.0–3.0) (McCrindle et al, 2013). Earlier studies have also reported the same finding.
3. Some centers recommend device closure of the fenestration 1 year or so after the Fontan procedure. However, about 20% to 40% of fenestration will close spontaneously over the first year or two postoperatively.
4. Patients should be encouraged to reside at sea level or elevation 400 feet or less. They should avoid vacationing in high altitude. Elevated altitude increases pulmonary and systemic vascular resistances, plasma catecholamine levels, and renin activity, which may lead to Fontan failure, Fontan complications (e.g., protein-losing enteropathy, liver dysfunction, and reduced rate of long-term survival; Johnson et al, 2013).
5. Antibiotic prophylaxis against SBE should be observed when indications arise.
6. Among patients with tricuspid atresia, the 5-year survival rate is 80%, and the 10-year survival rate is 70%. During years 11 to 16 after surgery, the majority of patients have shown acceptable results, with 48% in NYHA class I and 16% in class II (see Appendix A, Table A.3).

Evolution of the Fontan-Type Operation. The Fontan-type operation applies to many complex CHDs, most of which are otherwise uncorrectable. Therefore, this procedure can be considered a major advancement in pediatric cardiac surgery during the past 4 decades. Castaneda (1992) has written an excellent review article on the historical aspect of the Fontan-type operations. Many modifications have been made since the original Fontan operation in 1971. The results of animal experiments conducted in the 1940s and 1950s suggested that the RV could be successfully bypassed (i.e., systemic venous pressure was an adequate force for PBF). The Glenn shunt (1958), which is an end-to-end anastomosis of the SVC to the distal end of the right PA, was the first such example, although it involved only one lung.

The original Fontan operation consisted of a Glenn shunt, connection of the RA and the right PA with insertion of an aortic homograft, insertion of another allograft valve in the IVC–RA junction, and closure of the ASD (Fig. 14.41A). At that time, RA contractions were thought to be important in pulsatile assistance to the pulmonary circulation. It became evident later that inlet and outlet valves were more problematic than beneficial.

Kreutzer and associates (1973) made a direct anastomosis between the RA appendage and the PA trunk using either a homograft or the patient's own pulmonary valve. The ASD was closed (see Fig. 14.41B). Subsequently, modifications of the connection were made between the RA and RV (see Fig. 14.41C), as well as between the RA and the main or right PA (see Fig. 14.41D), by direct anastomosis of the two structures or by the use of patches or conduits with or without an interposed valve. It became evident later that a direct connection between the RA appendage and the right PA without an interposed valve provided equally good hemodynamic results and that the incorporation of a portion of the RV was not beneficial.

Kawashima and associates (1984) reported a new operation in four children with complex single ventricle. These children also had interrupted IVC with either azygous continuation to the right SVC or hemiazygous continuation to the left SVC, and they were palliated earlier with BT shunts. Either the right or left SVC, which received blood from the entire systemic venous system, was successfully connected end to side to the ipsilateral PAs (in Fig. 14.41D; azygous continuation is shown). This procedure proved for the first time that the entire systemic venous return could be put into the pulmonary circulation, completely bypassing the right side of the heart.

De Leval and associates (1988) have shown that the interposition of a compliant RA chamber between the systemic vein and the PA is a major cause of energy loss in the RA, and they have shown that a cavocaval baffle-to-PA anastomosis, the latest modification of the Fontan operation (see Fig. 14.41F), has significant hemodynamic advantages over earlier attempts to use the RA (as in Fig. 14.41D) as part of the venous pathway.

A two-stage Fontan operation was recommended for high-risk patients. Initially, a bidirectional Glenn shunt was performed. This was later followed by the completion of the cavocaval baffle-to-right PA anastomosis. After the first procedure, there was often a noticeable improvement in oxygen saturation and symptoms to the point that raised questions about the necessity of the second procedure.

A fenestrated Fontan operation has been recommended for high-risk patients (see Fig. 14.41G). Reported advantages of fenestration include a lower early surgical mortality rate; reduced incidence or duration of postoperative pleural effusion; shorter hospital stay; and right-to-left shunt through the fenestration, which may help maintain cardiac output if blood flow through the lungs decreases. The possible disadvantages are paradoxical embolization and stroke, lower arterial oxygen saturation, and the need to close the fenestration.

Extracardiac right heart bypass with an IVC-to-right PA Dacron conduit and SVC-to-PA PA anastomosis has also been performed (see Fig. 14.41H). This procedure is performed a little later than the standard intraatrial lateral tunnel operation to place a larger conduit. An extracardiac conduit appears to be better than the intraatrial lateral tunnel procedure with a very low operative mortality rate, a lower incidence of early and late arrhythmias, improved hemodynamics, and fewer postoperative complications (Backer et al, 2011), but the conduit does not have growth potential. However, a recent report by Rogers et al (2012) found an association between extracardiac conduit and prolonged period of pleural drainage.

Surgical approaches in tricuspid atresia are summarized in Fig. 14.42.

PULMONARY ATRESIA WITH INTACT VENTRICULAR SEPTUM

Prevalence

Pulmonary atresia with intact ventricular septum accounts for fewer than 1% of all CHDs. It accounts for 2.5% of the critically ill infants with CHDs.

Pathology

1. In 80% of these patients, the pulmonary valve is atretic with a diaphragm-like membrane. The infundibulum is atretic in 20% of these patients. The valve ring and the main PA are hypoplastic. The PA trunk is rarely atretic. The ventricular septum remains intact.
2. RV size varies and relates to survival. In 1982, Bull and associates divided this condition into three types based on the presence or absence of the three portions of the RV: inlet, trabecular, and infundibular portions (Fig. 14.43). The RV size is highly correlated with the size of the tricuspid valve.
   a. Tripartite type. All three of these portions are present, and the RV is almost normal in size.
   b. Bipartite type. The inlet and infundibular portions are present, but the trabecular portion is obliterated.
   c. Monopartite type. The inlet is the only portion present, and the RV size is diminutive. A rare type of pulmonary atresia that is not included in the classification is that associated with tricuspid insufficiency, less thickened but dilated RV cavity, and dilated RA.

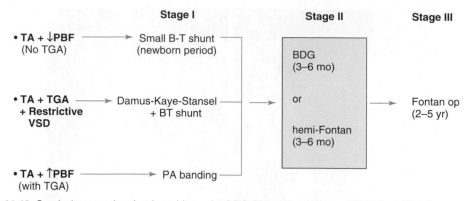

Fig. 14.42 Surgical approaches in tricuspid atresia. *BDG*, Bidirectional Glenn; *BT*, Blalock-Taussig; op, operation; *PA*, pulmonary artery; *PBF*, pulmonary blood flow; *TA*, tricuspid atresia; *TGA*, transposition of the great arteries; *VSD*, ventricular septal defect.

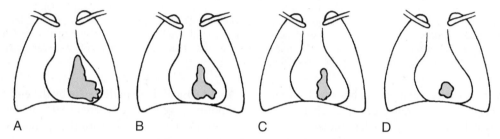

Fig. 14.43 Schematic diagrams of right ventriculograms that illustrate three types of pulmonary atresia with intact ventricular septum. **A**, Normal right ventricle (RV). **B**, Tripartite type that shows all three portions (inlet, trabecular, and infundibular) of the RV. **C**, Bipartite type in which only the inlet and infundibular portions are present. **D**, Monopartite type in which only the inlet portion of the RV is present.

3. This condition is frequently associated with important anomalies of the coronary arteries. The high pressure in the RV is decompressed through dilated coronary microcirculation (i.e., ventriculocoronary connection, coronary sinusoids, or RV-dependent coronary circulation) into the left or right coronary artery (see Fig. 14.44 for right ventriculograms showing coronary sinusoids). Often the proximal coronary arteries are obstructed (≈10%). Rarely, proximal portion(s) of the right or left coronary artery are absent. Sinusoid channels are demonstrable by a right ventriculogram in 30% to 50% of cases. If proximal coronary artery obstruction is present, coronary circulation is perfused entirely by desaturated RV blood (RV-dependent coronary circulation). Tricuspid valve z score less than −2.5 is a helpful predictor of coronary fistulas and RV-dependent coronary circulation. Such coronary sinusoids occur mostly only in patients with significantly hypertensive RV.
4. Confluent PAs are usually present with PBF provided through a PDA. Rarely, nonconfluent PAs are supplied by bilateral ductus arteriosus or multiple aortopulmonary collaterals.
5. An interatrial communication (i.e., either ASD or PFO) and PDA (or collateral arteries) are necessary for the patient to survive.
6. RV myocardium shows varying degrees of ischemia, infarction, fibrosis, and endocardial fibroelastosis, with poorly compliant RV, which may contribute to surgical mortality.

Clinical Manifestations
History

A history of severe cyanosis since birth is present.

Physical Examination

1. Severe cyanosis and tachypnea are seen in distressed neonates.
2. The S2 is single. A heart murmur is usually absent, but a soft murmur of either TR or a soft continuous murmur of PDA may be audible.
3. Inadequate interatrial communication causes hepatomegaly.

Electrocardiography

1. The QRS axis is normal (i.e., + 60 to + 140 degrees), in contrast to the superiorly oriented QRS axis seen in tricuspid atresia.
2. LVH is usually present. Occasionally RVH is seen in infants with a relatively large RV cavity. RAH is common, occurring in 70% of cases.

Radiography

The heart size may be normal or large, resulting from RA enlargement. Pulmonary vascular markings are decreased with dark lung fields. The main PA segment is concave.

Echocardiography

1. Diagnostic features of the condition include (a) a thickened, immobile, atretic pulmonary valve with no Doppler evidence of blood flow through it; (b) a hypertrophied

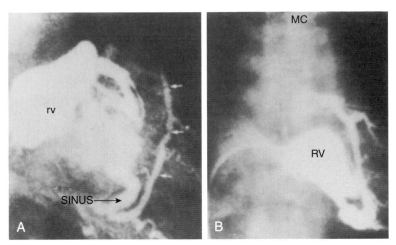

Fig. 14.44 Right ventriculograms in a patient with pulmonary atresia. **A,** Contrast medium filling the right ventricle (rv) passes into the ventricle-coronary fistula (sinus) and left anterior descending (LAD) coronary artery. Small white arrows point to multiple stenotic areas in the LAD. **B,** Massive filling of a dilated and irregular LAD coronary artery from the right ventricular injection (RV). (From Williams WG, Burrows P, Freedom RM, et al: Thromboexclusion of the right ventricle in children with pulmonary atresia and intact ventricular septum, *J Thorac Cardiovasc Surg* 101:222–229, 1991.)

RV wall with a small cavity; (c) a patent, but small, tricuspid valve; (d) a right-to-left atrial shunt through an ASD demonstrated by color flow and Doppler studies; and (e) ductus arteriosus running vertically from the aortic arch to the PA (i.e., "vertical ductus") (see Fig. 14.25).

2. The size of the tricuspid valve should be carefully measured because this measurement correlates well with the size of the RV cavity and thus determines whether a biventricular or univentricular repair is suitable (see Appendix D, Table D.5, for tricuspid and other valve annulus dimensions in the neonates). The most severely stenotic tricuspid valve is associated with the most underdeveloped RV and with likelihood of RV-dependent coronary circulation.

3. Images of the proximal coronary arteries help detect coronary artery anomalies. A coronary AV fistula is not easy to detect, but dilated or tortuous proximal coronary arteries suggest an RV-dependent coronary circulation. Color Doppler flow mapping may show retrograde flow in a proximal coronary artery. Absence of normal origin of a coronary artery may also suggest the presence of a fistulous connection to that coronary artery.

4. The right and left PA branches are usually well developed.

Cardiac Catheterization

Cardiac catheterization and angiocardiography are required for proper management in most patients with pulmonary atresia. A right ventriculogram demonstrates the size of the RV cavity and the presence or absence of coronary sinusoids (see Fig. 14.44). An ascending aortogram identifies stenosis or interruption of the coronary arteries. Both are important in surgical decision making, whether to go for univentricular or biventricular repair.

Natural History

Without appropriate management (which includes PGE$_1$ infusion and surgery), the prognosis is exceedingly poor.

About 50% of these patients die by the end of the first month if not managed properly; about 80% die by 6 months of age. Death usually coincides with the spontaneous closure of the ductus arteriosus.

Management
Medical

1. PGE$_1$ (Prostin VR Pediatric solution) infusion should begin as soon as the diagnosis is suspected or confirmed, so that the patency of the ductus arteriosus is maintained. Infusion is continued during cardiac catheterization and surgery. The starting dosage of Prostin is 0.05 to 0.1 μg/kg/min. When the desired effect is achieved, the dosage is gradually reduced to 0.01 μg/kg/min.

2. For small premature infants, a prolonged course of PGE$_1$ infusion may be necessary before surgery is undertaken.

3. In neonates with monopartite RV, who are not likely to be candidates for two-ventricular repair and are likely to require bidirectional Glenn operation or hemi-Fontan in a few months, some centers advocate using PDA stenting instead of the BT shunt. PDA stenting is less reliable and shorter lasting than the BT shunt but is likely to last to the time of bidirectional Glenn or hemi-Fontan procedure (Feltes et al, 2011).

4. In patients with membranous atresia, a laser-assisted pulmonary valvotomy with balloon pulmonary valvuloplasty may be a useful alternative to a surgical procedure that establishes an RV-to-PA continuity (Cheung et al, 2002). Infundibular atresia is unsuitable for catheter intervention.

Surgical

The size of the RV (or that of the tricuspid valve) and the presence or absence of coronary sinusoids or coronary artery anomalies dictate surgical procedures for infants with

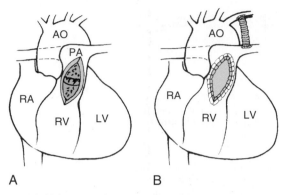

Fig. 14.45 Initial surgery for tripartite or bipartite type of pulmonary atresia. **A,** A longitudinal incision is made across the pulmonary annulus. The pulmonary valve is incised, and the right ventricular outflow tract is carefully widened. **B,** A piece of pericardium is used for the transannular patch. A left-sided Gore-Tex shunt is made between the left subclavian artery and the left pulmonary artery (PA). *AO,* Aorta; *LV,* left ventricle; *RA,* right atrium; *RV,* right ventricle.

pulmonary atresia with intact ventricular septum. Surgical options are as follows.

1. Two-ventricular repair, which is the ultimate goal whenever feasible, is possible only when there is an adequate size of the RV cavity with adequate RVOTs.
2. One and one-half ventricular repair may be chosen when the RV size is judged to be borderline for a two-ventricular repair but too good to be abandoned for Fontan-type repair.
3. One-ventricular repair (Fontan operation) is done when (1) an RV-dependent coronary circulation is present or (2) a monopartite RV (with a tricuspid valve z score <−4 to −5) is present.
4. Cardiac transplantation is a possible option.

Procedures

1. Staged two-ventricular repair: For the two-ventricular repair, the initial procedure consists of establishing a connection between the RV and the PA (to promote growth of the RV) and a systemic-to-PA shunt created at the same time. The second-stage operation consists of reconstruction of the RVOT.

a. First-stage operation: One of the following is done.
1) Placement of a transannular RV outflow patch and a systemic-to-PA shunt seems most promising for a two-ventricular repair at a later date (Fig. 14.45). Balloon atrial septostomy is not recommended with this approach, so that a high RA pressure is maintained to maximize the forward RV output.
2) For a patient with a well-formed pulmonary valve and adequate infundibulum, a closed transpulmonary valvotomy (without cardiopulmonary bypass) and a left-sided modified BT shunt procedure are performed. The mortality rate of these procedures is less than 5%.
3) An alternative to the closed surgical valvotomy is the use of laser wire and radiofrequency-assisted valvotomy and balloon dilatation during cardiac

catheterization (Cheung et al, 2002). The mortality rate of the procedure is about 5%.

b. Follow-up. After one of the above first stage procedures, the growth of the RV is monitored in the following manner.
1) Echo studies showing growth of the tricuspid valve size (to larger than z sore >−2), evidence of growth of the RV size, and stable O_2 saturation are positive signs for future two-ventricular repair.
2) Cardiac catheterization is performed within 6 to 18 months after the initial surgery. An arterial O_2 saturation greater than 70%, a greater RV volume, and evidence of a good forward flow through the pulmonary valve are all positive signs.
3) If the patient tolerates balloon occlusion of the shunt during cardiac catheterization, the patient is considered a candidate for a two-ventricular repair.
c. The second-stage operation: RVOT reconstruction and closure of the ASD are carried out under cardiopulmonary bypass. The systemic-to-PA shunt is closed at the time of surgery.

2. One and one-half ventricular repair

The one and one-half ventricular repair may be performed when the RV size is not quite large enough to have two-ventricular repair but the RV is too good to be abandoned for one-ventricular repair. This type of repair consists of the following.

a. A bidirectional Glenn anastomosis is created to bring the SVC blood directly to the PA, bypassing the RV.
b. The IVC blood goes to the lungs via the normal pathway through the RV, which is large enough to handle half of the systemic venous return.

After this procedure, the size of the tricuspid valve and the RV may actually increase with an adequate RV function. Complications associated with the Fontan procedure (e.g., arrhythmias, protein-losing enteropathy) do not occur after this procedure. The surgical mortality rate is between 0% and 12% (similar to the rate for the Fontan procedure).

3. One-ventricular repair (Fontan operation)

For patients with monopartite RV (with or without coronary sinusoids), a two-ventricular repair is not possible. These patients will need one-ventricular repair (Fontan operation).

a. A systemic-to-PA shunt without the RV outflow patch is recommended as the initial procedure. Some institutions use PDA stenting, instead of the BT shunt until the time of bidirectional Glenn or hemi-Fontan operation (at 3–6 months of age).
b. A staged Fontan operation is performed at a later time (see Tricuspid Atresia for a full description of the Fontan operation).
c. For patients who have rudimentary RV (with high RV pressure) and sinusoidal channels, there are two options.
1) The sinusoids are left alone without decompression, and a systemic-to-PA shunt is performed for a future Fontan-type operation. Decompression of the RV

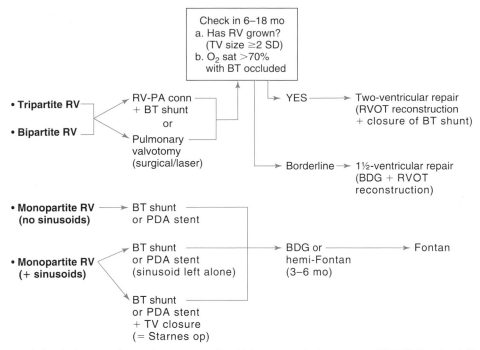

Fig. 14.46 Surgical approach to pulmonary atresia with intact ventricular septum. *BDG*, Bidirectional Glenn; *RT*, Blalock-Taussig; *op*, operation; *PDA*, patent ductus arteriosus; *RV*, right ventricle; *RVOT*, right ventricular outflow tract; *RV-PA conn*, right ventricle–to–pulmonary artery connection; *SD*, standard deviation; *TV*, tricuspid valve.

by valvotomy or an outflow patch cannot be done because it results in a reversal of coronary flow into the RV, thereby producing myocardial ischemia.

2) Alternatively, the tricuspid valve is closed (converting it to tricuspid atresia, the Starnes procedure), and a systemic-to-PA shunt is created for a future Fontan operation.

4. When the proximal portion of the coronary arteries is not identified or severe anomalies of the coronary circulation are present, surgical option is limited; cardiac transplantation may be an option.

Fig. 14.46 summarizes what has been discussed under the heading of Surgical Management.

Postoperative Follow-up. Most patients require close follow-up because none of the surgical procedures available are curative.

HYPOPLASTIC LEFT HEART SYNDROME

Prevalence

Hypoplastic left heart syndrome occurs in 1 in 5000 live births. About 2000 infants are born annually with the defect in the United States. About 10% of cases are associated with genetic syndromes such as Turner syndrome, trisomy 18, Jacobsen's syndrome (11q terminal deletion disorder), and others.

Pathology

1. HLHS includes a group of closely related anomalies characterized by hypoplasia of the LV, atresia or critical stenosis of the aortic or mitral valves, and hypoplasia of the

ascending aorta and aortic arch. The LV is small and nonfunctional or totally atretic.

2. The atrial septum may be intact with a normal foramen ovale, or the patient may have a true ASD (15%). A VSD appears in about 10% of patients. COA frequently is an associated finding (≤75%).

3. A high prevalence of brain abnormalities has been reported. Up to 29% of the patients had a CNS abnormality. Overt CNS malformations (e.g., agenesis of the corpus callosum, holoprosencephaly) were seen in 10% of these infants. Micrencephaly was found in 27% of the infants, and an immature cortical mantle was seen in 21% of the patients. The presence or absence of dysmorphic physical features did not predict CNS malformations (Glauser et al, 1990).

Pathophysiology

1. During fetal life, the PVR is higher than the SVR, and the dominant RV maintains normal perfusing pressure in the descending aorta and the placenta through the ductal right-to-left shunt. The proximal aorta and the coronary and cerebral circulations are adequately perfused retrogradely. Fetuses tolerate this serious cardiac anomaly well in utero.

2. Difficulties arise after birth for two reasons: reduction of PVR (with the onset of respiration) and closure of the ductus arteriosus. The result is a marked reduction in the aortic perfusing pressure and systemic hypoperfusion, producing circulatory shock and metabolic acidosis.

3. Maintenance of adequate systemic blood flow (and thus survival of these infants) depends on an adequate size of

the ductus arteriosus and maintenance of a high PVR to permit the RV to send an adequate amount of blood flow to the aorta. Large PBF increases pulmonary venous return to the LA. An adequate interatrial communication is necessary to decompress the LA. In the presence of a large ASD that permits a left-to-RA shunt, pulmonary edema is not severe, and the arterial oxygen saturation may be in the 80s. With an inadequate atrial septal communication, pulmonary edema is severe, and the arterial oxygen saturation is low. Without treatment, the infant usually dies shortly after birth.

Clinical Manifestations

1. A neonate with HLHS becomes critically ill within the first few hours to the first few days of life. Tachycardia, dyspnea, pulmonary crackles, weak peripheral pulses, and vasoconstricted extremities are characteristic. The patient may not have severe cyanosis but has a grayish blue color of the skin with poor perfusion.
2. The S2 is loud and single. Heart murmur usually is absent. Occasionally, a grade 1 to 2 of 6 nonspecific ejection systolic murmur may be heard over the precordium. Signs of CHF develop, with hepatomegaly and gallop rhythm.
3. The ECG almost always shows RVH. Rarely, the ECG suggests LVH with large R waves in V5 and V6 (because these leads are placed over the dilated RV, not over the hypoplastic LV).
4. Chest radiography characteristically shows pulmonary venous congestion or pulmonary edema (Fig. 14.47A). The heart is moderately or markedly enlarged.
5. Arterial blood gas levels reveal a slightly decreased Po_2 and a normal Pco_2. Severe metabolic acidosis out of proportion to the Pco_2 (caused by markedly decreased cardiac output) is characteristic of the condition.
6. Echocardiographic findings are diagnostic and usually obviate the need for cardiac catheterization and angiocardiography.

a. The LV cavity is diminutive, but the RV cavity is markedly dilated, and the tricuspid valve is large.
b. Imaging usually reveals severe hypoplasia of the aorta and aortic annulus and an absent or distorted mitral valve. COA frequently is an associated anomaly.
c. The patient may have an ASD or a PFO with a left-to-right shunt. The patient occasionally has a VSD with a relatively large LV, aortic annulus, and ascending aorta.
d. Imaging may show diffuse echodense endocardial thickening, endocardial fibroelastosis (EFE), suggestive of damaged myocardium secondary to continuously elevated LV wall tension.
e. Color-flow mapping and Doppler studies reveal retrograde blood flow in the aortic arch and ascending aorta (to perfuse the head and the coronary circulation).

Natural History

Pulmonary edema and CHF develop in the first week of life. Circulatory shock and progressive hypoxemia and acidosis result in death, usually in the first month of life.

Management
Presurgical Medical Management

1. IV infusion of PGE_1 (alprostadil, Prostin VR Pediatric) should be started as soon as the diagnosis is verified by echocardiogram (for the dosage, see Appendix E). This will keep or reopen the PDA, which is essential for systemic perfusion with right-to-left shunting at the PDA level.
2. Intubation is not necessary routinely unless patient has a respiratory indication (i.e., apnea). It is preferred to keep patient on an FiO_2 (fraction of inspired oxygen) of 21% to avoid pulmonary overcirculation.
3. Metabolic acidosis should be corrected.
4. Balloon atrial septostomy may be necessary in the case of severely restrictive PFO; however, mild restriction at the PFO level may be desirable to avoid significant pulmonary overcirculation until after surgery.

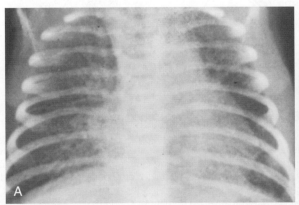 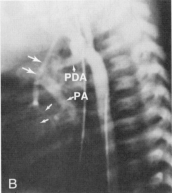

Fig. 14.47 Anteroposterior view of chest film (**A**) and lateral view of an aortogram (**B**) in a 1-day-old newborn with HLHS. The heart is enlarged, and the pulmonary vascularity is increased, with marked pulmonary venous congestion and pulmonary edema (**A**). The aortogram, obtained with injection of a radiopaque dye through an umbilical artery catheter, shows a hypoplastic ascending aorta *(thick arrows)* with small coronary arteries *(thin arrows)* filling retrogradely, a large patent ductus arteriosus (PDA), and pulmonary artery (PA) branches.

5. Support therapy only without surgical procedure is no longer acceptable in most parts of the world.
6. Infants with HLHS should have careful genetic, ophthalmologic, and neurologic evaluations, including imaging of their intracranial anatomy (MRI), and long-term follow-up because of a high prevalence of neurodevelopmental abnormalities seen with the condition.

Surgical

Three options are available in the management of these infants: (1) the Norwood operation (followed by a Fontan-type operation), (2) a hybrid operation (followed by a Fontan-type operation), and (3) cardiac transplantation. The surgical procedure of choice remains controversial, but the Norwood operation is more popular than cardiac transplantation. A hybrid operation is being done at some centers, but its long-term advantages are not clear at this time. A rare subgroup of patients with normal-sized LV (because of a large VSD) can have a two-ventricular repair rather than the Fontan operation.

Staged Surgical Approach. The first-stage (Norwood) operation is performed initially followed by the bidirectional Glenn or the hemi-Fontan and eventually by the Fontan-type operation.

1. The Norwood operation is performed in the neonatal period. The operation consists of the following procedures (Fig. 14.48).
    a. The main PA is divided, the distal stump is closed with a patch, and the ductus arteriosus is ligated and divided.
    b. Using an aortic or PA allograft, one connects the proximal PA and the hypoplastic ascending aorta and aortic arch.
    c. PBF is established by one of the following procedures.
        1) A right-side modified BT (BT) shunt is created (using a 4- to 5-mm Gore-Tex tube) to provide PBF while preventing CHF and pulmonary hypertension.

2) An RV-to-PA shunt (using polytetrafluoroethylene graft) was first used by Sano and colleagues (2003) (4 mm for patients weighing <2 kg and 5 mm for those weighing >2 kg) (Sano modification).

Sano central shunt may be an advantage over the modified BT shunt for the following reasons. Although the central shunt requires a right ventriculotomy to complete the shunt, (1) it promotes symmetrical growth of the PAs, and (2) it provides a higher aortic diastolic pressure (in the absence of diastolic run-off through the BT shunt) and thus a higher coronary artery perfusion pressure. The BT shunt, on the other hand, provides continuous forward flow to the PA during both systole and diastole, causing diastolic retrograde flow in the central aorta, which may cause "coronary steal" during diastole.

   f. The atrial septum is excised to allow adequate interatrial mixing.

Mortality. The Norwood procedure carries the highest surgical mortality rate among common cyanotic CHD, ranging from 7% to 19%. In addition, between the Norwood operation and the second stage operation, 4% to 15% of infants die. Ohye et al (2010) reported that survival rate after the first-stage (Norwood) operation was significantly higher in infants who had Sano modification than those who had modified BT shunt (74% vs 64%).

Post-Norwood Medical Management. Most patients are placed on the following medications after the Norwood operation (and most of them are continued throughout their lives even after the final Fontan operation).

   a. Small-dose diuretic therapy (not to produce hypovolemia) is given.
   b. Digoxin is given by some centers.
   c. ACE inhibitor (i.e., captopril, enalapril) as an afterload-reducing agent, is given to decrease strain on the systemic RV.
   d. Aspirin is given to prevent shunt thrombosis.

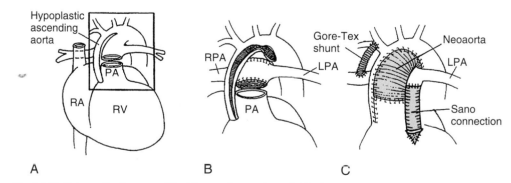

Fig. 14.48 Schematic diagram of the Norwood procedure. **A,** The heart with aortic atresia with a hypoplastic ascending aorta and aortic arch, along with a large pulmonary artery (PA) and ductus arteriosus, are shown. The main PA is transected. **B,** An incision that extends around the aortic arch to the level of the ductus is made in the ascending aorta. The distal PA is closed with a patch. The ductus arteriosus is ligated and divided. **C,** A modified right Blalock-Taussig shunt is created between the right subclavian artery and the right PA (RPA) as the sole source of pulmonary blood flow. Alternatively, a homograft conduit may be placed between the right ventricle (RV) and PA bifurcation as shown in the figure (Sano modification). Note that only one of these two procedures is performed but not both. By the use of an aortic or PA allograft *(striped area)*, the main PA is anastomosed to the ascending aorta and the aortic arch to create a large new arterial trunk. The Norwood procedure also includes widening of the atrial communication, which is not shown in the illustration. *LPA,* Left pulmonary artery; *PA,* pulmonary artery; *RA,* right atrium; *RV,* right ventricle.

e. Nutritional support is very important, if necessary, including nasogastric feeding or a gastrostomy tube feeding.

2. The second-stage operation for HLHS is either the bidirectional Glenn procedure or the hemi-Fontan procedure. These procedures are performed at 3 to 6 months of age.

a. Bidirectional Glenn operation (also called cavopulmonary shunt) is an end-to-side anastomosis of the superior vena cava to the right PA (see Fig. 14.38A) performed at 3 to 6 months of age in an effort to reduce the volume overload to the systemic RV. The mortality rate for this procedure is less than 5%.

b. The hemi-Fontan operation. This procedure includes augmentation of the central PA without dividing the SVC while excluding IVC blood from the PAs by means of a temporary intraatrial patch (see Fig. 14.39).

3. The third-stage operation is a modified Fontan operation performed at 2 to 5 years of age (see Fig. 14.38B). Five important hemodynamic and anatomic features considered essential to successful Fontan operation include (1) unrestrictive interatrial communication, (2) competence of the tricuspid valve, (3) unobstructed PA-to-descending aorta anastomosis (with pressure gradient <25 mm Hg), (4) undistorted PAs and low PVR, and (5) preservation of RV function.

Currently, the operative mortality rate of the Fontan procedure is less than 3%. Patients with HLHS have higher likelihood of prolonged pleural effusion and hospital stay than those with tricuspid atresia. Mean PA pressure of 15 mm Hg or greater was associated with prolonged hospital stay and unfavorable outcomes (Rogers et al, 2012). Significant TR appears to be an important predictor of poor outcome of the Fontan operation. The overall survival rate after the Fontan operation is better than 95% at follow-up of 50 months (Hirsch et al, 2008).

Hybrid Approach

Hybrid approach followed later by the Fontan-type operation was first reported in 2008 (Galantowicz et al, 2008). Some centers now use this procedure as an alternative to Norwood (stage 1) procedure for high-risk HLHS, for single-ventricle patients, or as a bridge to heart transplantation in infants with HLHS.

The advantages of this approach are that (1) it creates a stable, balanced circulation without the use of open-heart surgery using cardiopulmonary bypass (which carries a relatively high risk), and (2) it delays the open heart procedure until later in life when a bidirectional Glenn or hemi-Fontan operation can be safely performed (3–6 months of age).

1. Hybrid procedure is performed in the first weeks of life. The procedure consists of both:

a. Bilateral PA banding through a small median sternotomy, using a 1.0- to 2.0-mm ring from a 3.5-mm Gore-Tex tube graft (3.0-mm tube for patients <2.5 kg) to provide adequate PBF but without causing pulmonary hypertension or heart failure

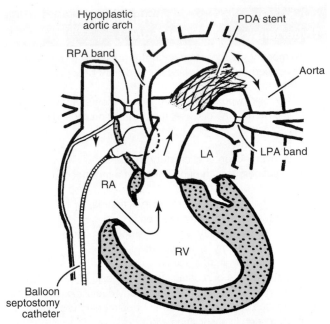

Fig. 14.49 Hybrid stage I intervention for hypoplastic left heart syndrome. Surgical bands around the right and left pulmonary arteries limit blood flow to the lungs, and a stent in the ductus arteriosus holds it open and maintains adequate blood flow to the body. A balloon atrial septostomy allows unobstructed return of pulmonary venous blood to the heart. *LA,* Left atrium; *LPA,* left pulmonary artery; *RA,* right atrium; *RPA,* right pulmonary artery.

b. Insertion of a PDA stent in the same setting through a sheath placed (through purse-string) in the main PA to ensure adequate systemic and coronary perfusion (Fig. 14.49)

c. As a separate procedure, balloon atrial septostomy with or without balloon dilatation is performed to establish a reliable atrial shunt.

2. The comprehensive stage 2 operation combines the Norwood operation and bidirectional Glenn operation. The surgery is performed at 3 to 6 months of age, with a surgical mortality rate of 8%. Thus, the stage 2 procedures include:

a. Removal of PDA stent and PA bands

b. Repair of aortic arch and the PAs (especially the LPA if necessary)

c. Reimplantation of the diminutive ascending aorta into the pulmonary root

d. Atrial septostomy

e. Bidirectional Glenn operation

3. A Fontan-type operation is performed at age of 2 to 5 years, the same as that described under the staged Norwood approach.

Other Surgical Approaches

1. Infants with aortic atresia and normal-sized LV caused by a large VSD can have a biventricular repair rather than a Fontan approach. The VSD is tunneled to the PA. The main pulmonary artery (MPA) is divided, and the proximal MPA is connected to the ascending aorta. The RV is

BOX 14.3 Causes of Persistent Pulmonary Hypertension of the Newborn

1. Pulmonary vasoconstriction in the presence of a normally developed pulmonary vascular bed may be caused by or seen in:
   a. Alveolar hypoxia (meconium aspiration syndrome, hyaline membrane disease, hypoventilation caused by CNS anomalies)
   b. Birth asphyxia
   c. LV dysfunction or circulatory shock
   d. Infections (e.g., group B hemolytic streptococcal infection)
   e. Hyperviscosity syndrome (polycythemia)
   f. Hypoglycemia and hypocalcemia
2. Increased pulmonary vascular smooth muscle development (hypertrophy) may be caused by:
   a. Chronic intrauterine asphyxia
   b. Maternal use of prostaglandin synthesis inhibitors (aspirin, indomethacin) resulting in early ductal closure
3. Decreased cross-sectional area of pulmonary vascular bed may be seen in association with:
   a. Congenital diaphragmatic hernia
   b. Primary pulmonary hypoplasia

CNS, Central nervous system; *LV,* left ventricle.

connected to the distal MPA using a valved conduit or a homograft.

2. Some centers considered cardiac transplantation the procedure of choice in the past. If the diameter of the ascending aorta is smaller than 2.5 mm, cardiac transplantation, rather than the Norwood operation, was believed to provide a better result. The surgical technique of cardiac transplantation is presented in Chapter 36.

For patients placed on a transplantation algorithm, it is necessary to keep the ductus open and to increase the size of the interatrial communication. A hybrid procedure may be used as a bridge to cardiac transplantation, in which an endovascular stent is placed in closing ductus to keep the ductus open and PA branches are banded to control PBF. Blade atrial septostomy followed by balloon dilatation has been performed for decompression of the LA.

At this time, not all cardiac centers offer orthotropic heart transplantation. The availability of the donor heart is limited, and the overall mortality rate while awaiting transplantation is 21% to 37%. Furthermore, this approach requires lifelong immunosuppression with the attendant risks of rejection, infection, graft atherosclerosis, and malignancies. Some patients may require subsequent retransplantation because of allograft vasculopathy and graft dysfunction.

Postsurgical Follow-up Plan. After the second-stage operation and the final Fontan operation, the follow-up plans are similar to those described for tricuspid atresia (also refer to Box 14.3).

Fig. 14.50 summarizes surgical approaches used in the management of patients with HLHS.

EBSTEIN'S ANOMALY

Prevalence

Ebstein's anomaly of the tricuspid valve occurs in fewer than 1% of all CHDs.

Pathology

1. There is downward displacement of the septal and posterior leaflets of the tricuspid valve into the RV cavity, so that a portion of the RV is incorporated into the RA (i.e., *atrialized* RV), and functional hypoplasia of the RV results (Fig. 14.51). Tricuspid regurgitation is usually present, and redundant tricuspid valve tissues can rarely obstruct the RVOT, which results in dilatation and hypertrophy of the RA.
2. An interatrial communication (e.g., PFO, true ASD) with a right-to-left shunt is present in all patients.
3. In addition to the structural abnormalities of the tricuspid valve, there is a global problem with RV myocardium, structurally and functionally, sometimes involving the LV as well. The RV free wall is often dilated and thin. Fibrosis is present in both RV and LV free walls; this may be responsible for severe symptoms early in life and LV dysfunction in later life.
4. WPW preexcitation is frequently associated with the anomaly and predisposes the patient to SVT.
5. PS, pulmonary atresia, TOF, VSD, and other defects are occasionally associated with the anomaly.

Clinical Manifestations

History

1. In severe cases, cyanosis and CHF develop during the first few days of life. Some subsequent improvement coincides with reduction of the PVR.
2. Children with milder cases may complain of dyspnea, fatigue, cyanosis, or palpitation on exertion.
3. A history of SVT is occasionally present.

Physical Examination

1. Mild to severe cyanosis is present, as well as clubbing of the fingers and toes in older infants and children.
2. Characteristic triple or quadruple rhythm is audible. This rhythm consists of a widely split S2, split S1, S3, and S4. A soft holosystolic (or early systolic) murmur of TR is usually audible at the lower left sternal border (Fig. 14.52). A soft, scratchy, mid-diastolic murmur is present at the same location.
3. Hepatomegaly is usually present.

Electrocardiography

1. Characteristic ECG findings of RBBB and RAH are present in most patients with this condition (Fig. 14.53).
2. First-degree AV block is frequent, occurring in 40% of patients. A WPW pattern of preexcitation is present in 15% to 20% of patients (with occasional episodes of SVT).

Radiography

In mild cases, the heart is almost normal in size and has normal pulmonary vascular markings. In severe cases, an

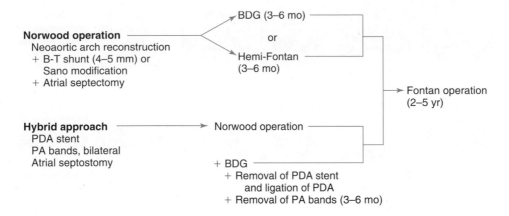

Fig. 14.50 Surgery for hypoplastic left heart syndrome. *BDG*, Bidirectional Glenn; *BT*, Blalock-Taussig; *PA*, pulmonary artery; *PDA*, patent ductus arteriosus.

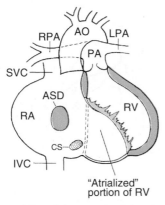

Fig. 14.51 Diagram of Ebstein's anomaly of the tricuspid valve. There is an apicalward displacement of the tricuspid valve, usually the septal and posterior leaflets, into the right ventricle (RV). Part of the RV is incorporated into the right atrium (RA) ("atrialized" portion of the RV). Regurgitation of the tricuspid valve results in RA enlargement. An atrial septal defect (ASD) is usually present. *CS*, Coronary sinus; *IVC*, inferior vena cava; *LPA*, left pulmonary artery; *PA*, pulmonary artery; *RPA*, right pulmonary artery; *SVC*, superior vena cava.

extreme cardiomegaly (principally involving the RA) with a balloon-shaped heart and decreased pulmonary vascular markings is present. Some of the largest heart sizes are found in newborns with this condition (Fig. 14.54).

Echocardiography

Two-dimensional echocardiography with color-flow Doppler study is the procedure of choice for the diagnosis and functional assessment of Ebstein's anomaly; cardiac catheterization and angiography are not needed.

1. The single most diagnostic feature is apical displacement of the hinge point of the septal leaflet of the tricuspid valve (Fig. 14.55). Normally, the septal leaflet of the tricuspid valve inserts on the ventricular septum slightly below the insertion of the mitral valve. In patients with Ebstein's anomaly, this normal displacement is exaggerated. A diagnosis of Ebstein's anomaly is made when the tricuspid valve is displaced toward the apex by more than 8 mm/m^2 of BSA from the mitral valve insertion. This displacement is best seen in the apical four-chamber view.

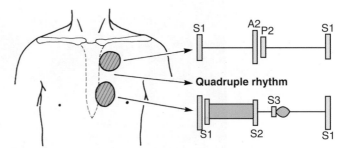

Fig. 14.52 Cardiac findings of Ebstein's anomaly. Quadruple rhythm and a soft, regurgitant systolic murmur (of tricuspid regurgitation) are characteristic of the defect.

2. The tricuspid valve leaflets are elongated, redundant, and dysplastic with abnormal chordal attachment.
3. A large RA, including the atrialized RV, and a small functional RV represent anatomic severity. Evidence of tricuspid valve regurgitation and tricuspid stenosis (TS) is present.
4. RVOT obstruction may occur owing to the redundant anterior leaflet of the tricuspid valve.
5. A nonrestrictive ASD is commonly imaged.
6. Other anomalies may include mitral valve prolapse and LV dysfunction.

Other Studies

Cardiac catheterization is rarely necessary in patients with Ebstein's anomaly. In the current era, echocardiography and MRI provide superior images.

Natural History

1. Some 18% of symptomatic newborns die in the neonatal period; 30% of patients die before the age of 10 years, usually from CHF.
2. Cyanosis tends to improve as the PVR falls during the newborn period. Cyanosis may reappear later.
3. Patients with a less severe anomaly may be either asymptomatic or mildly symptomatic.
4. Hemodynamic deterioration with increasing cyanosis, CHF, and LV dysfunction develops later in life. These developments foretell early death.

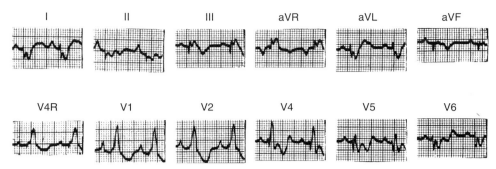

I   II   III   aVR   aVL   aVF

V4R   V1   V2   V4   V5   V6

Fig. 14.53 Tracing from a 5-year-old child with Ebstein's anomaly. The tracing shows right atrial hypertrophy, right bundle branch block, and first-degree atrioventricular block.

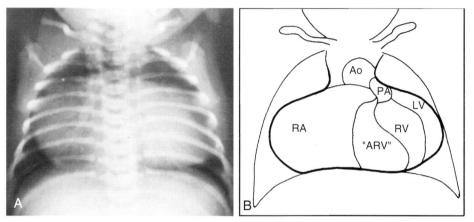

Fig. 14.54 Posteroanterior view (**A**) and diagram (**B**) of chest radiograph from a 2-week-old infant with severe Ebstein's anomaly. Note the extreme cardiomegaly involving primarily the right atrium (RA) and diminished pulmonary vascularity. *Ao,* Aorta; *ARV,* atrialized right ventricle; *LV,* left ventricle; *PA,* pulmonary artery; *RV,* right ventricle.

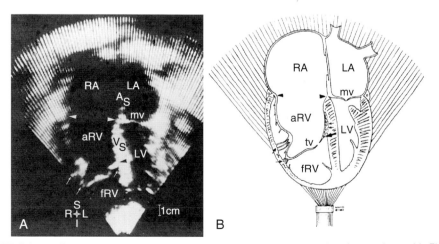

Fig. 14.55 Echocardiogram (**A**) and diagram (**B**) of an apical four-chamber view in a patient with Ebstein's anomaly. The septal leaflet is displaced into the right ventricle (RV; *large dark arrow*) and thus forms an atrialized RV (aRV). The anterior tricuspid leaflet is elongated. Both leaflets are tethered to underlying myocardium *(small arrows)*. The tricuspid annulus and the right atrium (RA) are dilated. *AS,* Atrial septum; *fRV,* functional right ventricle; *LA,* left atrium; *LV,* left ventricle; *mv,* mitral valve; *tv,* tricuspid valve; *VS,* ventricular septum. (From Shiina A, Serwer JB, Edwards WD, et al: Two-dimensional echocardiographic spectrum of Ebstein's anomaly: Detailed anatomic assessment, *J Am Coll Cardiol* 3:356–370, 1984.)

5. Attacks of SVT with associated WPW preexcitation occur in 15% to 20% of all patients. Sudden, unexpected death can occur, probably as a result of arrhythmias.

6. Other possible complications include infective endocarditis, brain abscess, and cerebrovascular accident.

Management
Medical

1. In severely cyanotic newborns, intensive treatment with mechanical ventilation, PGE_1 infusion, inotropic agents, and correction of metabolic acidosis may be necessary before proceeding with emergency surgery.

2. In infants who appear to have a mild form of Ebstein's anomaly and to be improving with the above management, treatment with PGE_1 and inotropic support is gradually withdrawn to observe the effect of ductal closure.

3. Asymptomatic children with mild Ebstein's anomaly require only regular observation. If CHF develops, anticongestive measures, including digoxin and diuretics, are indicated.

4. Acute episodes of SVT may be treated most effectively with adenosine (see Chapter 24). Beta-blockers are the most appropriate first-line preventive therapy for SVT. For patients with recurrent SVT caused by AV reentrant mechanism, radiofrequency catheter ablation techniques have been successful.

5. Varying degrees of activity restriction may be necessary for children with this condition.

Surgical

Indications. Although surgical indications for Ebstein's anomaly are not completely defined, they may include the following:

1. Critically ill neonates who show symptoms within the first week of life (after a period of intensive medical treatment)

2. Occurrence of moderately severe or progressive cyanosis (arterial saturation of ≤80%), polycythemia (hemoglobin level of ≥16 g/dL), or CHF

3. RVOT obstruction by redundant tricuspid valve

4. Severe activity limitation (i.e., NYHA functional class III or IV) (see Appendix A, Table A.3)

5. History of paradoxical embolus

6. Repeated, life-threatening arrhythmias in patients with associated WPW syndrome

Procedures. Controversy exists concerning the type and timing of surgical procedures.

1. **Palliative procedures.** For critically ill neonates, if medical management does not show signs of improvement, surgical intervention is indicated to avoid certain death.
   a. BT shunt (with enlargement of ASD). This procedure can be lifesaving when there are obstructive lesions between the RV and the PA or stenotic tricuspid valve. Good LV function (with an adequate LV size) is required to survive the procedure. A Fontan-type operation is performed later (see Fig. 14.38).
   b. If the LV is "pancaked" by large RV or RA, a procedure to reduce the RV or RA may be considered, such as the Starnes operation (pericardial closure of the tricuspid valve) or plication of large RA (atrialized RV), enlargement of ASD, and a BT shunt using a 4-mm tube. A Fontan-type operation (see Fig. 14.38) is performed later.
   c. Classic Glenn anastomosis (SVC to right PA end-to-end anastomosis) or its modification may be considered in severely cyanotic infants.

2. **Definitive procedures.** Children with good RV size and function are candidates for biventricular repair (with tricuspid valve repair or replacement). Inadequate RV size or function requires Fontan operation.
   a. **Two-ventricular repair.** Reconstruction of the tricuspid valve (e.g., Danielson and Carpentier procedure) is preferable to valve replacement. ASD is closed at the time of surgery.
      1) Danielson technique. For repair of the tricuspid valve, this technique is the most desirable and best tested, although it is frequently limited by anatomy. This technique can be applied in about 60% of patients (Fig. 14.56). It plicates the atrialized portion of the RV, narrows the tricuspid orifice in a selective manner, and results in a monoleaflet valve (by the anterior leaflet of the tricuspid valve). Two other leaflets are often severely hypoplastic and cannot be made to function as a leaflet. The mortality rate is about 5%, which is lower than that for valve replacement.
      2) Carpentier technique. As an alternative, Carpentier reconstructive surgery may be used. This repair also plicates the atrialized portion of the RV and the tricuspid annulus but in a direction that is at right angles to those used by Danielson. This repair can be applied in most patients with Ebstein's anomaly. The surgical mortality rate is 15%.
      3) Tricuspid valve replacement and closure of the ASD is a less desirable surgical approach but may be necessary for 20% to 30% of patients with Ebstein's anomaly who are not candidates for reconstructive surgery. The replacement valve of choice is a stented, antibiotically treated semilunar valve allograft or a heterograft valve. A pulmonary allograft valve mounted in a short Dacron sleeve can be used in younger children. The surgical mortality rate ranges from 5% to 20%.
   b. **One-ventricular repair.** For patients with inadequate size of the RV, a Fontan-type operation is usually performed in stages after the initial palliative procedures such as a bidirectional Glenn operation or hemi-Fontan operation (see Fig. 14.38).

3. **Other procedures.** For patients with WPW syndrome and recurrent SVT, surgical interruption at the time of surgery or radiofrequency ablation of the accessory pathway is recommended.

Complications

1. Complete heart block is a rare complication.

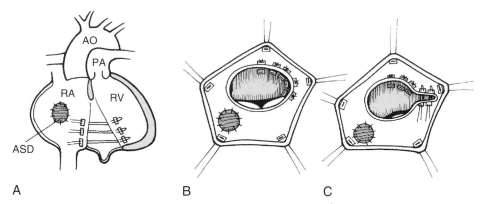

Fig. 14.56 Danielson technique for tricuspid valve repair. **A,** A series of interrupted mattress sutures are placed to obliterate the atrialized portion of the right ventricle (RV). The atrial septal defect (ASD) is closed with a patch. **B,** As the sutures are tied, the atrialized portion of the RV is obliterated (seen through a right atriotomy). **C,** Sutures are placed to further narrow the tricuspid orifice. The valve is now a monocusp valve (anterior leaflet of the tricuspid valve) that is mobile and opens widely during diastole. *AO,* Aorta; *PA,* pulmonary artery; *RA,* right atrium.

2. Supraventricular arrhythmias persist in 10% to 20% of patients after surgery.

Postoperative Follow-up

1. Frequent follow-up is necessary because of the persistence of arrhythmias after surgery, which occurs in 10% to 20% of patients, and because of possible problems associated with tricuspid valve surgery that require reoperation.
2. Some patients may need to be prohibited from participating in competitive or strenuous sports.

Surgical approaches for Ebstein's anomaly are shown in Fig. 14.57.

PERSISTENT TRUNCUS ARTERIOSUS

Prevalence

Persistent truncus arteriosus occurs in fewer than 1% of all CHDs.

Pathology

1. Only a single arterial trunk with a truncal valve leaves the heart and gives rise to the pulmonary, systemic, and coronary circulations. A large perimembranous, infundibular VSD is present directly below the truncus (Fig. 14.58). The truncal valve may be bicuspid, tricuspid, or quadricuspid, and it is often incompetent.
2. According to Collett and Edwards' classification, this anomaly is divided into four types by how the PAs arise from the truncus arteriosus (see Fig. 14.58 for the description of each type). Types I and II constitute 85% of cases. Type IV is not a true persistent truncus arteriosus; rather, it is a severe form of TOF with pulmonary atresia (i.e., pseudo-truncus arteriosus), with aortic collaterals supplying the lungs.
3. Van Praagh classification divides the defects into type A (with VSD) or type B (without VSD). Further subtypes include 1 through 4. Type A1 is the same as type I by Collett and Edwards. Type A2 corresponds to types II and III.

Type A3 reflects the absence of the origin of one of the PAs from the proximal trunk. Type A4 is truncus arteriosus with interrupted aortic arch.

4. The PBF is increased in type I, nearly normal in types II and III, and decreased in type IV.
5. Coronary artery abnormalities are common and may contribute to the high surgical mortality rate. The anomalies include stenotic coronary ostia, high and low takeoff of coronary arteries, and abnormal branching and course of the coronary arteries.
6. Interrupted aortic arch is seen in 13% of cases (type A4 of van Praagh classification). In this case, the interruption occurs distal to the takeoff of the left carotid artery (interrupted aortic arch type B) and lower extremity flow is accomplished through the PDA.
7. A right aortic arch is present in 30% of patients.
8. Evidence of DiGeorge syndrome with hypocalcemia is present in 33% of patients.

Clinical Manifestations

History

1. Cyanosis may be seen immediately after birth.
2. Signs of CHF develop within several days to weeks after birth.
3. A history of dyspnea with feeding, failure to thrive, and frequent respiratory infections is usually present in infancy.

Physical Examination

1. Varying degrees of cyanosis and signs of CHF with tachypnea and dyspnea are usually present.
2. The peripheral pulses are bounding, with a wide pulse pressure. The precordium is hyperactive, and the apical impulse is displaced laterally.
3. A systolic click is frequently audible at the apex and upper left sternal border. The S2 is single. A grade 2 to 4 of 6 systolic ejection murmur may be audible suggestive of truncal stenosis or PA branch stenosis. An apical diastolic rumble with or without gallop rhythm may be present when the

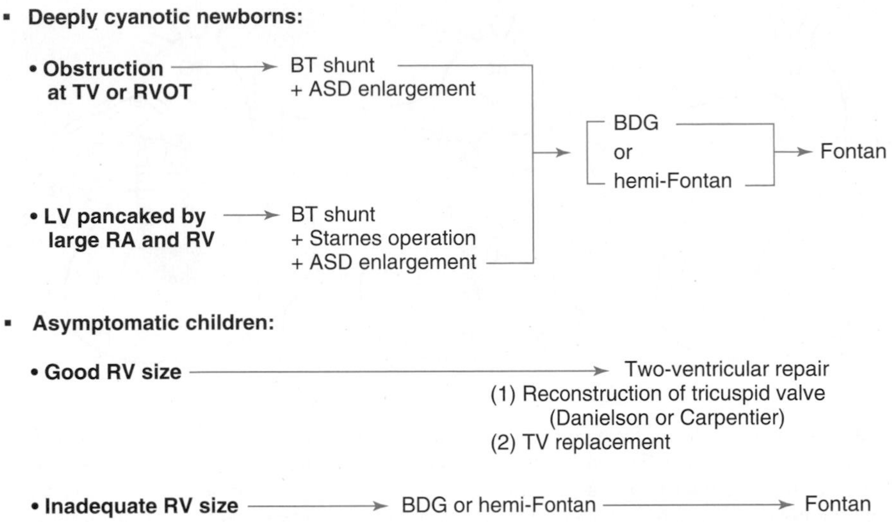

- **Deeply cyanotic newborns:**

  - **Obstruction** ⟶ BT shunt
    at TV or RVOT + ASD enlargement ⟶ ⟶ BDG or hemi-Fontan ⟶ Fontan

  - **LV pancaked by** ⟶ BT shunt
    large RA and RV + Starnes operation
    + ASD enlargement ⟶

- **Asymptomatic children:**

  - **Good RV size** ⟶ Two-ventricular repair
    (1) Reconstruction of tricuspid valve
    (Danielson or Carpentier)
    (2) TV replacement

  - **Inadequate RV size** ⟶ BDG or hemi-Fontan ⟶ Fontan

Fig. 14.57 Surgical approaches for Ebstein's anomaly of the tricuspid valve. *ASD,* Atrial septal defect; *BDG,* bidirectional Glenn; *BT,* Blalock-Taussig; *LV, left* ventricle; *RA,* right atrium; *RV,* right ventricle; *RVOT,* right ventricular outflow tract; *TV,* tricuspid valve.

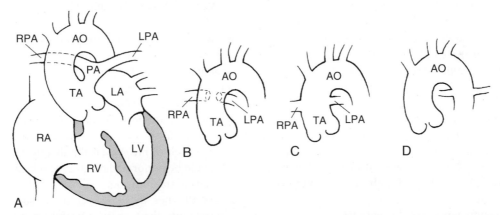

Fig. 14.58 The anatomic type of persistent truncus arteriosus (TA) is determined by the branching patterns of the pulmonary arteries. **A,** In type I, the main pulmonary artery (PA) arises from the truncus and then divides into the right (RPA) and left pulmonary artery (LPA) branches. **B,** In type II, the RPA and LPA arise separately from the posterior aspect of the truncus. **C,** In type III, the PAs arise separately from the lateral aspects of the truncus. **D,** In type IV, or pseudotruncus arteriosus, arteries arising from the descending aorta (AO) supply the lungs. *LA, Left* atrium; *LV,* left ventricle; *RA,* right atrium; *RV,* right ventricle.

PBF is large. A high-pitched, early diastolic, decrescendo murmur of truncal valve regurgitation may be audible.

Electrocardiography

The QRS axis is normal (+ 50 to + 120 degrees). BVH is present in 70% of cases; RVH or LVH is less common. Left atrial hypertrophy (LAH) is occasionally present.

Radiography

Cardiomegaly is usually present, with increased pulmonary vascularity. A right aortic arch is seen in 30% of cases.

Echocardiography

Two-dimensional and Doppler echocardiography show the following. The first three findings are diagnostic.

1. A large VSD is imaged directly under the truncal valve, similar to that seen in TOF.

2. A large, single great artery arises from the heart (i.e., truncus arteriosus). The type of persistent truncus arteriosus can be identified, and the size of the PAs can be determined. An artery, branching posteriorly from the truncus, is the PA.

3. The pulmonary valve cannot be imaged; only one semilunar valve (i.e., truncal valve) is imaged.

4. Cross-sectional imaging may determine the number of sinuses (usually three, although it may be two or four) of the truncal valve and the presence or absence of stenosis or regurgitation of the valve.

5. Right aortic arch is frequently present (in ≈35%). Interruption of the aortic arch is occasionally present.

Other Studies

Computed tomography or MRI may be necessary to evaluate arch anatomy or PA anatomy. Preoperative cardiac

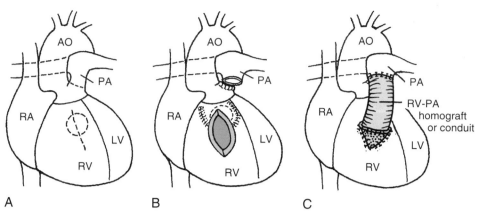

Fig. 14.59 Operative technique for type I truncus arteriosus. **A**, Truncus arteriosus type I is shown with a large ventricular septal defect (VSD; *broken circle*) directly under the truncal valve. The *vertical broken line* on the right ventricle (RV) is the site of the right ventriculotomy. **B**, The pulmonary artery (PA) trunk has been cut away from the truncal artery, and the opening in the truncal artery is sutured. Patch closure of the VSD (which is visible through the ventriculotomy) is completed in such a way that only left ventricular blood goes out to the truncal artery (creating the left ventricle [LV]–to–truncal artery pathway). **C**, A valved conduit or homograft is anastomosed to the pulmonary trunk. The posterior half of the proximal conduit is anastomosed to the upper end of the ventriculotomy. A small pericardial patch is trimmed and sutured into place to fill the defect between the allograft and the lower end of the right ventriculotomy. *AO*, Aorta; *RA*, right atrium.

catheterization is now rarely necessary in neonates. However, with late diagnosis of the condition, cardiac catheterization may be performed to evaluate PA pressure and PVR.

Natural History

1. Most infants present with CHF during the first 2 weeks. About 85% of untreated children die by 1 year of age.
2. Clinical improvement occurs if the infant develops pulmonary vascular obstructive disease, which may begin to occur by 3 to 4 months of age. Death occurs around the third decade of life.
3. Truncal valve insufficiency worsens with time.

Management
Medical

1. Vigorous anticongestive measures with diuretics and ACE inhibitors should be pursued before an operation is undertaken.
2. Because of the frequent association of DiGeorge (22q11.2 deletion) syndrome:
   a. Serum calcium and magnesium levels should be checked (because they may be low from hypoparathyroidism); their supplement may be indicated.
   b. Only irradiated blood products should be used (to prevent transfusion acquired acute graft-versus-host disease, which destroys lymphocytes) for an urgent surgery (because of an insufficient time for evaluation of immune status accurately).
3. Prophylaxis against SBE should be observed when indications arise.

Surgical

Palliative Procedures. Although PA banding was performed in the past in small infants with large PBF and CHF, primary repair of the defect is currently recommended by many centers. The banding produces distortion of the PAs and does not necessarily prevent pulmonary vascular obstructive disease. The procedure is associated with a high mortality rate, as high as 30%.

Definitive Procedure

1. Various modifications of the Rastelli procedure are performed. Ideally, surgery should be undertaken within the first week of life. When the diagnosis is delayed, surgery should be performed on an urgent basis after 2 to 3 days of medical stabilization.
2. For all types, the VSD is closed in such a way that the LV ejects into the truncus. Careful investigation of coronary artery anomalies and avoidance of surgical interruption of the coronary arteries are important.
   a. For type I, an aortic homograft (with internal diameter of 9–11 mm) is placed between the RV and the PA (Fig. 14.59).
   b. For types II and III, a circumferential band of the truncus, which contains both PA orifices, is removed. This cuff is tailored and then connected to the RV by the use of a homograft. Aortic continuity is restored with a tubular Dacron graft (Fig. 14.60). When associated with an interrupted aortic arch, aortic reconstruction is done by anastomosis of the proximal and distal aortas. Using a homograft, the RV and the PA are connected.
3. The regurgitant truncal valve is almost always amenable to various repair techniques. A prolapsing vestigial leaflet can be supported by suturing to the adjacent leaflet (closure of a commissure). Truncal valve replacement is indicated if there is significant truncal valve insufficiency. It has an extremely high mortality rate of 50% or greater

Postoperative Follow-up

1. Follow-up every 4 to 12 months is required to detect late complications, either natural or postoperative.

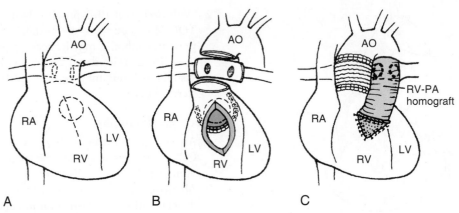

Fig. 14.60 Operative technique for types II and III truncus arteriosus. **A,** Two *broken lines* on the truncal artery indicate the sites of excision of the pulmonary arteries (PAs). The vertical broken line is the site of the right ventriculotomy. A ventricular septal defect (VSD) is under the truncal valve (broken circle). **B,** The VSD is closed with a patch through a right ventriculotomy (which is visible through the ventriculotomy) in such a way that the truncal artery receives blood only from the left ventricle (LV) (LV-to-truncus pathway). The cuff of truncal tissue, including the PA orifices, has been excised and trimmed. **C,** Continuity of the truncal artery, which is now the aorta (AO), has been restored with a Dacron graft. The lower end of a homograft has been anastomosed to the right ventriculotomy, and the upper end of the homograft has been anastomosed to the cuff containing the PAs. *RA,* Right atrium; *RV,* right ventricle.

a. Progressive truncal valve insufficiency may develop, and truncal valve repair or replacement may be needed.
b. A small conduit needs to be changed to a larger size, usually by 2 to 3 years of age.
c. Calcification of the valve in the conduit may occur within 1 to 5 years, which requires reoperation.
d. Ventricular arrhythmias may develop because of right ventriculotomy.
2. Balloon dilatation and stent implantation in the RV-to-PA conduit can prolong conduit longevity and delay the need to surgically replace the conduit.
3. For older children who had received a larger sized conduit and develop valvular regurgitation following balloon dilatation of the conduit valve, nonsurgical percutaneous pulmonary valve implantation technique developed by Bonhoeffer et al (2000) may be used (see further discussion under TOF with pulmonary atresia in this chapter).
4. SBE prophylaxis should be observed throughout the life.

SINGLE VENTRICLE

Prevalence

Single ventricle (double-inlet ventricle) occurs in less than 1% of all CHDs.

Pathology

1. Both AV valves are connected to a main, single ventricular chamber (i.e., double-inlet ventricle), and the main chamber is in turn connected to a rudimentary chamber through the BVF.
a. In about 80% of cases, the main ventricular chamber has anatomic characteristics of the LV (i.e., double-inlet LV). Occasionally, the main chamber has anatomic characteristics of the RV (i.e., double-inlet RV). Rarely does the ventricle have an intermediate trabecular pattern without a rudimentary chamber (i.e., common ventricle). Also, both atria rarely empty via a common AV valve into the main ventricular chamber with either LV or RV morphology (i.e., common-inlet ventricle).
b. One great artery arises from the main chamber, and the other arises from the rudimentary chamber. Either D-TGA or L-TGA is present in 85% of cases (Fig. 14.61).
2. The most common form of single ventricle is double-inlet LV with L-TGA with the aorta arising from the rudimentary chamber (see Fig. 14.61). This type occurs in 70% to 75% of cases of single ventricle. The mitral valve is right sided; the tricuspid valve is left sided. PS or pulmonary atresia is present in about 50% of cases. COA and interrupted aortic arch are also common. Less commonly, D-TGA is present with the aorta arising from the right and anterior rudimentary chamber.
3. The BVF is frequently obstructive.
4. Anomalies of the AV valves are common, which include stenosis, overriding, or straddling.

Pathophysiology

1. Because there is a complete mixing in the single ventricle, the systemic arterial saturation is determined primarily by the amount of PBF.
a. With PS, PBF is decreased and cyanosis is present (with arterial oxygen saturation <85%). With pulmonary atresia, cyanosis is intense at birth.
b. When the pulmonary valve is not stenotic, the PBF is large, and signs of CHF develop within days or weeks without cyanosis; arterial oxygen saturation is nearly 90%. When left untreated, pulmonary overcirculation can lead to pulmonary hypertension, which jeopardizes future Fontan operation.

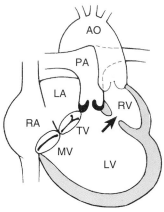

Fig. 14.61 Diagram of the most common form of single ventricle. The single ventricle is an anatomic left ventricle (double-inlet LV). The great arteries are transposed (L-transposition), with the aorta (AO) anterior to and left of the pulmonary artery (PA) and arising from the rudimentary right ventricle (RV). Both atrioventricular valves open into the single ventricle (double-inlet LV). The mitral valve is to the right of the tricuspid valve. The opening between the main and rudimentary ventricles is the bulboventricular foramen *(thick arrow)*. Stenosis of the pulmonary valve is present in about 50% of cases (shown as *thick valves*). This type accounts for 70% to 75% of cases of single ventricle. *AO,* Aorta; *LA,* left atrium; *LV,* left ventricle; *MV,* mitral valve; *PA,* pulmonary artery; *RA,* right atrium; *RV,* right ventricle; *TV,* tricuspid valve.

2. An obstructed BVF may either occur naturally with growth or, for unknown reasons, develop after PA banding. This condition occurs in 70% to 85% of patients who receive PA banding.
3. The occurrence of an obstructed BVF has a profound hemodynamic effect, as well as major surgical implications in patients with the aorta arising from the anterior rudimentary chamber. The obstruction increases PBF and decreases systemic perfusion.
4. The PA banding causes excessive hypertrophy of the main ventricle (LV), resulting in decreased compliance of the ventricle, which places the patient at risk for a future Fontan operation.

Clinical Manifestations
History
1. Cyanosis of varying degrees may be present from birth.
2. History of failure to thrive or pneumonia may be present in infants with increased PBF (signs of CHF).

Physical Examination
Physical findings depend on the magnitude of PBF.
1. With *increased* PBF, physical findings resemble those of TGA plus VSD or even those of large VSD. Mild cyanosis and CHF with growth retardation are present in early infancy. The S2 is single or narrowly split with a loud P2. A grade 3 of 4 of 6 long systolic murmur is audible along the left sternal border. An apical diastolic rumble may be audible. A diastolic murmur of PR may be present along the upper left sternal border as a result of pulmonary hypertension.

2. With *decreased* PBF, physical findings resemble those of TOF. Moderate to severe cyanosis is present. CHF is not present. Clubbing may be seen in older infants and children. The S2 is loud and single. A grade 2 of 4 of 6 ejection systolic murmur may be heard at the upper right or left sternal border.

Electrocardiography
1. An unusual ventricular hypertrophy pattern with similar QRS complexes across most or all precordial leads is common (e.g., RS, rS, or QR pattern).
2. Abnormal Q waves (representing abnormalities in septal depolarization) are also common and take one of the following forms: Q waves in the right precordial leads, no Q waves in any precordial leads, or Q waves in both the right and left precordial leads.
3. Either first- or second-degree AV block may be present.
4. Arrhythmias such as SVT or wandering pacemaker may occur.

Radiography
1. With increased PBF, the heart size enlarges, and the pulmonary vascularity increases.
2. When PBF is normal or decreased, the heart size is normal, and the pulmonary vascularity is normal or decreased.
3. A narrow upper mediastinum suggests TGA.

Echocardiography
1. The most important diagnostic sign of single ventricle is the presence of a single ventricular chamber into which two AV valves open.
2. The following anatomic and functional information is important from a surgical point of view. Efforts should be made to obtain information on all of these aspects in each patient with single ventricle:
   a. Morphology of the single ventricle (e.g., double-inlet LV, double-inlet RV)
   b. Location of the rudimentary outflow chamber, which is usually left and anterior
   c. Size of the BVF and whether there is an obstruction at the foramen. Obstruction of the foramen is considered present if the Doppler gradient is more than 1.5 m/sec or if the area of the foramen is less than 2 cm²/m². A foramen that is nearly as large as the aortic annulus is considered ideal.
   d. Presence or absence of D-TGA or L-TGA
   e. Presence or absence of stenosis of the pulmonary or aortic valve and size of the PAs
   f. Anatomy of the AV valves. The position of the mitral and tricuspid valves, in addition to the presence of stenosis, regurgitation, hypoplasia, or straddling of these valves, should be checked.
   g. The size of the ASD
   h. Associated defects such as interruption of IVC, COA, interrupted aortic arch, or PDA

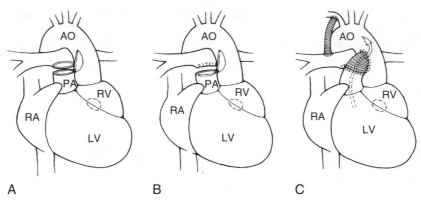

Fig. 14.62 Damus-Kaye-Stansel anastomosis for single ventricle and subpulmonary stenosis. **A,** The pulmonary artery (PA) is transected proximal to the bifurcation. An appropriately positioned and sized incision is made in the ascending aorta (AO). **B,** The distal end of the PA is oversewn, and the proximal end of the PA is anastomosed to the opening in the aorta. **C,** An appropriately shaped hood (Dacron tube, pericardium, allograft, or Gore-Tex) is added to the anastomosis. A Blalock-Taussig shunt has been completed. Sano shunt can be placed instead (see Fig. 14.48C). *LV,* Left ventricle; *RA,* right atrium; *RV,* right ventricle.

Other Studies

Echocardiographic and Doppler studies provide most of the anatomic and hemodynamic information needed for initial management of single ventricle. Cardiac catheterization is performed only when certain preoperative information is not available before the initial stage of surgical management. It is, however, routinely indicated before stages II and III surgical intervention.

Natural History

1. In patients without PS, CHF and growth failure develop in early infancy in association with pulmonary hypertension. Without surgery, about 50% of these patients die before reaching 1 year of age. The remainder of the patients with increased PBF develops pulmonary vascular obstructive disease after the first year of life with clinical improvement of CHF.
2. In patients with associated PS, cyanosis increases if PS worsens.
3. If the aorta arises from the rudimentary chamber, the BVF is often small or becomes obstructed. This results in increased PBF and decreased systemic perfusion.
4. Progressive AV valve regurgitation is poorly tolerated.
5. Complete heart block develops in about 12% of patients.
6. The cause of death can be CHF, arrhythmias, or sudden death.

Management
Initial Medical Management

1. Newborns with severe PS or pulmonary atresia and those with interrupted aortic arch or coarctation require PGE_1 infusion and other supportive measures before surgery.
2. Anticongestive measures are indicated if CHF develops.

Surgical

1. Initial surgical palliative procedures
The purpose of the first-stage operation is to make patients acceptable candidates for bidirectional Glenn or hemi-Fontan operation. The presence or absence of PS or of obstructive BVF results in one of the following four situations. PS (or pulmonary atresia) is present in about 50% of the patients.
   a. **No PS.** In patients with no PS and large PBF with resulting CHF and pulmonary edema, PA banding may be done. The major risk factor for the banding is the presence or development of an obstructed BVF. Most infants with obstructed foramen do not tolerate the banding well. Therefore, PA banding is performed only when the BVF is *normal* or *unobstructed*. In addition, these patients should be watched for the development of obstruction after the banding.
   b. **No PS + obstructed BVF.** In patients with no PS, if the BVF is too *small*, the Damus-Kaye-Stansel operation is performed rather than PA banding. The operation involves a PA-to-aorta anastomosis, which is accomplished by transection of the main PA and anastomosis of the proximal PA to the ascending aorta. This operation is combined with a right-sided BT shunt (Fig. 14.62) or a single ventricle–to–the main PA (Sano) shunt (not shown). A Fontan-type operation can be performed later (see Fig. 14.38B).
   1) **PS or pulmonary atresia.** If PS or pulmonary atresia is present (with O_2 saturation <85%), a BT shunt is necessary to improve cyanosis. Shunt to the right PA is preferable because any distortion of the RPA can be incorporated later in the Fontan anastomosis. The mortality rate is low (5%–10%). In PGE_1-dependent neonates, PDA is ligated after placement of the shunt.
   The hybrid procedure discussed under HLHS (consisting of PDA stenting, bilateral PA banding, and balloon atrial septostomy) can be used as an alternative to the BT shunt.
   2) **PS + obstructed BVF.** If PS is present and the BVF is obstructive, enlargement of the BVF by a transaortic approach and without cardiopulmonary bypass may be performed. The surgical mortality rate is about 15%.

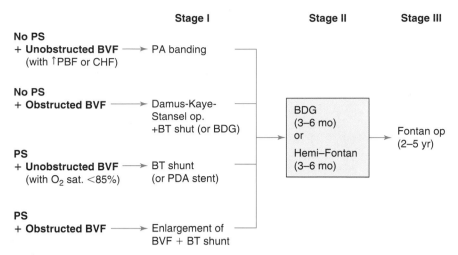

	Stage I	Stage II	Stage III
No PS **+ Unobstructed BVF** (with ↑PBF or CHF)	→ PA banding		
No PS **+ Obstructed BVF**	→ Damus-Kaye- Stansel op. +BT shut (or BDG)	BDG (3–6 mo) or Hemi–Fontan (3–6 mo)	→ Fontan op (2–5 yr)
PS **+ Unobstructed BVF** (with O₂ sat. <85%)	→ BT shunt (or PDA stent)		
PS **+ Obstructed BVF**	→ Enlargement of BVF + BT shunt		

Fig. 14.63 Surgical approach for single ventricle. *BDG*, Bidirectional Glenn; *BT*, Blalock-Taussig; *BVF*, bulboventricular foramen; *CHF*, congestive heart failure; *PA*, pulmonary artery; *PBF*, pulmonary blood flow; *PS*, pulmonary stenosis; *RPA*, right pulmonary artery.

An additional BT shunt may be needed to provide adequate PBF.

Medical Follow-up After the First-Stage Operation. The infant should be watched closely, until the time of the second stage palliation, for cyanosis (with O₂ saturation <75%) or signs of CHF (too large a PBF for which tightening of PA band should be considered).

2. Second-stage surgical palliative procedures
   a. Bidirectional Glenn operation (see Fig. 14.38) is carried out between the age of 3 month and 6 months, before proceeding with the Fontan operation. Alternatively, the hemi-Fontan procedure can be performed (see Fig. 14.39).
   b. After the second-stage surgical procedure, the child needs to be followed up with attention to the O₂ saturation. The follow-up plans are the same as those described in Box 14.2.
3. Definitive (Fontan) procedures

The Fontan-type operation is performed at 2 to 5 years of age. Many centers consider lateral tunnel Fontan procedure the procedure of choice (see Figs 14.38B and 14.40). Some centers make a 4- to 6-mm fenestration in the baffle, and others do not. Some centers prefer the extracardiac conduit modification of the Fontan procedure, which may reduce incidence of late atrial arrhythmias. If an AV valve is incompetent, it may need to be repaired as a separate surgery before the Fontan procedure or at the time of the Fontan procedure. The surgical mortality rate of the Fontan-type operation has been reduced to 5% to 10%, similar to that for tricuspid atresia.

The surgical approaches in single ventricle are summarized in Fig. 14.63.

Postoperative Follow-up

1. Close follow-up is necessary for early and late complications, which have been discussed in detail under the discussion of tricuspid atresia.
2. Some survivors of surgery, if performed late, remain symptomatic with cyanosis, dyspnea as a result of ventricular dysfunction, and arrhythmias. These symptoms require regular follow-up. Early surgery as outlined earlier tends to reduce unfavorable results.

DOUBLE-OUTLET RIGHT VENTRICLE

Prevalence

Double-outlet right ventricle occurs in fewer than 1% of all CHDs. DORV occurs frequently in patients with heterotaxy in association with other complex cardiac defects.

Pathology

1. Both the aorta and the PA arise from the RV. The only outlet from the LV is a large VSD.
2. The great arteries usually lie side by side. The aorta is usually to the right of the PA, although one of the great arteries may be more anterior than the other. The aortic and pulmonary valves are at the same level. Conus septum is present between the aorta and the PA. The subaortic and subpulmonary coni separate the aortic and pulmonary valves from the tricuspid and mitral valves, respectively. This means that there is no fibrous continuity between the semilunar valves and the AV valves. In a normal heart, the aortic valve is lower than the pulmonary valve, and the aortic valve is in fibrous continuity with the mitral valve.
3. The position of the VSD and the presence or absence of PS (or RVOT obstruction) influence hemodynamic alterations and form the basis for dividing the defect into the following types of DORV (Fig. 14.64):
   a. Subaortic VSD. The VSD is closer to the aortic valve than to the pulmonary valve and lies to the right of the conus septum (see Fig. 14.64A). This is the most common type, occurring in 55% to 70% of cases.
   b. Fallot type. In about 50% of patients with subaortic VSD, RVOT obstruction occurs (Fig. 14.64B). RVOT obstruction is most commonly caused by infundibular stenosis, but rarely pure valvular PS can occur with small annulus.

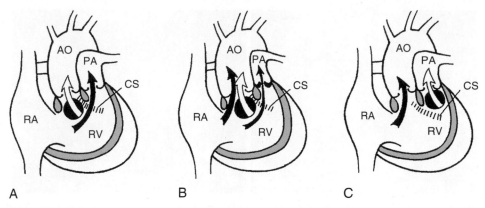

Fig. 14.64 Diagram of three representative types of double outlet right ventricle, viewed with the free wall of the right ventricle (RV) removed. **A,** Subaortic ventricular septal defect (VSD). **B,** Subaortic VSD with pulmonary stenosis (Fallot type). **C,** Subpulmonary VSD (Taussig-Bing anomaly). *Open arrows* represent highly oxygenated blood, and *black arrows* represent desaturated blood. Doubly committed and remote VSDs are not shown. *AO,* Aorta; *CS,* crista supraventricularis; *PA,* pulmonary artery; *RA,* right atrium; *RV,* right ventricle.

c. Subpulmonary VSD (i.e., Taussig-Bing anomaly) (see Fig. 14.64C). The VSD is closer to the pulmonary valve than to the aortic valve, and it usually lies above the crista supraventricularis and to the left of the conus septum. This type accounts for approximately 10% to 30% of cases.

d. Doubly committed VSD. The VSD is closely related to both semilunar valves and is usually above the crista supraventricularis (<5% of cases).

e. Noncommitted (or remote) VSD. The VSD is clearly away from the semilunar valves (≈10% of cases). It most commonly represents the AV canal-type VSD and occasionally an isolated muscular VSD. Atrial isomerism is commonly seen with this type.

4. Sometimes surgeons' and pathologists' definitions of DORV are different and are the source of confusion. Some cases of TOF with marked overriding of the aorta may be called DORV by surgeons because the mitral–aortic fibrous continuity is not always clear in the operating room. Surgeons use the so-called 50% rule: when the aortic annulus overlies the RV by at least 50%, it is called DORV.

Pathophysiology and Clinical Manifestations

The pathophysiology and clinical manifestations of DORV are determined primarily by the position of the VSD and the presence or absence of PS. Each type is presented separately.

1. **Subaortic VSD without PS.** In subaortic VSD, oxygenated blood from the LV is directed to the aorta, and desaturated systemic venous blood is directed to the PA, thereby producing mild or no cyanosis (see Fig. 14.64A). The PBF increases in the absence of PS, and CHF may result. Therefore, the clinical pictures of this type resemble those of a large VSD with pulmonary hypertension and CHF.
   a. Growth retardation, tachypnea, and other signs of CHF are usually present. A hyperactive precordium, a loud S2, and a VSD-type (holosystolic or early systolic) murmur are present. An apical diastolic rumble may be audible.

b. The ECG often resembles that of complete endocardial cushion defect (ECD). "Superior" QRS axis (i.e., −30 to −170 degrees) may be found in this type. RVH or BVH, as well as LAH, is common. Occasionally, first-degree AV block is present.

c. Chest radiography shows cardiomegaly with increased pulmonary vascular markings and a prominent PA segment.

2. **Subaortic VSD with PS (Fallot type).** Even though the VSD is subaortic, in the presence of PS (or RVOT obstruction), some desaturated blood goes to the aorta. This causes cyanosis and a decrease in PBF. The clinical pictures resemble those of TOF (see Fig. 14.64B).
   a. Growth retardation and cyanosis are common. The S2 is loud and single. A grade 2 to 4 of 6 midsystolic (ejection) murmur along the left sternal border is present, either with or without a systolic thrill.
   b. The ECG shows RAD, RAH, RVH, or RBBB. First-degree AV block is frequent.
   c. Chest radiography shows normal heart size with an upturned apex. Pulmonary vascularity is decreased.

3. **Subpulmonary VSD (Taussig-Bing malformation).** In subpulmonary VSD, or Taussig-Bing malformation, oxygenated blood from the LV is directed to the PA, and desaturated blood from the systemic vein is directed to the aorta. This results in severe cyanosis (see Fig. 14.64C). The PBF increases with the fall of the PVR. Clinical pictures resemble those of complete TGA.
   a. Growth retardation and severe cyanosis with or without clubbing are common findings. The S2 is loud, and a grade 2 to 3 of 6 systolic murmur is audible at the upper left sternal border. An ejection click and an occasional PR murmur (as a result of pulmonary hypertension) may be audible.
   b. The ECG shows RAD, RAH, and RVH. LVH may be seen during infancy.
   c. Chest radiography shows cardiomegaly with increased pulmonary vascular markings and a prominent PA segment.

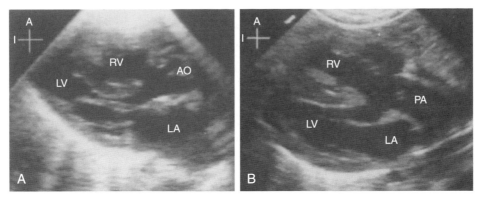

Fig. 14.65 Parasternal long-axis view of double outlet right ventricle. **A,** Subaortic ventricular septal defect (VSD). The VSD is closely related to the aorta (AO). The marked separation between the anterior mitral valve leaflet and the aortic valve can be seen. The aorta overrides the ventricular septum by more than 50%. **B,** Subpulmonary VSD. The great artery that is closely related to the VSD has an immediate posterior sweep, suggesting that it is a pulmonary artery (PA). Note the separation between the anterior mitral leaflet and the pulmonary valve. The PA overrides the ventricular septum by more than 50%. *LA,* Left atrium; *LV,* left ventricle; *RV,* right ventricle. (Part A from Snider AR, Serwer GA: *Echocardiography in Pediatric Heart Disease*, St. Louis, 1990, Mosby; part B from Snider AR: Two-dimensional and Doppler echocardiographic evaluation of heart disease in the neonate and fetus, *Clin Perinatol* 15:523–565, 1988.)

4. **Doubly committed or noncommitted ventricular septal defect.** With the VSD close to both semilunar valves (called *doubly committed VSD),* or remotely located from these valves (*noncommitted VSD),* cyanosis of a mild degree is present, and the PBF increases.

Echocardiography

Four diagnostic signs of DORV are (1) the presence of a large subaortic or subpulmonary VSD, (2) the origin of both great arteries from the anterior RV, (3) the absence of LV outflow other than the VSD, and (4) the discontinuity of the mitral and semilunar valves.

1. In the parasternal long-axis view, all four diagnostic features of DORV are imaged. Typical subaortic or subpulmonary VSD can be demonstrated in this view for most patients (Fig. 14.65). No great artery is seen to arise from the posterior ventricle. The great arteries arising from the anterior ventricle are seen in parallel orientation. In addition, a mass of echo-positive tissue, usually larger than 5 mm in length, is present between the mitral valve annulus and the semilunar valve (i.e., mitral–semilunar discontinuity).

2. In the parasternal short-axis view, a *double circle,* rather than the normal *circle and sausage* appearance of the great arteries, may be seen. The great arteries are side by side, with the aorta to the right or the aorta is anterior and slightly to the right of the PA.

3. The size and position of the VSD should be determined in relation to the great arteries.
   a. Typical subpulmonary or subaortic VSD can be demonstrated by parasternal long-axis scanning in most patients (see Fig. 14.65).
   b. In the subcostal four-chamber view, the subaortic VSD is located to the right of the conus septum just beneath the aortic valve. The subpulmonary VSD is located to the left of the conus septum just beneath the pulmonary valve.

   c. Doubly committed VSD is recognized in the parasternal or the apical long-axis view.
   d. Noncommitted (remote) VSDs, either endocardial cushion type or apical muscular VSD, are best recognized in the apical four-chamber view.

4. Associated anomalies such as valvular or subvalvular PS and other left-to-right shunt lesions (e.g., ASD, PDA) should be looked for.

5. Occasionally, differentiation of DORV from TOF with a marked overriding of the aorta or from TGA is necessary. There is mitral–semilunar continuity in TOF and TGA (i.e., mitral–aortic continuity in TOF and mitral–pulmonary continuity in TGA), but no mitral–semilunar continuity is present in DORV.

Other Studies

Cardiac catheterization and angiocardiography are not necessary for initial surgical management of the condition with PA banding or BT shunt. They are indicated to perform atrial septostomy in patients with Taussig-Bing malformation with inadequate atrial septal mixing. They are usually indicated before later stage operations.

Natural History

1. Infants without PS may develop severe CHF and later pulmonary vascular obstructive disease if left untreated. Spontaneous closure of VSD, which is fatal, is rare.

2. When PS is present, complications common to cyanotic CHDs (e.g., polycythemia, cerebrovascular accident) may develop.

3. In patients with the Taussig-Bing malformation, severe pulmonary vascular obstructive disease develops early in life, as seen in patients with D-TGA.

4. Associated anomalies (e.g., COA, LV hypoplasia) also contribute to the poor prognosis.

Management
Medical
Treatment of CHF with diuretics, ACE inhibitors, and digoxin is indicated.

Surgical
Palliative Procedures.
1. PA banding for symptomatic infants with increased PBF and CHF is occasionally performed in infants with multiple muscular VSD or a remote VSD. However, this procedure is not recommended for infants with subaortic VSD or doubly committed VSD. Primary repair is a better choice.
2. For infants with the Taussig-Bing type, enlarging the interatrial communication is important for better mixing and for decompressing the LA, which causes pulmonary venous congestion. Balloon or blade atrial septostomy should be considered.
3. In infants with PS and decreased PBF with cyanosis, a systemic-to-PA shunt procedure is occasionally indicated.

Definitive Surgeries
1. *Subaortic or doubly committed VSD.* An intraventricular tunnel between the VSD and the subaortic outflow tract is created by means of a Dacron patch. This procedure is performed early in life, preferably during the neonatal period or at least in early infancy, without preliminary PA banding. Sometimes the RVOT may have to be augmented with an outflow patch if the VSD-AO tunnel obstructs the RVOT. The mortality rate is less than 5% for simple subaortic VSD; it is slightly higher for doubly committed VSD.
2. **Fallot type.** There are three surgical options. Surgical repair is generally advised by 6 months of age, preferably during the neonatal period. However, if the patient's condition is poor or if there are major associated noncardiac anomalies, an initial shunt operation is an option.
   a. **Tunnel VSD closure + Rastelli operation.** An intraventricular tunnel between the VSD and the aorta is established and Rastelli operation is performed to relieve PS using either a pulmonary or aortic homograft conduit.
   b. **REV procedure.** So-called *réparation a l'étage ventriculare* (REV), which is similar to ASO, may be performed. In the REV procedure, the proximal ascending aorta and main PA are transected, and the proximal stump of the PA is oversewn (see Fig. 14.9, which is performed for D-TGA + VSD + PS, a situation very similar to this one). An intraventricular tunnel between the VSD and the aorta is established. The PAs are translocated anterior to the aorta (Lecompte maneuver), and the ascending aorta is reconnected. The distal PA is anastomosed directly to the upper margin of the infundibular incision. Autologous pericardium forms the anterior portion of the pathway. The hospital mortality rate is 18%.
   c. **Nikaidoh procedure.** This combines the principle of the Ross procedure and the Konno operation. The

aortic root, including the aortic valve, is detached in the same manner as done to the pulmonary root in the Ross procedure. The PA is divided, and the pulmonary valve is excised. The pulmonary root is divided, and the conal septum above the VSD is excised, which creates a large opening to the LV cavity. The aortic root is translocated posteriorly and sutured to the open orifice of the pulmonary annulus. A pericardial patch is used to connect the lower margin of the VSD and the anterior circumference of the harvested aortic root, completing LV to AO connection. A pericardial gusset completes the connection of the RV and the distal end of the MPA (see Fig. 14.10, which has been described for D-TGA + VSD + PS).

3. **Taussig-Bing anomaly (subpulmonary VSD).** There are two possible surgical approaches. These operations should be carried out by 3 to 4 months of age or sooner because of the rapid development of pulmonary vascular obstructive disease in this subtype.
   a. The procedure of choice is the creation of an intraventricular tunnel between the VSD and the PA (resulting in TGA), which is then corrected by the ASO. The mortality rate is between 5% and 15%.
   b. Creation of VSD-to-PA tunnel, followed by Damus-Kaye-Stansel operation and RV-to-PA conduit, is another possibility.
4. **Noncommitted VSD.** When possible, an intraventricular tunnel procedure between the AV canal-type VSD and the aorta is performed, but the mortality rate is high (30%–40%). PA banding is usually needed in infancy to control CHF, and the surgery may be delayed until 2 to 3 years of age. Some patients with noncommitted VSD may require Fontan operation.

The surgical approach for patients with DORV is summarized in Fig. 14.66.

Postoperative Follow-up
Long-term, regular follow-up at 6- to 12-month intervals is necessary to detect and manage late complications of surgery.
1. In general, patients who had subaortic VSD without PS have an excellent long-term outlook.
2. Ventricular arrhythmia should be treated because it may cause sudden death.
3. About 20% of patients require reoperation of the intraventricular tunnel.

HETEROTAXIA (ATRIAL ISOMERISM, SPLENIC SYNDROMES)

There is a failure of differentiation into right- and left-sided organs in heterotaxia (splenic syndrome or atrial isomerism), with resulting congenital malformations of multiple organs systems, including complex malformation of the cardiovascular system.
1. Asplenia syndrome (Ivemark's syndrome, RA isomerism) is associated with absence of the spleen, which is a left-sided organ, and a tendency for bilateral right-sidedness.

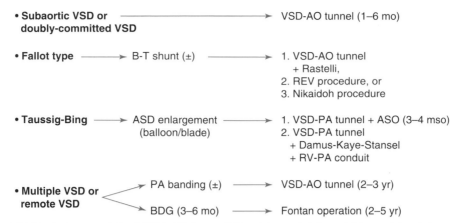

Fig. 14.66 Surgical approach for DORV. *AO,* Aorta; *ASD,* atrial septal defect; *ASO,* arterial switch operation; *BT,* Blalock-Taussig; *PA,* pulmonary artery; *REV, réparation à l'étage ventriculare; RV,* right ventricle; *RV-PA,* RV–to–pulmonary artery; *VSD,* ventricular septal defect; *VSD-AO,* VSD-to-aorta; *VSD-PA,* VSD–to–pulmonary artery.

2. In polysplenia syndrome (left atrial isomerism), multiple splenic tissues are present, with a tendency for bilateral left-sidedness.

There is a striking tendency for symmetrical development of normally asymmetrical organs or pairs of organs. Members of paired organs, such as the lungs, commonly show pronounced isomerism; unpaired organs, such as the stomach, seem to be located in a random fashion. In general, cardiovascular abnormalities are much more severe in patients with asplenia than in those with polysplenia.

Table 14.2 compares cardiovascular abnormalities in asplenia and polysplenia syndromes. Although the types and severity of cardiovascular malformations differ as a group between the two syndromes, the same types of defects are present in both. The abnormalities that help differentiate the two are shown with asterisks, but probably the most significant differential power is the IVC, which is almost always normal with asplenia syndrome but is interrupted (with azygous continuation) with polysplenia.

Some noncardiac findings suggest heterotaxia. Because of the symmetry of paired organs, normally different right- and left-sided organs show the same morphology. Some clinical findings available to general physicians that may lead to the recognition of heterotaxia include the following.
1. Symmetric "midline" liver (on palpation or radiography)
2. Discordant cardiac apex and stomach bubble (on chest radiography)
3. Biliary atresia in a neonate with CHDs
4. Symmetric mainstem bronchi on chest radiography
5. Superior P axis (or coronary sinus rhythm) on the ECG

It is important to know which type of isomerism one has from the point of prophylaxis against bacterial infection. Patients with asplenia syndrome are prone to fulminating sepsis and should be given daily antibiotic prophylaxis and vaccinated against pneumococcus, *Haemophilus influenzae* type b (Hib), and meningococcus (see later).

ASPLENIA SYNDROME

Prevalence

Asplenia syndrome occurs in 1% of newborns with symptomatic CHDs. This syndrome occurs more often in males than in females.

Pathology

1. The spleen is absent in asplenia syndrome. A striking tendency for bilateral right-sidedness characterizes malformations of the major organ systems. Bilateral, three-lobed lungs with bilateral, eparterial bronchi (Fig. 14.67); various gastrointestinal malformations (occurring in 20% of cases); a symmetrical, midline liver; and malrotation of the intestines are all present. The stomach may be located on either the right or the left.
2. Complex cardiac malformations are always present. Cardiovascular malformations involve all parts of the heart, systemic and pulmonary veins, and the great arteries. Two sinoatrial nodes are present (because of the presence of two right atria). Table 14.2 summarizes and compares these malformations with those of polysplenia syndrome. Cardiovascular anomalies that help distinguish asplenia syndrome from polysplenia syndrome include the following:
   a. A normal IVC is present in asplenia syndrome, but the hepatic portion of the IVC is commonly absent (with azygous continuation draining into the SVC) in 85% of patients with polysplenia syndrome.
   b. TGA with PS or pulmonary atresia occurs in about 80% of asplenia syndrome cases, thereby producing severe cyanosis during the newborn period. TGA is present in only 15% of patients with polysplenia syndrome.
   c. Single ventricle and common AV valve occur with greater frequency in asplenia syndrome. In polysplenia syndrome, two ventricles are usually present.
   d. TAPVR to *extracardiac* structures occurs in more than 75% of cases of asplenia syndrome, although it is

TABLE 14.2 Cardiovascular Malformations in Asplenia and Polysplenia Syndromes

Structure	Asplenia Syndrome (Bilateral Right-Sidedness)	Polysplenia Syndrome (Bilateral Left-Sidedness)
Systemic veins	Bilateral SVC (65%); single SVC usually right (35%) Normal IVC in all, but may be left sided (35%) (Interrupted IVC extremely rare) [b]IVC and aorta on the same side, either right or left Normal hepatic veins to IVC (75%)	Bilateral SVC (33%); single SVC right or left (66%) [a]Interrupted IVC with azygos continuation right or left (85%) Juxtaposition of the IVC and aorta occasionally Bilateral, common hepatic vein to RA or LA
Pulmonary veins	[a]TAPVR with *extracardiac* connection, supracardiac or infracardiac (>80%), often with PV obstruction	[b] Normal PV return (50%) Right PVs to right-sided atrium and left PVs to left-sided atrium (50%) (but not extracardiac)
Coronary sinus	Absent coronary sinus (30%)	Absent coronary sinus (80%)
Atrium and atrial septum	Bilateral right atria (with bilateral sinus node) [b]Absent atrial septum (common atrium) common Primum ASD (100%) Secundum ASD (66%)	Bilateral, left atria Single (or common) atrium, not common Primum ASD (60%), Secundum ASD (25%)
AV valve	[a]Common (single) AV valve (90%) Complete AV canal, usually complete	Normal AV valve (50%); single AV valve rare Partial ECD common (with large primum defect)
Ventricles and cardiac apex	VSD always present [b]Single ventricle (50%) usually morphologic RV or undetermined; two ventricles (50%) DORV (>80%) Left apex (60%); right apex (40%)	VSD frequent but not always [a]Two ventricles usually present; VSD (65%) DORV (20%) Left apex (60%); right apex (40%)
Semilunar valves	[b]PS or pulmonary atresia (80%)	Normal pulmonary valve (60%); PS or pulmonary atresia (40%)
Great arteries	[a]Transposition (70%), either D- or L-	[b]Normal great arteries (85%); transposition (15%)
ECG	Normal P axis or in the +90 to +180 degree quadrant (sinus rhythm)	[b]Superior P axis (nonsinus rhythm) (70%)

[a]Extremely important differentiating points.
[b]Important differentiating points.
ASD, Atrial septal defect; *AV*, atrioventricular; *DORV*, double-outlet right ventricle; *ECD*, endocardial cushion defect; *IVC*, inferior vena cava; *PS*, pulmonary stenosis; *PV*, pulmonary venous or vein; *RA*, right atrium; *RV*, right ventricle; *SVC*, superior vena cava; *TAPVR*, total anomalous pulmonary venous return; *VSD*, ventricular septal defect.

difficult to diagnose. Pulmonary venous return is normal in 50% of patients with polysplenia syndrome.

Pathophysiology

1. Complete mixing of systemic and pulmonary venous blood usually occurs because of the multiple cardiovascular abnormalities associated with this syndrome.
2. PBF is reduced because of stenosis or atresia of the pulmonary valve. This results in severe cyanosis shortly after birth.
3. Although rare, the absence of PS may result in CHF early in life.

Clinical Manifestations
Physical Examination

1. Cyanosis is usually the presenting sign and is often severe.
2. Auscultation of the heart is nonspecific. Heart murmurs of PS and VSD are frequently audible.

3. A symmetrical liver (midline liver) is palpable.

Electrocardiography

1. A "superior" QRS axis is present, as a result of the presence of ECD.
2. The P axis is either normal (0 to + 90 degrees) or alternating between the lower left and lower right quadrants. This occurs because two sinus nodes alternate the pacemaker function.
3. RVH, LVH, or BVH is present.

Radiography

1. The heart size is usually normal or slightly increased, with decreased pulmonary vascular markings.
2. The heart is in the right chest, left chest, or midline (mesocardia).
3. A symmetrical liver is a striking feature (see Fig. 4.8).
4. Tracheobronchial symmetry with bilateral, eparterial bronchi is usually identified.

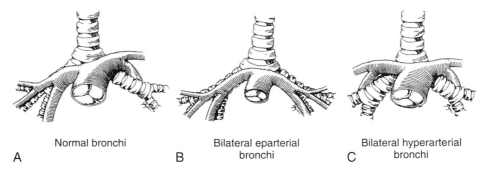

Normal bronchi	Bilateral eparterial bronchi	Bilateral hyperarterial bronchi
A	**B**	**C**

Fig. 14.67 Diagrams of normal bronchi (**A**); bilateral eparterial bronchi, usually seen in asplenia syndrome (**B**); and bilateral hyparterial bronchi, usually seen in polysplenia syndrome (**C**). (From Fyler DC, ed: *Nadas' Pediatric Cardiology*, St. Louis, 1992, Mosby.)

Echocardiography

When the systematic approach is used, 2D echo and color-flow Doppler studies can detect all or most of the anomalies described in the section on pathology. The anatomy of the IVC and great arteries and the presence or absence of PS (or pulmonary atresia) are important in differentiating the two splenic syndromes.

Other Imaging Modalities

Cardiac MRI or CT is usually indicated because almost all of the patients with asplenia syndromes have complex anomalies of pulmonary and systemic venous returns, which cannot be accurately imaged by echo studies.

Laboratory Studies

1. Howell-Jolly and Heinz bodies seen on the peripheral smear suggest asplenia syndrome. However, these bodies may be found in some normal newborns and in septic infants, too.
2. A splenic scan may be useful in older infants but is of limited value in extremely ill neonates.

Natural History

Without palliative surgical procedures, more than 95% of patients with asplenia syndrome die within the first year of life. Fulminating sepsis is one cause of death.

Management
Medical

1. In severely cyanotic newborns, PGE_1 infusion is given to reopen the ductus. (If obstructive anomalous pulmonary venous return is suspected, which is quite common in asplenia syndrome, pulmonary angiogram should be obtained while the ductus is open by PGE1 infusion.)
2. The risk of fulminating infection, especially by streptococcus pneumoniae, is high (*Red Book*, 2018). Continuous oral antibiotic therapy is recommended regardless of immunization status. Oral penicillin V (125 mg twice a day for children younger than 3 years and 250 mg twice a day for children 3 years or older) is recommended; some experts recommend amoxicillin (20 mg/kg/day). For children with anaphylactic allergy to penicillin, erythromycin

(250 mg, twice daily) can be given. Prophylactic penicillin can be discontinued at 5 years of age, but other experts continue prophylactic penicillin throughout childhood and into adulthood.

3. Asplenic infants and children have a high risk of fulminant bacteremia, especially associated with encapsulated bacteria (*Red Book*, 2018). *Streptococcus pneumoniae* is the most common pathogen causing septicemia in children with asplenia. Less common causes include Hib, *Neisseria meningitidis*, other streptococci, *Escherichia coli*, *Staphylococcus aureus*, and gram-negative bacilli, such as *Salmonella* spp., *Klebsiella* spp., and *Pseudomonas aeruginosa*.
   a. Pneumococcal conjugate and polysaccharide vaccines are vital for all children with asplenia (*Red Book*, 2018). After administration of appropriate number of doses of PCV13, pneumococcal polysaccharide vaccine (PPSV23) should be administered to children 24 month or older a minimum of 8 weeks after the last PCV13 dose. A second PPSV23 dose should be administered 5 years later. For children 2 through 18 years of age who have not received PCV13, even if they completed a PCV7 series or already received PPSV23 or both, one supplemental dose of PCV13 should be administered.
   b. Hib immunization should be initiated at 2 months of age, as recommended for otherwise healthy children. Previously unimmunized children younger than 5 years should receive Hib vaccine according to the catch-up schedule. Unimmunized children 5 years or older should receive a single dose of Hib vaccine.
   c. Meningococcal conjugate vaccine should be administered to all children with asplenia who are 2 month or older.
   d. Refer to *Red Book* 2018 for complete information regarding other immunizations.

Surgical

1. A systemic-to-PA shunt is usually necessary during the newborn period or infancy. The surgical mortality rate for the shunt is higher in asplenia patients than in those with other defects, and it is probably related to regurgitation of the common AV valve and undiagnosed obstructive TAPVR.

a. Patients with common AV valve, especially those with regurgitation of the valve, do not tolerate the volume overload that results from the shunt.

b. Patients with the obstructive type of TAPVR may show evidence of the anomalous return, with signs of pulmonary edema, only after the systemic-to-PA shunt.

c. Identification of infants with obstructive TAPVR by pulmonary angiography with PGE_1 infusion before surgery is important. In infants with the infracardiac type of TAPVR, a successful connection can be made between the pulmonary venous confluence and the RA with the use of a partial exclusion clamp and without cardiopulmonary bypass.

2. A Fontan-type operation can be performed. Regurgitation of the AV valve is a high-risk factor, requiring repair or replacement of the valve.

POLYSPLENIA SYNDROME

Prevalence

Polysplenia syndrome (left atrial isomerism) occurs in fewer than 1% of all CHDs. It occurs usually in females (70%).

Pathology

1. Multiple splenic tissues are present. A tendency for bilateral left-sidedness characterizes this syndrome. Noncardiovascular malformations include bilateral, bilobed lungs (i.e., two left lungs); bilateral, hyparterial bronchi (see Fig. 14.67); a symmetrical liver (25%); occasional absence of the gallbladder; and some degree of intestinal malrotation (80%).

2. Cardiovascular malformations are similar to those seen in asplenia syndrome but have a lower frequency of pulmonary valve stenosis or atresia. Occasionally, a normal heart or minimal malformation of the heart is present in patients with polysplenia syndrome (~13%). Cardiovascular malformations are summarized and compared with those of asplenia syndrome in Table 14.2. Important features of polysplenia syndrome that distinguish it from asplenia syndrome include the following:

a. Absence of the hepatic segment of the IVC with azygos (right side) or hemiazygos (left side) continuation is seen in 85% of patients. This abnormality is rarely present in asplenia syndrome.

b. Two ventricles are usually present. On the contrary, single ventricle with a common AV valve is common in asplenia syndrome.

c. TGA, PS or pulmonary atresia, and TAPVR occur less often than they do in asplenia syndrome.

d. The ECG shows a superiorly oriented P axis (i.e., ectopic atrial rhythm), resulting from absence of the sinus node (Fig. 14.68).

e. Polysplenia syndrome occurs more often in females (70%).

Pathophysiology

Because PS or pulmonary atresia occurs less frequently, cyanosis is not intense, if it is present at all. Rather, CHF often develops because of increased PBF.

Clinical Manifestations
Physical Examination

1. Cyanosis is either absent or mild. Signs of CHF may develop during the neonatal period.

2. Heart murmur of VSD may be audible. A symmetrical liver is usually palpable.

Electrocardiography (see Fig. 14.68)

1. Ectopic atrial rhythm with a superiorly oriented P axis (−30 to −90 degrees) is seen in more than 70% of patients because there is no sinus node when two left atria are present.

2. A "superior" QRS axis is present as a result of the presence of ECD.

3. RVH or LVH is common.

4. Complete heart block occurs in about 10% of patients.

Radiography

Mild to moderate cardiomegaly with increased pulmonary vascular markings; a midline liver (see Fig. 4.8); and bilateral, hyparterial bronchi may be present.

Laboratory Studies

1. Some patients with splenic hypoplasia and hypofunction may have Howell-Jolly bodies but not in an excessive number.

2. The radioactive splenic scan may show multiple splenic tissues.

Echocardiography

Two-dimensional and Doppler echo studies reveal all or most of the cardiovascular malformations listed in Table 14.2 and help differentiate this syndrome from asplenia syndrome.

Other Imaging Modalities

Cardiac MRI or CT is often indicated because many patients with polysplenia syndromes have complex anomalies of pulmonary and systemic venous returns.

Natural History

1. The first-year mortality rate is 60% compared with greater than 95% in asplenia syndrome.

2. Most infants with severe cardiac malformations die within the first year without surgical palliation or repair.

3. The heart rate is lower than in normal children (because of the absence of the sinus node). Excessive junctional bradycardia may develop, resulting in CHF.

Management
Medical

Congestive heart failure should be treated, if present. Although multiple splenic tissues may be present, they may be dysfunctional (functional asplenia). Their functionality needs to be confirmed by scintigraphy. In the case of functional asplenia, antibiotic prophylaxis is the same as with asplenia syndrome.

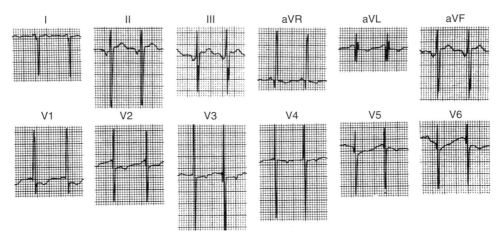

Fig. 14.68 Tracing from a 1-week-old neonate with polysplenia syndrome. Both the P and the QRS axes are superiorly oriented (−45 and −150 degrees, respectively). The QRS voltages indicate right ventricular hypertrophy and possible additional left ventricular hypertrophy.

Surgical

1. PA banding should be performed if intractable CHF develops with large PBF.
2. Occasionally, pacemaker therapy is required for children with excessive junctional bradycardia and CHF.
3. Total correction of the defect is possible in some children. If total correction is not possible, at least a Fontan-type operation can be performed. The surgical mortality rate of the Fontan-type operation in this group of children is about 25%, which is lower than that for asplenia but higher than that for tricuspid atresia.

   Postoperative Follow-up

Periodic follow-up is necessary because of continuing medical and surgical problems.

1. Although most patients are in NYHA class I or II (see Appendix A, Table A.3), persistent ascites or edema occurs frequently and requires medications such as digoxin, diuretics, and others for several years after the Fontan-type operation.
2. Cardiac arrhythmias, usually supraventricular, are present in 25% of patients. Some require antiarrhythmic medications.

PERSISTENT PULMONARY HYPERTENSION OF THE NEWBORN

Prevalence

Persistent PPHN (or persistence of the fetal circulation) occurs in approximately 1 in 1500 live births.

Pathology and Pathophysiology

1. This neonatal condition is characterized by persistence of pulmonary hypertension, which in turn causes a varying degree of cyanosis from a right-to-left shunt through the PDA or PFO. No other underlying CHD is present.
2. Various causes have been identified, but they can be divided into three groups by the anatomy of the pulmonary vascular bed:

   a. Intense pulmonary vasoconstriction in the presence of a normally developed pulmonary vascular bed
   b. Hypertrophy (of the medial layer) of the pulmonary arterioles
   c. Developmentally abnormal pulmonary arterioles with decreased cross-sectional area of the pulmonary vascular bed (see Box 14.3 for further description)

   In general, pulmonary hypertension caused by the first group is relatively easy to reverse, and that caused by the second group is more difficult to reverse than that caused by the first group. Pulmonary hypertension caused by the third group is most difficult or impossible to reverse.
3. Varying degrees of myocardial dysfunction often occur in association with PPHN.

Clinical Manifestations

1. Symptoms begin 6 to 12 hours after birth, with cyanosis and respiratory difficulties (with retraction and grunting). The idiopathic form usually affects full-term or postterm neonates. The patient usually has a history of meconium staining or birth asphyxia. A history of maternal ingestion of nonsteroidal antiinflammatory drugs (in the third trimester) may be elicited.
2. A prominent RV impulse and a single and loud S2 are usually found. Occasional gallop rhythm (from myocardial dysfunction) and a soft regurgitant systolic murmur of TR may be audible. Severe cases of myocardial dysfunction may manifest with systemic hypotension.
3. Arterial desaturation is found in blood samples obtained from an umbilical artery catheter. Arterial Po_2 may be lower in the descending aorta (the umbilical artery line) than in the preductal arteries (the right radial, brachial, or temporal artery) by 5 to 10 mm Hg because of a right-to-left ductal shunt. In severe cases, differential cyanosis may appear (with a pink upper body and a cyanotic lower body). If there is a prominent right-to-left intracardiac shunt, usually through the PFO, the preductal and postductal arteries may not show a Po_2 difference.

4. The ECG usually is normal for age, but occasional RVH is present. T-wave abnormalities suggestive of myocardial dysfunction may be seen.

5. Chest radiography reveals a varying degree of cardiomegaly. The lung fields may be free of abnormal findings or may show hyperinflation or atelectasis. The pulmonary vascular markings may appear normal, increased, or decreased.

6. Echocardiographic and Doppler studies are indicated to rule out CHDs and to identify patients with myocardial dysfunction. Patients with PPHN have no evidence of cyanotic or acyanotic CHDs. The only structural abnormality is the presence of a large PDA with a right-to-left or bidirectional shunt. The RV is enlarged with a flattened interventricular septum. There is evidence of increased RA pressures (with the atrial septum bulging toward the left) with or without an ASD or PFO. The LV dimension may be increased, and its systolic function (fractional shortening or ejection fraction) may be decreased.

7. Cardiac catheterization usually is not indicated. If the diagnosis is unclear or the patient does not respond to therapy, cardiac catheterization and pulmonary arteriography rarely are considered.

Management

The goals of therapy are to (1) lower the PVR and PA pressure through the administration of oxygen, the induction of respiratory alkalosis, and the use of pulmonary vasodilators; (2) correct myocardial dysfunction; and (3) stabilize the patient and treat associated conditions. Detailed description of management for each goal is beyond the scope of this book; only principles of management will be presented.

1. General supportive therapy includes monitoring oxygen saturation; detecting and treating acidosis, hypoglycemia, hypocalcemia, hypomagnesemia, and polycythemia; and maintaining body temperature between 98° and 99°F (36.6° and 37.2°C).

2. To increase arterial Po_2 levels, 100% oxygen is administered, initially without intubation. If this is not successful, intubation plus continuous positive airway pressure at 2 to 10 cm of water may be effective.

3. If the previous measures are not successful, mechanical ventilation is used to produce respiratory alkalosis. Because hyperoxia-induced lung damage high oxygen concentration should be avoided and FiO_2 should be adjusted to maintain preductal oxygen saturation of 90% to 95%. Ventilator settings are initially set to achieve Po_2 of 50 to 70 mm Hg and P_{CO2} of 40 to 50 mmHg. The patient is sedated (i.e., morphine, fentanyl) or even paralyzed with pancuronium (Pavulon) at 0.1 mg/kg IV. However, use of paralytic agents is controversial because it may promote atelectasis of dependent lung regions with resulting ventilation–perfusion mismatch.

4. Maintaining a normal or alkaline pH level can also be achieved with sodium acetate, which can be added to the IV fluids.

5. Inhalation nitric oxide (iNO) is a potent and selective pulmonary vasodilator. The usual dose is 20 ppm. Prolonged low-dose NO therapy has caused sustained improvement in oxygenation without systemic hypotension. Most newborn infants require iNO for fewer than 5 days. The use of iNO in PPHN has decreased the need for ECMO by approximately 40%. When administered by inhalation, NO diffuses to vascular smooth muscle, stimulating the production of cyclic guanosine monophosphate and causing vasodilatation. A high-frequency oscillatory ventilator is effective in patients with severe PPHN. Through the use of this device, about 40% of patients who would be candidates for extracorporeal membrane oxygenation (ECMO) can avoid this procedure. Sildenafil, a phosphodiesterase inhibitor type V, both as an IV or as an oral agent, can be added to patients with chronic pulmonary hypertension.

6. For myocardial dysfunction, dopamine is used with tolazoline to improve cardiac output. Correction of acidosis, hypocalcemia, and hypoglycemia helps improve myocardial function. Diuretics may be included in the regimen. For chronic myocardial dysfunction, digoxin may be added at a later stage.

7. ECMO has been shown to be effective in the management of selected patients with severe PPHN. However, this treatment may require ligation of a carotid artery and the jugular vein, and cerebrovascular accidents have been reported.

Prognosis

1. Prognosis generally is good for neonates with mild PPHN who respond quickly to therapy. Most of these neonates recover without permanent lung damage or neurologic impairment.

2. For those requiring a maximal ventilator setting for a prolonged time, the chance of survival is smaller, and many survivors develop bronchopulmonary dysplasia and other complications.

3. Patients with developmental decreases in cross-sectional areas of the pulmonary vascular bed usually do not respond to therapy, and their prognosis is poor.

4. Neurodevelopmental abnormalities may manifest. Patients have a high incidence of hearing loss ($\leq50\%$). Abnormal electroencephalogram findings ($\leq80\%$) and cerebral infarction (45%) have been reported.

15

Miscellaneous Congenital Cardiac Conditions

In this chapter, congenital heart defects with a relatively low prevalence that have not been discussed previously are presented briefly.

ANEURYSM OF THE SINUS OF VALSALVA

In aneurysm of the sinus of Valsalva (congenital aortic sinus aneurysm), there is a gradual downward protrusion of the aneurysm into a lower pressure cardiac chamber that eventually ruptures. Most of the aneurysm arises from the right coronary sinus (80%) and less frequently from the noncoronary cusp (20%). When a sinus of Valsalva aneurysm ruptures, a sinus of Valsalva fistula is formed. The fistula communicates most frequently with the right ventricle (RV) (75%) and less frequently with the right atrium (RA) (25%). Associated anomalies are common and include ventricular septal defect (VSD) (50%), aortic regurgitation (AR) (20%), and coarctation of the aorta. This rare anomaly has been reported primarily in the Asian population.

Unruptured aneurysm produces no symptoms or signs. A small sinus of Valsalva fistula may develop without symptoms. The aneurysm usually ruptures during the third or fourth decade of life. The rupture is often characterized by a sudden onset of chest pain, dyspnea, a continuous heart murmur over the right or left sternal border, and bounding peripheral pulses. Severe congestive heart failure (CHF) eventually develops. Chest radiography shows cardiomegaly and increased pulmonary vascularity. The ECG may show biventricular hypertrophy (BVH), first- or second-degree atrioventricular (AV) block, or junctional rhythm.

Patients with small- to moderate-sized unruptured aneurysms probably do not need surgery. Unruptured aneurysms of the sinus of Valsalva that produce hemodynamic derangement should be repaired. When the aneurysm of the congenital sinus of Valsalva has ruptured or is associated with a VSD with or without aortic regurgitation, prompt operation is advisable.

ANOMALOUS ORIGIN OF THE LEFT CORONARY ARTERY FROM THE PULMONARY ARTERY (BLAND-WHITE-GARLAND SYNDROME, ALCAPA SYNDROME)

In anomalous origin of the left coronary artery from the pulmonary artery (PA), the left coronary artery arises abnormally from the PA. Patients usually are asymptomatic in the newborn period until the PA pressure and pulmonary vascular resistance falls to a critical level after birth. The direction of blood flow is from the right coronary artery, through intercoronary collaterals retrogradely, to the left coronary artery, and into the PA. This results in left ventricular insufficiency or infarction.

Symptoms appear at 2 to 3 months of age and consist of recurring episodes of distress (anginal pain), marked cardiomegaly, and CHF. Significant heart murmur usually is absent, with a rare exception of a heart murmur of mitral regurgitation secondary to left ventricular dilation or myocardial infarction. The electrocardiogram (ECG) shows an anterolateral myocardial infarction pattern consisting of abnormally deep and wide Q waves, inverted T waves, and an ST-segment shift in leads I and aVL and the left precordial leads (see Fig. 3.27). Chest radiography may show cardiomegaly (of the left atrium [LA] and left ventricle [LV]) with or without pulmonary edema in advanced cases. Cardiac enzyme changes probably occur, but the relatively slow development of myocardial infarction and the uncertainty of the exact time of infarction may make it difficult to interpret laboratory data. However, knowledge of cardiac enzyme changes seen in adult cases of myocardial infarction helps in the diagnosis of this condition (see Appendix A, Fig A.3). Cardiac troponin I levels may also increase. The normal level of cardiac troponin I in children is 2 ng/mL or less and is frequently below the level of detection for the assay.

Two-dimensional echocardiography with color-flow mapping is diagnostic and has replaced cardiac catheterization. The presence of normal origin of both the right and left coronary arteries from the aorta should be routinely checked in every echocardiographic study, especially in newborns. The absence of a normal left coronary artery raises the possibility of the condition, so the diagnosis can be made in the newborn period before symptoms develop. Color Doppler examination may show retrograde flow into the proximal main PA (Fig. 15.1). The right coronary artery may be seen enlarged. The echocardiographic study also shows the size and function of the left heart. Increased echogenicity of papillary muscles and adjacent endocardium suggests fibrosis and fibroelastosis.

Computed tomography (CT) scans show high-resolution definition of coronary artery anatomy. The use of rapid acquisition scanners and pharmacologic slowing of the heart rate (with beta-blockers), especially in small infants, may be necessary to increase the ability to diagnose the condition.

Management

Medical treatment alone carries an unacceptably high mortality rate (80%–100%). Therefore, all patients with this diagnosis need operation. The optimal operation in infancy remains controversial, but most centers prefer definitive surgery unless the patient is critically ill.

Palliative Surgery

In critically ill infants, simple ligation of the anomalous left coronary artery close to its origin from the PA may be performed to prevent steal into the PA. This should be followed by a later elective bypass procedure (as described later).

Definitive Surgery

Even for infants who are critically ill, many centers prefer to create a two-coronary system by performing one of the following procedures.

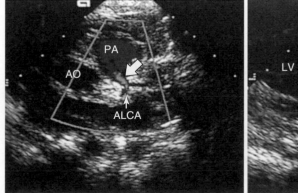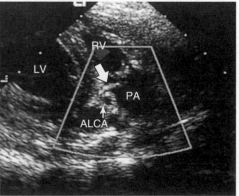

Fig. 15.1 Doppler examination in the high parasternal short-axis view *(left)* and in the high parasternal long-axis view of the right ventricular (RV) outflow tract *(right)* from an infant with anomalous left coronary artery (ALCA) arising from the pulmonary artery (PA) *(thin arrows)*. *Heavy white arrows* indicate retrograde *(red)* flow into the main PA from the ALCA as shown in both the frames. *AO,* Aorta; *LV,* left ventricle. (From Snider AR, Serwer GA, Ritter SB: *Echocardiography in Pediatric Heart Disease,* ed 2, Philadelphia, 1997, Mosby. Used with permission. (See Expert Consult for the color figure.))

Intrapulmonary Tunnel Operation (Takeuchi Repair). Intrapulmonary tunnel operation is the most popular among two-coronary repair surgeries (Fig. 15.2). Two circular openings are made in the contiguous wall of the aorta and the pulmonary trunk, and a 5- to 6-mm aortopulmonary window is created by suturing together these two openings. Two horizontal incisions are made in the anterior wall of the PA directly over the aortopulmonary window to create the flap of the PA wall. The flap is sutured in the posterior wall of the PA, and a tunnel is created that connects the opening of the aortopulmonary window and the orifice of the anomalous left coronary artery. The opening in the anterior wall of the PA is closed by a piece of pericardium. The mortality rate is near 0%, but as high as more than 20% has been reported. Late complications of the procedure include supravalvular PA stenosis (75%), baffle leak (52%) causing coronary–PA fistula, and aortic insufficiency.

Left Coronary Artery Implantation. Left coronary artery implantation, with direct transfer of the anomalous left coronary artery into the aortic root, appears to be the most advisable procedure, but it is not always possible. The anomalous coronary artery is excised from the PA along with a button of PA wall, and the artery is reimplanted into the anterior aspect of the ascending aorta. If the direct implantation may result in excessive tension in the coronary artery, flaps can be developed from the anterior main PA wall and ascending aorta. These flaps are sutured to form a tube extension for the left coronary artery, which is then implanted to the aorta. The early surgical mortality rate is 15% to 20%.

Tashiro Repair. Tashiro and colleagues (1993) reported a repair technique that was performed in adult patients. In this procedure, a narrow cuff of the main PA, including the orifice of the left coronary artery, is transected; the upper and lower edges of the cuff are closed to form a new left main coronary artery; and the aorta and the newly created left coronary artery are anastomosed side to end. The divided main PA is anastomosed end to end. This creates no obstruction to the PA. This technique has a potential application in the pediatric population, including small infants.

Subclavian–to–Left Coronary Artery Anastomosis. In subclavian–to–left coronary artery anastomosis, the end of the left subclavian artery is turned down and anastomosed end to side to the anomalous left coronary artery through a left thoracotomy approach. Aortic cross-clamping, which could be the source of ventricular impairment with postoperative low cardiac output and a high mortality rate, is avoided.

The need for simultaneous mitral valve reconstruction at the time of definitive surgery is controversial because spontaneous improvement of mitral regurgitation (MR) occurs after surgical revascularization. After successful two-coronary artery repair, LV systolic function and heart failure improve markedly, and the severity of the MR also decreases. Even the infarct pattern on ECG may eventually disappear.

AORTOPULMONARY SEPTAL DEFECT

In aortopulmonary septal defect (also known as aortopulmonary window or aortopulmonary fenestration), a large defect is present between the ascending aorta and the main PA (Fig. 15.3). This condition results from failure of the spiral septum to completely divide the embryonic truncus arteriosus.

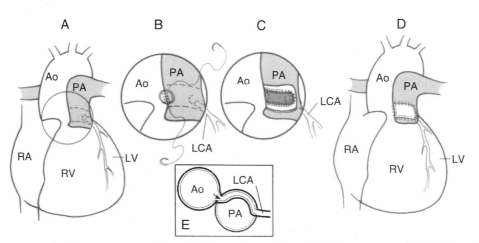

Fig. 15.2 Intrapulmonary artery tunnel repair for anomalous origin of the left coronary artery (LCA) from the pulmonary artery (PA) (Takeuchi repair). **A,** Two *dashed lines* on the anterior wall of the PA are the proposed incision sites to create a flap of the PA. **B,** An aortopulmonary shunt is created after a punch hole (5–6 mm in size) is made in the contiguous wall of the aorta (Ao) and PA. **C,** The flap of the PA is sutured in place to form the convex roof of a tunnel through which aortic blood passes to the anomalous orifice of the left coronary artery. **D,** A piece of pericardium is used to close the opening in the anterior wall of the PA. **E,** Cross-sectional view of the tunnel operation when completed. *LV,* Left ventricle; *RA,* right atrium; *RV,* right ventricle.

Hemodynamic abnormalities are similar to those of persistent truncus arteriosus and are more severe than those of patent ductus arteriosus (PDA). CHF and pulmonary hypertension appear in early infancy. Peripheral pulses are bounding, but the heart murmur is usually of the systolic ejection type (rather than continuous murmur) at the base.

The natural history of this defect is similar to that of a large untreated PDA, with development of pulmonary vascular disease in surviving patients. This defect has no known tendency to close spontaneously. Prompt surgical closure of the defect under cardiopulmonary bypass is indicated when the diagnosis is made. The surgical mortality rate is very low.

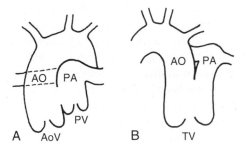

Fig. 15.3 Diagram of aortopulmonary window (**A**) and persistent truncus arteriosus (**B**). These two conditions are similar from a hemodynamic point of view. Anatomically, however, there are two separate semilunar valves (aortic valve [AoV] and pulmonary valve [PV]) without associated ventricular septal defect (VSD) in aortopulmonary window, but there is only one truncal valve (TV) with associated VSD in persistent truncus arteriosus. *AO,* Aorta; *PA,* pulmonary artery.

ARTERIOVENOUS FISTULA, CORONARY

Coronary artery fistulas are the most common congenital anomalies of the coronary artery, representing nearly half of all coronary artery anomalies. It can be isolated or associated with other CHDs, such as tetralogy of Fallot (TOF), atrial septal defect (ASD), PDA, and VSD. The right coronary artery is much more frequently involved than the left, and rarely both coronary arteries are involved.

These fistulas occur in one of two patterns.

1. **"True" coronary arteriovenous fistula.** This pattern occurs in only 7% of the cases of coronary fistulas (Fig. 15.4). This fistula involves a branching tributary from a coronary artery coursing along a normal anatomic distribution and eventually entering into the coronary sinus.
2. **Coronary artery fistula (or coronary-cameral fistula).** In the majority of cases (>90% of patients), the coronary fistula results from an abnormal coronary artery system with aberrant termination rather than true arteriovenous fistula. The right coronary is most commonly involved in coronary artery fistula. In more than 90% of reported cases, the fistula terminates in the right side of the heart (either to the RV or the PA; less commonly to the RA). It rarely terminates in the left side of the heart, but when it does, the majority enters the LA.

Patients usually are asymptomatic. However, CHF may develop if the shunt through the fistula is large. With a significant shunt, a continuous murmur, similar to the murmur of PDA, is audible over the precordium (rather than in the left infraclavicular area). The ECG usually is normal but may show right ventricular hypertrophy (RVH) or left ventricular

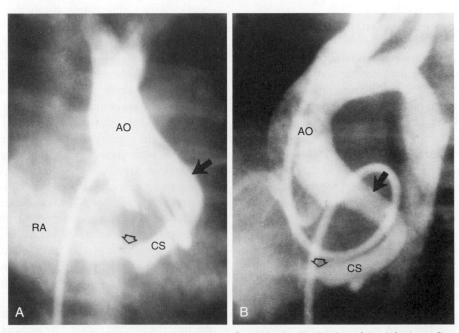

Fig. 15.4 Aortogram showing coronary arteriovenous fistula in the distribution of the left circumflex artery *(solid arrows).* **A,** Anteroposterior projection. **B,** Lateral projection. The fistula empties through the coronary sinus (cs) and eventually into the right atrium (RA). The point of entry into the RA is marked by an *open arrow. AO,* Aorta.

hypertrophy (LVH) if the fistula is large. Chest radiography shows a normal heart size.

Echocardiographic studies usually suggest the sites and types of the fistulas. The presence of a massively dilated proximal portion of one coronary artery while the other coronary artery is of normal size suggests coronary artery or arteriovenous fistula. The dilatation is usually uniform. One can follow the course of the dilated coronary artery to its site of entry. The site of entry can usually be located with the help of color Doppler echocardiography by the detection of either continuous or diastolic high-velocity flow. Often selective coronary artery angiography is necessary for an accurate diagnosis before the intended intervention. If the flow through the fistula is large, then the chamber or vessel receiving the fistula will be dilated.

A tiny coronary artery fistula to the PA (coronary artery–to–PA fistula) that produces no symptom can only be detected incidentally by an echocardiographic study. Most children with this condition are asymptomatic. Spontaneous closure may occur in small fistulae. However, some patients may present with symptoms of dyspnea on exertion, increased fatigability, and possibly signs of high-output CHF. Rarely, adult patients may present with angina, palpitation, or signs of exercise-related coronary insufficiency.

Small fistulous connections in the asymptomatic patient may be monitored. For a moderate or large coronary artery fistula, transcatheter occlusion is reasonable using coils or other occluding devices. Elective surgery is indicated if not amenable to catheter occlusion. Using cardiopulmonary bypass, the fistula is ligated as proximal as can be done without jeopardizing flow in the normal arteries, and it is ligated near its entrance to the cardiac chamber. The surgical mortality rate is 0% to 5%.

ARTERIOVENOUS FISTULA, PULMONARY

In this condition, the pulmonary arteries and veins communicate directly, bypassing the pulmonary capillary circulation. The fistulas may take the form of either multiple tiny angiomas (telangiectasis) or a large PA-to–pulmonary vein (PV) communication. About 60% of patients with pulmonary arteriovenous fistulas have hereditary hemorrhagic telangiectasis (Rendu-Osler-Weber syndrome), and 5% to 15% of patients with the syndrome have the fistula (see Table 2.1). Patients who have undergone a bidirectional Glenn operation are at risk of developing multiple pulmonary arteriovenous fistulas, although these malformations rarely occur after completion of a Fontan operation. This finding suggests that pulmonary circulation requires as yet undetermined hepatic factors, possibly vasoconstrictor prostaglandins, to suppress the development of arteriovenous malformations. Similarly, chronic liver disease can rarely be the cause of the arteriovenous fistula.

Desaturated systemic blood from the PAs reaches the PVs, bypassing the lung tissue, resulting in systemic arterial desaturation, cyanosis, and clubbing. The pulmonary blood flow and pressure remain unchanged, and there is no volume overload to the heart, unlike in systemic AV fistulas.

Physical examination may reveal cyanosis and clubbing. The peripheral pulses are not bounding. A faint systolic or continuous murmur may be audible over the affected lung in about 50% of patients. Polycythemia usually is present, and arterial oxygen saturation runs between 50% and 85%. Chest radiography shows normal heart size because there is no volume overload to the heart in pulmonary AV fistulas. One or more rounded opacities of variable size may be present in the lung fields. The ECG usually is normal. Occasional complications include stroke, brain abscess, rupture of the fistula with hemoptysis or hemothorax, and infective endocarditis.

The diagnosis can be made through contrast two-dimensional echocardiography by the appearance of microcavitations (bubbles) in the LA. In this technique, 4 to 10 mL of saline that has been agitated is injected into a peripheral vein while the appearance of bubbles in the atria is monitored. The bubbles appear first in the RA, and within two cardiac cycles, they appear in the LA. CT typically shows one or more enlarged arteries feeding a serpiginous or lobulated mass and one or more draining veins. Magnetic resonance imaging (MRI) has not been studied as much as CT in children. Pulmonary angiography remains the gold standard to determine the position and structure of abnormal vascular lesions in the lung before treatment.

Transcatheter occlusion is recommended for all symptomatic patients and for asymptomatic patients with discrete lesions with feeding arteries 3 mm or larger in diameter. Transcatheter occlusion has been proved to be effective with excellent long-term results. Diffuse microscopic pulmonary AV malformations are not amenable to transcatheter occlusion. Surgical resection of the lesions, with preservation of as much healthy lung tissue as possible, may be attempted in symptomatic children, but the progressive nature of the disorder calls for a conservative approach.

ARTERIOVENOUS FISTULA, SYSTEMIC

Systemic arteriovenous fistulas may be limited to small cavernous hemangiomas or may be extensive. In large AV fistulas, there is direct communication (either a vascular channel or angiomas) between the artery and a vein without the interposition of the capillary bed. The two most common sites of systemic arteriovenous fistulas are the brain and liver. In the brain, it is usually a large type occurring in newborns in association with a vein of Galan malformation. In the liver, either localized or generalized hemangioendotheliomas (densely vascular benign tumors) are more common than fistulous arteriovenous malformations. With a large fistula, because of decreased peripheral vascular resistance, an increase in stroke volume (with a wide pulse pressure) and tachycardia result, leading to increased cardiac output, volume overload to the heart, and even CHF.

Physical examination reveals a systolic or continuous murmur over the affected organ. An ejection systolic murmur may be present over the precordium because of increased blood flow through the semilunar valves. The peripheral pulses may be bounding during the high-output state but weak when

CHF develops. A gallop rhythm may be present with CHF. Chest radiography may show cardiomegaly and increased pulmonary vascular markings with a large fistula. The ECG may show hypertrophy of either or both ventricles.

Most patients with large cerebral arteriovenous fistulas and CHF die in the neonatal period, and surgical ligation of the affected artery to the brain is rarely possible without infarcting the brain. Surgical treatment of hepatic fistulas is often impossible because they are widespread throughout the liver. However, hemangioendotheliomas often eventually disappear completely. Patients with large liver hemangiomas have been treated with corticosteroids, aminocaproic acid, local radiation, or partial embolization, but the beneficial effects of these management options are not fully established. Catheter embolization is becoming the treatment of choice for many symptomatic patients with AV fistula.

ATRIAL SEPTAL ANEURYSM

An aneurysmal tissue is present in part or all of the atrial septum that shows phasic septal excursion (of 10–15 mm in an adult) protruding into either atria. Atrial septal aneurysm (ASA) is present in 4% of all the neonates using a different criterion (of marked mobility of the atrial septum). The prevalence of ASA varies between 0.2% and 1.9% of normal adult patients and up to 8% to 15% of adult stroke patients by transesophageal echocardiographic studies. It is commonly associated with patent foramen ovale (PFO), and together they might play a role in cryptogenic stroke in adult patients. ASA may prove to be a cause of atrial arrhythmias in some patients. See the section on PFO later in this chapter for further discussion of PFO or ASA versus stroke.

CERVICAL AORTIC ARCH

In this rare anomaly, the aortic arch is elongated, usually into the neck above the level of the clavicle. The aortic arch is usually right sided and sometimes with the descending aorta on the left, producing an anatomical vascular ring. Sometimes it is associated with arch hypoplasia or abnormal branching of the arch (e.g., anomalous subclavian artery, separate origin of the internal and external carotid arteries, and common origin of both carotid arteries). Rarely, discrete aortic coarctation or stenosis or atresia of the left subclavian artery is seen.

Infants with this condition may present with stridor, dyspnea, or repeated lower respiratory infection, similar to the signs of vascular ring. In adults, dysphagia is a common presenting complaint. A pulsating mass with associated thrill is present in the right supraclavicular fossa. A presumptive diagnosis of cervical aortic arch is made by noting loss of femoral pulses during brief compression of the pulsating mass. Chest radiographs may show a wide upper mediastinum with absence of the aortic knob. Echocardiography, CT, and MRI may be diagnostic. However, an aortogram is often necessary to make an accurate diagnosis of the condition with arch vessel abnormalities.

Treatment is necessary if the cervical arch is complicated by arch hypoplasia; symptomatic vascular ring; or rarely, aneurysm of the cervical arch itself.

CLEFT MITRAL VALVE

Isolated cleft of the mitral valve is a very uncommon defect. There is a cleft in the septal leaflet of the mitral valve, not associated with endocardial cushion defect (ECD). About two thirds of cases are associated with other cardiac defects such as VSD (50%), left ventricular outflow tract (LVOT) obstructive lesions including aortic stenosis (AS) and subaortic stenosis (40%), secundum ASD (20%), and others. About 60% of the patients have syndromes, including trisomy 21, CHARGE association (coloboma, heart defects, choanal atresia, growth or mental retardation, genitourinary anomalies, ear anomalies; see Table 2.1), heterotaxia, and others.

On the parasternal short-axis view of two-dimensional echocardiography, the cleft is seen in the septal mitral leaflet, directed toward the LVOT (11 o'clock direction) and associated with a varying degree of MR. This contrasts with the cleft associated with ECD that is directed toward the inlet (or posterior) septum (9 o'clock direction) in the same view.

More than half of these patients require surgical repair of the cleft because of an increasing severity of MR. During surgery, the cleft is usually buttressed by means of a Kaye annuloplasty or an annuloplasty band, depending on the age of the patient (Zhu et al, 2009).

COMMON ATRIUM (OR SINGLE ATRIUM)

In common atrium (single atrium, cor triloculare biventriculare), either the atrial septum is completely absent or only the vestigial element of a poorly developed atrial septum is present. This is a form of ECD with cleft mitral valve. Patients with asplenia syndrome (with other complex heart defects) have common atrium. This condition is also commonly seen with Ellis–van Creveld syndrome (see Table 2.1).

Symptoms may include shortness of breath and easy fatigability. Occasional infants may be critically ill with heart failure. Cyanosis varies from obvious to very mild, presenting only with exertion. The ECG shows left anterior hemiblock ("superior QRS axis"), as in ECD, and an rsR' pattern in the right precordial leads, as in ASD. Surgery should be performed early in life because the patients usually have symptoms and are at risk for developing pulmonary vascular obstructive disease. Successful creation of a polyvinyl septum is possible.

COR TRIATRIATUM

Cor triatriatum is a rare congenital cardiac anomaly in which the LA is divided into two compartments by an abnormal fibromuscular septum with an opening (Fig. 15.5A), producing varying degrees of obstruction of pulmonary venous return. Pulmonary venous and pulmonary arterial hypertension may result. Embryologically, this condition results from failure of incorporation of the embryonic common PV into

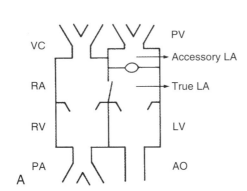

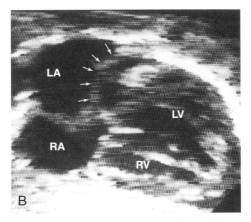

Fig. 15.5 Cor triatriatum. **A,** Diagram of cor triatriatum. **B,** Subcostal four-chamber view of an echocardiogram demonstrating a membrane *(small arrows)* in the left atrium (LA). *AO,* Aorta; *LV,* left ventricle; *PA,* pulmonary artery; *PV,* pulmonary vein; *RA,* right atrium; *RV,* right ventricle; *VC,* vena cava.

the LA. Therefore, the upper compartment (accessory LA) is a dilated common PV, and the lower compartment is the true LA. Hemodynamic abnormalities of this condition are similar to those of mitral stenosis in that both conditions produce pulmonary venous and pulmonary arterial hypertension (see Chapter 10).

Important physical findings include dyspnea, basal pulmonary crackles, a loud S2, and a nonspecific systolic murmur. The ECG shows right-axis deviation and severe RVH and occasional right atrial hypertrophy. Chest radiography shows evidence of pulmonary venous congestion or pulmonary edema, a prominent PA segment, and right-sided heart enlargement. Echocardiography demonstrates a linear structure within the LA cavity (Fig. 15.5B). Surgical correction is always indicated. Pulmonary hypertension regresses rapidly in survivors if the correction is made early.

DOUBLE-CHAMBERED RIGHT VENTRICLE

Double-chambered RV (anomalous muscle bundle of the RV) is characterized by aberrant hypertrophied muscle bands that divide the RV cavity into a proximal high-pressure chamber and a distal low-pressure chamber. In the majority of patients, VSD or pulmonary valve stenosis is also present.

Clinical manifestations closely resemble those of pulmonary valvular or infundibular stenosis: a loud, grade 3 to 5 of 6 ejection systolic murmur along the upper and mid-left sternal border is present. Two-dimensional echocardiography is usually diagnostic in this lesion. The anomalous muscle bundle can be visualized best from either the subcostal or parasternal view. Color-flow Doppler assesses the severity and identifies the site of the obstruction. MRI may provide the same information as two-dimensional echocardiography. Surgical resection of the bundle, as well as repair of other anomalies, is usually indicated as soon as the diagnosis is made.

ECTOPIA CORDIS

In this extremely rare condition, the heart is partially or totally outside the thorax. Most reported cases of ectopia

cordis are either thoracic (60%) or thoracoabdominal (40%); rarely, a case may be cervical or abdominal. The thoracic type is characterized by a sternal defect, absence of the parietal pericardium, cephalic orientation of the cardiac apex, epigastric omphalocele, and a small thoracic cavity. The thoracoabdominal type (Pentalogy of Cantrell) has partial absence or cleft of the lower sternum, an anterior diaphragmatic defect through which a portion of the ventricle protrudes into the abdominal cavity, a defect of the parietal pericardium, and an omphalocele. Intracardiac abnormalities are very common but not invariable; ASD, VSD, TOF, and tricuspid atresia are the most common intracardiac defects. One reported case of the abdominal type (1806) was an otherwise healthy French soldier, the father of three children, who died of pyelonephritis.

The treatment and prognosis of the defect are determined by the location of the defect, the extent of the cardiac displacement, and the presence or absence of intracardiac anomalies. Simple sternal cleft with minimal cardiac protrusion can be successfully treated in early infancy. However, in more severe cases, most surgical efforts to put the heart into the thorax have failed because of the smallness of the thorax and kinking of the blood vessels. Patients without omphalocele or intracardiac defects may remain largely asymptomatic and can undergo surgical repair later in childhood.

HEMITRUNCUS ARTERIOSUS

In hemitruncus arteriosus (origin of one PA from the ascending aorta), one of the PAs, usually the right PA, arises from the ascending aorta (Fig. 15.6). Associated defects such as PDA, VSD, and TOF are occasionally present. Hemodynamically, one lung receives blood directly from the aorta, as in PDA, with resulting volume or pressure overload, and the other lung receives the entire RV output, resulting in volume overload of that lung. Therefore, pulmonary hypertension of both lungs develops. CHF develops early in infancy, with respiratory distress and poor weight gain. A continuous murmur and bounding pulses may be present. The ECG shows BVH,

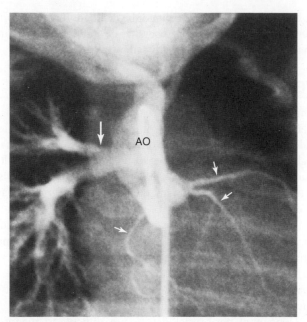

Fig. 15.6 Hemitruncus. Aortogram showing the right pulmonary artery *(large arrow)* originating anomalously from the ascending aorta (AO). Coronary arteries are also opacified *(small arrows).*

and chest radiography shows cardiomegaly and increased pulmonary vascular markings.

Definitive diagnosis is made by echocardiography, angiography, or other imaging modalities. Cardiac catheterization is needed to define the anatomy and assess pulmonary vascular resistance. Early surgical correction (anastomosis of the anomalous PA to the main PA) is indicated.

IDIOPATHIC DILATATION OF THE PULMONARY ARTERY

In idiopathic dilatation of the PA (congenital pulmonary insufficiency), pulmonary regurgitation is present in the absence of pulmonary hypertension in asymptomatic children or adolescents. Many regard this as a very mild pulmonary valve stenosis with resulting poststenotic dilatation but subsequent loss of pressure gradient across the pulmonary valve.

A characteristic auscultatory finding is a grade 1 to 3 of 6 low-frequency, decrescendo diastolic murmur at the upper and mid-left sternal borders. The S2 is normal. The ECG usually is normal, but occasional right bundle branch block is present. Chest radiography shows a prominent main PA segment with normal peripheral pulmonary vascularity. Echocardiographic studies reveal a poststenotic dilatation of the main PA and varying degree of pulmonary regurgitation with little or no pressure gradient across the pulmonary valve but with a whirling of blood flow in the PA. The prognosis is generally good, but right-sided heart failure may occur in adult life.

KARTAGENER SYNDROME

Kartagener syndrome consists of the triad of situs inversus (with dextrocardia), paranasal sinusitis, and bronchiectasis. This disorder is inherited as an autosomal recessive trait;

males and females are affected with equal frequency. The dextrocardia is a mirror image of normal and is functionally normal. Bronchiectasis is believed to result from a functional defect of the mucociliary epithelium with immotility of the cilia. In addition, affected males are infertile as a result of immobile spermatozoa.

PARACHUTE MITRAL OVALE

Parachute mitral valve is a severe form of congenital mitral valve stenosis. In this anomaly, all chordae tendineae are thickened and shortened, and they attach to a single posteriorly located papillary muscles, producing severe mitral stenosis. The anterior papillary muscle is usually absent. The diagnosis can be suspected by two-dimensional echocardiography on the parasternal views. In the parasternal short-axis view, only one papillary muscle is imaged. Commonly associated conditions include supramitral ring, subvalvular or valvular AS and COA, or the complete "Shone complex," which is the combination of all or some of these abnormalities.

PATENT FORAMEN OVALE

Patent foramen ovale is a tunnel between the septum secundum and the superior margin of the septum primum. The septum secundum is a thick, concave, muscular structure that expands from the posterosuperior wall and partially partitions the atria. The septum primum, a thin flap, extends from inferiorly and makes a tunnel. During fetal life, the tunnel (foramen ovale) is open and allows a direct flow of inferior vena cava (IVC) blood into the LA, sending blood with higher oxygen saturation to the LA (and eventually to the brain and coronary circulation).

Postnatally, lung expansion promotes increase in pulmonary flow and therefore increase in pulmonary venous return and with it an increase in LA pressure. When the pressure in the LA exceeds that in the RA, the thin flap of the superior end of the septum primum is forced to shut against the septum secundum, thereby resulting in functional closure of the foramen. In most individuals, the foramen ovale is sealed shortly after birth, but for some reason, functional closure does not always occur, resulting in a small left-to-right atrial shunt detectable by color Doppler study. This condition is called "incompetent foramen ovale" (IFO) and is quite common in newborns, presenting in 75% of neonates. Probe patency of a competent foramen ovale is found in 25% of normal adults. In recent years, paradoxical embolization through PFO has been proposed as a potential cause of cryptogenic stroke in adults.

Patent Foramen Ovale Versus Strokes in Adults

There have been controversies regarding the management of PFO, which has been proposed as a potential cause of cryptogenic stroke in adult patients. Some retrospective observational reports have shown a strong association (but not cause-and-effect relationship) between cryptogenic strokes and both PFO and ASA in adults. The prevalence of PFO was four times higher in stroke patients (40%) than in control participants (10%), and it was much higher (33 times) in patients with both PFO and ASA. Thus, paradoxical embolism via a PFO has been postulated as a possible cause of stroke. The proponents of the hypothesis of paradoxical embolization have advocated closing PFO for secondary prevention of stroke in patients with PFO and in high-risk adult patients without stroke.

However, evidence is casting doubts about the above hypothesis and thus the rational of closing PFO to prevent recurrence of stroke remains controversial. In these early observational studies, causes of stroke other than paradoxical embolization through PFO were not considered, such as transient atrial fibrillation (with left atrial thrombus formation), emboli from aortic atherosclerotic plaques, and the hypercoagulable state were not ruled out. Several recent studies, including a meta-analysis, a prospective case control study, and a prospective population study, concluded that PFO alone or in combination with ASA does not appear to substantially increase the odd ratio for stroke. Patients with ASA have been found to have a higher vulnerability to atrial fibrillation than those without it (Berthet et al, 2000). Atrial fibrillation, even transient one, is a known cause of cardiogenic embolism. Unless the RA pressure is elevated and frequent venous thrombus formation is demonstrated, hemodynamics does not favor paradoxical embolization in normal individuals with normal RA pressure.

Besides the causative relationship between PFO and cryptogenic stroke, controversies remain in the management of the stroke patients; is the device closure of PFO superior to medical management (aspirin, warfarin, or both) in preventing recurrence of strokes? A guideline from the American Heart Association and American Stroke Association (Goldstein et al, 2006) does not support closure of PFO for prevention of recurrent stroke. Rather, it recommends antithrombotic therapy with aspirin or warfarin. PFO closure may be considered for patients with recurrent cryptogenic stroke despite medical therapy.

In a recent review article by Mojadidi et al (2018) which included two randomized controlled trials of PFO closure versus medical therapy, to the authors Mojadidi et al concluded that PFO closure was associated with a significantly lower risk of recurrent stroke than those maintained on antiplatelet therapy. However, in both studies, PFO closure was associated with a higher risk of atrial fibrillation. Two other international studies found that the risk of subsequent stroke was lower among those assigned to PFO closure plus antiplatelet therapy than among those assigned to antiplatelet therapy alone. However, PFO closure was associated with higher rates of device complications and atrial fibrillation (Mas et al, 2017; Soendergaard et al, 2017). Thus, it remains unknown how PFO closure compares with systemic anticoagulation (e.g., with novel oral anticoagulations) for the prevention of recurrent ischemic stroke.

In the absence of convincing evidence for PFO as a cause of paradoxical embolization in adult patients and the absence of a superiority of PFO closure to medical therapy in adult patients, the rationale for closing PFOs in pediatric patients is at best controversial and may not be justified. It appears prudent to wait until this controversy is cleared before adopting the practice of closing PFOs in pediatric patients.

PERICARDIAL DEFECT, CONGENITAL

This rare congenital anomaly of the pericardium may be partial or complete. The majority of these cases occur on the left side (85%), and they are more often complete (65%) than partial. About 30% to 50% of cases are associated with congenital anomalies of the heart (PDA, ASD, TOF, and mitral stenosis), lung, chest wall, or diaphragm. Pleural defect is almost always present.

Unless an associated cardiac anomaly is present, most patients are asymptomatic. Occasionally, a *partial* defect may produce chest pain, syncope, or systemic embolism secondary to herniation and strangulation of the left atrial appendage. A *complete* defect may produce vague positional discomfort in the supine or left lateral position.

Congenital pericardial defects are difficult to diagnose preoperatively. Occasionally, chest radiography may show a prominence of the left hilum or the PA caused by herniation of these structures through the partial defect. Complete absence of the left pericardium may be characterized by leftward displacement of the heart and aortic knob or a prominent PA. Echocardiography findings of complete absence of the left pericardium include an unusual cardiac hypermobility (cardioptosis), abnormal swing motion of the heart with each cardiac beat, and an abnormal systolic anterior motion of the ventricular septum (on M-mode echocardiography). (These findings are similar to the echocardiographic findings of a transplanted heart, in which the donor heart is untethered and is placed in a large potential space.) Traditionally, the appearance of pneumopericardium after the introduction of air into the left pleural cavity was diagnostic. CT or MRI now permits better visualization of absence of the pericardium.

Surgical treatment is recommended only for symptomatic patients. Surgical procedures used in this condition include longitudinal pericardiotomy; partial pericardiectomy; primary closure; partial appendectomy (of the left atrial appendage); and pericardioplasty with pleural flaps, Teflon, or porcine pericardium.

PSEUDOCOARCTATION OF THE AORTA

Pseudocoarctation of the aorta is a condition in which the distal portion of the aortic arch and the proximal portion of the descending aorta are abnormally elongated and tortuous, with narrowing of the aortic isthmus but without significant obstruction. The elongation of the arch frequently produces an increased distance between the origin of the left common carotid and the left subclavian artery. Unlike cervical aortic arch, the aortic arch stays below the level of the clavicle. A variety of CHDs have been reported in association with pseudocoarctation. Physical examination and the ECG are normal when it is not associated with other cardiac defects.

Pseudocoarctation is not a benign entity as once believed because there is tendency for dilatation and aneurysm formation related to turbulent flow across the kink, and it may progress to show a substantial obstruction. Therefore, close follow-up is required for asymptomatic patients who are without any associated anomalies. Cardiac catheterization (with measurement of pressure gradient) and angiography provide a definitive diagnosis for this condition. Similarly, CT is very helpful in the diagnosis. Surgical intervention may be required if dilatation compresses surrounding structures (e.g., esophagus) or aneurysm formation is present.

PULMONARY ARTERY STENOSIS

Incidence

Pulmonary artery stenosis accounts for more than 3% of all CHDs.

Pathology

1. Stenosis of the PA occurs either at the main PA or in the peripheral pulmonary arteries. The most frequent site of stenosis is near the bifurcation as an isolated anomaly. More often it is seen with other CHDs such as valvular pulmonary stenosis, ASD, VSD, PDA, or TOF (in which 20% of the patients have associated peripheral PA stenosis).
2. When associated with cyanotic CHDs (e.g., pulmonary atresia with intact ventricular septum or TOF with pulmonary atresia), the stenosis usually involves multiple branches and multiple sites.
3. It may also be seen in association with other conditions such as rubella syndrome, Williams syndrome, and Alagille syndrome.
4. Some PA stenosis is secondary to surgical procedures, such as previous systemic-to-PA shunts.

Clinical Manifestation

1. Mild stenosis of the PAs causes no symptoms. If the stenosis is severe, the RV may hypertrophy.
2. An ejection systolic murmur grade 2 to 3 of 6 is audible at the upper left sternal border, with good transmission to the ipsilateral axilla and back. Occasionally, a continuous murmur is audible with severe stenosis. The S2 is either normal or more obviously split.
3. The ECG is normal with mild stenosis, but it shows RVH with severe stenosis.
4. Chest radiography findings usually are normal.
5. The echocardiogram may show stenosis in the main PA or near the bifurcation, but those in smaller branches cannot be imaged by echocardiography.
   a. Significant PA stenosis is clearly present when (1) there is measurable pressure gradient greater than 20 to 30 mm Hg, (2) RV or main PA pressure is higher than 50% of systemic pressure, or (3) lung perfusion scan shows relative flow discrepancy between two lungs of 35%/65% or worse. (The normal right–left perfusion ratio was found to be 52.5%/47.5% (+/− 2.1%) rather than the often quoted 55%/45% split, which was found to be more than 1 standard deviation greater than the mean; Cheng et al, 2006.)
   b. Many significant stenoses may not be demonstrable by pressure gradient because of discrepant blood flow away from the stenotic area or because of low pulmonary flow situation (e.g., with Glenn shunt and Fontan circulation).
6. Lung perfusion scintigraphy had been a useful noninvasive method for determining relative pulmonary flows. Currently, MRI represents the gold standard for assessing differential blood flow to the lungs as derived by flow calculation in the branch pulmonary arteries. In patients with multiple previous stenting of the pulmonary tree, contrast-enhanced CT imaging is preferred. Angiocardiography is the best invasive tool in the diagnosis of peripheral PA stenosis.

Management

1. Mild to moderate PA stenosis usually does not require treatment, but severe cases require some form of treatment.
2. The central (extraparenchymal) type is surgically amenable, but the peripheral (intraparenchymal) type is not correctable by surgery; catheter therapy is often the only option.
3. For peripheral PA stenosis, treatment modalities include the use of standard balloon angioplasty, a cutting balloon, and the placement of endovascular stent.
   a. Balloon angioplasty using low-pressure inflations has only a limited success rate (~50%, with a 16% recurrence rate). Using high-pressure balloons (that can be inflated to 20–25 atm) appears to improve the effectiveness.
   b. Using cutting balloons: Vessels resistant to high-pressure balloon angioplasty respond to either cutting balloon angioplasty alone or that followed by high-pressure ballooning. These techniques are best suited for small, lobar PA branches not amenable to stenting. Cutting balloons have three or four microsurgical blades with a cutting depth of 0.15 mm, which are activated when the balloons are inflated.
   c. In contrast, stainless-steel balloon-expandable stents can overcome an obstruction, with an acute success rate close to 100% and a recurrence rate of only 2% to 3%. These stents are balloon dilatable to potential adult diameters of the vessel. This technique has become the primary mode of therapy for branch PA stenosis.

PULMONARY VEIN STENOSIS

Pulmonary vein stenosis is a very rare anomaly that can be either congenital (or "primary") or acquired. The primary type is one that occurs without any inciting event, and the acquired type follows either a surgical or interventional procedure.

Congenital ("Primary") Pulmonary Vein Stenosis

The congenital or "primary" form of stenosis can be isolated to a single PV but most often occurs in multiple veins simultaneously, and the severity can be progressive, leading to partial or even total obstruction of flow.

The stenosis can be a localized narrowing at its junction with the LV, a longer segment of narrowing, or a diffuse hypoplasia of pulmonary veins. It can be associated with other CHD (Ebstein's anomaly or common AV canal), but nearly half of the patients have no associated cardiac anomalies (Latson et al, 2007).

Obstruction to pulmonary venous return results in pulmonary edema, pulmonary arterial hypertension, and increased pulmonary vascular resistance, similar to mitral stenosis. The number and severity of the stenosis of the PVs involved determine the timing and severity of symptoms. Most patients with the primary form of the disease present early in infancy with a history of significant respiratory symptoms (with tachypnea and recurrent pneumonias). If only one or two veins are involved, the manifestation may be delayed, or the patient may remain asymptomatic for a long time. As the disease progresses, signs of pulmonary hypertension appear. Chest radiography may show localized or diffuse pulmonary edema depending on the number of PVs involved. Hemoptysis may develop in older surviving children.

Diagnosis

Signs of pulmonary hypertension in the absence of a readily recognizable cause should raise the possibility of PV stenosis (Latson et al, 2007).

1. Echocardiographic study can visualize all PVs in nearly all patients. The finding of turbulent flow on color Doppler should raise the suspicion of PV stenosis. Monophasic flow or flow velocities above 1.7 m/sec indicate functionally significant stenosis. Normally, early diastolic flow velocity is less than 1 m/sec, and systolic flow velocity is much less than that.
2. MRI has been shown to be very useful in evaluation of PVs, although its applicability is limited by long acquisition time.
3. Multidetector CT angiography is an excellent technique for detailed analysis of the PVs.
4. Angiography provides the most selective detailed views of the PVs. It can be done by selective injection of contrast dye into the major branch or small branches of the PA.
5. Radionuclide imaging may demonstrate reduced flow to the affected portion of the lung that drains by affected PV(s).

Treatment and Prognosis

Prognosis is exceedingly poor in patients with involvement of most or all of the pulmonary veins, and long-term survival is rare without treatment. Most of the deaths are caused by pulmonary hypertensive crisis. Patients with only one or two PVs involved have much more benign courses. Patients with involvement of only one PV survive much longer.

Surgical as well as catheter intervention have a uniformly bad long-term outcome. Surgery can widen the narrowed veins, and interventional procedures can stretch the vessels, but the result is usually a short-term solution because the stenosis typically recurs within a month to 6 weeks.

1. Surgical relief of stenosis by various techniques has not improved survival significantly because of progression of the disease. Only 50% of patients survive for 5 years after surgery.
2. Catheter intervention offers only limited success. Balloon angioplasty with low-pressure dilatation follows quick recurrence in most of the patients. High-pressure balloon angioplasty or angioplasty with a cutting balloon may offer a better result. Use of stent has reported no better medium- or long-term results than cutting balloon angioplasty.

Acquired Pulmonary Vein Stenosis

Pulmonary vein stenosis may be secondary to surgery for anomalous pulmonary venous return. Significant stenosis of the PVs occurs in about 10% of patients after surgical repair of total anomalous pulmonary venous return. Rare causes of PV stenosis in adults include neoplasm growth, sarcoidosis, or fibrosing mediastinitis. Most common cause of PV stenosis in adults is radiofrequency ablation procedures done for treatment of atrial fibrillation. Various treatment modalities used in adult patients are also disappointing.

SCIMITAR SYNDROME

All or some of the pulmonary veins from the lower lobe and sometimes the middle lobe of the right lung drain anomalously into the IVC, either just above or below the diaphragm. The appearance of chest radiography resembles a curved Turkish sword, a scimitar, with vertical radiographic shadow along the lower right cardiac border.

Infants

1. Symptomatic infants frequently have associated cardiac anomalies (e.g., ASD, PDA), hypoplasia of the right lung and right PA, pulmonary venous obstruction, and pulmonary sequestration of right lung tissue (receiving systemic arterial supply from the aorta). Left-sided obstructive lesions (e.g., hypoplastic LV, subaortic stenosis, aortic arch obstruction) also are frequently present. Dextrocardia or mesocardia also is frequently found secondary to hypoplasia of the right lung.
2. For symptomatic infants, embolization or ligation of the systemic arterial supply to the right lung, if present, may result in improvement of pulmonary hypertension and signs of CHF. In infants with associated ASD, a pericardial tunnel of synthetic patch may be used to direct flow from the scimitar vein through the RA and into the LA. For most symptomatic infants with additional associated defects, the surgical mortality rate is high (up to near 50%).

Older Children and Adults

1. Children (and adults) with the syndrome are either minimally symptomatic or asymptomatic, probably because they have a low incidence of associated anomalies.
2. For older children, the anomalous pulmonary venous return can be redirected to the LA, but in patients with associated pulmonary sequestration, the involved lobes of the right lung may need to be resected. In selected older children and adult patients, the anomalous pulmonary venous return can be connected to the LA through a right thoracotomy without the use of cardiopulmonary bypass (Schwill et al, 2010).

SYSTEMIC VENOUS ANOMALIES

A wide variety of abnormalities appears in the systemic venous system; some of these have little physiologic importance, and others produce cyanosis. Recent developments in the diagnosis and treatment of patients with cardiovascular disorders have brought these anomalies to the attention of cardiologists and thoracic surgeons. Some of these abnormalities produce difficulties in the manipulation of catheters during cardiac catheterization, and preoperative knowledge of systemic venous anomalies is important in cardiac surgery. Therefore, the search for common abnormalities of the systemic veins has become routine in the evaluation of pediatric cardiac patients during echo and cardiac catheterization.

Two well-known anomalies of systemic veins are persistent left superior vena cava (SVC) and infrahepatic interruption of the IVC with azygos continuation. Very rarely, either persistent left SVC or interrupted IVC drains into the LA, producing cyanosis.

Anomalies of the Superior Vena Cava

Persistent left SVC occurs in 3% to 5% of children with CHDs. It is connected to the RA in 92% of cases and to the LA (producing cyanosis) in the remainder.

Persistent Left Superior Vena Cava Draining Into the Right Atrium

In the most common type, the left SVC is connected to the coronary sinus. As a rule, bilateral SVC is present in this type (Fig. 15.7A). Rarely, the right SVC is absent, and the blood from the right upper part of the body drains through the right innominate vein (Fig. 15.7B).

Isolated persistent left SVC (see Fig. 15.7A and B) does not produce symptoms or signs. Cardiac examination is entirely normal. Chest radiography films may show the shadow of the left SVC along the upper left border of the mediastinum. A high prevalence of leftward P axis (+15 degrees or less) has been reported on the ECG. Imaging of an enlarged coronary sinus by echo study is often the first clue to the diagnosis of persistent left SVC. Echo study usually provides accurate diagnosis of the condition. Treatment for isolated persistent left SVC is not necessary.

Persistent Left Superior Vena Cava Draining Into the Left Atrium

Rarely (in 8% of cases), persistent left SVC drains into the LA, resulting in systemic arterial desaturation (see Fig. 15.7C and D). This is caused by failure of invagination between the left sinus horn and LA; therefore, the coronary sinus is absent. Associated cardiac anomalies are almost invariably present. Complex defects, such as cor biloculare, conotruncal abnormalities, and asplenia syndrome, are commonly found. Defects of the atrial septum (single atrium, secundum ASD, primum ASD) are also frequently found.

Clinical manifestations are dominated by the associated complex cardiac defects. In the absence of complex defects, cyanosis is more marked when there is no atrial communication (see Fig. 15.7C) than when there is an ASD. When there is an ASD (see Fig. 15.7D), clinical findings resemble those of ASD with left-to-right shunt, with only mild cyanosis. Echo study with color-flow mapping usually provide adequate diagnosis. MRI is increasingly used to establish the diagnosis of the condition. Cardiac catheterization and selective left SVC angiography establish the diagnosis.

Surgical correction is necessary. When there is an adequate-size bridging vein that connects two SVCs, simple ligation of the left SVC is performed. If the right SVC is absent or a bridging vein is inadequate, the left SVC is transposed to the RA.

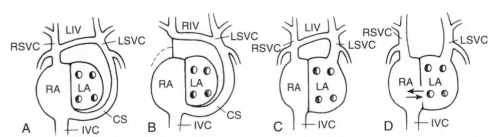

Fig. 15.7 Schematic diagram of persistent left superior vena cava (LSVC). **A,** The left SVC drains via the coronary sinus (CS) into the right atrium (RA). The left innominate vein (LIV) and the right SVC (RSVC) are adequate. **B,** Uncommonly, the RSVC may be atretic. The coronary sinus is large because it receives blood from both the right and left upper parts of the body. **C,** The coronary sinus is absent, and the LSVC drains directly into the left atrium (LA). It connects to the RSVC through LIV. The atrial septum is intact. **D,** The LSVC connects to the LA, and there is a posterior atrial septal defect, which allows a predominant left-to-right atrial shunt. *IVC,* Inferior vena cava; *RIV,* right innominate vein.

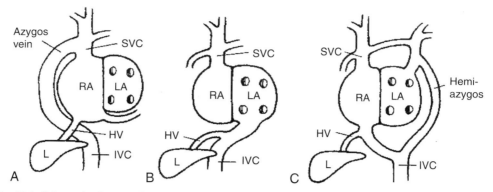

Fig. 15.8 Schematic diagram of selected abnormalities of the inferior vena cava (IVC). **A,** Interrupted IVC with azygos continuation, the most common abnormality of the IVC. The hepatic veins (HVs) connect directly to the right atrium (RA). **B,** Right IVC draining into the left atrium (LA). **C,** The left-sided IVC drains into the LA through the left hemiazygous system and the left SVC. **D,** Complete absence of the right IVC with communicating vein draining to the azygos vein. *L,* Liver.

Anomalies of the Inferior Vena Cava

Among the significant anomalies of the IVC are infrahepatic interruption of the IVC with azygos continuation and anomalous drainage of the IVC into the LA, producing cyanosis (Fig. 15.8).

Interrupted Inferior Vena Cava with Azygos Continuation

This anomaly has been reported in about 3% of children with congenital heart defects (see Fig. 15.8A). The IVC below the level of the renal veins is normal, but the hepatic portion of the IVC is absent. Instead of receiving the hepatic veins and entering the RA, the IVC drains via an enlarged azygos system into the right SVC and eventually to the RA. The hepatic veins connect directly to the RA. Bilateral SVC also is common. Azygos continuation of the IVC often is associated with complex cyanotic heart defects, such as polysplenia syndrome, double-outlet RV, cor biloculare, and anomalies of pulmonary venous return. Less often, a simple cardiac defect

is associated. No case has been reported in association with asplenia syndrome. This defect creates difficulties during cardiac catheterization and interventional procedures and can complicate surgical correction of an underlying cardiac defect.

This anomaly does not result in clinical manifestations. This condition is readily diagnosed by echo studies as well as by MRI. No specific treatment of this condition is indicated.

Inferior Vena Cava Connecting to the Left Atrium

In this extremely rare condition, the IVC receives the hepatic vein, curves toward the LA, and makes a direct connection with the chamber (see Fig. 15.8B). In another rare subtype of the IVC abnormalities, the lower end of the right IVC is absent, and the dominant left IVC drains into the LA through the (left-sided) hemiazygos system and persistent left SVC (see Fig. 15.8C).

This group of IVC anomalies produces cyanosis. IVC blood is surgically redirected into the RA.

Vascular Ring

PREVALENCE

Vascular ring reportedly represents fewer than 1% of all congenital cardiovascular anomalies, but this may be an underestimate because some conditions are asymptomatic.

PATHOLOGY

Vascular ring refers to a group of anomalies of the aortic arch that cause respiratory symptoms or feeding problems. A rare anomaly of the left pulmonary artery (LPA) that causes symptoms is also included in this group, although it does not involve the aortic arch. The vascular ring may be divided into two groups, complete (or true) and incomplete.

1. **Complete vascular ring** refers to conditions in which the abnormal vascular structures or their remnants form a complete circle around the trachea and esophagus. Double aortic arch and right aortic arch with left ligamentum arteriosum are examples of complete vascular ring.

2. **Incomplete vascular ring** refers to vascular anomalies that do not form a complete circle around the trachea and esophagus but do compress the trachea or esophagus. These include anomalous innominate artery, aberrant right subclavian artery, and anomalous LPA ("vascular sling" or "pulmonary sling").

Five major vascular rings are discussed in this chapter:

1. **Double aortic arch is the most common vascular ring** (40%) (Fig. 16.1). This anomaly is caused by a failure of regression of both the right and left fourth branchial arches, resulting in right and left aortic arches, respectively. These two arches completely encircle and compress the trachea and esophagus, producing respiratory distress and feeding problems in early infancy. The right arch gives off two arch vessels, the right common carotid and the right subclavian arteries, and the left arch gives off the left common carotid and left subclavian arteries (see Fig. 16.1). The right aortic arch is usually larger than the left arch (seen in 75% of patients), but on rare occasions, partial obstruction or complete atresia of the left arch (with a ligamentous remnant) may occur. Double aortic arch is commonly an isolated anomaly but is rarely associated with a variety of congenital heart defects (CHDs) such as transposition of the great arteries, ventricular septal defect (VSD), persistent truncus arteriosus, tetralogy of Fallot (TOF), and coarctation of the aorta (COA).

2. **Right aortic arch with left ligamentum arteriosum.** One of the major components of most vascular rings is a right aortic arch. Vascular ring with a right arch with left ligamentum arteriosum has several different forms; two common types are described here. Although rare, right aortic arch may occur without forming a vascular ring if the aorta stays and descends on the right of the vertebrae.

   a. In the most frequent form of vascular ring with right aortic arch with left ligamentum arteriosum (occurring in ≈65% of cases), the right arch first gives off the left carotid artery; then the right carotid artery followed by the right subclavian artery; and last, the left subclavian artery (see Fig. 16.1). The aberrant left subclavian artery often arises from a retroesophageal diverticulum (called diverticulum of Kommerell). The ring is completed by a left-sided ductus arteriosus (or its remnant ligamentum arteriosum) passing from the subclavian artery to the proximal LPA (see Fig. 16.1). The descending aorta usually courses to the left of the vertebral column to pass through the diaphragm in the usual location of the aortic hiatus. About 10% of this type of vascular ring is associated with an intracardiac defect.

	Anatomy	Ba-Esophag.	Chest Film	Symptoms	Treatment
Double aortic arch	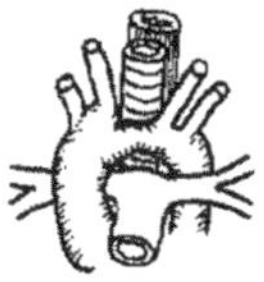	PA lat 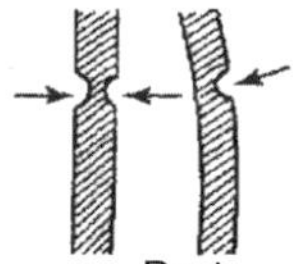 →□← □← Post. →	Anterior compression of trachea	Respiratory difficulties in early infancy Swallowing dysfunction	Surgical division of a smaller arch
Right aortic arch with left lig. arteriosum	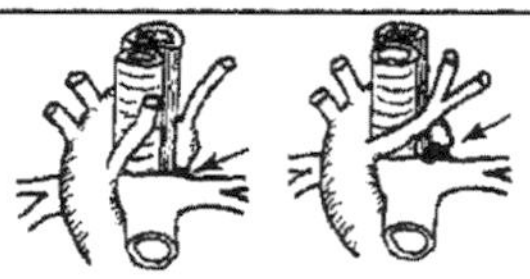 Aber. rt. subclav. Mirror image	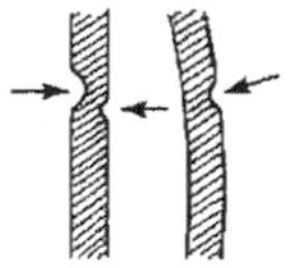 →□← □←	Right aortic arch	Mild respiratory difficulties late in infancy Swallowing dysfunction	Surgical division of left lig. arteriosum
Anomalous innominate artery	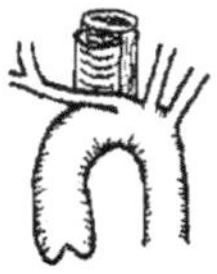	Normal	Anterior compression of trachea	Stridor or cough in infancy	Conservative management Surgical suturing of the artery to the sternum (±)
Aberrant right subclavian	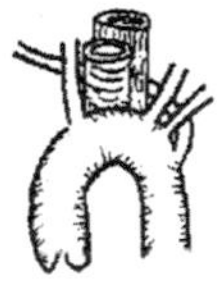	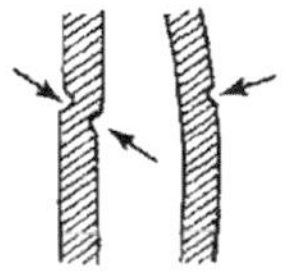 →□ □←		Occasional swallowing dysfunction	Usually no treatment is necessary
"Vascular sling"	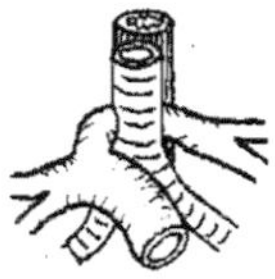	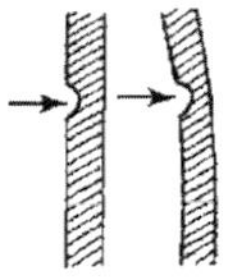 →□→ □	Right-sided emphysema or atelectasis Posterior compression of trachea	Wheezing and cyanotic episodes since birth	Surgical division of the anomalous LPA (from the RPA) and anastomosis to the MPA

Fig. 16.1 Clinical summary of vascular ring. In the anatomy of right aortic arch with left ligamentum arteriosum (in the *second row*), thick short black bands (indicated by *thick arrows*) are left-sided ductal ligaments. *Aber.*, Aberrant; *Ba-Esophag.*, barium esophagogram; *Lat.*, lateral view; *Lig.*, ligamentum; *LPA*, left pulmonary artery; *MPA*, main pulmonary artery; *P-A*, posteroanterior view; *Post.*, posterior; *RPA*, right pulmonary artery; *Rt.*, right; *Subclav.*, subclavian.

As a rare variant of this type, an aberrant innominate artery, rather than subclavian artery, may arise from the upper descending, and the ligamentum arteriosum connects the base of the innominate artery and the proximal LPA, completing a vascular ring. Clinical manifestations are similar to the one described earlier.

  b. In the second type of vascular ring with right aortic arch and ligamentum arteriosum (occurring in ≈35%), the left innominate artery originates from the right arch in mirror image fashion as the first branch followed by the right carotid and right subclavian arteries. A left-sided ductus or ligamentum arteriosum passes between the descending aorta and the proximal LPA (see Fig. 16.1). More than 90% of patients with this type of vascular ring have associated intracardiac defects, notably TOF and truncus arteriosus.

3. Anomalous innominate artery occurs in about 10% of patients with vascular ring (see Fig. 16.1). If the innominate artery takes off too far to the left from the aortic arch or more posteriorly, it may compress the trachea, producing mild respiratory symptoms. This anomaly is commonly associated with other CHDs such as VSD.

4. Aberrant right subclavian artery is the most common arch anomaly (accounting for 0.5% of the general population, but its true incidence may be higher if asymptomatic patients are included). Most cases are asymptomatic. When the right subclavian artery arises independently from the descending aorta, it courses behind the esophagus, compressing the posterior aspect of the esophagus and producing mild feeding problems (Figs. 16.1 and 16.2). Often, a larger compression is found behind the esophagus by an aortic diverticulum at the take-off of the right subclavian artery. This anomaly usually is an isolated anomaly, but it has a high association with coarctation of the aorta or interrupted aortic arch. Its incidence is very high (38%) in patients with Down syndrome with CHDs.

5. Anomalous LPA (also called "vascular sling") is a rare anomaly in which the LPA arises from the right pulmonary

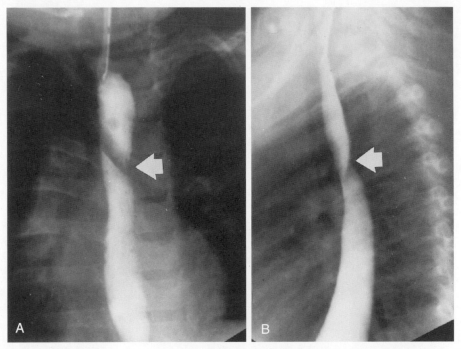

Fig. 16.2 Barium esophagogram in a child with aberrant right subclavian artery. **A,** Anteroposterior view shows an oblique indentation of the esophagus *(arrow)* at the level slightly higher than the carina produced by the subclavian artery. The indentation proceeds upward and to the right toward the right shoulder. **B,** Lateral projection shows a relatively shallow, long retroesophageal impression produced by the aberrant artery.

artery (PA) (Figs. 16.1 and 16.3). To reach the left lung, the anomalous artery courses over the proximal portion of the right mainstem bronchus, behind the trachea, and in front of the esophagus to the hilum of the left lung. Therefore, both respiratory symptoms and feeding problems (e.g., coughing; wheezing; stridor; episodes of choking, cyanosis, or apnea) may occur. About 10% to 20% of patients with this anomaly have associated cardiac defects, such as patent ductus arteriosus, VSD, atrial septal defect (ASD), atrioventricular canal, single ventricle, or aortic arch anomalies.

CLINICAL MANIFESTATIONS

History

1. Inspiratory stridor and feeding problems of varying severity are present, beginning at different ages. In double aortic arch, symptoms tend to appear in the newborn period or in early infancy (before 3 months of age), and they are more severe than those in right aortic arch with left ligamentum arteriosum. Symptoms often are made worse by feeding. Affected infants frequently hyperextend their necks to reduce tracheal compression.
2. Respiratory symptoms or feeding problems are milder with incomplete forms of vascular ring than with the complete form.
3. A history of pneumonia frequently is elicited.
4. A history of atelectasis, emphysema, or pneumonia of the right lung is found with "vascular sling."

Physical Examination

1. Physical examination is not revealing except for a varying degree of rhonchi when the vascular ring is an isolated anomaly.
2. Cardiac examination is usually normal except in about 25% of patients in whom associated cardiac anomalies are present.

Electrocardiography

The electrocardiography findings are normal unless the vascular ring is associated with other CHDs.

DIAGNOSIS

The diagnosis of vascular ring is accomplished by using the following imaging techniques; some are routinely available, and others are specialized.

1. **Chest radiography:** Because patients usually present with symptoms of respiratory difficulty, chest radiography is always the first and most commonly performed test.
   a. One looks for right aortic arch. In right aortic arch, the trachea is deviated to the left of the midline rather than to the right as seen in the presence of a normal left arch. If a right aortic arch is identified, a vascular ring is highly likely. If only a left arch is identified, a vascular right is much less likely but not excluded.
   b. An ill-defined aortic arch location is often observed in patients with double aortic arch.
   c. With the complete form of vascular ring, compression of the air-filled trachea may be visible on posteroanterior or lateral chest radiography.

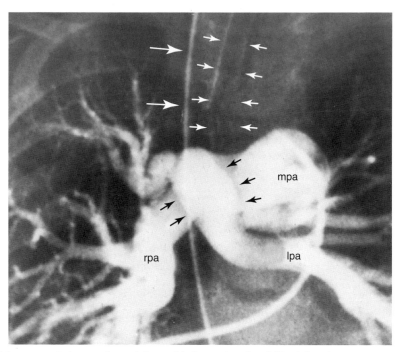

Fig. 16.3 Pulmonary arteriogram in an infant with "vascular sling." The left pulmonary artery (lpa) arises from the posterosuperior aspect of the right pulmonary artery (rpa) *(black arrows)* rather than from the main pulmonary artery (mpa). The origin of the left pulmonary artery (lpa) is to the right of the trachea, which is easily identifiable by an endotracheal tube (two rows of *white arrows*). The esophagus is directly behind the proximal portion of the aberrant left pulmonary artery, which caused an anterior indentation on the barium esophagogram. The esophagus is identifiable by an orogastric tube that was inserted at the time of cardiac catheterization *(large white arrows)*.

d. Aspiration pneumonia may be present. Hyperinflation or atelectasis of the right lung may be a suggestive sign of anomalous LPA ("vascular sling").

2. **Barium esophagography:** If plain chest radiography suggests vascular rings and when access to computed tomography (CT) scan is not possible, barium esophagography is the next logical step, which is usually diagnostic of most vascular rings (see Fig. 16.1). Patients with normal esophagography findings do not have a significant vascular ring.

   a. In double aortic arch, two large indentations are present in both sides (with the right one usually larger) on the posteroanterior view, and a large posterior indentation is seen on the lateral view (see Fig. 16.1).

   b. In right aortic arch with left ligamentum arteriosum, a large right-sided indentation and a much smaller left-sided indentation are present. A posterior indentation, either small or large, also is present on the lateral view. A large posterior indentation suggests the presence of diverticulum of Kommerell (see Fig. 16.1).

   c. In aberrant right subclavian artery, there is a small oblique indentation extending toward the right shoulder on the posteroanterior view. There is a small posterior indentation on the lateral view (see Figs. 16.1 and 16.2). Indentations may be large if the compression is made by an aortic diverticulum.

   d. In "vascular sling," an anterior indentation of the esophagus seen in the lateral view at the level of the

carina is characteristic. This is the only vascular ring that produces an anterior esophageal indentation (see Fig. 16.1). A right-sided indentation usually is seen on the posteroanterior view. The right lung is either hyperlucent or atelectatic with pneumonic infiltrations.

   e. Barium esophagography findings are normal in anomalous left innominate artery.

3. **Echocardiography and color-flow Doppler:** Echo and color-flow Doppler studies are very helpful, both for diagnosing vascular ring and for excluding associated intracardiac defects. One should perform a careful segmental investigation of the aortic arch and arch vessels. The suprasternal notch views are especially useful in establishing the diagnosis.

   However, there are limitations to echo study in the diagnosis of vascular ring. Structures without a lumen, such as a ligamentum arteriosum or an atretic arch, have no blood flow and are difficult to identify with color-flow echocardiography. Also, identification of compressed midline structures and their relationship to encircling vascular anomalies is difficult to detect with echo studies.

4. **CT scan, magnetic resonance imaging (MRI), and digital subtraction angiography:** These radiologic studies are often used in the diagnosis of vascular rings and may eliminate the need for invasive aortography.

   a. CT and MRI are useful diagnostic tools because they reveal not only the position of vascular structures but also of the tracheobronchial and esophageal structures and their relationships to the vascular structures. These studies do not show ligamentum arteriosum either. MRI has been proposed as an excellent substitute for angiography.

b. These radiologic techniques have advantages and disadvantages. The major advantage of CT is the rapidity with which data can be acquired, in many cases without the need for sedation. Its disadvantage is the use of radiation and need for intravenous (IV) contrast media. MRI, on the other hand, does not use radiation or iodinated IV contrast media but does have longer imaging times, requiring sedation in most pediatric patients; sedation may be particularly risky in young children with airway obstruction, and general anesthesia with intubation might be required.

5. **Aortic angiography and cardiac catheterization:** In the past, diagnostic aortography was performed in delineating anomalous arch vasculatures. However, it is more invasive and does not have tomographic or multiplanar capability. Echo with color Doppler studies, CT, or MRI can usually provide the required information before surgery. Therefore, when a choice is available, MRI and CT angiography are preferable for detailed diagnosis and preoperative assessment.

6. Tracheography and bronchoscopy usually add little information and may be hazardous in some patients. However, these tests may be useful in delineating tracheobronchial malacia associated with vascular ring in some patients.

MANAGEMENT

Medical

1. Asymptomatic patients need no surgical treatment even when the anomalies are found incidentally.

2. Medical management for infants with mild symptoms includes careful feeding with soft foods and aggressive treatment of pulmonary infections.

Surgical

Indications and Timing

Respiratory distress and a history of recurrent pulmonary infections and apneic spells are indications for surgical intervention. The timing of surgery depends on the severity of symptoms, and surgery may be performed during infancy.

Procedures and Mortality

1. **Double aortic arch.** Division of the smaller of the two arches (usually the left) is performed through a left thoracotomy. Knowing which arch is the dominant arch is very important because thoracotomy is typically performed on the side of the nondominant arch. The surgical mortality rate is less than 5%.

2. **Right aortic arch and left ligamentum arteriosum.** Ligation and division of the ligamentum are performed through a left thoracotomy. If a Kommerell diverticulum is found, the diverticulum is resected, and the left subclavian artery is transferred to the left carotid artery. The mortality rate is less than 5%.

3. **Anomalous innominate artery.** Through a right anterolateral thoracotomy, the innominate artery is suspended to the posterior sternum. Asymptomatic patients do not require surgery; only 10% of the patients with the anomaly require surgery.

4. **Aberrant right subclavian artery.** Surgical interruption of the aberrant artery is performed rarely only in symptomatic patients with dysphagia. The procedure consists of division of the aberrant artery and translocation to the right common carotid artery.

5. **Anomalous LPA.** Surgical division and reimplantation of the LPA to the main PA is performed, usually through a median sternotomy and with the use of cardiopulmonary bypass. The surgical mortality rate is near 0%.

Complications

In infants who have had surgery for severe symptoms, airway obstruction may persist for weeks or months. Careful respiratory management is required in the postoperative period. A period of months to 1 year may be required before disappearance of the noisy respiration, which is caused by preexisting tracheomalacia. This fact should be anticipated and clearly explained to the parents preoperatively. This complication is more likely in patients who have had double aortic arch, vascular sling, or right aortic arch with left ligamentum arteriosum.

VARIANTS OF AORTIC ARCH BRANCHING

Although the most common aortic arch branching pattern is three-vessel branching pattern in humans, up to about 30% of patients have a two-vessel branching pattern, which is a normal variant. The two-vessel branching pattern has incorrectly been called the "bovine aortic arch" in humans. True bovine aortic arch branching has no resemblance to the two-vessel branching patterns seen in humans. Thus, the use of misnomers such as "bovine arch" should be avoided. Instead, one should use descriptive branching patterns as described below or simply call it a two-vessel branching pattern if further branching information is not known (Layton etal, 2006).

The following describes standard aortic arch branching and its normal variants in humans (Fig. 16.4).

1. The most common aortic arch branching pattern (standard aortic arch branching) in humans consists of three great arteries originating from the aortic arch. The first branch is the innominate artery, the second one the left common carotid artery, and the third one the left subclavian artery (see Fig. 16.4A). This pattern is present in about 70% of patients.

2. A common variant of the standard aortic arch is the one in which two great arteries originate from the aortic arch. This occurs in about 30% of patients, more commonly observed in Africans. In one group of these patients, the innominate artery and the left carotid artery share the common trunk, which occurs in about 13% of patients (correctly described as "common origin of the innominate artery and left common

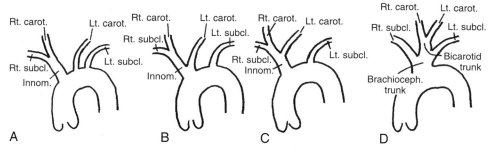

Fig. 16.4 Variants in the aortic arch branching pattern in humans and the bovine aortic arch. **A,** The most common branching pattern found in humans. **B,** The second most common pattern in humans. **C,** Less common branching pattern in humans in which the left carotid artery originates from the innominate artery. **D,** True bovine aortic arch. *Brachioceph.,* Brachiocephalic; *carot.,* carotid; *Innom.,* innominate. *Lt.,* left; *Rt.,* right; *subcl.,* subclavian.

carotid artery") (see Fig. 16.4B). In the other group of the two-vessel branching variant, the left common carotid artery branches from the innominate artery (rather than sharing the common trunk). This variant occurs in about 9% of patients (correctly described as "origin of the left carotid artery from the innominate artery") (see Fig. 16.4C).

In the true bovine aortic arch, there is only one great artery originating from the arch. It has no resemblance to any of the branching patterns seen in humans. The single trunk, called the "brachiocephalic trunk," gives rise to both subclavian arteries and a bicarotid trunk. The bicarotid trunk then bifurcates into the left and right common carotid arteries (see Fig. 16.4D).

Chamber Localization and Cardiac Malposition

In this chapter, clinical methods of locating cardiac chambers using chest radiography, electrocardiography (ECG), and echocardiography are discussed. This is followed by application of a principle that may aid in the anatomic diagnosis of the heart in the right chest (dextrocardia) or in the midline (mesocardia). Although these methods are valid, many false-positive and false-negative results are possible. Two-dimensional echocardiography usually reveals the correct diagnosis, but occasionally, additional studies such as magnetic resonance imaging (MRI) or angiography may be needed.

CHAMBER LOCALIZATION

The heart and great arteries can be viewed as three separate segments: the atria, the ventricles, and the great arteries. These three segments can vary from their normal positions either independently or together, resulting in many possible sets of abnormalities. The *segmental approach* of Van Praagh is useful in determining the relationship at each segment. This approach also simplifies the description of complex cardiac defects and abnormal positions of the heart (e.g., dextrocardia, levocardia, mesocardia).

Localization of the Atria

The atria can be localized accurately by three noninvasive methods: chest radiography, ECG, and echocardiography. The radiographic method relies on the fact that the atrial situs is almost always the same as the type of visceral situs; the right atrium (RA) is on the same side as the liver or on the opposite side of the stomach bubble. The ECG method is based on the principle that the sinus node is always located in the RA and that the site of the sinus node can be determined by the P axis. Echocardiography clarifies the relationship between systemic and pulmonary veins and the atria.

Chest Radiography

The clinician should locate the liver shadow and the stomach bubble.
1. A right-sided liver shadow and left-sided stomach bubble (situs solitus) indicate situs solitus of the atria (with the RA on the right of the left atrium [LA], as in normal) (Fig. 17.1A). A left-sided liver shadow and right-sided stomach bubble (situs inversus) indicate situs inversus of the atria (with the RA on the left of the LA) (Fig. 17.1B).
2. A midline (symmetrical) liver shadow with a variable location of stomach bubble suggests heterotaxia (or splenic syndromes) in which either two RAs or two LAs (situs ambiguus) and other associated complex cardiac anomalies are present (Fig. 17.1C; see also sections on heterotaxia in Chapter 14).

Electrocardiography

The sinus node is always located in the anatomic RA. Therefore, the P axis of the ECG can be used to locate the atria; the RA is located on the opposite side of the P axis.
1. When the P axis is in the lower left quadrant of the hexaxial reference system (0 to +90 degrees), the RA is on the right side (with the RA to the right of the LA, or situs solitus of the atria) (Fig. 17.2).
2. When the P axis is in the lower right quadrant (+90 to +180 degrees), the RA is on the left side (with the RA on the left of the LA, or situs inversus of the atria) (see Fig. 17.2).
3. With heterotaxia, the P axis may be superiorly directed (as seen with polysplenia syndrome) or may change between the lower left quadrant and lower right quadrant from time to time (as seen with asplenia syndrome, in which two sinus nodes are present).

Two-Dimensional Echocardiography and Other Methods

Two-dimensional echocardiography identifies the inferior vena cava (IVC), pulmonary veins, or both. The atrial chamber that is connected to the IVC is the morphologic RA, and the atrium that receives the pulmonary veins is usually the morphologic LA. The morphology of the atrial appendages further specifies and differentiates the atria, with right atrial appendage being broad and triangular and left atrial appendage being narrow and fingerlike. Cardiac MRI, angiocardiography, surgical inspection, and autopsy findings aid further in the diagnosis of atrial situs.

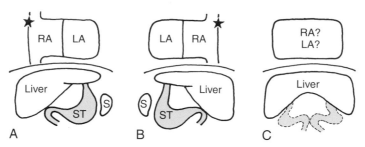

Fig. 17.1 The visceroatrial relationship. **A,** Situs solitus. **B,** Situs inversus. **C,** Situs ambiguus. The right atrium (RA) is either on the same side as the liver or on the opposite side of the stomach (ST). The sinoatrial node *(star)* is always in the RA. *LA,* Left atrium; *S,* spleen.

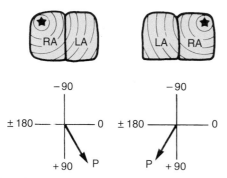

Fig. 17.2 Locating the atria by the use of the P axis. When the right atrium (RA) is on the right side, the P axis is in the left lower quadrant (0 to +90 degrees). When the RA is on the left side, the P axis is in the right lower quadrant (+90 to +180 degrees). *LA,* Left atrium. (From Park MK, Guntheroth WG: *How to Read Pediatric ECGs*, ed 4, Philadelphia, 2006, Mosby.)

Localization of the Ventricles

Ventricles can be localized noninvasively by the ECG and two-dimensional echocardiography (or by MRI or angiocardiography).

Electrocardiography

The ECG method of localizing the ventricle is based on the fact that the depolarization of the ventricular septum moves from the embryonic left ventricle (LV) to the right ventricle (RV). This produces Q waves in the precordial leads that lie over the anatomic LV.

1. If Q waves are present in V5 and V6 but not in V1, D-loop of the ventricle, as in the normal person, is likely (Fig. 17.3A).
2. If Q waves are present in V4R, V1, and V2 but not in V5 and V6, L-loop of the ventricles is likely (ventricular inversion) (see Fig. 17.3B).

Two-Dimensional Echocardiography

The anatomic RV and LV are identified by the facts that the tricuspid valve leaflet usually inserts on the interventricular septum in a more apical position than the mitral septal leaflet and that the LV is invariably attached to the mitral valve and the RV to the tricuspid valve. A ventricular chamber that has two papillary muscles is the LV. Furthermore, the

trabeculations in the RV are more coarse and in the LV endocardial surface is more smooth.

Magnetic Resonance Imaging or Ventriculography

The anatomic RV is coarsely trabeculated and triangular, and the anatomic LV is finely trabeculated and ellipsoid.

Localization of the Great Arteries

One can accurately determine the relationship between the two great arteries and the relationship of the great arteries to the ventricles noninvasively through echocardiography or MRI (and invasively through angiocardiography). The ECG and chest radiography are not very helpful in determining the relationship between the great arteries and the ventricles. In many cases, however, one can deduce the relationship through the *loop rule* (of Van Praagh). The loop rule states that the D-loop of the ventricle (with the anatomic RV to the right of the LV) usually is associated with normally related great arteries or with complete transposition of the great arteries (D-looped ventricles, thus D-TGA). The L-loop of the ventricle (with the anatomic RV to the left of the anatomic LV) usually is associated with the mirror image of normally related great arteries or with congenitally corrected transposition of the great arteries (L-looped ventricles, thus L-TGA).

There are four types of relationships between the two great arteries: (1) solitus, (2) inversus, (3) D-transposition, and (4) L-transposition (Fig. 17.4). One can deduce the relationship of the great artery. For example, when the situs solitus of the atria and the D-loop of the ventricle are confirmed, a situs solitus relationship is present if the patient is not cyanotic; if the patient is cyanotic, a D-TGA is present.

Segmental Expression

The following symbols are used in describing the segmental relationship of cardiac chambers and great arteries:

1. Visceroatrial relationship: S (solitus), I (inversus), or A (ambiguus)
2. Ventricular loop: D (D-loop), L (L-loop), or X (uncertain or indeterminate)
3. Great arteries: S (solitus), I (inversus), D (D-transposition), or L (L-transposition)

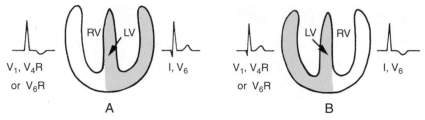

Fig. 17.3 Locating the ventricles from the electrocardiogram (ECG). The left ventricle (LV) is usually located on the same side as the precordial leads that show Q waves. If V6 shows a Q wave, the LV is on the left side (**A**). If V4R and V1 show a Q wave, the LV is to the right of the anatomic right ventricle (RV) (**B**). Note that Q waves are also present in V1 in severe right ventricular hypertrophy. (From Park MK, Guntheroth WG: *How to Read Pediatric ECGs*, ed 4, Philadelphia, 2006, Mosby.)

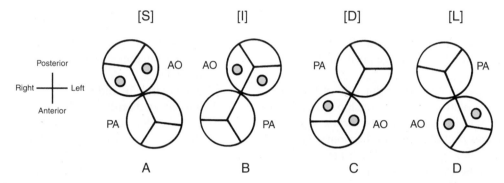

Fig. 17.4 Four types of relationships between the great arteries, viewed in the horizontal section. **A**, Solitus (S) relationship is present when the aortic valve is posterior and to the right of the pulmonary valve. **B**, In inversus (I) relationship, the aortic valve is posterior to and left of the pulmonary valve (mirror image of normal). **C**, Complete transposition (D) is present when the aortic valve is anterior and to the right of the pulmonary valve. **D**, Congenitally corrected transposition (L) is present when the aortic valve is anterior and to the left of the pulmonary valve. *AO*, Aorta; *PA*, pulmonary artery.

With these symbols, the segmental relationship of the heart can be expressed by three letters. The first letter signifies the visceroatrial relationship; the second letter, the ventricular loop; and the third letter, the relationship of the great arteries. The segmental approach to the diagnosis of cardiac malposition is independent of the location of the cardiac apex. Consequently, this approach applies to normally located hearts (levocardia in situs solitus) as well as to abnormally located hearts, such as dextrocardia and mesocardia. A few examples of normal and well-known abnormal segmental relationships can be expressed as follows:

Normal heart with situs solitus: S, D, S

Normal heart with situs inversus (mirror image of normal): I, L, I

D-TGA: S, D, D

D-TGA with situs inversus: I, L, L

L-TGA with situs solitus: S, L, L

A normally formed heart that is displaced to the right side of the chest secondary to hypoplasia of the right lung ("dextroversion"): S, D, S

DEXTROCARDIA AND MESOCARDIA

Dextrocardia refers to a condition in which the apex of the heart is located on the right side of the chest. Mesocardia indicates that the apex of the heart is located approximately on the

midline of the thorax; that is, the heart lies predominantly neither to the right nor to the left on the posteroanterior chest radiograph. The terms *dextrocardia* and *mesocardia* express the position of the heart as a whole but do not specify the segmental relationship of the heart. *Dextroposition* refers to the position of the heart in the right hemithorax (i.e. in cases of congenital left diaphragmatic hernia, in which the heart is pushed to the right with the apex of the heart pointing to the left).

The four common types of dextrocardias are classic mirror-image dextrocardia (Fig. 17.5A), normal heart displaced to the right side of the chest (Fig. 16.5B), L-TGA (Fig. 17.5C), and single ventricle. Less commonly, asplenia and polysplenia syndromes with situs ambiguus and complicated cardiac defects cause dextrocardia (Fig. 17.5D). All of these abnormalities may result in mesocardia.

With chest radiography studies and the ECG, one can deduce the location of the atria and the ventricles in dextrocardia (as well as in mesocardia). One can gain a more conclusive diagnosis of the segmental relationship through two-dimensional echocardiography or MRI (or invasively with angiocardiography).

1. Classic mirror-image dextrocardia (I, L, I) (see Fig. 17.5A) shows:
   a. The liver shadow on the left and the stomach bubble on the right on radiography and the P axis between +90 and +180 degrees on the ECG (situs inversus)

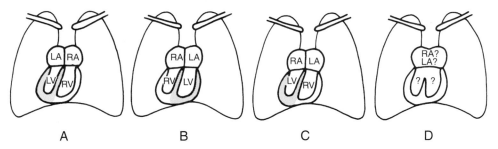

Fig. 17.5 Examples of common conditions in which the apex of the heart is in the right chest. **A,** Classic mirror-image dextrocardia. **B,** A normally formed heart shifted toward the right side of the chest. **C,** Congenitally corrected transposition of the great arteries (L-TGA) with situs solitus. **D,** Situs ambiguus seen with splenic syndromes. *LA,* Left atrium; *LV,* left ventricle; *RA,* right atrium; *RV,* right ventricle. (From Park MK, Guntheroth WG: *How to Read Pediatric ECGs,* ed 4, Philadelphia, 2006, Mosby.)

b. Q waves in V5R and V6R (V5R and V6R are right-sided precordial leads, the mirror-image positions of V5 and V6, respectively)

2. Normal heart shifted toward the right side of the chest with the normal right-to-left relationship maintained (dextroversion) (S, D, S) (see Fig. 17.5B) shows:
   a. The liver shadow on the right and the stomach bubble on the left on radiography and the P axis between 0 and +90 degrees on the ECG (situs solitus)
   b. Q waves in V5 and V6

3. L-TGA with situs solitus (S, L, L) (see Fig. 17.5C) shows:

   a. Situs solitus of abdominal viscera on radiography and the P axis in the normal quadrant (0 to +90 degrees) on the ECG
   b. Q waves in V5R and V6R

4. Undifferentiated cardiac chambers (see Fig. 17. D) are often associated with complicated cardiac defects and may show:
   a. Midline liver on radiography and shifting P axis or superiorly oriented P axis on the ECG
   b. Abnormal Q waves in the precordial leads (similar to those described for single ventricle; see Chapter 14)

PART 5

Acquired Heart Disease

Among acquired heart diseases, emphasis is placed on the more common pediatric diseases, such as cardiomyopathies; cardiovascular infections, including myocarditis and infective endocarditis; acute rheumatic fever; and valvular heart disease. Although the cause of Kawasaki's disease is not entirely clear, it is discussed in the chapter on cardiovascular infection. Mitral valve prolapse is discussed in the chapter on valvular heart disease. A chapter on cardiac involvement in some systemic diseases also is presented.

Cardiomyopathies are structural or functional abnormalities of the myocardium not secondary to congenital, valvular, hypertensive, pulmonary, or coronary heart diseases. Cardiomyopathy has traditionally been classified into three types based on anatomic and functional features: hypertrophic, dilated, and restrictive (Fig. 18.1). In 1995, two other categories were added by the World Health Organization (WHO), namely, arrhythmogenic right ventricular cardiomyopathy/dysplasia (ARVC/ARCD) and unclassified cardiomyopathies. Over the ensuing years, however, other organizations have proposed or classified cardiomyopathies that emphasize the genetic aspect of the disease.

The original three types of cardiomyopathies are functionally different from one another, and demands of therapy also are different. Table 18.1 summarizes clinical characteristics and treatment of the original three types of cardiomyopathies.

1. In hypertrophic cardiomyopathy (HCM), there is massive ventricular hypertrophy with a smaller than normal ventricular cavity. Contractile function of the ventricle is enhanced, but ventricular filling is impaired by relaxation abnormalities.
2. Dilated cardiomyopathy (DCM) is characterized by decreased contractile function of the ventricle associated with ventricular dilatation. Endocardial fibroelastosis (seen in infancy) and doxorubicin cardiomyopathy (seen in children who have received chemotherapy for malignancies) have clinical features similar to those of DCM.
3. Restrictive cardiomyopathy denotes a restriction of diastolic filling of the ventricles (usually infiltrative disease). Contractile function of the ventricle may be normal, but there is marked dilatation of both atria.
4. Two other cardiomyopathies, namely, ARVD/ARVC, first described in 1977, and left ventricular (LV) noncompac-

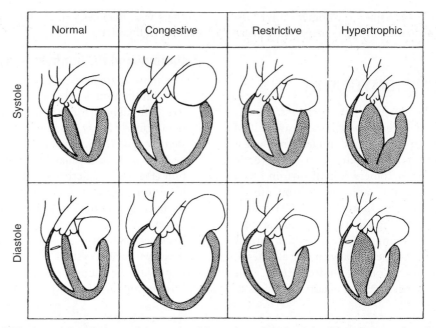

Fig. 18.1 Diagram of the 50-degree left anterior oblique view of the heart in different types of cardiomyopathies at end-systole and end-diastole. "Congestive" corresponds to "dilated" cardiomyopathy as used in the text. (From Goldman MR, Boucher CA: Values of radionuclide imaging techniques in assessing cardiomyopathy, *Am J Cardiol* 46:1232–1236, 1980.)

TABLE 18.1 Summary of Clinical Characteristics of Cardiomyopathies

Clinical Features	Hypertrophic	Dilated	Restrictive
Cause	Inherited (AD in ~50%) Sporadic (new mutation ±)	Pluricausal (e.g., toxic, metabolic, infectious, alcohol, doxorubicin) Inherited form (20%–35% of idiopathic forms)	Myocardial fibrosis, hypertrophy, or infiltration (amyloid, hemochromatosis)
Hemodynamic dysfunction	Diastolic dysfunction (with normal systolic function; abnormally stiff LV with impaired ventricular filling)	Systolic contractile dysfunction (↓ cardiac output, ↓ stroke volume, ↑ LVEDP)	Diastolic dysfunction (rigid ventricular walls impede ventricular filling)
Echocardiography (morphology)	Thickened LV (and *occasionally* RV) wall	Biventricular dilatation (↑ LVDD, ↑ LVSD)	Biatrial enlargement
	Small or normal LV chamber dimension	Atrial enlargement in proportion to ventricular enlargement	Normal LV and RV volume
	Supernormal LV contractility	Decreased LV contractility	Normal LV systolic function until advanced stage
	HOCM, ASH, or both	Apical thrombus (±)	Atrial thrombus (±)
Doppler	Reduced relaxation pattern (see Fig. 18.6)	Reduced relaxation pattern (see Fig. 18.6)	"Restrictive" pattern (see Fig. 18.6)
Treatment	Beta-adrenoreceptor blockers	Vasodilator therapy	Diuretics
	Calcium antagonists	Digitalis plus diuretics	Anticoagulants (±)
	(Digitalis/catechols and nitrates contraindicated)	Beta-adrenoceptor blockers (±)	Corticosteroids (±)
		Anticoagulants	Permanent pacemaker for advanced heart block (±)
	(Diuretics may worsen symptoms)	Antiarrhythmics (±)	
	ICD implantation to prevent sudden death in high-risk patients	Cardiac transplantation (±)	Cardiac transplantation (±)

AD, Autosomal dominant; *ASH,* asymmetrical septal hypertrophy; *HOCM,* hypertrophic obstructive cardiomyopathy; *ICD,* intracardiac cardioverter–defibrillator; *LV,* left ventricle; *LVDD,* left ventricular diastolic dimension; *LVEDP,* left ventricular end-diastolic pressure; *LVSD,* left ventricular systolic dimension; *RV,* right ventricle.

tion cardiomyopathy (unclassified cardiomyopathy), first described as an isolated entity in 1984, are presented later in this chapter.

HYPERTROPHIC CARDIOMYOPATHY

Hypertrophic cardiomyopathy is a heterogeneous, usually familial disorder of heart muscle. In about 50% of cases, HCM is inherited as a Mendelian autosomal dominant trait and is caused by mutations in one of 10 genes encoding protein components of the cardiac sarcomere (e.g., β-myosin heavy chain, myosin binding protein C, and cardiac troponin-T). The remainder of the cases occur sporadically. HCM usually is seen in adolescents and young adults, with equal gender distribution. It is the most common cause of sudden cardiac death in teens and young adults, especially among athletes. It may be seen in children with Noonan syndrome (see Table 2.1). A usually transient form of HCM occurs in infants of mothers with diabetes, which is presented under a separate heading in this chapter.

Pathology and Pathophysiology

1. The most characteristic abnormality is a hypertrophied LV, with the ventricular cavity usually small or normal in size. Although asymmetrical septal hypertrophy, a condition formerly known as idiopathic hypertrophic subaortic stenosis (Fig. 18.2), is most common, the hypertrophy may be concentric or localized to a small segment of the septum (Fig. 18.3). Microscopically, an extensive disarray of hypertrophied myocardial cells, myocardial scarring, and abnormalities of the small intramural coronary arteries are present.

2. In some patients, an intracavitary pressure gradient develops during systole, either at subaortic or rarely at midcavity. This subset is called hypertrophic obstructive cardiomyopathy (HOCM).

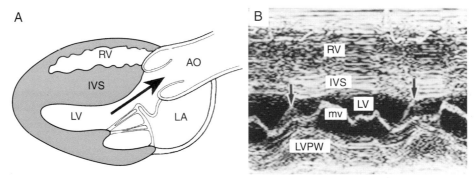

Fig. 18.2 Systolic anterior motion of the mitral valve. **A,** Diagram of systolic anterior motion in the presence of an asymmetrical septal hypertrophy. The Venturi effect may be important in the production of systolic anterior motion. **B,** M-mode echocardiography of the mitral valve in a patient with hypertrophic cardiomyopathy. Systolic anterior motion of the anterior leaflet of the mitral valve is indicated by *arrows. AO,* Aorta; *IVS,* interventricular septum; *LA,* left atrium; *LV,* left ventricle; *LVPW,* LV posterior wall; *mv,* mitral valve; *RV,* right ventricle.

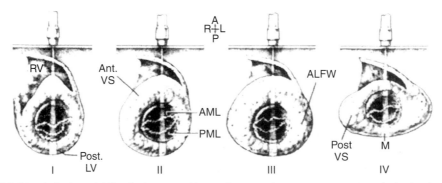

Fig. 18.3 Morphologic variability in hypertrophic cardiomyopathy seen on parasternal short-axis view of two-dimensional echo. In type I hypertrophy, relatively mild left ventricular hypertrophy confined to the anterior portion of the ventricular septum (VS) is present. In type II, hypertrophy of the anterior and posterior septum is present in the absence of free wall thickening. In type III, there is diffuse hypertrophy of substantial portions of both the ventricular septum and the anterolateral free wall (ALFW). In type IV, the M-mode echocardiography beam (M) does not traverse the thickened portions of the left ventricle (LV) in the posterior septum and anterolateral free wall. A or ANT, Anterior; AML, anterior mitral leaflet; L, left; LVFW, left ventricular free wall; P or Post, posterior; PML, posterior mitral leaflet; R, right. (From Maron BJ: Asymmetry in hypertrophic cardiomyopathy: the septal to free wall thickness ratio revisited [editorial], *Am J Cardiol* 55:835–838, 1985.)

a. The subaortic obstruction is commonly caused by systolic anterior motion (SAM) of the mitral valve against the hypertrophied septum (see Fig. 18.2). The SAM probably is created by the high outflow velocities and Venturi forces with frequent association of mitral regurgitation (MR).

b. In some patients, midcavity obstruction is caused by anomalous insertion of anterolateral papillary muscle into the anterior mitral leaflet, rather than SAM.

3. In so-called apical HCM, hypertrophy is confined to the LV apex without intracavitary obstruction (and with giant negative T waves on the electrocardiogram [ECG]). This subtype is present in about 25% of patients in Japan and fewer than 10% in other parts of the world.

4. The myocardium itself has an enhanced contractile state, but diastolic ventricular filling is impaired by abnormal stiffness of the LV, which may lead to left atrial enlargement and pulmonary venous congestion, producing congestive symptoms (exertional dyspnea, orthopnea, paroxysmal nocturnal dyspnea).

5. A unique aspect of HOCM is the variability of the degree of obstruction from moment to moment; the intensity of the heart murmur varies from time to time. Because the obstruction of the left ventricular outflow tract (LVOT) results from SAM of the mitral valve against the hypertrophied ventricular septum, any influence that reduces the LV systolic volume (e.g., positive inotropic agents, reduced blood volume, or lowering of the systemic vascular resistance) increases the obstruction. On the other hand, any influence that increases the LV systolic volume (e.g., negative inotropic agents, leg raising, blood transfusion, or increasing systemic vascular resistance) lessens the obstruction.

6. A large portion of the stroke volume (~80%) is ejected during the early part of systole when there is little or no obstruction, producing a sharp upstroke in the arterial pulse, a characteristic finding of HOCM. The obstruction occurs late in systole, producing a late systolic murmur.

7. Patients with severe hypertrophy and obstruction may experience anginal chest pain, lightheadedness, near syncope, or syncope. Patients also are prone to develop arrhythmias, which may lead to sudden death (presumably from ventricular tachycardia [VT] or ventricular fibrillation [VF]). Nearly 30% of children with HCM have myocardial bridging[a] (seen on coronary angiograms) with narrowing of the anterior descending coronary artery, which may have a key role in the development of ventricular arrhythmias. These patients may be more prone to sudden death.

---

[a]Normally, the large epicardial coronary arteries run on the surface of the heart, with only their terminal branches penetrating the myocardium. When parts of the epicardial artery dip beneath the epicardial muscle so that there is a muscle bridge over the artery, they are called myocardial bridges.

Clinical Manifestations

History

1. Easy fatigability, dyspnea, palpitation, dizziness, syncope, or anginal pain may be present.
2. Family history is positive for the disease in 30% to 60% of patients.

Physical Examination

1. A sharp upstroke of the arterial pulse is characteristic (in contrast to a slow upstroke seen with fixed aortic stenosis [AS]). An LV lift and a systolic thrill at the apex or along the lower left sternal border may be present.
2. The S2 is normal, and an ejection click is generally absent. A grade 1 to 3 of 6 ejection systolic murmur of medium pitch is most audible at the mid- and lower left sternal borders or at the apex. A soft holosystolic murmur of MR is often present. The intensity and even the presence of the murmur vary from examination to examination.

Electrocardiography

The ECG is abnormal in the majority of patients. Common ECG abnormalities include left ventricular hypertrophy (LVH), ST-T changes, and abnormally deep Q waves (owing to septal hypertrophy) with diminished or absent R waves in the left precordial leads (Fig. 18.4). Occasionally, "giant" negative T waves are seen in the left precordial leads, which may suggest apical HCM. Other ECG abnormalities may include cardiac arrhythmias and first-degree atrioventricular (AV) block.

Radiography

Mild LV enlargement with a globular-shaped heart may be present. The pulmonary vascularity usually is normal.

Echocardiography

1. Echocardiography is diagnostic. Two-dimensional echocardiography demonstrates the wide morphologic spectrum of the disease, including concentric hypertrophy (Fig. 18.5), localized segmental hypertrophy, and asymmetrical septal hypertrophy (see Fig. 18.3). Apical HCM may be missed by two-dimensional echocardiography. (If apical HCM is suspected, cardiac magnetic resonance imaging [MRI] should be obtained.)
2. A diastolic LV wall thickness of 15 mm or larger (or on occasion, 13 or 14 mm), usually with LV dimension smaller than 45 mm, is accepted for the clinical diagnosis of HCM in adults. For children, z-score of 2 or more relative to body surface area is theoretically compatible with the diagnosis.

The heart of some highly trained athletes may show hypertrophy of the LV wall, making the differentiation between the physiologic hypertrophy and HCM difficult. An LV wall thickness of 13 mm or larger is very uncommon in highly trained athletes, and it is always associated with an enlarged LV cavity (with LV diastolic dimension >54 mm, with ranges

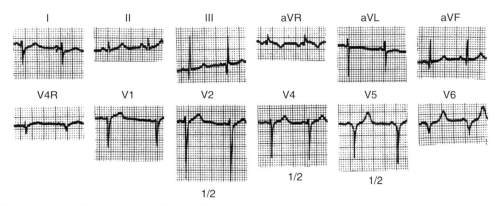

Fig. 18.4 Tracing from a 17-year-old girl with hypertrophic obstructive cardiomyopathy with marked septal hypertrophy. Note the prominent Q waves with absent R waves in V5 and V6.

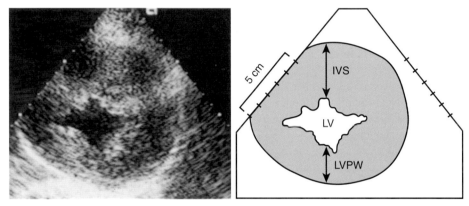

Fig. 18.5 Parasternal short-axis view of a 14-year-old boy with hypertrophic cardiomyopathy. Marked hypertrophy of the interventricular septum (IVS) as well as the posterior wall of the left ventricle (LVPW) is present. The left ventricle (LV) cavity is small. The IVS is approximately 39 mm, and the LV posterior wall is 26 mm thick. The thickness of both structures does not exceed 10 mm in normal persons.

55–63 mm). Therefore, athletes with LV wall thickness greater than 16 mm and a nondilated LV cavity are likely to have HCM (Pelliccia et al, 1991).

3. M-mode echocardiography may demonstrate an asymmetrical septal hypertrophy of the interventricular septum (with the septal thickness 1.4 times greater than the posterior LV wall) and occasionally SAM of the anterior mitral valve leaflet in the obstructive type (see Fig. 18.2).

4. Mitral inflow Doppler tracing demonstrates diastolic dysfunction with decreased E-wave velocity, increased deceleration time, and decreased E/A ratio of the mitral valve (usually <0.8) (Fig. 18.6). LV systolic function is normal or supernormal.

5. Doppler peak gradient in the LVOT of 30 mm Hg or greater indicates an obstructive type.

Natural History

1. The obstruction may be absent, stable, or slowly progressive. Genetically predisposed individuals often show striking increases in wall thickness during childhood.

2. Death is often sudden and unexpected and typically is associated with sports or vigorous exertion. Sudden death may occur most commonly in patients between 10 and 35 years of age. The incidence of sudden death may be as high as 4% to 6% a year in children and adolescents and 2% to 4% a year in adults. VF is the cause of death in the majority of sudden deaths. Even brief episodes of asymptomatic VT on ambulatory ECG may be a risk factor for sudden death. Patients with myocardial bridging (occurring in ~30%) may be at risk for sudden death.

3. Atrial fibrillation (AF) may cause stroke or heart failure. AF results from left atrium (LA) enlargement with loss of the atrial "kick" needed for filling the thick LV.

4. In a minority of patients, heart failure with cardiac dilation ("burned-out" phase of the disease) may develop later in life.

Management

The goal of treatment is to reduce ventricular contractility, increase ventricular volume, increase ventricular compliance, and increase LVOT dimensions. In the obstructive form of the condition, reduction of the LVOT pressure gradient is important. However, unfortunately, most of the therapeutic modalities used do not appear to significantly reduce the mortality rate. Surgical implantation of an automatic defibrillator may prove to be a very important modality to reduce sudden death.

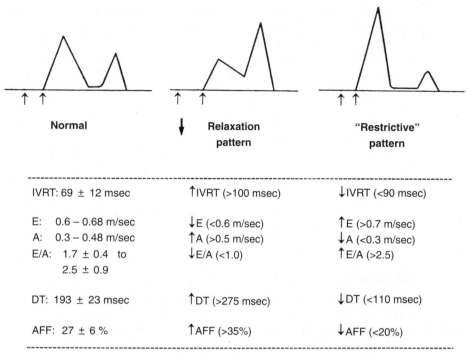

Fig. 18.6 Examples of diastolic dysfunction seen in various forms of cardiomyopathy. (See Chapter 5 and Fig. 5.12 for further discussion.) *A*, A-wave velocity (the velocity of a second wave that coincides with atrial contraction); *AFF*, atrial filling fraction; *DT*, deceleration time; *E*, E-wave velocity (the velocity of an early peak); *E/A*, ratio of E-wave to A-wave velocity; *IVRT*, isovolumic relaxation time.

General Management

1. Moderate restriction of physical activity is recommended. Patients with a diagnosis of HCM should avoid strenuous exercise and competitive sports, regardless of age, gender, symptoms, LVOT obstruction, or treatment.
2. Cardiac arrhythmias detected in patients with HCM should be treated appropriately.
   a. Ventricular arrhythmias. Special attention must be paid to ventricular arrhythmias; they are related to sudden death in patients with HCM. They may be treated with propranolol, amiodarone, and other standard antiarrhythmic agents guided by serial ambulatory ECG monitoring.
   b. AF occurs more often in patients with LA enlargement. It can possibly trigger ventricular arrhythmias in certain patients. For new-onset AF, electrical cardioversion followed by anticoagulation with warfarin (superior to aspirin) is recommended. Amiodarone is generally considered as the most effective agent for preventing the recurrence of AF.
3. Digitalis is contraindicated because it increases the degree of obstruction. Other cardiotonic drugs and vasodilators should be avoided because they tend to increase the pressure gradient. Diuretics usually are ineffective and can be harmful. However, judicious use can help improve congestive symptoms (e.g., exertional dyspnea, orthopnea) by reducing LV filling pressure.
4. Prospective screening of first-degree relatives and other family members should be encouraged and should begin at age 12 years with physical examination, ECG, echo study, and MRI.
5. Annual evaluation of adolescents (12–18 years of age) is recommended, regardless of symptoms, with physical examination, ECG, and two-dimensional echo studies.
6. Genetic testing for HCM sequencing and deletion/duplication panels are available from blood, oral rinse, or buccal (cheek) swabs.

Patients with Symptoms (Dyspnea, Chest Discomfort, Disability)

Exertional dyspnea and disability are caused by diastolic dysfunction with impaired filling caused by increased LV stiffness. Chest pain is probably caused by myocardial ischemia of severely hypertrophied LV. Beta-blockers and calcium channel blockers are effective therapies in children with HCM. These agents reduce hypercontractile systolic function and improve diastolic filling.

1. A beta-adrenergic blocker (e.g., propranolol, atenolol, or metoprolol) appears to be a preferred drug for symptomatic patients with outflow gradient, which develops only with exertion. Beta-blockers reduce the degree of outflow tract obstruction, decrease the incidence of anginal pain, and have antiarrhythmic effects.

In small children, propranolol is the drug of choice because of its liquid formulation and low side-effect profile. The dosage is 2 to 4 mg/kg/day given in three divided doses, with the heart rate goal of 80 to 100 beats/min. In older children, atenolol is typically used. In patients with excessive LVH and severe LVOT obstruction, a combination therapy with atenolol and verapamil may be considered.

2. Calcium channel blockers (principally verapamil) may be equally effective in both the nonobstructive and obstructive forms. Adverse hemodynamic effects may occur presumably as the result of vasodilating properties predominating over negative inotropic effects.

Asymptomatic Patients

Prophylactic therapy with either beta-adrenergic blockers or the calcium channel blocker verapamil is controversial in asymptomatic patients without LV obstruction. Some favor prophylactic administration of these drugs to prevent sudden death or to delay progression of the disease process; others limit prophylactic drug therapy to young patients with a family history of premature sudden death and those with particularly marked LVH. The efficacy of empiric prophylactic drug treatment with the above agents is unresolved.

Drug-Refractory Patients with Obstruction

When standard pharmacologic therapy fails, there are limited options. In small children with persistent LVOT obstruction, the Morrow's myectomy is the only option. In adults, alcohol septal ablation has been used, but it has not been used in children. In patients with syncope, ventricular arrhythmias, or other high-risk factors, implantable cardioverter–defibrillator (ICD) implantation should be considered.

1. **Morrow's myotomy–myectomy.** Transaortic LV septal myotomy–myectomy (the Morrow operation) is the procedure of choice for drug-refractory patients with LVOT obstruction. This operation is performed through an aortotomy without the benefit of complete direct visualization. Two vertical and parallel incisions are made (1 cm apart, 1–1.5 cm deep) into the hypertrophied ventricular septum. A third transverse incision connects the two incisions at their distal extent, and the bar of rectangular septal muscle is excised. Indication for the procedure is the presence of a resting pressure gradient of greater than 50 mm Hg by continuous-wave Doppler study in patients who are symptomatic despite medical management.

   The mortality rate, including for children, is 1% to 3%. Partial or complete left bundle branch block (LBBB) always results. Symptoms improve in most patients, but patients may later die of congestive symptoms and arrhythmias caused by the cardiomyopathy. Serious complications of the surgery such as complete heart block requiring permanent pacemaker and surgically induced ventricular septal defect (VSD) have become uncommon (1%–2%).

2. **Percutaneous alcohol septal ablation.** For adult patients with persistent LVOT obstruction, the introduction of absolute alcohol into a target septal perforator branch of the left anterior descending coronary artery produces myocardial infarction within the proximal ventricular septum. This is analogous to surgical myomectomy. A decrease in pressure gradient occurs after 6 to 12 months. A large proportion of patients demonstrate subjective improvement in symptoms and in quality of life. Increasing popularity of the procedure is probably unjustifiable. This procedure should not be considered a routine invasive procedure

because selection of the appropriate perforator branch is crucially important.

The procedure-related mortality rate is 1% to 4%. Permanent pacemaker implantation occurs in 1% to 4%. This procedure commonly results in right bundle branch block (RBBB) rather than LBBB seen with surgical myotomy.

3. **Pacemaker implantation.** Dual-chamber pacing was shown in earlier studies to reduce symptoms and the pressure gradient across the LVOT, but more recent studies did not support earlier findings. There are currently no data to support the contention that pacing improves survival or quality of life.

Implantable Cardioverter–Defibrillators

Recently, HCM has become one of the most frequent indications for ICD implantation in children with proven efficacy to prevent sudden death from arrhythmias. ICD reliably senses VT and VF and restores sinus rhythm by delivering appropriate defibrillation shock. Special consideration may be given to adolescents for ICD implantation because it is the period of life consistently showing the greatest predilection for sudden death. The strategy to implant ICD must be weighed against the distinct possibilities of device-related complications (including inappropriate shock and lead malfunction).

Implantable cardioverter–defibrillator implantation is warranted when the risk for sudden death is judged to be unacceptably high. The following are risk factors for sudden death in patients with HCM:

1. Prior cardiac arrest (VF)
2. Spontaneous sustained VT (3 beats or more or at least 120 beats/min)
3. Family history of premature sudden death
4. Unexplained syncope, particularly in young patients
5. LV thickness of 30 mm or greater, particularly in adolescents and young adults
6. Abnormal exercise blood pressure (attenuated response or hypotension)
7. Nonsustained VT

Mitral Valve Replacement

Mitral valve replacement with a low-profile prosthetic valve may be indicated in selected patients with symptomatic mitral regurgitation. The operative mortality rate is about 6%. About 70% of patients show symptomatic improvement, but complications related to the prosthetic valve occur.

INFANTS OF MOTHERS WITH DIABETES

Prevalence

At least 1.3% of pregnancies are complicated by diabetes mellitus.

Pathology

1. The teratogenic action of diabetes mellitus is generalized, affecting multiple organ systems. The prevalence of major congenital malformations in infants of mothers with diabetes is as high as 6% to 9% (i.e., three to four times that

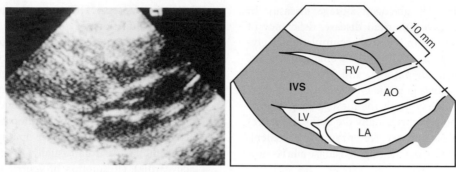

Fig. 18.7 Parasternal long-axis view of a two-dimensional echocardiogram of an infant of a mother with diabetes. There is asymmetrical hypertrophy of the interventricular septum (IVS), which is at least two times as thick as the posterior wall of the left ventricle (LV). *AO,* Aorta; *LA,* left atrium; *RV,* right ventricle.

found in the general population). Neural tube defects (anencephaly, myelomeningocele), congenital heart defects, and sacral dysgenesis or agenesis are common ones. Infants born to mothers with insulin-dependent diabetes are at highest risk for developing congenital malformations; infants born to mothers with non–insulin-dependent, well-controlled diabetes do not appear to have an increased risk of congenital malformations.

2. Infants of mothers with diabetes have a high prevalence of congenital heart defects, cardiomyopathy, and persistent pulmonary hypertension of the newborn (PPHN).

    a. The risk of congenital heart defect is three to four times greater than that in the general population, with VSD, transposition of the great arteries, truncus arteriosus, tricuspid atresia, and coarctation of the aorta (COA) among the more common defects.

    b. HCM with or without obstruction is seen in 10% to 20% of these infants. The weight of the heart is increased by the increased myocardial fiber size and number (rather than by excess glycogen, as once thought); the hypertrophy is thought to be caused by hyperinsulinemia. Although free walls of both ventricles and the ventricular septum are hypertrophied, the ventricular septum characteristically is more hypertrophied than the LV posterior wall (asymmetrical septal hypertrophy) (Fig. 18.7).

    c. Infants of mothers with diabetes also have an increased risk of PPHN. They often are affected by conditions that promote the persistence of pulmonary hypertension, such as hypoglycemia, perinatal asphyxia, respiratory distress, and polycythemia.

Clinical Manifestations

The clinical manifestations of only cardiomyopathy are presented in this section. Congenital heart defects and PPHN are discussed under specific headings.

1. The history usually reveals gestational or insulin-dependent diabetes mellitus in the mother. The patient often has a history of progressive respiratory distress with tachypnea (80–100 breaths/min) from birth.

2. These large-for-gestational-age babies often are plethoric and mildly cyanotic and may have tachypnea and

tachycardia (>160 beats/min). Signs of congestive heart failure (CHF) with gallop rhythm may be found in 5% to 10% of these babies. The patient may have a systolic murmur along the left sternal border, which may be caused by an outflow tract obstruction or an associated defect.

3. Chest radiography may reveal a varying degree of cardiomegaly. Pulmonary vascular markings are normal or mildly increased because of pulmonary venous congestion.

4. The ECG usually is nonspecific, but a long QT interval caused by a long ST-segment secondary to hypocalcemia may be found. Occasionally, RVH, LVH, or biventricular hypertrophy may be seen.

5. Echocardiography may show the following:

    a. The ventricular septum often is disproportionately thicker than the LV free wall, but even free walls are thicker than normal (see Fig. 18.7).

    b. Supernormal contractility of the LV and evidence of LVOT obstruction appear in about 50% of infants with cardiomyopathy.

    c. Rarely, the LV is dilated, and its contractility is decreased.

Management

1. General supportive measures are provided, such as intravenous fluids, correction of hypoglycemia and hypocalcemia, and ventilatory assistance, if indicated.

2. In most cases, the hypertrophy spontaneously resolves within the first 6 to 12 months of life. Beta-adrenergic blockers, such as propranolol, may help the LVOT obstruction, but treatment usually is not necessary. Digitalis and other inotropic agents are contraindicated because they may worsen the obstruction.

3. If the LV is dilated with decreased LV contractility, the usual anticongestive measures (e.g., digoxin, diuretics) are indicated.

OTHER RARE FORMS OF HYPERTROPHIC CARDIOMYOPATHIES

The following are some examples of HCM that manifest in syndromic forms.

1. **Pompe disease** (type II glycogen storage disease). In this autosomal recessive inherited disease, deficiency of α-1,4-glucosidase results in massive accumulation of glycogen in various organs, leading to an enlarged tongue, striking hepatomegaly, hypotonia, and HCM and CHF. The ECG typically shows gigantic QRS voltages and short PR interval. The disease typically manifests during the first 5 months of life, and patients usually die before their second year of life unless they receive enzyme replacement. Enzyme therapy with Myozyme (alglucosidase alfa) is now possible.

2. **Fabry disease.** Fabry disease is an X-linked recessive disorder with skin manifestations (angiokeratomas), corneal clouding, peripheral neuropathy, renal failure, and anhidrosis. It is caused by mutations in the gene encoding the enzyme α galactosidase A. Deposits of glycosphingolipids on various tissues, particularly the kidneys and coronary arteries, cause the most important disease manifestations. The diagnosis of the condition is often delayed until the adolescence or adulthood; the average age of first symptoms is 11 years, but the diagnosis is usually further delayed. Primary cardiac manifestations in affected males are HCM and MR. The ECG shows a short PR interval. Replacement enzyme infusion is now approved by the US Food and Drug Administration for treatment of this condition. This treatment resulted in clearance of pathological globotriaosylceramide deposits in the kidneys.

DILATED CARDIOMYOPATHY

Prevalence

Dilated cardiomyopathy, previously called congestive cardiomyopathy, is the most common form of cardiomyopathy in children, with an estimated incidence of 0.56 cases per 100,000 children per year. Although some children with the condition completely recover from the disease, it carries a high risk of mortality with many of them needing treatment for advanced heart failure therapies.

Cause

1. The causes of DCM are heterogeneous. The most common cause of DCM is idiopathic (~50%). About 20% to 35% of patients with idiopathic cardiomyopathy have been shown to have inherited familial DCM (Judge, 2009). Among the familial type, an autosomal dominant inheritance pattern is most frequent (occurring in 30%–50%); X-linked, autosomal recessive, and mitochondrial inheritance patterns are less common. There are at least 35 different genes in which mutation have been reported to cause DCM (Judge, 2009).

2. The most common known causes of DCM are myocarditis (46%) and neuromuscular diseases (~25%) followed by familial cardiomyopathy, active myocarditis, and other causes. Some cases of idiopathic DCM may be the result of subclinical myocarditis.

3. The most frequently recognized familial form is Duchenne muscular dystrophy.

4. Other rare causes of DCM include infectious causes other than viral infection (bacterial, fungal, protozoan, rickettsial), as well as endocrine and metabolic disorders (hyper- and hypothyroidism, excessive catecholamines, diabetes, hypocalcemia, hypophosphatemia, glycogen storage disease, mucopolysaccharidoses) and nutritional disorders (kwashiorkor, beriberi, carnitine deficiency).

5. Some of the patients with idiopathic type may have tachycardia-induced cardiomyopathy, which is related to chronic tachycardia (usually atrial or supraventricular tachycardia). (Resolution of ventricular dysfunction in 3 weeks after successful therapy may suggest the diagnosis, but echo improvement may take 3 to 20 weeks.)

6. Cardiotoxic agents such as doxorubicin and systemic diseases such as connective tissue diseases can also cause DCM.

Pathology and Pathophysiology

1. In DCM, a weakening of systolic contraction is associated with dilatation of all four cardiac chambers. Dilatation of the atria is in proportion to ventricular dilatation. The ventricular walls are not thickened, although heart weight is increased.

2. Intracavitary thrombus formation is common in the apical portion of the ventricular cavities and in atrial appendages and may give rise to pulmonary and systemic emboli.

3. Histologic examinations from endomyocardial biopsies show varying degrees of myocyte hypertrophy and fibrosis. Inflammatory cells are usually absent, but a varying incidence of inflammatory myocarditis has been reported.

Clinical Manifestations

History

1. A history of fatigue, weakness, and symptoms of left-sided heart failure (dyspnea on exertion, orthopnea) may be elicited.

2. A history of prior viral illness occasionally is obtained.

Physical Examination

1. Signs of CHF (tachycardia, pulmonary crackles, weak peripheral pulses, distended neck veins, hepatomegaly) are present. The apical impulse usually is displaced to the left and inferiorly.

2. The S2 may be normal or narrowly split with accentuated P2 if pulmonary hypertension develops. A prominent S3 is present with or without gallop rhythm. A soft regurgitant systolic murmur (caused by MR or tricuspid regurgitation [TR]) may be present.

Electrocardiography

1. Sinus tachycardia, LVH, and ST-T changes are the most common findings. Left or right atrial hypertrophy (left atrial hypertrophy [LAH] or right atrial hypertrophy [RAH]) may be present. Rarely, a healed anterior myocardial infarction pattern may be present.

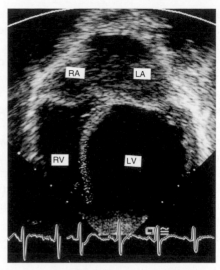

Fig. 18.8 Apical four-chamber view of two-dimensional echocardiogram showing a massively dilated left ventricular cavity in a 12-year-old child with dilated cardiomyopathy. *LA,* Left atrium; *LV,* left ventricle; *RA,* right atrium; *RV,* right ventricle.

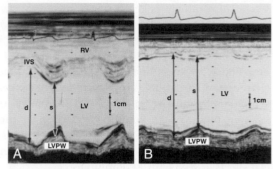

Fig. 18.9 M-mode echocardiogram in a child with dilated cardiomyopathy (DCM). **A,** M-mode echocardiogram from a 9-year-old normal child. The left ventricular (LV) diastolic dimension (d) is 36 mm, and the LV systolic dimension (s) is 24 mm, with resulting fractional shortening of 33%. **B,** M-mode echocardiogram from an 8-year-old child with DCM with a markedly decreased LV contractile function. The LV diastolic dimension (62 mm) and LV systolic dimension (52 mm) are markedly increased, with a marked decrease in the fractional shortening (16%). *IVS,* Interventricular septum; *LVPW,* LV posterior wall; *RV,* right ventricle.

2. Atrial or ventricular arrhythmias and AV conduction disturbances may be seen.

Radiography

Generalized cardiomegaly is usually present, with or without signs of pulmonary venous hypertension or pulmonary edema.

Echocardiography

Echocardiography is the most important tool in the diagnosis of the condition and is important in the longitudinal follow-up of patients.

1. Two-dimensional echocardiography shows a marked LV enlargement and poor contractility (Fig. 18.8). The LA may also be enlarged. Occasionally, an intracavitary thrombus may be found, especially in the left atrial appendage and cardiac apex. Pericardial effusion may be seen.
2. On M-mode echocardiography, the end-diastolic and end-systolic dimensions of the LV are increased, with a markedly reduced fractional shortening and ejection fraction (EF) of the LV (Fig. 18.9). The M-mode measurement provides a valuable technique for serial assessment of patients with DCM.
3. Mitral inflow Doppler tracing demonstrates a reduced E velocity and a decreased E/A ratio (ratio of E-wave to A-wave velocity) (see Fig. 18.6).

Other Laboratory Tests

1. Urine for organic and amino acids. 3-methylglutaconic acid (i.e., Barth syndrome)
2. Blood studies for complete blood count, comprehensive metabolic panel, lactate, calcium, magnesium, carnitine/acylcarnitine, thyroid function, creatine kinase and its MB fraction (CK-MB), troponin, brain natriuretic peptide (BNP) or its N-terminal fragment (NT-proBNP)
3. Genetic testing for DCM sequencing and deletion/duplication panels are available from blood, oral rinse, or buccal (cheek) swabs.

Cardiac Catheterization

Catheterization can be helpful to (1) exclude anomalous coronary artery; (2) predict etiology and prognosis by obtaining endomyocardial biopsy; and (3) evaluate for cardiac transplantation, including measurement of pulmonary vascular resistance. Endomyocardial biopsy typically shows varying degrees of myocyte hypertrophy and fibrosis without significant lymphocytic infiltration.

Natural History

1. Progressive deterioration is the rule rather than the exception. About two thirds of patients die from intractable heart failure within 4 years after the onset of symptoms of CHF. In one report in children, the 1- and 5-year rates of death or transplantation were 31% and 46%, respectively.
2. Atrial and ventricular arrhythmias develop with time (in ~50% of patients studied by 24-hour Holter) but are not predictive of outcome.
3. Systemic and pulmonary embolism resulting from dislodgment of intracavitary thrombi occurs in the late stages of the illness.
4. Causes of death are CHF, sudden death resulting from arrhythmias, and massive embolization.

Management

If no identifiable and treatable cause of DCM is found, therapy is supportive and consists of (1) an anticongestive regimen, (2) control of significant arrhythmias, and (3) minimizing the risk of thromboembolic complications.

1. Integral part of anticongestive regimen for DCM consists of inhibition of the renin–angiotensin–aldosterone system, diuretics, and digoxin, as well as bed rest or restriction of activity. Recently, beneficial effects of the combined use of angiotensin-converting enzyme (ACE) inhibitors and beta-blockers have been reported (Viollet et al, 2012).

a. Use of ACE inhibitors is a cornerstone of heart failure management in children. ACE inhibitors (captopril, enalapril) are the first line of drug to use, along with pulsed use of diuretics, according to guidelines recommended by the Canadian Cardiovascular Society (Kanto et al, 2013). ACE inhibitors reduce congestive symptoms by moving the Frank-Starling curve to the left and upward with resulting reduction in cardiac afterload and increase in stroke volume (see Fig. 27.2). Angiotensin receptor blockers may have similar beneficial effects as seen with ACE inhibitors.

b. The beneficial effects of beta-adrenergic blocking agents (somewhat unorthodox, given poor contractility) have been reported in adult patients with improvement in LV EF. Similar beneficial effects of beta-blockers have been reported in children with DCM of various causes. Carvedilol is a beta-adrenergic blocker with additional vasodilating action. Recent evidence suggests that activation of the sympathetic nervous system may have deleterious cardiac effects (rather than being an important compensatory mechanism, as traditionally thought). Beta-adrenergic blockers may exert beneficial effects by a negative chronotropic effect with reduced oxygen demand, reduction in catecholamine toxicity, inhibition of sympathetically mediated vasoconstriction, or reduction of potentially lethal ventricular arrhythmias. Further discussion on the use of beta-adrenergic blockers is presented in Chapter 27.

c. Diuretics (furosemide) remain as important medications in the treatment of congestion.

d. Digoxin, one of the old orally effective inotropic agents, is still commonly used.

e. Aldosterone antagonists (spironolactone) have also been shown to be beneficial with a 30% decrease in the risk of death at 24 months.

3. Antiplatelet agents (aspirin) should be initiated. The propensity for thrombus formation in patients with dilated cardiac chambers and blood stasis may prompt use of anticoagulation with warfarin. If thrombi are detected, they should be treated aggressively with heparin initially and later switched to long-term warfarin therapy.

4. Patients with arrhythmias may be treated with amiodarone or other antiarrhythmic agents. Amiodarone is effective and relatively safe in children. An ICD may be considered for high-risk patients. Children who are considered to have risk factors for sudden death in DCM include those with (a) LV end-diastolic dimension Z-score >2.6, (b) age at diagnosis before 14 years, and (c) an LV posterior wall thickness to end-diastolic dimension ratio of less than 0.14 (Pahl et al, 2012). For symptomatic bradycardia, a cardiac pacemaker may be necessary.

5. If carnitine deficiency is considered as the cause for the cardiomyopathy, carnitine supplementation should be started.

6. Beneficial effects of growth hormone (for 3–6 months' duration) were reported in adult patients with DCM, with increased LV wall thickness, reduction of the chamber size, and improved cardiac output. A small study involving children (McElhinney et al, 2004) has reported that administration of recombinant human growth hormone (0.025–0.04 mg/kg/day for 6 months) showed a trend toward improved LVEF, along with significant acceleration of somatic growth. Whether growth hormone treatment will finally find a place in the treatment of congestive cardiomyopathy remains to be established.

7. Children with severe decompensation may require mechanical circulatory support therapy with a ventricular assist device, intraaortic balloon counterpulsation, or extracorporeal membrane oxygenation (ECMO). In children, mechanical circulatory support commonly is a bridge to transplantation.

8. Many of these children with DCM may become candidates for cardiac transplantation.

Prognosis

The long-term outcomes of DCM vary depending on the underlying etiology but overall remain poor. Review of literature in children suggests that approximately one third die, one third recover completely, and one third improve with some residual cardiac dysfunction.

ENDOCARDIAL FIBROELASTOSIS

Prevalence

The prevalence of the nonfamilial form of endocardial fibroelastosis is extremely rare. The prevalence has declined in the past 3 decades for unknown reasons; in the past, it accounted for 4% of cardiac autopsy cases in children.

Pathology

1. Primary endocardial fibroelastosis is a form of DCM seen in infants. The condition is characterized by diffuse changes in the endocardium with a white, opaque, glistening appearance. The heart chambers, primarily the LA and LV, are notably dilated and hypertrophied. Involvement of the right-sided heart chambers is rare. Deformities and shortening of the papillary muscles and chordae tendineae (resulting in MR) are often present late in the course. Similar pathology appears secondary to severe congenital obstructive lesions of the left heart, such as AS, COA, and hypoplastic left heart syndrome (called *secondary fibroelastosis*).

2. The cause of primary fibroelastosis is not known. It may be the result of a process of reaction to many different insults rather than a specific disease. Viral myocarditis and a sequela to interstitial myocarditis have received more attention than other proposed causes, including systemic carnitine deficiency and genetic factors. The mumps virus genome has been found in the myocardium in a significant number of patients with the diagnosis, suggesting that endocardial fibroelastosis is a complication of myocarditis caused by the mumps virus; the decrease of the incidence of this condition is believed to be in accord of decline with worldwide disappearance of mumps.

Clinical Manifestations

1. Symptoms and signs of CHF (feeding difficulties, tachypnea, sweating, irritability, pallor, failure to thrive) develop in the first 10 months of life.
2. Patients have tachycardia and tachypnea. No heart murmur is audible in the majority of patients, although a gallop rhythm usually is present. Occasionally, a heart murmur of MR is audible. Hepatomegaly frequently is present.
3. The ECG typically shows LVH with "strain." Occasionally, myocardial infarction patterns, arrhythmias, and varying degrees of AV block may be seen.
4. Chest radiographs show marked generalized cardiomegaly with normal or congested pulmonary vascularity.
5. Echocardiography characteristically shows a markedly dilated and poorly contracting LV in the absence of structural heart defects. The LA also is markedly dilated. Bright endocardial echoes are typical of the condition.
6. Cardiac MRI has also been used to diagnose this condition by emission of hyperintense signals during myocardial delayed-enhancement sequences.

Management

1. Early diagnosis and long-term (for years) treatment with digoxin, diuretics, and afterload-reducing agents are mandatory. Digoxin is continued for a minimum of 2 to 3 years and is then gradually discontinued if symptoms are absent, heart size is normal, and the ECG has reverted to normal.
2. An afterload-reducing agent may be beneficial.

Prognosis

When proper treatment is instituted, about one third of patients deteriorate and die of CHF. Another third survive but experience persistent symptoms. The remaining third exhibit complete recovery. Operative procedures are not available.

DOXORUBICIN CARDIOMYOPATHY

Prevalence

Anthracyclines remain among the most widely used and effective anticancer agents. Unfortunately, life-threatening anthracycline cardiomyopathy continues to develop among survivors of cancer. Its prevalence is nonlinearly dose related, occurring in 2% to 5% of patients who have received a cumulative dose of 400 to 500 mg/m^2 of doxorubicin (Adriamycin) and up to 50% of patients who have received more than 1000 mg/m^2 of the drug. It may be seen occasionally in patients who received only 220 mg/m^2. When radiation therapy is combined with doxorubicin, the risk of cardiac damage is even greater.

Cause

1. C-13 anthracycline metabolites, which are inhibitors of adenosine triphosphatases of sarcoplasmic reticulum, mitochondria, and sarcolemma, have been implicated in the mechanism of cardiotoxicity causing cardiomyopathy.
2. Risk factors for developing doxorubicin cardiomyopathy may include the following.

a. Cumulative dose of anthracyclines greater than 360 mg/m^2 are 40 times more likely to die than those who received less than 240 mg/m^2.
b. Age younger than 4 years
c. A dosing regimen with larger and less frequent doses has been raised as a risk factor but not proved.
d. Concomitant cardiac irradiation

Pathology and Pathophysiology

1. Dilated LV, decreased contractility, elevated filling pressures of the LV, and reduced cardiac output characterize pathophysiologic features.
2. Microscopically, interstitial edema without evidence of inflammatory changes, loss of myofibrils within the myocyte, vacuolar degeneration, necrosis, and fibrosis are present.

Clinical Manifestations

1. Patients are usually asymptomatic until signs of heart failure develop. Patients have a history of receiving doxorubicin, with the onset of symptoms 2 to 4 months, and rarely years, after completion of therapy. Tachypnea and dyspnea made worse by exertion are the usual presenting complaints. Occasionally, palpitation, cough, and substernal discomfort are complaints.
2. Signs of CHF develop, with hepatomegaly and distended neck veins. Gallop rhythm may be present, with occasional soft murmur of MR or TR.
3. Radiography shows cardiomegaly with or without pulmonary congestion or pleural effusion.
4. The ECG shows sinus tachycardia. T-wave flattening or inversion is nonspecific evidence of cardiac involvement.
5. Echocardiographic abnormalities of DCM occur within 1 year after doxorubicin treatment and may include the following:
   a. The LV size is slightly increased, and the LV wall thickness slightly decreased.
   b. LV contractility (either EF or fractional shortening) is decreased. Cardiotoxicity is defined as an LVEF decline of 5% or greater to less than 55% with heart failure symptoms or an asymptomatic decrease of LVEF 10% or greater to less than 55% (Curigliano et al, 2012).
6. During doxorubicin therapy, an acute ECG changes may include a prolonged QT interval occurring in 40% of patients immediately after a single dose. Echo may show reduced LV systolic function (EF or fractional shortening) during therapy. Stopping therapy based on these changes may not be justified.

Management

1. Attempts to prevent anthracycline cardiomyopathy have been directed toward (a) anthracycline dose limitation, (b) method of drug administration, (c) developing less cardiotoxic analogs, (d) concurrently administering cardioprotective agents to attenuate the cardiotoxic effects of anthracycline to the heart, and (e) secondary prevention strategies of early detection of cardiotoxicity and early initiation of therapy.

a. Restriction of the total dose is controversial. Limiting the total cumulative dose to 400 to 500 mg/m^2 reduces the incidence of CHF to 5%, but this dose may not be effective in treating some malignancies.

b. Continuous slow infusion therapy may reduce cardiac injury by avoiding peak levels. At least one study recommends infusion over 6 hours. However, a more recent study (Lipshultz et al, 2012) has reported no long-term cardioprotection of continuous infusion over bolus infusion.

c. Liposomal doxorubicin (which contains doxorubicin wrapped up in a fatty covering called liposome) preserves anticancer properties of the drug but reduces cardiotoxicity.

d. Concurrent administration of the cardioprotective agents, such as dexrazoxane (an iron chelator), carvedilol (a beta-receptor antagonist with antioxidant property), and enalapril (an ACE inhibitor) have shown varying levels of protective effects. Among these, dexrazoxane appears to be most cardioprotective, and some authorities recommend dexrazoxane to be included in the pediatric oncology protocol.

e. Early detection of cardiotoxicity by echo study (LVEF <55%) and early initiation of drug therapy with enalapril plus carvedilol appear to make LV systolic function recovery more likely.

2. When anthracycline cardiomyopathy is diagnosed, management is the same as discussed earlier for DCM in general. Currently, the following medications are used.

a. Afterload-reducing agents (ACE inhibitors, e.g., enalapril), diuretics, and digoxin are useful.

b. Beta-blockers have been shown to be beneficial in some children with chemotherapy-induced cardiomyopathy, similar to what has been reported in adults. Carvedilol, a nonselective beta-blocker, also has vasodilator effect and antioxidant activity.

3. Cardiac transplantation may be an option for selected patients.

Prognosis

Symptomatic cardiomyopathy carries a high mortality rate. The 2-year survival rate is about 20%, and all patients die by 9 years after the onset of the illness.

CARNITINE DEFICIENCY

Carnitine deficiency is a rare cause of cardiomegaly in infants and small children. Carnitine is an essential cofactor for transport of long-chain fatty acids into mitochondria, where oxidation takes place. Carnitine deficiency leads to depressed mitochondrial oxidation of fatty acids, resulting in storage of fat in muscle and functional abnormalities of cardiac and skeletal muscle. It is synthesized predominantly in the liver.

Primary carnitine deficiency is an uncommon inherited disorder. The condition has been classified as either systemic or myopathic.

The systemic form of the disease manifests with low concentrations of carnitine in plasma, muscle, and liver. Symptoms are variable but include muscle weakness, cardiomyopathy, abnormal liver function, encephalopathy, impaired ketogenesis, and hypoglycemia during fasting. In systemic carnitine deficiency, patients may present with acute hepatic hypoglycemia and encephalopathy during the first year of life before the cardiomyopathy becomes symptomatic. Both hypertrophic and DCMs have been reported with carnitine deficiency.

Myopathic disease is characterized primarily by muscle weakness. Fatty infiltration of muscle fiber is found at biopsy. The most common manifestation of myopathic carnitine deficiency is progressive cardiomyopathy, with or without skeletal muscle weakness that begins at 2 to 4 years of age.

Patients with cardiomyopathy may show bizarre T wave spiking on the ECG. These children may die suddenly, presumably from arrhythmias.

Secondary forms of carnitine deficiency have been reported in renal tubular disorders (with excessive excretion of carnitine), chronic renal failure (excessive loss of carnitine from hemodialysis), inborn errors of metabolism with increased concentrations of organic acids, and occasional patients receiving total parental nutrition. Diagnosis of the condition is established by extremely low level of carnitine in plasma and skeletal muscle.

Treatment

1. Treatment with oral carnitine (L-carnitine: 50–100 mg/kg/day orally, divided twice or thrice a day; maximum daily dose, 3 g) may improve myocardial function, reduce cardiomegaly, and improve muscle weakness.

2. A recent multicenter study has shown that treatment of various forms of cardiomyopathy with L-carnitine, especially those with suggestive evidence of disorders of metabolism, provided clinical benefits.

3. Benefits of carnitine administration has been reported for other conditions with myocardial dysfunction, including prevention of diphtheric myocarditis in children and potential protective and therapeutic effects on doxorubicin-induced cardiomyopathy in rats.

BARTH SYNDROME

Barth syndrome is a sex-linked cardioskeletal myopathy with abnormal mitochondria and neutropenia. This disorder typically presents in male infants as CHF associated with neutropenia (cyclic) and 3-methylglutaconic academia. Echocardiography shows LV dysfunction with LV dilation, endocardial fibroelastosis, or a dilated hypertrophic LV. Some infants die from CHF, VT, or sepsis caused by leukocyte dysfunction. Most children survive infancy and do well clinically, although CDM usually persists. Some require cardiac transplantation.

RESTRICTIVE CARDIOMYOPATHY

Prevalence and Cause

Restrictive cardiomyopathy is an extremely rare form of cardiomyopathy, accounting for 5% of cardiomyopathy cases in children. It may be idiopathic or may be associated with a systemic infiltrative disease (e.g., scleroderma, amyloidosis, and sarcoidosis) or an inborn error of metabolism (mucopolysaccharidosis). Malignancies or radiation therapy may result in restrictive cardiomyopathy.

Pathology and Pathophysiology

1. This condition is characterized by markedly dilated atria and normal or decreased volume of both ventricles. Ventricular diastolic filling is impaired, resulting from excessively stiff ventricular walls. Systolic function of the ventricle is normal (or near normal). Therefore, this condition resembles constrictive pericarditis in clinical presentation and hemodynamic abnormalities.
2. There are areas of myocardial fibrosis and hypertrophy of myocytes, or the myocardium may be infiltrated by various materials. Infiltrative restrictive cardiomyopathy may be caused by conditions such as amyloidosis, sarcoidosis, hemochromatosis, glycogen deposit, Fabry's disease (with deposition of glycosphingolipids), or neoplastic infiltration.
3. Development of pulmonary hypertension caused by diastolic dysfunction is a significant problem in children as it is in adults.

Clinical Manifestations

1. Patients may have a history of exercise intolerance, weakness and dyspnea, or chest pain.
2. Jugular venous distention, hepatomegaly, a loud pulmonary component of S2 (P2), gallop rhythm, and a systolic murmur of AV valve regurgitation may be present.
3. Chest radiography shows cardiomegaly, pulmonary venous congestion, and occasional pleural effusion.
4. The ECG usually shows LAH, RAH, or both. It may show AF and paroxysms of supraventricular tachycardia. AV block may be present in familial restrictive cardiomyopathy.
5. Echocardiographic studies reveal:
   a. Marked dilated atria with normal dimension of the LV and right ventricle (RV) is almost diagnostic.
   b. LV systolic function is normal or near normal (until the late stage of the disease).
   c. Atrial thrombus may be present.
   d. Findings of diastolic dysfunction are present; the mitral inflow Doppler tracing shows an increased E velocity, shortened deceleration time, and increased E/A ratio (see Fig. 18.6).
   e. Differentiation from constrictive pericarditis can pose difficulties. In constrictive pericarditis, echocardiography shows a thickened pericardium, and Doppler studies show a marked respiratory variation in the filling phase. Doppler studies also show similar findings of diastolic dysfunction as those seen in restrictive cardiomyopathy.
6. Cardiac catheterization should be performed. It shows elevated LV and RV end-diastolic pressures and frequent pulmonary hypertension (with elevated pulmonary vascular resistance). Endomyocardial biopsy reveals myocyte hypertrophy and interstitial fibrosis; it may also reveal a specific cause.

Management

Treatment is nonspecific and directed at alleviating symptoms. In general, medical therapy does not improve survival. The prognosis is poor.

1. Diuretics are beneficial to relieve congestive symptoms, but they should be used judiciously because they can reduce end-diastolic pressure, making symptoms worse. Digoxin is not indicated because systolic function is unimpaired. ACE inhibitors may reduce systemic blood pressure without increasing cardiac output and therefore should probably be avoided.
2. Calcium channel blockers may be used to increase diastolic compliance.
3. Anticoagulants (warfarin) and antiplatelet drugs (aspirin and dipyridamole) may help prevent thrombosis.
4. Most classes of drugs used to treat pulmonary hypertension are not useful and some are harmful.
5. A permanent pacemaker is indicated for complete heart block.
6. Because current medical therapy appears ineffective, the development of pulmonary hypertension is common, and the mortality rate is high, cardiac transplantation is the definite therapy. Early transplantation is preferable before severe pulmonary hypertension develops. In patients with systemic disease (e.g., sarcoidosis), recurrence is a major concern after transplantation and it may not be a viable option.

ARRHYTHMOGENIC CARDIOMYOPATHY

This cardiomyopathy is also known as arrhythmogenic RV dysplasia, arrhythmogenic RV cardiomyopathy, RV dysplasia, or RV cardiomyopathy.

Cause

1. Most cases appear to be sporadic, although familial occurrences have been reported. Arrhythmogenic cardiomyopathy is caused by genetic defects of the myocardial desmosomes, mostly affecting the RV which may occur in the LV as well. The mode of inheritance is autosomal dominant.
2. An inflammatory process, possibly infection (by coxsackievirus B3 and adenovirus), has been implicated as a cause as well.
3. The prevalence of the disease is not known, but it is estimated to range from 1 in 1000 to 1 in 5000 population.

Pathology

1. This is a rare abnormality in which the myocardium of the RV is partially or totally replaced by fibrous or adipose tissue. The RV wall may assume a paper-thin appearance because of the total absence of myocardial tissue, but in others, RV wall thickness is normal or near normal. The LV is also often affected.
2. Histologic sections show a variable reduction in myofibrils and inflammation associated with interstitial infiltration by histocytes and lymphocytes.

Clinical Manifestations

1. The onset is in infancy, childhood, or adulthood (but usually before the age of 20 years) with a history of palpitation,

syncopal episodes, or both. Sudden or aborted cardiac death may be the first sign of the disease.

2. The physical examination is usually normal. An irregular rhythm or signs of heart failure may occasionally be present.

3. The ECG is helpful. Tall P waves in lead II (right atrial hypertrophy) and decreased RV forces may be present. Inverted T waves in the right precordial leads (V1–V4) may be significant (although this pattern is normally seen in young children). Postexcitations (epsilon waves), which occur secondary to slowed intraventricular depolarization, may be seen on ECG; the visualization of these late potentials could be enhanced by signal-averaged ECG (SAECG), a technique that suppresses the electrical interference and augments small segments of electrical activities of the standard ECG. ECG may show premature ventricular contractions or VT with LBBB morphology. An incomplete RBBB pattern may be present (in >30% of the cases).

4. Chest radiography usually show no or minimal cardiomegaly. Pulmonary vascular markings are usually normal.

5. Echocardiography shows selective RV enlargement and often systolic bulging or areas of akinesia or dyskinesia.

6. Cardiac MRI can visualize RV enlargement, aneurysm, systolic bulging of the RV free wall, myocardial fibrosis, and inflammation. Cardiac MRI is emerging as a more definite diagnostic tool than endomyocardial biopsy because the ventricular septum may lack the characteristic histologic changes.

7. Cardiac catheterization may show an elevated right atrial "a" wave. An RV angiogram usually shows RV systolic dysfunction. The hallmark of the disease is systolic bulging of the RV free wall. Endomyocardial biopsy of the RV septum shows classic pathologic changes in more than 90% of the patients but with a high false-negative rate.

8. A substantial portion of patients die before 5 years of age from CHF and intractable VT.

Management

1. Various antiarrhythmic agents may be tried, but they are often unsuccessful in abolishing VT.

2. Surgical intervention (ventricular incision or complete electrical disarticulation of the RV free wall) may be tried if antiarrhythmic therapy is unsuccessful.

3. An ICD may be indicated in selected cases.

NONCOMPACTION CARDIOMYOPATHY

Noncompaction cardiomyopathy, also known as LV noncompaction, LV hypertrabeculation, or spongy myocardium, has been suggested to be the result of an intrauterine arrest of normal compaction of the loose interwoven meshwork of the ventricular myocardium (which normally occurs during the first month of fetal life). Several gene mutations in patients with noncompaction cardiomyopathy have been reported; thus, the genetic testing of the relatives of an index case has been recommended by the Heart Rhythm Society when a mutation-specific gene has been identified.

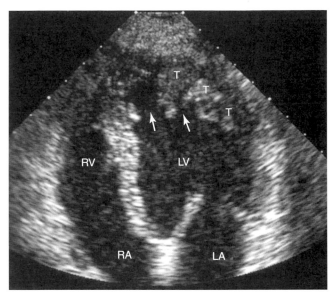

Fig. 18.10 Noncompaction cardiomyopathy. Apical four-chamber view of a two-dimensional echocardiogram showing characteristic increase in trabeculation (T) and deep recesses *(arrows)* in the left ventricular apical area. (From Connolly HM, Oh JK: Echocardiography. In Bonow RO, Mann DL, Zipes DP, Libby P (eds): *Braunwald's Heart Disease*, ed 9, Philadelphia, 2012, Saunders. Used with permission.)

Clinical Manifestations

1. Most of the patients with this disorder are asymptomatic. Occasionally, they may present with signs and symptoms of heart failure during infancy. Familial occurrence has been reported in up to 25% with a less severe form of the disease.

2. Physical examination findings may be entirely normal in some patients. Associated dysmorphic facial features may be seen in 14%. Nearly 30% of the patients have neurologic disorders, including seizures, hypotonia, myopathy, or mental or motor retardation. Patients with dysmorphic features or neuromuscular disorders may have associated metabolic disorders. It may coexist with various congenital heart defects. Signs of LV dysfunction may be present when the diagnosis is made; if not, most of them eventually develop CHF.

3. The ECG may show giant QRS complexes, sometimes with Wolff-Parkinson-White preexcitation. Chest radiography findings are usually normal.

4. Echocardiography findings
   a. Characteristic echocardiography findings are segmental thickening of the LV wall consisting of two layers with a thin, compacted epicardial layer and an extremely thickened noncompacted endocardial layer with prominent trabeculations and deep recesses. The apical and midventricular segment of both the inferior and lateral walls are most commonly affected (Fig. 18.10).
   b. The LV is uniformly affected, resulting in systolic and diastolic dysfunction and clinical heart failure. The RV is rarely affected, but it is difficult to demonstrate by echocardiographic study. In pediatric patients, LV systolic dysfunction is seen in 35% to 90% at diagnosis and during follow-up.

5. When echocardiography studies are inconclusive, cardiac MRI should be obtained. MRI not only helps establish the diagnosis but can also find RV dysfunction in 16% of patients.

6. The disease is usually progressive with worsening of heart failure despite optimal treatment. Arrhythmias and thromboembolic events are mostly seen in adults, but they may also be seen in children.

Treatment

Treatment should be directed toward its complications. The most common complication of the disease is heart failure. Less common complications are thromboembolic events and ventricular arrhythmias, more frequently seen in adult patients.

1. Anticongestive measures with digoxin, diuretics, and afterload-reducing agents are usually used.

2. In addition to the usual anticongestive measures, the use of carvedilol, a beta-blocker, should be considered in patients with LV dysfunction. Carvedilol has been shown to improve LV dysfunction.

3. All patients should be on an antiplatelet dose of aspirin. If thrombosis is detected, anticoagulation with warfarin should be started.

4. Appropriate antiarrhythmic therapy is indicated. Implantation of an ICD may be considered for life-threatening ventricular arrhythmias.

5. Patients with dysmorphic features or neurologic manifestations may need detailed metabolic screening (e.g., fatty acid oxidation disorder or mitochondrial disease).

6. Heart transplantation is a possible option for selected patients.

Cardiovascular Infections

Included in this chapter are infective endocarditis (IE), myocarditis, pericarditis, Lyme carditis, and postperfusion syndrome. Other conditions in which the cause is not well established but the host's immune response to an infective agent is thought to play a role are also included, such as Kawasaki's disease (KD) and postpericardiotomy syndrome.

INFECTIVE ENDOCARDITIS

Prevalence

Infective endocarditis (excluding postoperative endocarditis) accounts for 0.5 to 1 of every 1000 hospital admissions.

Pathogenesis

1. Two factors are important in the pathogenesis of IE: (a) a damaged area of endothelium and (b) bacteremia, even transient. The presence of structural abnormalities of the heart or great arteries, with a significant pressure gradient or turbulence, produces endothelial damage. Such endothelial damage induces thrombus formation with deposition of sterile clumps of platelet and fibrin (nonbacterial thrombus). Prosthetic valve or prosthetic materials used in surgery also promote deposition of sterile thrombus. Nonbacterial thrombus provides a nidus for bacteria to adhere and eventually form infected vegetation. Platelets and fibrin are deposited over the organisms, leading to the enlargement of the vegetation.

2. Almost all patients who develop IE have a history of congenital or acquired heart disease. Drug addicts may develop endocarditis in the absence of known cardiac anomalies.

3. All congenital heart defects, with the exception of secundum-type atrial septal defect (ASD), predispose to endocarditis. More frequently encountered defects are tetralogy of Fallot (TOF), ventricular septal defect (VSD), aortic valve disease, transposition of the great arteries (TGA), and systemic–to–pulmonary artery (PA) shunt. Those with a prosthetic heart valve or prosthetic material in the heart are at particularly high risk of developing endocarditis. Patients with mitral valve prolapse (MVP) with mitral regurgitation (MR) and those with rheumatic MR also are vulnerable to IE.

4. Bacteremia resulting from dental procedures can cause IE (Table 19.1). Bacteremia also occurs with activities such

as chewing or brushing the teeth. Chewing with diseased teeth or gums may be the most frequent cause of bacteremia. Therefore, good dental hygiene is very important in the prevention of IE.

Pathology

Vegetation of IE is usually found on the low-pressure side of the defect, either around the defect or on the opposite surface of the defect where endothelial damage is established by the jet effect of the defect. For example, vegetations are found in the PA in patent ductus arteriosus (PDA) or systemic-to-PA shunts, on the atrial surface of the mitral valve in MR, on the ventricular surface of the aortic valve and mitral chordae in aortic regurgitation (AR), and on the superior surface of the aortic valve or at the site of a jet lesion in the aorta in patients with aortic stenosis (AS).

Microbiology

1. In the past, *Streptococcus viridans*, enterococci, and *Staphylococcus aureus* were responsible for more than 90% of the cases. In recent years, this frequency has decreased to 50% to 60%, with a concomitant increase in cases caused by fungi and HACEK organisms (*Haemophilus, Actinobacillus, Cardiobacterium, Eikenella,* and *Kingella* spp.). HACEK organisms are particularly common in neonates and immunocompromised children, accounting for 17% to 30% of cases.
2. Alpha-hemolytic streptococci (*S. viridans*) are the most common causes of endocarditis in patients who have had dental procedures or in those with carious teeth or periodontal disease.
3. Staphylococci (*S. aureus* and coagulase-negative staphylococci) account for more cases than *S. viridans* in developed countries, usually health care–associated infections.
   a. The organisms most commonly found in postoperative endocarditis are staphylococci.
   b. IE associated with indwelling vascular catheters, prosthetic material, and prosthetic valve is frequently caused by *S. aureus* or coagulase-negative staphylococci.

c. Among newborn infants, *S. aureus* and coagulase-negative staphylococci (and *Candida* spp.) are the most common causes of IE.
   d. Intravenous (IV) drug abusers are at risk for IE from *S. aureus*.
4. Enterococci are the organisms most often found after genitourinary (GU) or gastrointestinal (GI) surgery or instrumentation.
5. Fungal endocarditis (which has a poor prognosis) may occur in sick neonates, in patients who are on long-term antibiotic or steroid therapy, or after open-heart surgery. Fungal endocarditis is often associated with very large friable vegetations; emboli from these vegetations frequently produce serious complications.
6. Culture-negative endocarditis. A diagnosis of culture-negative endocarditis is made when a patient has clinical or echocardiographic evidence of endocarditis but persistently negative blood cultures. The most common cause of culture-negative endocarditis is current or recent antibiotic therapy or infection caused by a fastidious organism that grows poorly in vitro. Fungal endocarditis is a rare cause of culture-negative endocarditis. At times, the diagnosis can be made only by removal of vegetation (during surgery). In the United States, about 5% to 7% are culture-negative endocarditis.

Clinical Manifestations
History

1. Most patients have a history of an underlying heart defect. However, some patients with bicuspid aortic valve may not have been diagnosed with the defect before the onset of the endocarditis.
2. A history of a recent dental procedure or tonsillectomy is occasionally present, but a history of toothache (from dental or gingival disease) is more frequent than a history of a procedure.
3. A history of recent cardiovascular procedures or surgeries or hospital care may be present.
4. Endocarditis is rare in infancy; at this age, it usually follows open-heart surgery.

TABLE 19.1	**Prophylactic Regimens for Dental Procedures**		
		SINGLE DOSE 30-60 MIN BEFORE PROCEDURE	
Situation	**Agent**	**Children**	**Adults**
Oral	Amoxicillin	50 mg/kg	2 g
Unable to take oral medications	Ampicillin, or	50 mg/kg (IM, IV)	2 g (IM, IV)
	Cefazolin or ceftriaxone	50 mg/kg (IM, IV)	1 g (IM, IV)
Allergic to penicillin or ampicillin (PO)	Cephalexin[a,b] or	50 mg/kg	2 g
	Clindamycin or	20 mg/kg	600 mg
	Azithromycin or	15 mg/kg	500 mg
	Clarithromycin	15 mg/kg	500 mg
Allergic to penicillin or ampicillin and unable to take oral medication	Cefazolin or ceftriaxone	50 mg/kg (IM, IV)	1 g (IM, IV)
	Clindamycin	20 mg/kg (IM, IV)	600 mg (IM, IV)

[a]Or other first- or second-generation oral cephalosporin in equivalent adult or pediatric dosage.
[b]Cephalosporins should not be used in an individual with a history of anaphylaxis, angioedema, or urticaria with penicillin or ampicillin.
IM, Intramuscular; *IV,* intravenous; *PO,* oral.

5. The onset is usually insidious with prolonged low-grade fever and somatic complaints, including fatigue, weakness, loss of appetite, pallor, arthralgia, myalgias, weight loss, and diaphoresis.

Physical Examination

1. Heart murmur is universal (100%). The appearance of a new heart murmur and an increase in the intensity of an existing murmur are important. However, many innocent heart murmurs are also of new onset.
2. Fever is common (80%–90%). Fever fluctuates between 101° and 103°F (38.3° and 39.4°C).
3. Splenomegaly is common (70%).
4. Skin manifestations (50%) (either secondary to microembolization or as an immunologic phenomenon) may be present in the following forms:
   a. Petechiae on the skin, mucous membranes, or conjunctivae are the most frequent skin lesions.
   b. Osler's nodes (tender, pea-sized red nodes at the ends of the fingers or toes) are rare in children.
   c. Janeway's lesions (small, painless, hemorrhagic areas on the palms or soles) are rare.
   d. Splinter hemorrhages (linear hemorrhagic streaks beneath the nails) also are rare.
5. Embolic or immunologic phenomena in other organs are present in 50% of cases:
   a. Pulmonary emboli may occur in patients with VSD, PDA, or a systemic-to-PA shunt.
   b. Seizures and hemiparesis are the result of embolization to the central nervous system (CNS) (20%) and are more common with left-sided defects such as aortic and mitral valve disease or with cyanotic heart disease.
   c. Hematuria and renal failure may occur.

d. Roth's spots (oval, retinal hemorrhages with pale centers located near the optic disc) occur in fewer than 5% of patients.
6. Carious teeth or periodontal or gingival disease is frequently present.
7. Clubbing of fingers in the absence of cyanosis develops rarely in more chronic cases.
8. Signs of heart failure may be present as a complication of the infection.
9. The clinical manifestations in a neonate with IE are nonspecific (respiratory distress, tachycardia) and may be indistinguishable from septicemia or congestive heart failure (CHF) from other causes. Embolic phenomena (e.g., osteomyelitis, meningitis, pneumonia) are common. Patients may have neurologic signs and symptoms (seizures, hemiparesis, apnea).

Laboratory Studies

1. Positive blood cultures are found in more than 90% of patients in the absence of previous antimicrobial therapy. Antimicrobial pretreatment reduces the yield of positive blood culture to 50% to 60%.
2. A complete blood cell count shows anemia, with hemoglobin levels lower than 12 g/100 mL (present in 80% of patients), and leukocytosis with a shift to the left. Patients with polycythemia preceding the onset of IE may have normal hemoglobin.
3. The sedimentation rate is increased unless there is polycythemia.
4. Elevated C-reactive protein (CRP)
5. Microscopic hematuria is found in 30% of patients.

Echocardiography

Two-dimensional echocardiography is the main modality for detecting endocardial infection (Fig 19.1). It detects the

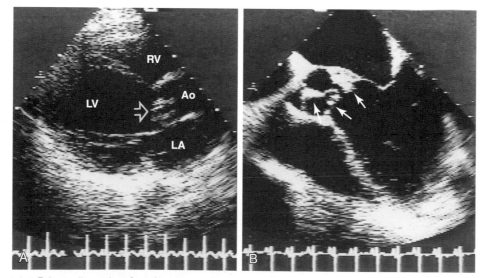

Fig. 19.1 Echocardiography of aortic valve vegetation. **A,** Parasternal long-axis view of a young adult patient with a bicuspid aortic valve demonstrating vegetation on the aortic valve *(arrow)*. Severe aortic regurgitation was present, with a dilated left ventricle (LV). **B,** Five-chamber transverse plane of a transesophageal echocardiographic image in the same patient that demonstrates vegetations and aortic valve anatomy more clearly than the ordinary two-dimensional echocardiography. *Ao,* Aorta; *LA,* left atrium; *RV,* right ventricle.

site of infection, extent of valvular damage, and cardiac function. Baseline evaluation of ventricular function and cardiac chamber dimension is important for comparison later in the course of the infection. Color Doppler is a sensitive modality for detection of valvular regurgitation.

1. Certain echo findings are included as major criteria in the modified Duke criteria. They include:
   a. Oscillating intracardiac mass on valve or supporting structures, in the path of regurgitation jets, or on implanted material
   b. Abscesses
   c. New partial dehiscence of prosthetic valve
   d. New valvular regurgitation

2. Although standard transthoracic echocardiography (TTE) is sufficient in most clinical circumstances, transesophageal echocardiography (TEE) may be an important adjunct to TTE in the obese or very muscular adolescents, in post-cardiac surgery patients, or in the presence of compromised respiratory function or pulmonary hyperinflation. TEE may be superior to TTE in identifying vegetations on prosthetic valves, detecting complications of left ventricular (LV) outflow tract endocarditis (either valvular or subvalvular), and detecting aortic root abscess and involvement of sinus of Valsalva.

3. The absence of vegetations on echo does not in itself rule out IE. Both TTE and TEE may produce false-negative results if vegetations are small or have already embolized, and they may miss initial perivalvular abscess. Repeat examinations are indicated if suspicion exists without diagnosis of IE or worrisome clinical course during early treatment of IE.

4. Conversely, a false-positive diagnosis is possible. An echogenic mass may represent a sterile thrombus, sterile prosthetic material, normal anatomic variation, an abnormal uninfected valve (previous scarring, severe myxomatous changes), or improper gain of the echo machine. Echo evidence of vegetation may persist for months or years after bacteriologic cure.

5. Certain echo features suggest a high risk case or a need for surgery:
   a. Large vegetations (greatest risk when the vegetation is >10 mm)
   b. Severe valvular regurgitation
   c. Abscess cavities
   d. Pseudoaneurysm
   e. Valvular perforation or dehiscence
   f. Decompensated heart failure

Diagnosis

The diagnosis of IE would be easy in the presence of classical features such as fever, heart murmur, skin manifestations, splenomegaly, and positive blood culture. Unfortunately, in everyday clinical practice, this presentation is rarely seen these days, and an atypical presentation occurs more frequently. At present time, the clinical diagnosis of IE relies on integration of clinical presentation, microbiological results, echocardiographic findings, and laboratory findings. In 2005,

---

BOX 19.1 Definition of Infective Endocarditis According to the Modified Duke Criteria

Definite Infective Endocarditis
A. Pathological criteria
   1. Microorganisms demonstrated by culture or histologic examination of a vegetation, a vegetation that has embolized, or an intracardiac abscess specimen *or*
   2. Pathological lesions; vegetation or intracardiac abscess confirmed by histologic examination showing active endocarditis
B. Clinical criteria
   1. Two major criteria *or*
   2. One major criterion and three minor criteria *or*
   3. Five minor criteria

Possible Infective Endocarditis
1. One major criterion and one minor criterion *or*
2. Three minor criteria

Rejected
1. Firm alternative diagnosis explaining evidence of IE *or*
2. Resolution of IE syndrome with antibiotic therapy for <4 days *or*
3. No pathological evidence of IE at surgery or autopsy, with antibiotic therapy for <4 days *or*
4. Does not meet criteria for possible IE as above

IF, infective endocarditis
Adapted from Baddour LM, Wilson WR, Bayer AS, et al: Infective endocarditis: diagnosis, antimicrobial therapy, and management of complications: a statement for healthcare professionals from the Committee on Rheumatic Fever, Endocarditis, and Kawasaki Disease, Council on Cardiovascular Disease in the Young, and the Councils on Clinical Cardiology, Stroke, and Cardiovascular Surgery and Anesthesia, American Heart Association: endorsed by the Infectious Diseases Society of America, *Circulation* 111(23):e394–e433, 2005.

---

the American Heart Association (AHA) (Baddour et al, 2005) recommended the modified Duke criteria in the diagnosis and management of IE. The usefulness of the criteria has been validated in clinical studies.

There are three categories of diagnostic possibilities using the modified Duke criteria: definite, possible, and rejected (Box 19.1).

1. A diagnosis of "definite" IE is made by pathological evidence *and* fulfillment of certain clinical criteria.
   a. Pathological evidence of IE includes (1) demonstration of microorganism by culture or (2) histology in a vegetation or from an embolic site or an intracardiac abscess or histologic evidence of active endocarditis demonstrated in vegetation or intracardiac abscess.
   b. Fulfillment of clinical criteria is met by the presence of two major criteria, one major and three minor criteria, or five minor criteria as described in Box 19.2. Major clinical criteria are (1) positive blood cultures for acceptable microorganism and (2) evidence of endocardial involvement, demonstrated by echo findings. A positive echo finding is considered as a major criterion.

BOX 19.2   Definition of Terms Used in the Modified Duke Criteria for the Diagnosis of Infective Endocarditis

Major Criteria

A. Blood culture positive for IE
1. Typical microorganisms consistent with IE from two separate blood cultures: *Viridans* streptococci, *Streptococcus bovis*, HACEK group, *Staphylococcus aureus*; or community-acquired enterococci in the absence of a primary focus *or*
2. Microorganisms consistent with IE from persistently positive blood cultures defined as follows: at least two positive cultures of blood samples drawn >12 hr apart or all of three or a majority of four separate cultures of blood (with first and last sample drawn at least 1 hr apart)
3. Single positive blood culture for *Coxiella burnetii* or anti–phase 1 IgG antibody titer >1:800

B. Evidence of endocardial involvement

Echocardiogram positive for IE (TEE recommended for patients with prosthetic valves, rated at least "possible IE" by clinical criteria, or complicated IE [paravalvular abscess]; TTE as first test in other patients) defined as follows:
1. Oscillating intracardiac mass on valve or supporting structures, in the path of regurgitant jets, or on implanted material in the absence of an alternative anatomic explanation *or*
2. Abscess; *or*
3. New partial dehiscence of prosthetic valve; *or*
4. New valvular regurgitation (worsening or changing or pre-existing murmur not sufficient)

Minor Criteria
1. Predisposition, predisposing heart condition, or IDUs
2. Fever, temperature >38°C
3. Vascular phenomena: major arterial emboli, septic pulmonary infarcts, mycotic aneurysm, intracranial hemorrhage, conjunctival hemorrhages, and Janeway's lesions
4. Immunologic phenomena: glomerulonephritis, Osler's nodes, Roth's spots, and rheumatoid factor
. Microbiological evidence: positive blood culture but does not meet a major criterion as noted above[a] or serologic evidence of active infection with organism consistent with IE

[a] Excludes single positive cultures for coagulase-negative staphylococci and organisms that do not cause endocarditis.
HACEK, Haemophilus, Actinobacillus, Cardiobacterium, Eikenella, and *Kingella* spp.; *IE,* infective endocarditis; *IDU,* injection drug user; *TEE,* transesophageal echocardiography; *TTE,* transthoracic echocardiography.
Baddour LM, Wilson WR, Bayer AS, et al: Infective endocarditis: diagnosis, antimicrobial therapy, and management of complications: a statement for healthcare professionals from the Committee on Rheumatic Fever, Endocarditis, and Kawasaki Disease, Council on Cardiovascular Disease in the Young, and the Councils on Clinical Cardiology, Stroke, and Cardiovascular Surgery and Anesthesia, American Heart Association: endorsed by the Infectious Diseases Society of America, *Circulation* 111(23):e394–e433, 2005.

2. The category of "possible" IE is made when the following are present:
   a. One major criterion and one minor criterion or
   b. Three minor criteria

3. The other category of diagnosis is "rejected" IE which is made:
   a. When an alternative diagnosis is established,
   b. When clinical manifestations of IE have resolved within 4 days of antibiotic therapy, or
   c. No pathological evidence is found on direct examination of the vegetation obtained from surgery or autopsy after antibiotic therapy for less than 4 days
   d. When criteria for possible IE are not met

Management

1. Blood cultures are indicated for all patients with fever of unexplained origin and a pathologic heart murmur, a history of heart disease, or previous endocarditis.
   a. Usually three blood cultures are drawn by separate venipunctures over 24 hours unless the patient is very ill. In 90% of cases, the causative agent is recovered from the first two cultures.
   b. If there is no growth by the second day of incubation, two more may be obtained. There is no value in obtaining more than five blood cultures over 2 days unless the patients received prior antibiotic therapy.
   c. It is not necessary to obtain the cultures at any particular phase of the fever cycle.
   d. Adequate volume of blood must be obtained; 1 to 3 mL in infants and young children and 5 to 7 mL in older children are optimal.
   e. Aerobic incubation alone suffices because it is rare for IE to be caused by anaerobic bacteria.

2. It is highly recommended that consultation from an infectious disease specialist be obtained when IE is suspected or confirmed because antibiotics of choice are continually changing and there may be special situation pertaining to the local area.

3. Initial empirical therapy is started with the following antibiotics while awaiting the results of blood cultures.
   a. The usual initial regimen is an antistaphylococcal semisynthetic penicillin (nafcillin, oxacillin, or methicillin) and an aminoglycoside (gentamicin). This combination covers against *S. viridans, S. aureus,* and gram-negative organisms. Some experts add penicillin to the initial regimen to cover against *S. viridans,* although a semisynthetic penicillin is usually adequate for initial therapy.
   b. If a methicillin-resistant *S. aureus* is suspected, vancomycin should be substituted for the semisynthetic penicillin.
   c. Vancomycin can be used in place of penicillin or a semisynthetic penicillin in penicillin-allergic patients.

4. The final selection of antibiotics depends on the organism isolated and the results of an antibiotic sensitivity test.
   a. Streptococcal IE
      1) In general, native cardiac valve IE caused by a highly sensitive *S. viridans* can be successfully treated with IV penicillin (or ceftriaxone given once daily) for 4 weeks. Alternatively, penicillin, ampicillin, or ceftriaxone combined with gentamicin for 2 weeks may be used.
      2) For IE caused by penicillin-resistant streptococci, 4 weeks of penicillin, ampicillin, or ceftriaxone combined with gentamicin for the first 2 weeks is recommended.
   b. Staphylococcal endocarditis

1) The drug of choice for native valve IE by methicillin-susceptible staphylococci is one of the semisynthetic beta-lactamase-resistant penicillin (nafcillin, oxacillin, and methicillin) for a minimum of 6 weeks (with or without gentamicin for the first 3–5 days).

2) Patients with methicillin-resistant native valve IE are treated with vancomycin for 6 weeks (with or without gentamicin for the first 3–5 days).

c. Enterococcus-caused native valve endocarditis usually requires a combination of IV penicillin or ampicillin together with gentamicin for 4 to 6 weeks. If patients are allergic to penicillin, vancomycin combined with gentamicin for 6 weeks is required.

d. HACEK organisms have begun to become resistant to ampicillin. Ceftriaxone or another third-generation cephalosporin alone or ampicillin plus gentamicin for 4 weeks is recommended. Patients with IE caused by other gram-negative bacteria (e.g., *E. coli, Pseudomonas aeruginosa,* or *Serratia marcescens*) are treated with piperacillin or ceftazidime together with gentamicin for a minimum of 6 weeks.

e. Fungal endocarditis (usually caused by *Candida* spp.) is very difficult to treat. Amphotericin B, with or without Flucytosine, is the most often used, but surgical replacement of the infected valve (native or prosthetic) is usually required. The prognosis is very poor.

f. Culture-negative endocarditis Treatment is directed against staphylococci, streptococci, and the HACEK organisms using ceftriaxone and gentamicin. When staphylococcal IE is suspected, nafcillin should be added to the therapy.

5. Patients with prosthetic valve endocarditis should be treated for 6 weeks based on the organism isolated and the results of the sensitivity test. Operative intervention may be necessary before the antibiotic therapy is completed if the clinical situation warrants (e.g., progressive CHF, significant malfunction of prosthetic valves, persistently positive blood cultures after 2 weeks' therapy). Bacteriologic relapse after an appropriate course of therapy also calls for operative intervention.

Prognosis

The overall recovery rate is 80% to 85%; it is 90% or better for *S. viridans* and enterococci and about 50% for *Staphylococcus* organisms. Fungal endocarditis is associated with a very poor outcome.

Prevention

Until 2007, antibiotic prophylaxis for IE was routinely recommended before dental procedures for almost all congenital heart diseases (CHDs) (with exception of ASD), rheumatic and other valvular diseases, hypertrophic cardiomyopathy, mitral valve prolapse with MR, and all other conditions included in the current recommendation. In 2007, the AHA made a major change in the antibiotic prophylaxis against IE (Wilson et al, 2007). The same has been recommended jointly by the American College of Cardiology (ACC) and AHA in 2008 in a focused practice guideline (Nishimura et al, 2008). The following are the main reasons

for the change in the long-standing tradition of antibiotic prophylaxis in patients with almost all of the CHDs.

1. An exceedingly small numbers of IE that could be caused by bacteremia-producing dental procedures. The estimated frequency of bacteremia during routine daily activities (e.g., chewing, tooth brushing, flossing, used of toothpicks, use of water irrigation devices, and other activities) far exceeds that occurring during dental procedures. For example, tooth brushing and flossing results in bacteremia in 20% to 40% of the time and chewing food in 7% to 51% of the time. Cumulative risk over time of bacteremia from routine daily activities is estimated to be greater than 100,000 times compared with that resulting from dental procedures.

2. Besides, the ability of antibiotic therapy to prevent or reduce bacteremia is controversial, and nonfatal adverse reactions (e.g., rash, diarrhea, and gastrointestinal upset) also occur frequently.

Therefore, an emphasis should be on maintaining good oral hygiene and eradicating dental disease to decrease the frequency of bacteremia from routine daily activities. The 2008 new guidelines recommended antibiotic prophylaxis only for selected cardiac conditions. This recommendation was updated in 2017, and the cardiac conditions for which IE prophylaxis is indicated are listed in Box 19.3. Procedures for which antibiotic prophylaxis is recommended and those for which it is not recommended are listed in Box 19.4. Note that prophylaxis is no longer recommended for routine bronchoscopy; it is recommended for tonsillectomy and adenoidectomy only in high-risk patients (see Box 19.4). Prophylaxis is no longer recommended for GI or GU procedures, such as diagnostic esophagogastroduodenoscopy or colonoscopy.

Special Situations.

1. Patients already receiving antibiotics
   a. Rheumatic fever prophylaxis. Rather than using a higher dose of the same antibiotic, use other antibiotics, such as clindamycin, azithromycin, or clarithromycin.
   b. If possible, delay a dental procedure until at least 10 days after completion of the antibiotic therapy.

2. Patients who undergo cardiac surgery

A careful preoperative dental evaluation is recommended so that required dental treatment may be completed whenever possible before cardiac valve surgery or replacement or repair of CHD. Prophylaxis at the time of surgery should be directed primarily against staphylococci and should be of short duration. Prophylaxis should be initiated immediately before the operative procedure, repeated during prolonged procedures to maintain serum concentrations intraoperatively, and continued for no more than 48 hours postoperatively.

MYOCARDITIS

Prevalence

Myocarditis severe enough to be recognized clinically is rare, but the prevalence of mild and subclinical cases is probably much higher.

Box 19.3 **2017 American Heart Association/American College of Cardiology Updated Recommendation on Cardiac Conditions for Which Prophylaxis with Dental Procedures is Recommended**

Prophylaxis against IE is reasonable before dental procedures that involve manipulation of gingival tissue, manipulation of the peripheral region of teeth, or perforation of the oral mucosa in patients with the following.
1. Prosthetic cardiac valves, including transcatheter-implanted prostheses and homografts
2. Prosthetic material used for cardiac valve repair, such as annuloplasty rings and chords
3. Previous IE
4. Unrepaired cyanotic congenital heart disease or repaired CHD, with residual shunts or valvular regurgitation at the site of or adjacent to the site of a prosthetic patch or prosthetic device
5. Cardiac transplant with valve regurgitation caused by a structurally abnormal valve.[a]

[a]The risk of infective endocarditis (IE) is highest in the first 6 months after transplantation because of endothelial disruption, high-intensity immunosuppressive therapy, frequent central venous catheter access, and frequent endomyocardial biopsies.
CHD, congenital heart disease.
Modified from Nishimura RA, Otto CM, Bonow RO, et al: 2017 AHA/ACC focused update of the 2014 AHA/ACC guideline for the management of patients with valvular heart disease: a report of the American College of Cardiology/American Heart Association Task Force on Clinical Practice Guidelines, *Circulation* 135(25):e1159–e1195, 2017.

BOX 19.4 **Procedures for Which Endocarditis Prophylaxis is Recommended**

1. Dental procedures
   All dental procedures that involve manipulation of gingival tissue of the periapical region of teeth or perforation of the oral mucosa. Antibiotic choices and dosages for dental procedures are shown in Table 19.1.
2. Respiratory tract procedures
   a. Prophylaxis is recommended for the procedures that involve incision or biopsy of the respiratory mucosa, such as tonsillectomy and adenoidectomy.
   b. Prophylaxis is not recommended for bronchoscopy (unless it involves incision of the mucosa, such as for abscess or empyema).
3. GI and GU procedures
   a. No prophylaxis for diagnostic esophagogastroduodenoscopy or colonoscopy.
   b. Prophylaxis is reasonable in patients with infected GI or GU tract (with amoxicillin or ampicillin to cover against enterococci).
4. Skin, skin structure, or musculoskeletal tissue
   a. Prophylaxis is recommended for surgical procedures that involve infected skin, skin structure, or musculoskeletal tissue (with antibiotics against staphylococcus and beta-hemolytic streptococcus, such as antistaphylococcal penicillin or a cephalosporin).
   b. Vancomycin or clindamycin is administered if unable to tolerate beta-lactam or if infection is caused by MRSA.

GI, Gastrointestinal; *GU,* genitourinary; *MRSA,* methicillin-resistant *Staphylococcus aureus.*

Pathology

1. The principal mechanism of cardiac involvement in viral myocarditis is believed to be a cell-mediated immunologic reaction, not merely myocardial damage from viral replication. Isolation of virus from the myocardium is unusual at autopsy.
2. The inflamed myocardium is soft, flabby, and pale, with areas of scarring on gross examination. Microscopic examination reveals patchy infiltrations by plasma cells, mononuclear leukocytes, and some eosinophils during the acute phase and giant cell infiltration in the later stages.

Cause

1. In North America, viruses are probably the most common causes of myocarditis. Among viruses, enterovirus (particularly adenovirus and coxsackieviruses A and B) and adenovirus, more recently human herpes virus 6, and parvovirus B19 are the most common agents. Many other viruses (e.g., cytomegalovirus, Epstein-Barr virus, hepatitis C virus, influenza A virus, human immunodeficiency virus (HIV), poliomyelitis, mumps, measles, rubella, and influenza) can cause myocarditis.
2. Myocarditis secondary to a bacterial infection is rare. A wide variety of bacteria (e.g., *Mycoplasma pneumoniae, Listeria monocytogenes, Staphylococcus* spp., *Streptococcus* spp., *Mycobacterium* spp.) have been associated with myocarditis.

3. In South America, Chagas' disease (caused by *Trypanosoma cruzi,* a protozoan) is a common cause of myocarditis.
4. Rarely, rickettsia, fungi, and parasites are the causative agents.
5. Autoimmune disorders (sarcoidosis, systemic lupus erythematosus) are associated with significant myocarditis.
6. Immune-mediated diseases, including acute rheumatic fever and KD, may be the cause.

Clinical Manifestations
History

1. Older children may have a history of an upper respiratory infection.
2. The illness may have a sudden onset in newborns and small infants, with anorexia, vomiting, lethargy, and occasionally circulatory shock.

Physical Examination

1. The presentation depends on the patient's age and the acute or chronic nature of the infection. In neonates and infants, signs of CHF may be present; these include poor heart tone, tachycardia, gallop rhythm, tachypnea, and, rarely, cyanosis. In older children, a gradual onset of CHF and arrhythmia are commonly seen.
2. A soft, systolic heart murmur and irregular rhythm caused by supraventricular or ventricular ectopic beats may be audible.
3. Hepatomegaly (evidence of viral hepatitis) may be present.

Electrocardiography

Any one or a combination of the following may be seen: low QRS voltages, ST-T changes, PR prolongation, prolongation of the QT interval, and arrhythmias, especially premature contractions.

Radiography

Cardiomegaly of varying degrees is the most important sign of myocarditis.

Echocardiography

The common echocardiography findings include ventricular systolic dysfunction, often regional in nature, dilatation, and changes in wall thickness or wall motion. Occasionally, LV thrombi are found.

Laboratory Studies.

1. Cardiac troponin levels (troponin I and T) and myocardial enzymes (creatine kinase [CK], MB isoenzyme of CK [CK-MB]) may be elevated. In children, the normal value of cardiac troponin I has been reported to be 2 ng/mL or less, and it is frequently below the level of detection for the assay. Troponin levels may be more sensitive than the cardiac enzymes.
2. BNP and NT-proBNP levels are usually elevated in patients with dilated cardiomyopathy secondary to myocarditis.
3. Radionuclide scanning (after administration of gallium-67 or technetium-99m pyrophosphate) may identify inflammatory and necrotic changes characteristic of myocarditis.
4. Myocarditis can be confirmed by an endomyocardial biopsy.

Natural History

1. The mortality rate is as high as 75% in symptomatic neonates with acute viral myocarditis.
2. The majority of patients, especially those with mild inflammation, recover completely.
3. Some patients develop subacute or chronic myocarditis with persistent cardiomegaly (with or without signs of CHF) and electrocardiographic (ECG) evidence of LV hypertrophy or biventricular hypertrophy. Clinically, these patients are indistinguishable from those with dilated cardiomyopathy (DCM). Myocarditis may be a precursor to idiopathic DCM in some cases.
4. The transplant-free survival rate is 80% to 90%. Some patients develop refractory heart failure and may become candidates for heart transplantation.

Management

Patients with myocarditis are mainly treated with supportive and symptomatic care.

1. Oxygen and bed rest are recommended. Use of a "cardiac chair" or "infant seat" relieves respiratory distress.
2. Bed rest and limitation in activities are recommended during the acute phase (because exercise intensifies the damage from myocarditis in experimental animals).

3. For symptomatic but stable patients with heart failure, the following anticongestive medications may be used.
   a. Rapid-acting diuretics (furosemide or ethacrynic acid, 1 mg/kg, each one to three times a day)
   b. Angiotensin-converting enzyme inhibitors, such as captopril, or angiotensin receptor blockers may prove beneficial in the acute phase.
   c. Rapid-acting inotropic agents, such as dobutamine or dopamine, and the inodilator milrinone are useful in critically ill children; however, they have the potential for arrhythmia. Use of digoxin is not recommended because some patients with myocarditis are found to be exquisitely sensitive to the drug.
   d. Beta-blockers are not recommended in the acute phase but may be required as long-term maintenance drug. Nonsteroidal antiinflammatory agents are not recommended during acute and subacute phases. The role of corticosteroids is unclear at this time, except in the treatment of severe rheumatic carditis.
4. Recently, beneficial effects of intravenous immunoglobulin (IVIG) (2 g/kg over 24 hours) have been reported. IVIG was associated with better survival during the first year after presentation, echo evidence of smaller LV diastolic dimension, and higher fractional shortening compared with the control group. Myocardial damage in myocarditis is mediated in part by immunologic mechanisms, and a high dose of gamma globulin is an immunomodulatory agent shown to be effective in myocarditis secondary to KD.
5. Arrhythmias should be treated aggressively and may require the use of IV amiodarone. In patients with significant atrioventricular (AV) conduction disturbance, permanent pacemaker may be necessary.

PERICARDITIS

Cause

1. Viral infection is probably the most common cause of pericarditis in the developed world, particularly in infancy. Viral causes include coxsackievirus, herpesvirus, mumps virus, and HIV, among others.
2. Bacterial infection (purulent pericarditis) is a rare, serious form of pericarditis. Commonly encountered are *S. aureus, Streptococcus pneumoniae, Haemophilus influenzae, Neisseria meningitidis,* and streptococci.
3. Tuberculosis is a common cause in developing counties. Tuberculous pericarditis is an occasional cause of constrictive pericarditis, with an insidious onset.
4. Acute rheumatic fever is a common cause of pericarditis, especially in certain parts of the world (see also Chapter 20).
5. Heart surgery is a possible cause (see Postpericardiotomy Syndrome).
6. Collagen disease such as rheumatoid arthritis (see Chapter 23) can cause pericarditis.
7. Pericarditis can be a complication of oncologic disease or its therapy, including radiation.
8. Uremia (uremic pericarditis) is a rare cause.

Pathology

1. The parietal and visceral surfaces of the pericardium are inflamed. Pericardial effusion may be serofibrinous, hemorrhagic, or purulent. Effusion may be completely absorbed or may result in pericardial thickening or chronic constriction (constrictive pericarditis).
2. Findings of myocarditis are also present in about one third of the patients.

Pathophysiology

The pathogenesis of symptoms and signs of pericardial effusion is determined by two factors: the speed of fluid accumulation and the competence of the myocardium.

1. A rapid accumulation of a large amount of pericardial fluid produces more serious circulatory embarrassment.
2. A slow accumulation of a relatively small amount of fluid may result in serious circulatory embarrassment (cardiac tamponade) if the extent of myocarditis is significant.
3. Slow accumulation of a large amount of fluid may be accommodated by stretching of the pericardium, if the myocardium is intact.
4. When the pericardial effusion builds up, resulting in compression of the heart, it is called *cardiac tamponade*. The onset may be rapid or gradual. With the development of pericardial tamponade, several compensatory mechanisms are triggered, including systemic and pulmonary venous constriction to improve diastolic filling, an increase in systemic vascular resistance to raise falling blood pressure, and tachycardia to improve cardiac output.

Clinical Manifestations

History

1. The patient may have a history of upper respiratory tract infection.
2. Precordial or substernal pain (sharp, dull, aching, or stabbing) with occasional radiation to the shoulder and neck may be a presenting complaint. The pain may be relieved by leaning forward and may be made worse by a supine position or deep inspiration.
3. Fever of varying degrees may be present.

Physical Examination

1. Pericardial friction rub (a grating, to-and-fro sound in phase with the heart sounds) is the pathognomonic physical sign.
2. The heart is quiet and hypodynamic in the presence of a large amount of pericardial effusion.
3. Pulsus paradoxus is characteristic of pericardial effusion with tamponade (see Chapter 2 and Fig. 2.2).
4. Heart murmur is usually absent, although it may be present in acute rheumatic carditis (see Chapter 20).
5. In children with *purulent pericarditis,* septic fever (101°–105° F [38.3°–40.5°C]), tachycardia, chest pain, and dyspnea are almost always present.
6. Signs of *cardiac tamponade* may be present; these include distant heart sounds, tachycardia, pulsus paradoxus, hepatomegaly, venous distention, and occasional hypotension with peripheral vasoconstriction. Cardiac tamponade

occurs more commonly in purulent pericarditis than in other forms of pericarditis.

Electrocardiography

1. The low-voltage QRS complex caused by pericardial effusion is characteristic but not a constant finding.
2. The following time-dependent changes secondary to myocardial involvement may occur (see Fig. 3.25):
   a. Initial ST-segment elevation
   b. Return of the ST segment to the baseline with inversion of T waves (2–4 weeks after onset)

Chest Radiography

1. A varying degree of cardiomegaly is present.
2. A pear-shaped or water-bottle-shaped heart is characteristic of a large effusion.
3. Pulmonary vascular markings may be increased if cardiac tamponade develops. Tamponade may occur without enlargement of the cardiac silhouette if it develops quickly.

Echocardiography

Echocardiography is the most useful tool in establishing the diagnosis of pericardial effusion. It appears as an echo-free space between the epicardium (visceral pericardium) and the parietal pericardium.

1. Pericardial effusion first appears posteriorly in the dependent portion of the pericardial sac. The presence of small amount of effusion posteriorly without anterior effusion suggests a small pericardial effusion. A small amount of fluid, which appears only in systole, is normal.
2. With larger effusion, the fluid also appears anteriorly. The larger the echo-free space, the larger is the pericardial effusion. With very large effusions, the swinging motion of the heart may be imaged.
3. In patients with chronic effusion, fibrinous strands and other organized materials can be seen in the pericardial fluid, which may lead to fluid loculations.
4. Echocardiography is very helpful in detecting *cardiac tamponade.* Helpful two-dimensional (2D) echo findings of tamponade are as follows:
   a. Collapse of the right atrium (RA) in late diastole (see Fig. 19.2) (because the pressure in the pericardial sac exceeds the pressure within the RA at end-diastole when the atrium has emptied)
   b. Collapse or indentation of the right ventricular (RV) free wall, especially the outflow tract

Management

1. Pericardiocentesis or surgical drainage to identify the cause of the pericarditis is mandatory, especially when purulent or tuberculous pericarditis is suspected. A drainage catheter may be left in place with intermittent low-pressure drainage.
2. Pericardial fluid studies include cell counts and differential, glucose, and protein concentrations; histologic examination of cells; Gram and acid-fast stains; and viral, bacterial, and fungal cultures.

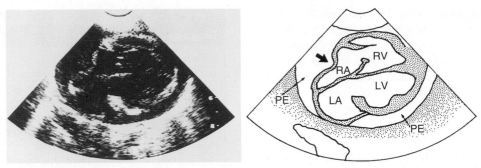

Fig. 19.2 Subcostal four-chamber view demonstrating pericardial effusion (PE) and collapse of the right atrial wall *(large arrow)*, a sign of cardiac tamponade. *LA,* Left atrium; *LV,* left ventricle; *RA,* right atrium; *RV,* right ventricle.

3. For cardiac tamponade, urgent decompression by surgical drainage or pericardiocentesis should be carried out. While getting ready for the procedure, fluid push with crystalloids and colloids should be given to increase central venous pressure and thereby improve diastolic filling, which can provide temporary emergency stabilization. Medications that decrease systemic pressure such as vasodilators and diuretics should be avoided.
4. Urgent surgical drainage of the pericardium is indicated when purulent pericarditis is suspected. This must be followed by IV antibiotic therapy for 4 to 6 weeks.
5. There is no specific treatment for viral pericarditis.
6. Treatment focuses on the basic disease itself (e.g., uremia, collagen disease).
7. Salicylates are given for precordial pain and nonbacterial or rheumatic pericarditis.
8. Corticosteroid therapy may be indicated in children with severe rheumatic carditis or postpericardiotomy syndrome.

CONSTRICTIVE PERICARDITIS

Although rare in children, constrictive pericarditis may be associated with an earlier viral pericarditis, tuberculous pericarditis, incomplete drainage of purulent pericarditis, hemopericardium, mediastinal irradiation, neoplastic infiltration, or connective tissue disorders. In this condition, a fibrotic, thickened, and adherent pericardium restricts diastolic filling of the heart.

Diagnosis of constrictive pericarditis is suggested by the following clinical findings:

1. Signs of elevated jugular venous pressure occur.
2. Hepatomegaly with ascites and systemic edema may be present.
3. Auscultation of the heart may reveal diastolic pericardial knock, which resembles the opening snap, often heard along the left sternal border in the absence of heart murmur.
4. Chest radiograph may show calcification of the pericardium, enlargement of the superior vena cava and left atrium (LA), and pleural effusion.
5. The ECG may show low QRS voltages, T-wave inversion or flattening, and LA hypertrophy. Atrial fibrillation occasionally is seen.

6. Echocardiography
   a. M-mode echo may reveal two parallel lines representing the thickened visceral and parietal pericardia or multiple dense echoes.
   b. 2D echo shows (1) a thickened pericardium, (2) dilated inferior vena cava and hepatic vein, and (3) paradoxical septal motion and abrupt displacement of the interventricular septum during early diastolic filling ("septal bounce") (not specific for this condition).
   c. Doppler examination of the mitral inflow reveals findings of diastolic dysfunction (see Fig. 18.6) and a marked respiratory variation in diastolic inflow tracings.
7. Cardiac catheterization may document the presence of constrictive physiology.
   a. The RA and LA pressures, ventricular end-diastolic pressures, and PA wedge pressure are all elevated and usually equalized.
   b. Ventricular pressure waveforms demonstrate the characteristic "square root sign" (in which there is an early rapid fall in diastolic pressure followed by a rapid rise to an elevated diastolic plateau).

The treatment for constrictive pericarditis is complete resection of the pericardium; symptomatic improvement occurs in 75% of patients.

KAWASAKI'S DISEASE

Kawasaki's disease is an acute, self-limited febrile illness of unknown cause that predominantly affects children younger than 5 years of age. The major concern with this illness is its predilection to affect coronary arteries with aneurysm formation.

Cause and Epidemiology

1. The cause of KD (also called *mucocutaneous lymph node syndrome*) is not known. Most investigators believe that the disease is related to, if not caused by, an infectious disease. The disease is probably driven by abnormalities of the immune system initiated by the infectious insult.
2. Children of all racial and ethnic groups are affected, although it is more common in Asians and Pacific islanders, especially in Japanese. The male-to-female ratio is 1.5 to 1.

3. It affects predominantly young children, with 76% occurring in children younger than 5 years of age. Its peak incidence is between 1 and 2 years of age; 80% of patients are younger than 4 years of age, and 50% are younger than 2 years of age. Cases in children older than 8 years and younger than 3 months of age are uncommon.

4. In the United States, KD is more common during the winter and early spring months.

5. Possibility of recurrence and familial occurrence have been documented in Japan; the recurrence rate is around 3%, and the relative risk in siblings is 10-fold higher.

6. Coronary artery aneurysms from KD account for 5% of acute coronary syndrome in adults younger than 40 years of age.

Pathology

1. During the first 10 days after the onset of fever, generalized microvasculitis occurs throughout the body, with a predilection for the coronary arteries. Other arteries such as the iliac, femoral, axillary, and renal arteries are less frequently involved.

2. Coronary artery aneurysm develops in 15% to 20% during the acute phase and persists for 1 to 3 weeks. It tends to develop most frequently in the proximal segment of the major coronary arteries and may assume fusiform, saccular, cylindrical, or beads-on-a-string appearance.

3. During the acute phase, there is pancarditis, with inflammation of the AV conduction system (which can produce AV block), myocardium (myocardial dysfunction, CHF), pericardium (pericardial effusion), and endocardium (with aortic and mitral valve involvement).

4. Late changes (after 40 days) consist of healing and fibrosis in the coronary arteries, with thrombus formation and stenosis in the postaneurysmal segment and myocardial fibrosis from old myocardial infarction (MI).

5. The elevated platelet count seen in this condition contributes to coronary thrombosis.

6. Fate of aneurysms. Mildly dilated arteries may be able to return to normal. Large saccular aneurysms have lost their intima, media, and elastica, which cannot be regenerated. Fusiform aneurysms with partially preserved media can thrombose or develop progressive stenosis. Large or giant coronary artery aneurysms (>8 mm) do not resolve, regress, or remodel. They rarely rupture and always contain thrombi that can become occlusive.

Clinical Manifestations

The clinical course of the disease can be divided into three phases: acute (first 10 days), subacute (11-25 days), and convalescent. Each phase of the disease is characterized by unique symptoms and signs. Only clinical features seen in acute phase are important in making the diagnosis of the disease and they are discussed in depth.

Acute Phase (First 10 Days)

1. Six signs that compose the **principal clinical features** of KD are present during the acute phase (Box 19.5).

> ### BOX 19.5   Diagnosis of Classic Kawasaki's Disease
>
> a. Fever persisting ≥5 days
> b. Presence of at least four of the following principal features
>   1. Erythema and cracking of lips, strawberry tongue, or erythema of the oral and pharyngeal mucosa
>   2. Bilateral bulbar conjunctival injection without exudates
>   3. Rash: maculopapular, diffuse erythroderma, or erythema multiforme–like
>   4. Erythema and edema of the hands and feet in acute phase or periungual desquamation in the subacute phase
>   5. Cervical lymphadenopathy (>1.5 cm in diameter), usually unilateral
>   • Exclusion of other diseases with similar findings (see Differential Diagnosis)

Adapted from McCrindle BW, Rowley AH, Newburger JW, et al: Diagnosis, treatment, and long-term management of Kawasaki disease: a scientific statement for health professionals from the American Heart Association, *Circulation* 135:e927–e999, 2017.

a. The onset of illness is abrupt, with a high fever, usually higher than 39°C (102°F) and in many cases higher than 40°C (104°F). Fever persists for a mean of 11 days without treatment. With appropriate therapy, the fever usually resolves within 2 days of treatment. Within 2 to 5 days after the onset of fever, other principal features develop.

b. Conjunctivitis occurs shortly after the onset of fever. It is not associated with exudate, being different from that seen in other conditions such as measles, Stevens-Johnson syndrome, or viral conjunctivitis. Conjunctivitis resolves rapidly.

c. Changes in the lips and oral cavity include (1) erythema, dryness, fissuring, peeling, cracking, and bleeding of the lips; (2) "strawberry tongue" that is indistinguishable from scarlet fever; and (3) diffuse erythema of the oropharyngeal mucosa. Oral ulceration and pharyngeal exudates are not seen.

d. Changes in the hands and feet consist of erythema of the palms and soles, firm edema, and sometimes painful induration. Desquamation of hands and feet takes place within 2 to 3 weeks.

e. The rash usually appears within 5 days of the onset of fever and may take many forms (except bullous and vesicular eruptions), even in the same patient. The most common is a nonspecific, diffuse maculopapular eruption. Its distribution is extensive, involving the trunk and extremities, with accentuation in the perineal region (where early desquamation may occur); desquamation usually occurs by days 5 to 7.

f. Cervical lymph node enlargement is the least common of the principal clinical features, occurring in approximately 50% of patients. The firm swelling is usually unilateral, involves more than one measuring more than 1.5 cm in diameter, and is confined to the anterior cervical triangle.

2. **Cardiovascular abnormalities** results from involvement of the pericardium, myocardium, endocardium, valves, and coronary arteries, with some or all of the following manifestations.
   a. Tachycardia, gallop rhythm, or other signs of heart failure
   b. LV dysfunction with cardiomegaly (myocarditis)
   c. Pericardial effusion
   d. Mitral valve regurgitation murmur
   e. Chest radiographs may show cardiomegaly if myocarditis or significant coronary artery abnormality or valvular regurgitation is present.
   f. ECG changes may include arrhythmias, prolonged PR interval (occurring in ≤60%), and nonspecific ST-T changes. Abnormal Q waves (wide and deep) in the limb leads or precordial leads suggest MI.
   g. Coronary artery abnormalities are seen initially at the end of the first week through the second week of illness (see below for further discussion).

3. **Clinical findings of other systems.** Signs of involvement of other organ systems are frequent during the acute phase. This may lead physicians to consider a diagnosis other than KD.
   a. Musculoskeletal system: arthritis or arthralgia of multiple joints (30%) involving small as well as large joints
   b. Gastrointestinal system: abdominal pain with diarrhea (20%), liver dysfunction (40%), hydrops of the gallbladder (10%, demonstrable by abdominal ultrasound) with jaundice
   c. GU system: sterile pyuria (60%), urethritis, hydrocele
   d. CNS: extreme irritability, lethargy or semicoma, aseptic meningitis (25%), facial nerve palsy, and sensory neuronal hearing loss
   e. Other systems: desquamating rash in the groin, retropharyngeal phlegmon

4. **Laboratory studies.** Even though laboratory results are nonspecific, they provide support for a diagnosis of KD in patients with nonclassic but suggestive clinical features.
   a. Marked leukocytosis with a shift to the left and anemia are common during acute phase. Leukopenia and lymphocyte predominance suggest a viral illness.
   b. Acute-phase reactant levels (CRP, erythrocyte sedimentation rate [ESR]) are always elevated, which are uncommon with viral illnesses. An elevated ESR (but not CRP) can be caused by IVIG infusion therapy. The CPR is more useful as a marker of inflammation in patients with KS.
   c. Thrombocytosis (usually >450,000 /mm³) is a characteristic feature of KD but generally does not occur until the second week, peaking in the third week (reaching mean of 700,000 to >1 million/mm³) and normalizes by 4 to 6 weeks after the onset. A low platelet count suggests viral illnesses.
   d. Pyuria (caused by urethritis) is seen in up to 80% of children.
   e. Liver enzymes (transaminases) are moderately elevated (more than two times the upper limit of normal) in 40% of patients; hypoalbuminemia and mild hyperbilirubinemia may be present in 10%.
   f. Elevated serum cardiac troponin I may occur, which suggests myocardial damage.
   g. Lipid abnormalities are common. Decreased levels of high-density lipoprotein are present during the illness and follow-up for more than 3 years, especially in patients with persistent coronary artery abnormalities. The total cholesterol level is normal, but the triglyceride level tends to be high.

5. **Echocardiography.** The main purpose of an echo study during acute phase is to detect coronary artery aneurysm and other cardiac dysfunction. The initial study serves as baseline for follow-ups.
   a. Coronary artery aneurysm rarely occurs before day 10 of illness. During this period, other echo findings may suggest cardiac involvement.
      1) Perivascular brightness and ectasia (dilatation) may represent coronary arteritis (before aneurysm formation).
      2) Decreased LV systolic function with increased LV dimensions
      3) Mild mitral valve regurgitation (presumably from myocarditis, MI, or coronary artery occlusion)
      4) Pericardial effusion
   b. During the acute phase, detection of dilated proximal coronary artery segments is important in the diagnosis of the disease. All major proximal coronary artery segments (left main coronary artery [LMCA], left anterior descending [LAD], and right coronary artery [RCA]) should be measured and compared with normal values (see Appendix D, Table D.6). A coronary dimension that is greater than a standard deviation (SD) of +3 in one of the three proximal segments (LMCA, LAD, and RCA) or one that is greater than +2.5 SD in two proximal segments are highly unusual in the normal population (Kurotobi et al, 2002). One must measure the dimension at a specific point as shown in the figure in Table D.6. The LMCA is measured at a point between the ostium and the first bifurcation of the artery, the LAD distal to and away from the bifurcation of the branch from the LMCA, and the RCA in the relatively straight section of the artery just after rightward turn from the initial anterior course of the artery.
   c. Configuration (saccular, fusiform, ectatic), size, and number of aneurysms, and presence or absence of intraluminal or mural thrombi should be assessed. Aneurysms are classified as saccular (nearly equal axial and lateral diameters), fusiform (symmetric dilatation with gradual proximal and distal tapering), and ectatic (dilated without segmental aneurysm). "Giant" aneurysm is present when the diameter of the aneurysm is 8 mm or greater or the Z score is 10 or greater. Fig. 19.3 shows a large saccular aneurysm of the RCA.

Clinical findings seen during the subacute phase and convalescent phase are not important in diagnosis or planning management, but they are more or less useful in confirming the diagnosis at a later time.

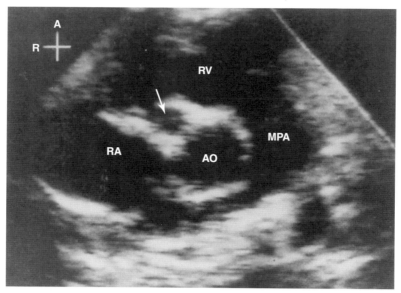

Fig. 19.3 Parasternal short-axis view from a patient with Kawasaki's disease. There is a large saccular aneurysm *(arrow)* of the right coronary artery. *A*, Anterior; *AO*, aorta; *MPA*, main pulmonary artery; *R*, right; *RA*, right atrium; *RV*, right ventricle. (From Snider AR, Serwer GA: *Echocardiography in Pediatric Heart Disease*, St. Louis, 1990, Mosby.)

Subacute Phase (11 to 25 Days After Onset)

1. Desquamation of the tips of the fingers and toes is characteristic.
2. Rash, fever, and lymphadenopathy disappear.
3. Significant cardiovascular changes, including coronary aneurysm, pericardial effusion, CHF, and MI, occur in this phase. Approximately 20% of patients manifest coronary artery aneurysm on echo.
4. Thrombocytosis also occurs during this period, peaking at 2 weeks or more after the onset of the illness.

Convalescent Phase

This phase lasts until the elevated ESR and platelet count return to normal. Deep transverse grooves (Beau's lines) may appear across the fingernails and toenails.

Diagnosis

Timely and correct diagnosis of KD is very important because early treatment with IVIG can reduce damages to the coronary arteries. Unfortunately, there is no specific diagnostic test or pathognomonic clinical feature of KD. The diagnosis of KD relies on clinical criteria. Box 19.5 lists the principal clinical features that establish the diagnosis. In cases with less than full criteria for the disease (incomplete KD), other clinical and laboratory findings (as discussed earlier) may aid physicians in making the decision to initiate treatment.

1. The presence of fever of 5 days' duration or more and at least four of the five principal criteria (see Box 19.5) are required to make the diagnosis of classic KD. More than 90% of patients have fever plus the first four of the five signs, but only about 50% of patients have lymphadenopathy. A careful history may reveal that one or more principal clinical features were present during the illness but resolved by the time of presentation.

2. However, patients with fever for 5 days' duration or more and fewer than four criteria can be diagnosed as having KD when coronary artery abnormality is detected. Indeed, a substantial fraction of children with KD with coronary artery anomalies never meet the diagnostic criteria. However, coronary aneurysm rarely occurs before day 10 of KD. During this period, perivascular brightness or ectasia (dilatation) of the coronary artery, decreased LV systolic function, mild MR, or pericardial effusion may be present instead.

3. **Incomplete KD** with two or three principal clinical features creates a management problem. Incomplete KD is more common in young infants than older children. Given the potential serious consequences of missing the diagnosis of KD in patients with incomplete manifestations of the principal clinical features, together with the efficiency and safety of early treatment with IVIG, physicians should not wait for full manifestations of the disease but should consider other laboratory findings and abnormal echo findings in deciding whether or not to initiate treatment. Fig. 19.4 is an algorithm recently proposed by the AHA (2017) that helps physicians to evaluate suspected incomplete KD. The algorithm includes abnormal echocardiographic findings and some laboratory test results that are commonly found in complete cases of KD, which help in deciding to give treatment.

Abnormal acute-phase reactants (CRP ≥3.0 mg/dL and ESR ≥40 mm/hr) are very helpful. Other helpful supplemental laboratory tests include (with their abnormal values shown in parenthesis) (1) anemia for age, (2) platelets after 7 days (≥450,000/mm³), (3) serum albumin (≤3.0 g/dL), (4) alanine aminotransferase (>50 or 60 U/L), (5) white blood cell count (≥15,000/mm³), and (6) urine white blood cell count (≥10 cells/high-power field). Patients with positive

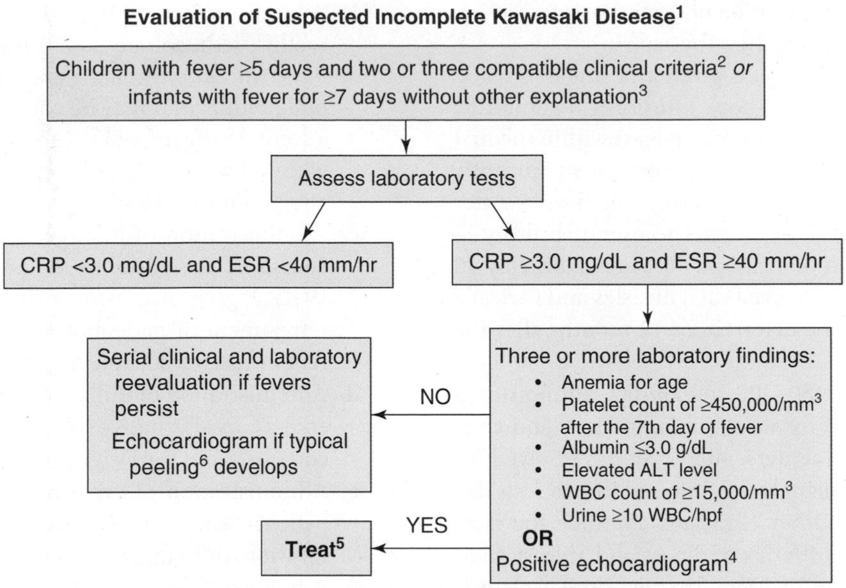

Evaluation of Suspected Incomplete Kawasaki Disease[1]

Fig. 19.4 Algorithm for evaluation of suspected incomplete Kawasaki's disease (KD). The algorithm is not evidence based; it represents the informed opinion of the expert committee. *(1)* Clinical findings of KD are listed in Box 19.5. Characteristics suggesting that another diagnosis should be considered include exudative conjunctivitis, exudative pharyngitis, ulcerative intraoral lesions, bullous or vesicular rash, generalized adenopathy, or splenomegaly. *(2)* Infants 6 months of age or younger are the most likely to develop prolonged fever without other clinical criteria or KD; these infants are at particularly high risk of developing coronary artery abnormalities. *(3)* Echocardiography is considered positive for purposes of this algorithm if any of three conditions are met: Z score of left anterior descending coronary artery (CA) or right CA of 2.5 or greater; CA aneurysm is observed; or three or more other suggestive features exist, including decreased left ventricular function, mitral regurgitation, pericardial effusion, or Z score in the left anterior descending CA or right CA of 2 to 2.5. *(4)* If the echocardiogram is positive, treatment should be given within 10 days of fever onset or after the 10th day of fever in the presence of clinical and laboratory signs (C-reactive protein [CRP] or erythrocyte sedimentation rate [ESR]) of ongoing inflammation. *(5)* Typical peeling begins under the nail beds of the fingers and toes. *ALT,* Alanine aminotransferase; *WBC,* white blood cell. (Reprinted with permission Circulation.2017;135:e927–e999 © 2017 American Heart Association, Inc)

acute-phase reactants plus three or more abnormal supplemental laboratory tests may be given treatment along with echo studies. Even if there are fewer than three abnormal laboratory test results, patients with abnormal echocardiographic findings (see earlier) qualify for treatment (see Fig. 19.4).

Differential Diagnosis

One must rule out diseases with similar manifestations through appropriate cultures and the use of laboratory tests (Box 19.6), because the principal clinical findings that fulfill the diagnostic criteria for KD are not specific. Measles and group A beta-hemolytic streptococcal infection most closely mimic KD. Children with KD are extremely irritable (often inconsolable). In addition, children with KD are less likely to have exudative conjunctivitis, pharyngitis, generalized lymphadenopathy, or discrete intraoral lesions (Koplik's spot) and are more likely to have a perineal distribution of their rash. Other diseases with findings similar to KD, such as viral exanthems, drug reactions, juvenile rheumatoid arthritis, and Rocky Mountain spotted fever, require differentiation. Viral illness is more likely if acute-phase reactants and platelet counts are normal after 7 days of the illness.

BOX 19.6 Differential Diagnosis of Kawasaki's Disease

Measles
Other viral infections (e.g., adenovirus, enterovirus)
Staphylococcal and streptococcal toxin-mediated diseases (e.g., scarlet fever and toxic shock syndrome)
Drug hypersensitivity reactions, including Stevens Johnson syndrome
Systemic onset juvenile idiopathic arthritis
With epidemiologic risk factors:
- Rocky Mountain spotted fever or other rickettsial infections
- Leptospirosis

Modified from McCrindle BW, Rowley AH, Newburger JW, et al: Diagnosis, treatment, and long-term management of Kawasaki disease: a scientific statement for health professionals from the American Heart Association, *Circulation* 135:e927–e999, 2017.

Management
Initial Treatment

The standard treatment of patients with KD is high-dose IVIG together with aspirin. Two goals of therapy are reduction of inflammation within the coronary artery and the myocardium (by high-dose IVIG) and prevention of thrombosis formation by inhibition of platelet aggregation (by aspirin).

1. A high dose of IVIG (2 g/kg) is given as a single infusion (given slowly in a 10- to 12-hour infusion). It should be given ideally by 7 days of illness but at least within the first 10 days of illness. IVIG has been shown to significantly reduce the incidence of coronary artery aneurysm. After IVIG infusion, two thirds of patients become afebrile by 24 hours after completion of infusion; 90% are afebrile by 48 hours. In patients who receive IVIG, measles and varicella immunization should be deferred for 11 months after the treatment.

2. Aspirin in high dose (80–100 mg/kg/day, administered every 6 hours) is given for its antiinflammatory and antipyretic effects. In most centers, after fever has resolved for 48 to 72 hours, the aspirin dose is lowered to 3 to 5 kg/day given in single dose. Other clinicians continue the high dose aspirin until the 14th day of illness and at least 48 to 72 hours after cessation of fever. The low-dose aspirin is continued for 6 to 8 weeks when no evidence of coronary changes exists. For children who develop coronary abnormalities, aspirin may be continued indefinitely.

   In Japan and Western Europe, the antiplatelet dose (3–5 mg/kg/day) of aspirin is given from the onset because high-dose aspirin does not have antiplatelet effect; does not appear to reduce coronary aneurysm; and may result in increased frequency of hepatotoxicity, GI irritation and bleeding, and Reye's syndrome.

3. Other antiinflammatory agents, such as corticosteroids, abciximab, infliximab, have been reported to have varying levels of beneficial effects on the coronary artery aneurysm. Because the data on IVIG efficacy are so clear, these antiinflammatory agents are not considered reasonable monotherapy. Some of them may be used in select patients with special problems (as discussed next).

Special Situations in the Treatment of Kawasaki's Disease

1. Late diagnosis and recurrence
   a. It is reasonable to administer IVIG to children presenting after the 10th day of illness (i.e., in whom the diagnosis is missed earlier) if they have persistent fever without other explanation or coronary artery abnormalities together with systemic inflammation (as manifested by elevation of ESR or CRP).
   b. Patients with recurrent KD (defined as a repeat episode of complete or incomplete KD after complete resolution of the previous episode) should receive IVIG.

2. **IVIG-resistant patients.** Approximately 10% to 20% of patients with KD develop recrudescent or persistent fever at least 36 hours after the end of their IVIG infusion and are termed IVIG resistant. The following are the 2017 AHA recommendations (McCrindle et al, 2017).
   a. It is reasonable to administer a second dose of IVIG (2 g/kg) to patients with persistent or recrudescent fever at least 36 hours after the end of the first IVIG infusion.
   b. Administration of high-dose pulse steroids (usually methylprednisolone 20–30 mg/kg intravenously for 3 days, with or without a subsequent course and taper of oral prednisone) may be considered as an alternative to a second infusion of IVIG or for retreatment of patients with KD who have had recurrent or recrudescent fever after additional IVIG.
   c. Administration of a longer (e.g., 2–3 weeks) tapering course of prednisolone or prednisone, together with IVIG 2 g/kg and aspirin, may be considered in the retreatment of patients with KD who have had recurrent or recrudescent fever after initial IVIG treatment.
   d. Administration of infliximab (5 mg/kg) may be considered as an alternative to a second infusion of IVIG or corticosteroid for IVIG-resistant patients.
   e. Administration of cyclosporine may be considered in patients with refractory KD in whom a second IVIG infusion, infliximab, or a course of steroids has failed.
   f. Administration of immunomodulatory monoclonal antibody therapy (except tumor necrosis factor–α blockers), cytotoxic agents or (rarely) plasma exchange may be considered in highly refractory patients who have failed to respond to a second infusion of IVIG, an extended course of steroids, or infliximab.

3. Prevention of thrombosis during the acute illness (McCrindle et al, 2017)
   a. Low-dose ASA (3–5 mg/kg/day) should be administered to patients without evidence of coronary artery changes until 4 to 6 weeks after onset of illness.
   b. For patients with rapidly expanding coronary artery aneurysms or a maximum Z score of 10 or greater, systemic anticoagulation with low-molecular-weight heparin (LMWH) or warfarin (international normalized ratio target, 2.0–3.0) in addition to low-dose ASA is reasonable.
   c. For patients at increased risk of thrombosis, for example, with large or giant aneurysms (≥8 mm) or Z score ≥10) and a recent history of coronary artery thrombosis, "triple therapy" with ASA, a second antiplatelet agent (e.g., dipyridamole [Persantine] or clopidogrel [Plavix]), and anticoagulation with warfarin or LMWH may be considered.

4. Treatment of coronary artery thrombosis
   a. Coronary artery thrombosis with actual or impending occlusion of the arterial lumen should be treated with thrombolytic therapy or in patients of sufficient size by mechanical restoration of coronary artery blood flow at cardiac catheterization.
   b. Thrombolytic agents should be administered together with low-dose ASA and low-dose heparin with careful monitoring for bleeding.

Natural History

Kawasaki's disease is a self-limited disease for most patients. Cardiovascular involvement is the most serious complication.

1. Coronary aneurysm develops in 15% to 25% of untreated patients and is responsible for MI (<5%) and death (1%–5%). A significantly higher temperature (101.3°F [38.5°C] on days 9 to 12) and longer duration of fever (>14 days) appear to be risk factors for coronary aneurysm. Despite prompt treatment with high-dose IVIG, at least transient coronary artery abnormalities develop in 5% of the patients and giant aneurysm in 1%.

2. Angiographic resolution of aneurysm 1 to 2 years after the illness occurs in 50% to 67% of the patients, but these arteries do not dilate in response to exercise or coronary vasodilators. In some patients, stenosis, tortuosity, and thrombosis of the coronary arteries result. The resolution appears to be more likely to occur with a smaller aneurysm, age at onset before 1 year, fusiform rather than saccular aneurysm, and aneurysm located at a distal coronary segment.

3. More than 70% of MIs occur in the first year after onset of the disease without warning symptoms or signs. Giant aneurysm (>8 mm) is associated with greater morbidity and mortality (because of thrombotic occlusion or stenotic obstruction and subsequent MI). Ring calcification of giant coronary artery aneurysms may be visible on routine chest films indicative of an ongoing process that leads to irreversible changes even years after the initial onset of KD.

4. If the coronary arteries remain normal throughout the first month after the onset, subsequent development of a new coronary lesion is extremely unusual.

Long-Term Follow-up

Serial cardiology follow-up is important for evaluation of the cardiac status. The recommendations of the Committee on Rheumatic Fever, Endocarditis, and Kawasaki Disease of the AHA (2004) are summarized in Table 19.2.

1. For children with no or transient coronary abnormalities, aspirin is discontinued after 6 to 8 weeks. No follow-up diagnostic tests are indicated. Only a periodic counseling is recommended.

2. If there is coronary aneurysm, low-dose aspirin is continued indefinitely. With large aneurysm, a combination of aspirin and warfarin is indicated.

3. Varying levels of activity restriction is indicated in patients who have coronary artery aneurysm (see Table 19.2).

4. Echocardiography. In the absence of coronary artery abnormalities in the first 6 to 8 weeks, follow-up echocardiography is not indicated. If significant abnormalities of the coronary vessels, LV dysfunction, or valvular regurgitation are found, echocardiography should be repeated at 6 to 12 month intervals.

5. Exercise stress testing or myocardial perfusion evaluation is indicated in children with coronary artery aneurysms at 1 to 2 year intervals.

6. Occasionally, coronary angiography may be indicated in infants with large aneurysms or stenosis, in patients with symptoms suggestive of ischemia, in patients with positive exercise tests or thallium studies, or in those with evidence of MI.

7. Rarely, for patients with evidence of reversible ischemia from coronary artery stenosis (demonstrable on stress-imaging tests), percutaneous intervention, such as balloon angioplasty, rotational atherectomy, stenting, or a combination of these procedures, may be indicated (Ishii et al, 2002). On rare occasions, coronary artery bypass surgery may be indicated. The internal mammary artery graft may be used for bypass surgery.

LYME CARDITIS

Prevalence

Lyme carditis occurs in about 10% of patients with Lyme disease.

Cause and Pathology

1. Lyme disease is the leading tick-borne illness in North America and Europe. The disease is endemic in three US regions: the Northeast (most commonly in coastal areas from Maryland to northern Massachusetts), the upper Midwest (Wisconsin and Minnesota), and the Far West (California and Oregon). The disease has been reported from every part of the world, including most of the United States. The disease is named after the town of Old Lyme, Connecticut, where a number of cases were identified in 1975.

2. It is caused by the spirochete *Borrelia burgdorferi,* carried by hard-bodied ticks (e.g., *Ixodes dammini*). The spirochete initially produces a characteristic skin lesion (erythema chronicum migrans) and then spreads through the lymphatics and bloodstream and disseminates to other organs, including the heart and the central and peripheral nervous systems.

3. The organism can be found in the heart and other parts of the body and is responsible for clinical symptoms and signs.

Clinical Manifestations

1. Most cases are identified during the summer months, and a history of tick bites may be elicited.

2. Lyme disease can be divided into three stages.

   a. *Stage 1* (localized erythema migrans) begins 3 to 30 days after the tick bite with the onset of influenza-like symptoms (fever, headache, myalgia, arthralgias, malaise) and the characteristic rash, *erythema chronicum migrans.* The skin lesion, seen in 60% to 80% of patients at the site of the tick bite, begins as a macule or papule followed by progressive expansion of an erythematous ring over approximately 7 days. The ring may be as large as 15 cm with red borders and central clearing, most often appearing on the thigh, groin, or axilla. Erythema migrans lesions usually fade within 3 to 4 weeks, but they may recur.

   b. *Stage 2* (disseminated infection) starts 2 to 12 weeks after the tick bite; neurologic (10% to 15%) and cardiac (10%) manifestations occur in this stage. The classic triad of Lyme neuroborreliosis includes aseptic meningitis, cranial nerve palsies (most commonly, unilateral

TABLE 19.2   Follow-up Recommendations According to the Degree of Coronary Artery Involvement

Risk Level	Pharmacologic Therapy	Physical Activity	Follow-up and Diagnostic Testing	Invasive Testing
I (no coronary artery changes at any stage of illness)	None beyond first 6–8 wk (aspirin for first 6–8 wk only)	No restrictions beyond first 6–8 wk	Cardiovascular risk assessment, counseling at 5-yr intervals	None recommended
II (transient coronary artery ectasia disappears within first 6–8 wk)	None beyond first 6–8 wk (aspirin for first 6–8 wk only)	No restrictions beyond initial 6–8 wk	Cardiovascular risk assessment and counseling at 3- to 5-yr intervals	None recommended
III (one small to medium coronary artery aneurysm on major coronary artery)	Low-dose aspirin (3–5 mg/kg/day) at least until aneurysm regression documented	For patients younger than 11 yr, no restrictions beyond initial 6–8 wk Patients 11–20 yr old: physical activity guided by stress test or myocardial perfusion scan every 2 years Contact and high-impact sports are discouraged for patients taking antiplatelet agents	Annual cardiology follow-up with echocardiogram + ECG Cardiovascular risk assessment and counseling Stress test with myocardial perfusion scan every 2 yr in patients older than 10 yr	Angiography if noninvasive test suggests ischemia
IV (≥one large or giant coronary artery aneurysm or multiple or complex aneurysm in same coronary artery without obstruction)	Long-term aspirin (3–5 mg/kg/day) and warfarin (target: INR, 2.0–2.5) or LMWH (target antifactor Xa level, 0.5–1.0 U/mL) should be combined in giant aneurysm	Contact and high-impact sports should be avoided because of risk of bleeding Other physical activity recommendations guided by annual stress test or myocardial perfusion evaluation	Cardiology follow-up with echocardiogram + ECG every 6 months Annual stress test with myocardial perfusion evaluation For women of childbearing age, reproductive counseling is recommended	First angiography at 6–12 mo or sooner if clinically indicated Repeat angiography if noninvasive test, clinical, or laboratory findings suggest ischemia Elective repeat angiography under some circumstances (e.g., atypical anginal pain, inability to do stress testing)
V (coronary artery obstruction)	Long-term low-dose aspirin (3–5 mg/kg/day) Warfarin LMWH if giant aneurysm persists Consider use of beta-blocker to reduce myocardial oxygen consumption	Contact and high-impact sports should be avoided because of risk of bleeding Other physical activity recommendations guided by stress test or myocardial perfusion scan results	Cardiology follow-up with echocardiogram and ECG every 6 mo Annual stress test or myocardial perfusion scan For women of childbearing age, reproductive counseling is recommended	Angiography recommended to address therapeutic options of bypass grafting or catheter intervention

ECG, Electrocardiography; *INR*, international normalized ratio; *LMWH*, low-molecular-weight heparin.
Modified from Newburger JW, Takahashi M, Gerber MA, et al: Diagnosis, treatment, and long-term management of Kawasaki disease: a statement for health professionals from the Committee on Rheumatic Fever, Endocarditis, and Kawasaki Disease, Council on Cardiovascular Disease in the Young, American Heart Association, *Pediatrics* 114:1708–1733, 2004.

or bilateral Bell's palsy), and peripheral radiculoneuropathy. The most common cardiac manifestation is fluctuating AV block (see later discussion), although myocarditis, pericarditis, and LV dysfunction can occur.

c. *Stage 3* (persistent infection) manifests as large-joint arthritis weeks to years after stage 2 and is seen in about

50% of the patients not previously treated. In general, joint manifestation is self-limited but may recur in patients who do not receive appropriate antibiotic therapy.

3. Cardiac manifestations occur in about 10% of cases. They generally appear 4 to 8 weeks after the initial illness, but

their appearance can vary from 4 days to 7 months. The most common cardiac manifestation is varying degrees of AV block, occurring in up to 87% of cases. More than 95% of these patients show first-degree AV block at some time in their course. Up to 50% develop complete heart block, and some of them develop permanent heart block. First-degree AV block can change to complete heart block within minutes.

Diagnosis

1. The diagnosis is suggested by the presence of the distinctive erythema chronicum migrans and other features of Lyme disease. A history of tick exposure (e.g., travel to an endemic area) and any of the manifestations of stages 2 and 3 are important clues to the disease. The presence of AV block alone is not specific for Lyme carditis; it can be caused by other infective agents, such as viral infections (coxsackie virus A and B, echovirus, mumps, polio), rickettsial infections, *Treponema pallidum*, *Yersinia enterocolitica*, toxoplasmosis, diphtheria, and Chagas' disease.
2. Although cultivation or visualization of *B. burgdorferi is* the most reliable technique to confirm the diagnosis, the test result is rarely positive.
3. Enzyme-linked immunosorbent assays (ELISAs) are probably more accurate than indirect immunofluorescence assays. The diagnosis of Lyme disease is confirmed if there is a single titer greater than 1:256 or a fourfold increase in antibody titer over time and compatible clinical symptoms.

Management

1. Doxycycline (100 mg twice a day, orally, for 14–21 days) is the drug of choice for children older than 8 years of age. For children younger than 8 years of age, amoxicillin (25–50 mg/kg/day orally, divided into two doses, for 2–3 weeks) is the drug of choice. For patients allergic to penicillin, cefuroxime axetil is an alternative.
2. If antibiotic therapy is begun in stage 1, the duration of the skin lesion is shortened, and subsequent complications can be averted. Antibiotic treatment also improves cardiac and neurologic symptoms.
3. Heart block responds to antibiotic treatment, usually within 6 weeks, and has a good prognosis.
4. For high-level AV block, temporary pacing may be indicated (in up to one third of patients).
5. Recently, a Lyme disease vaccine (LYMErix, SmithKline Beecham) was licensed by the US Food and Drug Administration for persons 15 to 70 years of age. The vaccine seems to be safe and effective, but its cost effectiveness has yet to be determined.

POSTPERICARDIOTOMY SYNDROME

Postpericardiotomy syndrome is a febrile illness with inflammatory reaction of the pericardium and pleura that develops after surgery involving pericardiotomy. It is believed to be an autoimmune response to damaged myocardium or pericardium or blood in the pericardial sac. There is also possibility of anti-heart antibodies created idiopathically or caused by concurrent cross-reactivity of the antibodies produced against viral antigens. However, the latter assumption is not fully proven because of conflicting studies. The incidence is about 25% to 30% of patients who receive pericardiotomy. A nonsurgical example of this syndrome is seen after MI (Dressler's syndrome) and traumatic hemopericardium. It can occur after percutaneous coronary intervention or after pacemaker or pacemaker wire placement.

Clinical Manifestations

1. The onset of the syndrome is a few weeks to a few months (median, 4 weeks) after cardiac surgery that involves pericardiotomy. It is rare in infants younger than 2 years of age.
2. The syndrome is characterized by fever and chest pain. Fever may be sustained or spike up to 104°F (40°C). Chest pain may be severe, caused by both pericarditis and pleuritis. Chest pain resulting from pericardial effusion radiates to the left side of the chest and shoulder and worsens in a supine position. Pleural pain worsens on deep inspiration. On physical examination, pericardial and pleural friction rubs and hepatomegaly are usually present. Tachycardia, tachypnea, rising venous pressure, and falling arterial pressure with a paradoxical pulse are signs of cardiac tamponade.
3. Chest x-ray films show an enlarged cardiac silhouette and pleural effusion, especially on the left. The ECG shows persistent ST-segment elevation and flat or inverted T waves in the limb leads and left precordial leads.
4. Echocardiography is the most reliable test in confirming the presence and amount of pericardial effusion and in evaluating evidence of cardiac tamponade.
5. Leukocytosis with a shift to the left and an elevated ESR are present. Levels of acute-phase reactants (ESR, CRP) are elevated.
6. Although the disease is self-limited, its duration is highly variable; the median duration is 2 to 3 weeks. Recurrences are common, appearing in 21% of patients.

Management

1. Bed rest is all that is needed for mild cases.
2. Nonsteroidal antiinflammatory agents, such as ibuprofen or indomethacin, may be effective in most cases.
3. In severe cases, moderate doses of corticosteroids may be indicated for a few days if the diagnosis is secure and infection has been ruled out. A more prompt response is seen with steroid therapy, but a serious drawback is the tendency for the condition to rebound after withdrawal of the drug, with some patients becoming steroid bound.
4. Emergency pericardiocentesis may be required if signs of cardiac tamponade are present.
5. Diuretics may be used for pleural effusion.
6. Pericardiectomy may be necessary in patients with recurrent effusion.

Acute Rheumatic Fever

PREVALENCE

Acute rheumatic fever (ARF) is a relatively uncommon disease in the United States and other developed countries, but it is a common cause of heart disease in less developed countries and among specific ethnic and socioeconomic groups. In the past few decades, however, new outbreaks have occurred, and new sporadic cases are being reported in the United States.

CAUSE

1. ARF is believed to be an immunologic response that occurs as a delayed sequela of group A streptococcal (GAS) infection of the pharynx but not of the skin (Parks, 2012). The attack rate ARF after streptococcal infection varies with the severity of the infection, ranging from 0.3% to 3%.
2. Important predisposing factors include family history of rheumatic fever indicative of genetic disposition as well as low socioeconomic status (poverty, poor hygiene, medical deprivation) and age between 6 and 15 years (with a peak incidence at 8 years of age).

PATHOLOGY

1. The inflammatory lesion is found in many parts of the body, most notably in the heart, brain, joints, and skin.
2. Although rheumatic carditis was considered to be pancarditis, valvulitis is much more important than myocardial and pericardial involvements. The dominant and most important abnormality with rheumatic carditis is the valvulitis, specifically mitral regurgitation (MR) or aortic regurgitation (AR). MR occurs in about 95% of the patients and AR in 20% to 25% of the patients. In rheumatic myocarditis, myocardial contractility is rarely impaired, and the serum level of troponin is not elevated.
3. The mitral valve is most frequently and most severely involved. It is not only the valve leaflets that are heavily involved with fibrinous vegetations on the coapting surfaces, but the entire mitral valve apparatus is involved (with annular dilatation and stretching of chordae tendineae).
4. Aschoff bodies in the atrial myocardium are believed to be characteristic of rheumatic fever. These consist of inflammatory lesions associated with swelling, fragmentation of collagen fibers and alterations in the staining characteristics of connective tissue, now believed to be necrotic myocardial cells.

CLINICAL MANIFESTATIONS

History

1. History of streptococcal pharyngitis, 1 to 5 weeks (average, 3 weeks) before the onset of symptoms, is common. The latent period may be as long as 2 to 6 months (average, 4 months) in cases of isolated chorea.
2. Pallor, malaise, easy fatigability, and other history, such as epistaxis (5%–10%) and abdominal pain, may be present.

Major Manifestations

Among the five major manifestations of ARF, carditis (50%–79%), and arthritis (35%–66%) are more common than the others. These are followed by chorea (10%–30%), which is seen more frequently in females, followed by subcutaneous nodules (0%–10%) and erythema marginatum (<6%). Five major criteria of ARF are discussed next.

Carditis

1. Carditis is the most common manifestation of ARF (50%–79%).
2. Tachycardia (out of proportion to the degree of fever) is common; its absence makes the diagnosis of myocarditis unlikely.
3. A heart murmur of MR or AR is almost always present.

4. Echo examination can determine the presence and severity of MR and AR more objectively than auscultation can. Inclusion of echocardiography and Doppler findings can enhance correct diagnosis of acute rheumatic carditis, including those with *subclinical carditis* (see later for further discussion).

5. Other abnormal echo findings may include pericardial effusion, increased left ventricular (LV) dimension, or impaired LV function. Pericardial effusion is usually of small amount and almost never causes cardiac tamponade. Pericarditis does not occur without mitral valve involvement in rheumatic fever. Cardiac chamber enlargement is indicative of severity of valvulitis or congestive heart failure (CHF); valvulitis is the most important determinant of the cardiac status.

6. Clinical presentation may be quite variable from the asymptomatic patients with characteristic heart murmur to the critically ill patients presenting in heart failure (occurring in 15%–25%).

7. The severity of carditis and valvular involvement often decreases as the inflammation subsides. Mild cardiac involvement may completely resolve, but moderate to severe involvement is more likely to experience persistent rheumatic heart disease.

   Concept of Subclinical Carditis. In the past, clinical evidence of carditis was based solely on the presence of heart murmur of MR or AR on auscultation. Auscultation would have missed some heart murmur of MR and AR in part because of declining skills of auscultation. With increasing availability of echocardiography and Doppler studies, more cases of cardiac involvement are being detected than previously. *Subclinical carditis* refers to the circumstance in which auscultatory findings of MR or AR are not recorded, but echocardiography and Doppler studies reveal evidence of mitral or aortic valvulitis. The prevalence of subclinical carditis may reach as high as 50%. Accordingly, all the studies overwhelmingly support the use of echocardiography and Doppler results as part of evidence of carditis (i.e., subclinical carditis).

   Therefore, echocardiography and Doppler studies should be performed in all cases of confirmed and suspected cases of ARF. Echocardiography and Doppler studies should be performed strictly fulfilling the findings noted in Box 20.1 to assess whether carditis is present in the absence of auscultatory findings. Echocardiography and Doppler findings not consistent with carditis should exclude that diagnosis in patients with a heart murmur thought to indicate rheumatic carditis.

Arthritis

Arthritis is the second most common manifestation of ARF (occurring in 35%-66%). Arthritis of ARF is typically a migratory polyarthritis, and the joints most frequently involved are large ones, including the knees, ankles, elbows, and wrists. Swelling, heat, redness, severe pain, tenderness, and limitation of motion are common. If the patient was given salicylate-containing analgesics, these signs of inflammation may be mild or

---

BOX 20.1 Echocardiography and Doppler Findings in Rheumatic Valvulitis

Morphological Findings	Doppler Findings
<ul><li>Acute mitral valve changes</li><ul><li>Annular dilation</li><li>Chordal elongation</li><li>Chordal rupture resulting in flail leaflet with severe MR</li><li>Anterior (or less commonly posterior) leaflet tip prolapse</li><li>Beading or nodularity of the leaflet tips</li></ul><li>Chronic mitral valve changes: not seen in acute carditis</li><ul><li>Leaflet thickening</li><li>Chordal thickening and fusion</li><li>Restricted leaflet motion</li><li>Calcification</li></ul><li>Aortic valve changes in either acute or chronic carditis</li><ul><li>Irregular or focal leaflet thickening</li><li>Coaptation defect</li><li>Restricted leaflet motion</li><li>Leaflet prolapse</li></ul></ul>	<ul><li>Pathological mitral regurgitation (all four criteria met)</li><ul><li>Seen in at least two views</li><li>Jet length ≥2 cm in at least one view</li><li>Peak velocity >3m/sec</li><li>Pansystolic jet in at least one envelope</li></ul><li>Pathologic aortic regurgitation (all four criteria met)</li><ul><li>Seen in at least 2 views</li><li>Jet length ≥1 cm in at least one view</li><li>Peak velocity >3m/sec</li><li>Pandiastolic jet in at least one envelope</li></ul></ul>

MR, Mitral regurgitation.
Reprinted with permission Circulation. 2015;131:1806–1818 © 2012 American Heart Association, Inc.

---

resolved. The arthritis responds dramatically to salicylate therapy; if patients treated with salicylates (with documented therapeutic levels) do not improve in 48 hours, the diagnosis of ARF probably is incorrect. Generally, the arthritis in ARF runs a self-limited course, even without therapy, lasting about 4 weeks.

Sydenham's Chorea

Sydenham's chorea (St. Vitus' dance) is found in 10% to 30% of patients with ARF. It occurs more often in prepubertal girls (8–12 years) than in boys. Evidence of a recent GAS infection may be difficult or impossible to document because of the long latent period between the inciting infection and the onset of chorea.

Sydenham's chorea is a neuropsychiatric disorder consisting of both neurologic (choreic movement and hypotonia) and psychiatric signs (e.g., emotional lability, hyperactivity, separation anxiety, obsessions and compulsions). It begins with emotional lability and personality changes. These are soon replaced (in 1–4 weeks) by the characteristic spontaneous, purposeless movement of chorea (which lasts 4–18 months) followed by motor weakness. The distractibility and inattentiveness outlast the choreic movements. The adventitious movements, weakness, and hypotonia continue for an average of 7 months

(≤17 months) before slowly waning in severity. Recently, elevated titers of "antineuronal antibodies" recognizing basal ganglion tissues have been found in more than 90% of patients. The levels of the antineuronal antibody titer are positively related to the severity of choreic movements. These findings suggest that chorea may be related to dysfunction of basal ganglia and cortical neuronal components.

Subcutaneous Nodules

Subcutaneous nodules are found in 2% to 10% of patients, particularly in cases with recurrences; it is almost never present as a sole manifestation of rheumatic fever. They are firm, painless, nonpruritic, freely movable, swelling, and 0.2 to 2 cm in diameter. They usually are found symmetrically, singly or in clusters, on the extensor surfaces of both large and small joints, over the scalp, or along the spine. They are not transient, lasting for weeks, and have a significant association with carditis. Subcutaneous nodules are not exclusive to rheumatic fever. They occur in 10% of children with rheumatoid arthritis, and benign subcutaneous nodules have been described in children and adults. In adults, they occur with rheumatoid arthritis, systemic lupus erythematosus, and other diseases.

Erythema Marginatum

Erythema marginatum occurs in fewer than 10% of patients with ARF. It is the unique, evanescent, pink rash seen with pale centers and rounded or serpiginous margin. They are most prominent on the trunk and the inner proximal portions of the extremities; they are never seen on the face. The rashes are evanescent, disappearing on exposure to cold and reappearing after a hot shower or when the patient is covered with a warm blanket. They seldom are detected in air-conditioned rooms.

Minor Manifestations

The following are four minor criteria for the diagnosis of ARF.

1. Polyarthralgia refers to multiple joint pain without the objective changes of arthritis.
2. Fever (usually with a temperature of ≥101.3°F [38.5°C]) is present early in the course of untreated rheumatic fever.
3. In laboratory findings, elevated acute-phase reactants (elevated C-reactive protein [CRP] levels and elevated erythrocyte sedimentation rate [ESR]) are objective evidence of an inflammatory process.
4. A prolonged PR interval on the electrocardiogram (ECG) is neither specific for ARF nor an indication of active carditis.

Other Clinical Features

1. Abdominal pain, rapid sleeping heart rate, tachycardia out of proportion to fever, malaise, anemia, epistaxis, and precordial pain are relatively common but not specific.
2. A positive family history of rheumatic fever also may heighten the suspicion.

BOX 20.2 **Revised Jones Criteria**[a]

Major Criteria
- Carditis (clinical or subclinical)
- Arthritis (polyarthritis only)
- Chorea
- Erythema marginatum
- Subcutaneous nodules

Minor Criteria
- Polyarthralgia
- Fever ≥38.5°C
- ESR ≥60 mm/hr and/or CRP ≥3.0 mg/dL
- Prolonged PR interval for age

Evidence of Preceding Group A Streptococcal Infection (Any One of the Following)
- Increased or rising ASO titer (or anti–DNASE B)
- Positive throat culture for group A beta-hemolytic streptococci
- Positive rapid group A streptococcal carbohydrate antigen

Diagnosis
Initial ARF: Two major or one major + two minor
Recurrent ARF: Two major, 1 major + two minor, or three minor
+ Evidence of preceding GAS infection

[a] For low-risk population only. Note that for moderate or high-risk population areas, a lighter requirement for the diagnosis of acute rheumatic fever (ARF) exists.
ASO, Antistreptolysin O; *CRP,* C-reactive protein; *ESR,* erythrocyte sedimentation rate; *GAS,* group A streptococcal.
Modified from Gewitz MH, Baltimore RS, Tani LY, et al: Revision of the Jones Criteria for the diagnosis of acute rheumatic fever in the era of Doppler echocardiography. A scientific statement from the American Heart Association, *Circulation* 131:1806–1818, 2015.

Evidence of Antecedent Group A Streptococcal Infection

Because other illness may closely resemble ARF, laboratory evidence of antecedent GAS infection is needed whenever possible, and the diagnosis is in doubt when such evidence is not available. The exception to this includes chorea, which usually has a long latent period and insidious onset of the illness.

Any one of the following can serve as evidence of preceding infection according to a recent AHA statement.

1. Increased or rising antistreptolysin O (ASO) titer or other streptococcal antibodies (anti–DNASE B)
2. Positive throat culture for group A beta-hemolytic streptococcus
3. A positive rapid group A streptococcus carbohydrate antigen test result in a child whose clinical presentation suggests a high pretest probability of streptococcal pharyngitis

DIAGNOSIS

Acute rheumatic fever is diagnosed by the use of revised Jones criteria (updated in 2015; Box 20.2). The criteria are three groups of important clinical and laboratory findings: (1) five major criteria, (2) four minor criteria, and (3) supporting evidence of preceding GAS infection.

1. A diagnosis of ARF is highly probable when either two major criteria or one major and two minor criteria plus evidence of antecedent streptococcal infection are present.

2. For recurrent ARF (in individuals with previous history of ARF or those with RHD), less rigid criteria is used because they are at high risk for recurrent attacks if reinfected with GAS. In addition to the same criteria as mentioned earlier, only three minor criteria in the presence of evidence of preceding GAS infection suffice.

3. The following tips help in applying the Jones criteria:
   a. The absence of supporting evidence of a previous GAS infection makes the diagnosis doubtful (except when chorea is present).
   b. Two major criteria are always stronger than one major plus two minor criteria.
   c. Polyarthralgia or a prolonged PR interval cannot be used as a minor criterion when using arthritis and carditis, respectively, as major criterion.
   d. The vibratory innocent (Still's) murmur is often misinterpreted as a murmur of MR and thereby is a frequent cause of misdiagnosis (or overdiagnosis) of ARF. The murmur of MR is a *regurgitant-type* systolic murmur (starting with the S1) caused by MR, but the innocent murmur is low pitched and an *ejection* type. A cardiology consultation and echocardiography and Doppler study during the acute phase will minimize the frequency of misdiagnosis.
   e. The possibility of the early suppression of full clinical manifestations should be sought during the history taking. Subtherapeutic doses of aspirin or salicylate-containing analgesics (e.g., Bufferin, Anacin) may suppress full manifestations.

4. Exceptions to the Jones criteria include the following two specific situations:
   a. Chorea may occur as the only manifestation of ARF.
   b. Indolent carditis may be the only manifestation in patients who come to medical attention months after the onset of rheumatic fever.

DIFFERENTIAL DIAGNOSIS

1. Juvenile rheumatoid arthritis is often misdiagnosed as ARF. The following findings suggest juvenile rheumatoid arthritis rather than ARF: involvement of peripheral small joints, symmetrical involvement of large joints without migratory arthritis, pallor of the involved joints, a more indolent course, no evidence of preceding streptococcal infection, and the absence of prompt response to salicylate therapy within 24 to 48 hours.

2. Other collagen vascular diseases (systemic lupus erythematosus, mixed connective tissue disease); reactive arthritis, including poststreptococcal arthritis; serum sickness; and infectious arthritis (such as gonococcal) occasionally require differentiation.

3. Virus-associated acute arthritis (rubella, parvovirus, hepatitis B virus, herpesviruses, enteroviruses) is much more common in adults.

4. Hematologic disorders, such as sicklemia and leukemia, should be considered in the differential diagnosis.

CLINICAL COURSE

1. Only carditis can cause permanent cardiac damage. Signs of mild carditis disappear rapidly in weeks, but those of severe carditis may last for 2 to 6 months.

2. Arthritis subsides within a few days to several weeks, even without treatment, and does not cause permanent damage.

3. Chorea gradually subsides in 6 to 7 months or longer and usually does not cause permanent neurologic sequelae.

MANAGEMENT

1. When ARF is suggested by history and physical examination, one should obtain the following laboratory studies: complete blood count, acute-phase reactants (ESR and CRP), throat culture, ASO titer (and a second antibody titer, particularly with chorea), chest x-ray films, and ECG. Cardiology consultation is indicated to clarify whether there is cardiac involvement; two-dimensional echo and Doppler studies are usually performed at that time.

2. Benzathine penicillin G, 0.6 to 1.2 million units intramuscularly, is given to eradicate streptococci. This serves as the first dose of penicillin prophylaxis as well (see later discussion). In patients allergic to penicillin, erythromycin, 40 mg/kg/day in two to four doses for 10 days, may be substituted for penicillin.

3. Antiinflammatory or suppressive therapy with salicylates or steroids must not be started until a definite diagnosis is made. Early suppressive therapy may interfere with a definite diagnosis of ARF by suppressing full development of joint manifestations and suppressing acute-phase reactants.

4. When the diagnosis of ARF is confirmed, one must educate the patient and parents about the need to prevent subsequent streptococcal infection through continuous antibiotic prophylaxis.

5. Bed rest of varying duration is recommended. The duration depends on the type and severity of the manifestations and may range from a week (for isolated arthritis) to several weeks for severe carditis. Bed rest is followed by a period of indoor ambulation of varying duration before the child is allowed to return to school. The ESR is a helpful guide to the rheumatic activity and therefore to the duration of restriction of activities. Full activity is allowed when the ESR has returned to normal, except in children with significant cardiac involvement. Table 20.1 is a general guide to the period of bed rest and indoor ambulation.

6. Therapy with antiinflammatory agents should be started as soon as ARF has been diagnosed.
   a. For mild to moderate carditis, aspirin alone is recommended in a dosage of 90 to 100 mg/kg/day in four to six divided doses. An adequate blood level of salicylates is 20 to 25 mg/100 mL. This dose is continued for 4 to 8 weeks, depending on the clinical response. After improvement, the therapy is withdrawn gradually over 4 to 6 weeks while monitoring acute-phase reactants.

TABLE 20.1   General Guidelines for Bed Rest and Indoor Ambulation

	Arthritis Alone	Mild Carditis[a]	Moderate Carditis[b]	Severe Carditis[c]
Bed rest	1–2 wk	3–4 wk	4–6 wk	As long as CHF is present
Indoor ambulation	1–2 wk	3–4 wk	4–6 wk	2–3 mo

CHF, Congestive heart failure.
[a]Questionable cardiomegaly.
[b]Definite but mild cardiomegaly.
[c]Marked cardiomegaly or heart failure.

b. For severe carditis, prednisone (2 mg/kg/day in four divided doses) for 2 to 6 weeks is indicated. The dose of prednisone should be tapered and aspirin started during the final week of prednisone to prevent rebound.

c. For arthritis, aspirin therapy is continued for 2 weeks and gradually withdrawn over the following 2 to 3 weeks. Rapid resolution of joint symptoms with aspirin within 24 to 36 hours is supportive evidence of the arthritis of ARF.

7. Treatment of CHF includes the following (also see Chapter 27).
   a. Complete bed rest with orthopneic position and moist, cool oxygen
   b. Prednisone for severe carditis of recent onset
   c. Furosemide, 1 mg/kg every 6 to 12 hours, if indicated
   d. Afterload reduction may be beneficial.

8. Management of Sydenham's chorea:
   a. Reduce physical and emotional stress and use protective measures as indicated to prevent physical injuries.
   b. Give benzathine penicillin G, 1.2 million units, initially for eradication of streptococcus and also every 28 days for prevention of recurrence, just as in patients with other rheumatic manifestations. Without the prophylaxis, about 25% of patients with isolated chorea (without carditis) develop rheumatic valvular heart disease in 20-year follow-up.
   c. Antiinflammatory agents are not needed in patients with isolated chorea.
   d. For severe cases, any of the following drugs may be used: phenobarbital (15–30 mg every 6–8 hours), haloperidol (starting at 0.5 mg and increasing every 8 hours to 2 g), valproic acid, chlorpromazine (Thorazine), diazepam (Valium), or steroids.
   e. Results of plasma exchange (to remove antineuronal antibodies) and intravenous immune globulin therapy (to inactivate the effects of the antineuronal antibodies) are promising in decreasing the severity of chorea and they were better than prednisone (Garvey et al, 2005).

PROGNOSIS

The presence or absence of permanent cardiac damage determines the prognosis. The development of residual heart disease is influenced by the following three factors.

1. Cardiac status at the start of treatment: The more severe the cardiac involvement at the time the patient is first seen, the greater the incidence of residual heart disease.
2. Recurrence of rheumatic fever: The severity of valvular involvement increases with each recurrence.
3. Regression of heart disease: Evidence of cardiac involvement at the first attack may disappear in 10% to 25% of patients 10 years after the initial attack. Valvular disease resolves more frequently when prophylaxis is followed.

PREVENTION

Primary Prevention

Group A streptococcal infection of the pharynx is the precipitating cause of rheumatic fever. Primary prevention of rheumatic fever is possible by appropriate antibiotic treatment of streptococcal pharyngitis in most cases. However, primary prevention is not possible in all patients because about 30% of the patients develop subclinical pharyngitis and therefore do not seek medical treatment. In addition, some symptomatic patients do not seek medical care. In these instances, rheumatic fever is not preventable.

Throat culture or a rapid antigen detection test is required for the diagnosis of GAS pharyngitis. Streptococcal skin infection (impetigo or pyoderma) have not been proven to lead to ARF. After positive throat culture result for GAS, either oral penicillin V or intramuscular benzathine penicillin G is the treatment of choice, because it is cost effective, has a narrow spectrum of activity, and has long-standing proven efficacy, and GAS resistant to penicillin have not been documented. For individuals allergic to penicillin, cephalosporin, clindamycin, azithromycin, or clarithromycin may be given.

Secondary Prevention

An individual with a previous attack of rheumatic fever in whom GAS pharyngitis develops is at high risk of a recurrent attack of rheumatic fever. Prevention of recurrent rheumatic fever requires continuous antimicrobial prophylaxis rather than recognition and treatment of acute episode of streptococcal pharyngitis.

1. Who should receive prophylaxis?
   Patients with documented histories of rheumatic fever, including those with isolated chorea and those without evidence of rheumatic heart disease, must receive prophylaxis.
2. For how long?
   Ideally, patients should receive prophylaxis indefinitely. For patients who had ARF without carditis, the prophylaxis should continue for at least 5 years or until the person is 21 years of age, whichever is longer. Patients who have history of carditis or persistent valvular disease (clinical or echocardiographic evidence) should receive secondary prophylaxis for a longer period of time (Table 20.2).

TABLE 20.2   Recommended Duration of Secondary Rheumatic Fever Prophylaxis

Category	Duration After Last Attack
Rheumatic fever with carditis and residual heart disease (persistent valvular disease[a])	10 yr or until 40 yr of age (whichever is longer)
Rheumatic fever with carditis but no residual heart disease (no valvular disease[a])	10 yr or until 21 yr of age (whichever is longer)
Rheumatic fever without carditis disease)	5 yr or until 21 yr of age (whichever is longer)

[a]Clinical or echocardiographic evidence.

From Gerber MA, Baltimore RS, Eaton CB, et al: Prevention of rheumatic fever and diagnosis and treatment of acute streptococcal pharyngitis: a scientific statement from the American Heart Association Rheumatic Fever, Endocarditis, and Kawasaki Disease Committee of the Council on Cardiovascular Disease in the Young, the Interdisciplinary Council on Functional Genomics and Translational Biology, and the Interdisciplinary Council on Quality of Care and Outcome Research, Reprinted with permission Circulation. 2009;119:1541-1551©2009 American Heart Association, Inc.

3. Choice of antibiotics
   a. Benzathine penicillin G, 600,000 U units given intramuscularly every 28 days (not once a month) for children weighing less than 27 kg (60 lb) and 1.2 million units for children weighing more than 60 lb is the drug of choice.
   b. Alternatively, penicillin V (250 mg twice a day, oral) or sulfadiazine (oral), 0.5 g once daily for children weighing less than 27 kg (60 lb) or 1.0 g once a day for children weighing more than 60 lb, is given.
   c. For individuals allergic to penicillin and sulfadiazine, a macrolide or azalide may be given.

21

Valvular Heart Disease

Valvular heart diseases are either congenital or acquired in origin. Pathophysiology and clinical manifestations are similar for both entities and are discussed in Chapter 10. Congenital stenoses of the aortic and pulmonary valves are discussed in depth in the section on Obstructive Lesions in Chapter 13.

In this chapter, mitral stenosis (MS), mitral regurgitation (MR), and aortic regurgitation (AR) of both congenital and acquired etiology are discussed if they are isolated or the major lesion. Although the cause of mitral valve prolapse (MVP) is not entirely clear, it is discussed in this chapter because it involves a cardiac valve. Isolated congenital pulmonary regurgitation (PR), tricuspid regurgitation (TR), and tricuspid stenosis of significance are exceedingly rare and therefore are not discussed. PR after tetralogy of Fallot (TOF) surgery is discussed under TOF in Chapter 14. TR is most frequently seen with Ebstein's anomaly and is discussed under that condition.

Mitral stenosis of rheumatic etiology is rare in the developed countries, although it still occurs in developing countries, frequently affecting young adult population. Among rheumatic heart disease, mitral valve involvement occurs in about three fourths and aortic valve involvement in about one fourth of the cases. Stenosis and regurgitation of the same valve usually occur together. Isolated aortic stenosis (AS) of rheumatic origin without mitral valve involvement is extremely rare. Rheumatic involvement of the tricuspid and pulmonary valves almost never occurs.

MITRAL STENOSIS

Prevalence

1. Congenital MS occurs in 0.2 to 0.6% of congenital heart diseases (CHDs), usually as part of other defects. Isolated congenital MS is very rare. It is usually associated with other anomalies such as Shone complex.
2. MS of rheumatic origin is rare in children (because it requires 5–10 years from the initial attack to develop the condition), but it is the most common valvular involvement in adult rheumatic patients in areas where rheumatic fever is still prevalent.

Pathology and Pathophysiology

In children, MS is mostly congenital and very rarely caused by rheumatic heart disease.

1. Congenital MS encompasses different types of obstructions occurring at different levels near the mitral valve position. The stenosis may be caused by obstruction at the mitral valve level (fusion of the leaflets), at the papillary muscle level (single papillary muscle seen with parachute mitral valve), at the chordae (thickened and fused chordae seen in single papillary muscle), or at the supravalvar region (supravalvar mitral ring), and it may be caused by the hypoplasia of the valve ring itself (as seen with hypoplastic left heart syndrome). Some of these anomalies are associated with other CHDs.

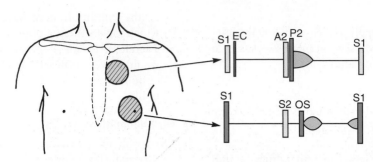

Fig. 21.1 Cardiac findings of mitral stenosis. Abnormal sounds are shown in *black* and include a loud S1, an ejection click (EC), a loud S2, and an opening snap (OS). Also note the mid-diastolic rumble and presystolic murmur. The murmur of pulmonary regurgitation indicates long-standing pulmonary hypertension.

2. Rheumatic MS is extremely rare in the pediatric age group. In rheumatic MS, thickening of the leaflets and fusion of the commissures dominate the pathologic findings. Calcification with immobility of the valve results over time.
3. Regardless of the etiology, a significant MS results in the enlargement of the left atrium (LA), pulmonary venous hypertension, and pulmonary artery hypertension with resulting enlargement and hypertrophy of the right side of the heart.
4. In patients with severe pulmonary venous hypertension, pulmonary congestion and edema, fibrosis of the alveolar walls, hypertrophy of the pulmonary arterioles, and loss of lung compliance result.

Clinical Manifestations
History
1. Patients with mild MS are asymptomatic.
2. In infants with severe MS, symptoms develop early in life with shortness of breath and failure to thrive.
2. Dyspnea with or without exertion is the most common symptom in older children. Orthopnea, nocturnal dyspnea, or palpitation is present in more severe cases.

Physical Examination (Fig. 21.1)
1. An increased right ventricular impulse is palpable along the left sternal border. Neck veins are distended if right-sided heart failure supervenes.
2. A loud S1 at the apex and a narrowly split S2 with accentuated P2 are audible if pulmonary hypertension is present. In older children with rheumatic MS, an opening snap (a short snapping sound accompanying the opening of the mitral valve) may be audible in rheumatic MS. A low-frequency mitral diastolic rumble is present at the apex (see Fig. 21.1). A crescendo presystolic murmur may be audible at the apex. Occasionally, a high-frequency diastolic murmur of PR (Graham Steell's murmur) is present at the upper left sternal border, but it is difficult to distinguish from AR.

Electrocardiography
Right-axis deviation, left atrial hypertrophy (LAH), and right ventricular hypertrophy (RVH) (caused by pulmonary hypertension) are common. Atrial fibrillation is rare in children.

Chest Radiography
1. The LA and right ventricle (RV) are usually enlarged, and the main pulmonary artery (PA) segment is usually prominent.
2. Lung fields show pulmonary venous congestion, interstitial edema shown as Kerley's B lines (dense, short, horizontal lines most commonly seen in the costophrenic angles), and redistribution of pulmonary blood flow with increased pulmonary vascularity to the upper lobes.

Echocardiography
Echocardiography is the most accurate noninvasive tool for the detection of MS.
1. A two- or three-dimensional echo study should define structural abnormalities of the valve, supravalvar region, chordae, and papillary muscles.
2. It shows a dilated LA. The main PA, RV, and right atrium (RA) also are dilated.
3. Doppler studies can estimate the pressure gradient and thus the severity of stenosis. A mean Doppler gradient of less than 4 to 5 mm Hg results from mild stenosis, 6 to 12 mm Hg is seen with moderate stenosis, and a mean gradient greater than 13 mm Hg is seen with severe stenosis.
4. RV systolic pressure can be estimated from the TR jet velocity (by Bernoulli equation), which may be elevated.
5. In patients with rheumatic MS, an M-mode echo may show a diminished E to F slope (reflecting a slow diastolic closure of the anterior mitral leaflet), anterior movement of the posterior leaflet during diastole, multiple echoes from thickened mitral leaflets, and large LA dimension.

Natural History
1. Infants with significant MS with failure to thrive require either balloon or surgical intervention.
2. Most children with mild MS are asymptomatic but become symptomatic with exertion.
3. For rheumatic MS, recurrence of rheumatic fever worsens the stenosis.
4. Atrial flutter or fibrillation and thromboembolism (related to the chronic atrial arrhythmias) are rare in children.
5. Hemoptysis can develop from the rupture of small vessels in the bronchi as a result of long-standing pulmonary venous hypertension.

Management

Different management plans apply to the two distinctly different forms of MS: congenital MS seen in infants versus rheumatic MS seen in adolescents or adults.

For Congenital Mitral Stenosis

1. Patients with mild or moderate stenosis usually do not warrant surgery or catheter intervention.
   a. Diuretic therapy may be beneficial.
   b. Varying degrees of restriction of activity may be indicated.
   c. Watch for secondary complications, such as failure to thrive, development of pulmonary hypertension, atrial fibrillation, and respiratory infection.
   d. If atrial fibrillation develops, propranolol, verapamil, or digoxin is the initial treatment to slow the atrioventricular (AV) conduction. Intravenous procainamide may be used for conversion to sinus rhythm in hemodynamically stable patients. For patients with chronic atrial fibrillation, anticoagulation with warfarin should be started 3 weeks before cardioversion to prevent systemic embolization of atrial thrombus. Anticoagulation is continued for 4 weeks after restoration of sinus rhythm (see Chapter 24 for further discussion). Quinidine may prevent recurrence. Recurrent atrial fibrillation, thromboembolic phenomenon, and hemoptysis may be indications for surgery in children.
2. Patients with severe MS require relief of obstruction. Options of intervention include balloon mitral valvuloplasty, surgical valvuloplasty, or surgical valve replacement.
   a. Balloon valvuloplasty could be considered for children with typical valvular stenosis, double orifice mitral valve, or parachute mitral valve. Significant MR is a concerning complication of the procedure. If the balloon procedure fails or significant MR develops, one of the surgical options should be considered in 10% to 25% of the patients.
   b. Surgical mitral valvuloplasty, rather than the balloon procedure, may be indicated in children with supravalvar ring, parachute mitral valve, or those with other associated CHDs (e.g., ventricular septal defect [VSD], coarctation of the aorta, subaortic stenosis). Supravalvar mitral ring is resected, and thickened and fused chordae may be split to make fenestration for a parachute mitral valve.
   c. Mitral valve replacement with mitral prosthesis is usually placed in the supra-annular position. After a mechanical prosthesis placement (but not after placement of a bioprosthesis), anticoagulation is required.
3. Surgical management of children with congenital MS is challenging. The limited lifespan of the prosthesis (particularly bioprosthesis) and the fixed size of the prosthesis require reintervention later in life with significant morbidity and mortality. The need for anticoagulation with warfarin for mechanical prosthesis is also a major challenge, especially in young children. Some survivors of the condition may have pulmonary hypertension, which makes them a poor candidate for transplantation. Therefore, in some infants with severe pathology that would be very difficult for surgical repair, it might be an option to consider a Norwood or hybrid approach early in life.

For Rheumatic Mitral Stenosis

1. For patients with rheumatic MS, secondary prevention of rheumatic fever with penicillin or sulfonamide is indicated (see Chapter 20).
2. The 2014 American Heart Association/American College of Cardiology (AHA/ACC) guidelines recommend the following for patients with rheumatic MS. (Refer to the publication Nishimura et al, 2014, for detailed guidelines.)
   a. Anticoagulation with warfarin or heparin is indicated in patients with (1) MS and atrial fibrillation, (2) MS and a prior embolic event, or (3) MS and an LA thrombus.
   b. Percutaneous mitral balloon commissurotomy is recommended for symptomatic patients with severe MS (defined as mitral valve area ≤1.5 cm^2, stage D) and favorable valve morphology in the absence of LA thrombus or moderate to severe MR.
   c. Mitral valve surgery (repair, commissurotomy, or valve replacement) is indicated in severely symptomatic patients with severe MS (as defined earlier) who are not high risk for surgery and who are not candidates for or who have failed previous percutaneous mitral balloon commissurotomy.
3. **Mitral valve replacement surgery.** A prosthetic valve (Starr-Edwards, Bjork-Shiley, St. Jude) is inserted either in the annulus or in a supra-annular position. The surgical mortality rate is 0% to 19%. All mechanical valves require anticoagulation with warfarin with its long-term risk, and reoperation may become necessary because of valve entrapment by pannus formation. The bioprostheses (porcine valve, heterograft valve) do not require anticoagulation therapy but require low-dose aspirin. Bioprostheses tend to deteriorate more rapidly because of calcific degeneration in children.

Postintervention Follow-up

1. Regular checkups every 6 to 12 months with echo and Doppler studies should be done for possible dysfunction of the repaired or replaced valve.
2. After replacement with a *mechanical valve* with no risk factors, warfarin is indicated to achieve an international normalized ratio (INR) of 2.5 to 3.5. Low-dose aspirin is also indicated.
3. After replacement with a bioprosthesis, if there are risk factors (e.g., atrial fibrillation, a prior embolic event, and LA thrombus), warfarin is also indicated. When there are no risk factors after bioprosthesis placement, aspirin alone is indicated at 75 to 100 mg/day (see ACC/AHA 2014 guidelines).

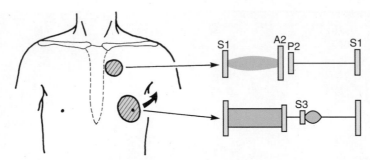

Fig. 21.2 Cardiac findings of mitral regurgitation. The *arrow* near the apex indicates the direction of radiation of the murmur toward the left axilla.

MITRAL REGURGITATION

Prevalence

Mitral regurgitation is more common than MS. Isolated congenital MR is rare; it is most often associated with AV canal defect. MR of rheumatic origin is rare but is the most common valvular involvement in children with rheumatic heart disease.

Pathology

1. Mitral valve regurgitation associated with AV canal occurs frequently through the cleft in the mitral valve (with eccentric regurgitation). When the valve annulus is dilated from any causes that dilate the left ventricle (LV) (e.g., AR or dilated cardiomyopathy), central regurgitation occurs.
2. In rheumatic heart disease, mitral valve leaflets are shortened because of fibrosis, resulting in MR.
3. With increasing severity of MR, dilatation of the LA and LV results, and the mitral valve ring may become dilated. Pulmonary hypertension may eventually develop as with MS.

Clinical Manifestations
History

1. Patients are usually asymptomatic with mild MR.
2. With increasing severity of MR, shortness of breath, tachypnea, fatigue (caused by reduced forward cardiac output), and palpitation (caused by atrial fibrillation) develop.

Physical Examination (Fig. 21.2)

1. The jugular venous pulse is normal in the absence of congestive heart failure (CHF). A heaving, hyperdynamic apical impulse is palpable in severe MR.
2. The S1 is normal or diminished. The S2 may split widely as a result of shortening of the LV ejection and early closure of the aortic valve. The S3 commonly is present and loud. The hallmark of MR is a regurgitant systolic murmur starting with S1, grade 2 to 4 of 6, at the apex, with good transmission to the left axilla (best demonstrated in the left decubitus position). A short, low-frequency diastolic rumble may be present at the apex (see Fig. 21.2).

Electrocardiography

1. Electrocardiography (ECG) is normal in mild cases.

2. Left ventricular hypertrophy (LVH) or LV dominance, with or without LAH, is usually present.
3. Atrial fibrillation is rare in children but often develops in adults.

Radiography (Fig. 21.3)

1. The LA and LV are enlarged to varying degrees.
2. Pulmonary vascularity usually is within normal limits, but a pulmonary venous congestion pattern may develop if CHF supervenes.

Echocardiography

1. Two-dimensional echo shows dilated LA and LV; the degree of dilatation is related to the severity of MR. Regurgitant fraction of 50% or greater is considered severe.
2. Color-flow mapping of the regurgitant jet into the LA and Doppler studies can assess the severity of the regurgitation.
3. The echocardiogram can distinguish eccentric regurgitation through the cleft mitral valve from central regurgitation (associated with annular dilatation).

Natural History

1. Patients are relatively stable for a long time with mild regurgitation.
2. LV failure and consequent pulmonary hypertension may occur in adult life.

Management
Medical

1. Afterload-reducing agents are particularly useful in maintaining the forward cardiac output.
2. Anticongestive therapy (with diuretics) is provided if CHF develops.
3. Activity need not be restricted in most mild cases.
4. If atrial fibrillation develops (rare in children), propranolol, verapamil, or digoxin is indicated to slow the ventricular response.

Surgical
Indications

1. It is generally advised to delay surgery in infants and small children until the onset of severe symptoms, such as intractable CHF or progressive cardiomegaly with symptoms. It appears that such a delay is not associated with late LV dysfunction.

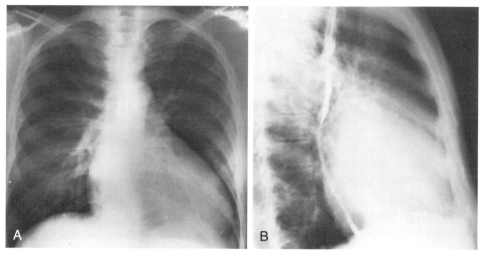

Fig. 21.3 Posteroanterior (**A**) and lateral (**B**) views of chest radiographs in a patient with moderately severe mitral regurgitation of rheumatic origin. The lateral view was obtained with barium swallow. The cardiothoracic ratio is increased (0.64), and the apex is displaced downward and laterally in the posteroanterior view. The lateral view shows an indentation of the barium-filled esophagus by an enlarged left atrium, and the left ventricle is displaced posteriorly.

2. Surgical repair is preferable to valve replacement whenever possible. The following conservative surgical techniques have been used: cleft repair, annuloplasty, chordal shortening, commissuroplasty, and accessory office closure.

3. According to the ACC/AHA 2014 guidelines (Nishimura et al, 2014), indications for mitral valve surgery in adult patients with severe MR are as follows. Similar indication may apply for adolescents and children. For detailed indications for surgery, readers are advised to read the 2014 AHA/ACC guidelines.

   a. Mitral valve surgery is recommended for symptomatic patients with severe MR and left ventricular ejection fraction (LVEF) greater than 30%.

   b. Mitral valve surgery is recommended for asymptomatic patients with severe AR and LV systolic dysfunction (LVEF 30%–60% or LV end-systolic dimension ≥40 mm).

   c. Mitral valve repair is recommended in preference to valve replacement when surgical treatment is indicated on the anterior, posterior, or both leaflets.

Procedures and Mortality

Mitral valve repair or replacement is performed under cardiopulmonary bypass.

1. Valve repair surgery is preferred over valve replacement, performed usually beyond infancy and during childhood. For cleft leak, repair of the cleft is performed. For central regurgitation with dilated annulus, annuloplasty is performed by commissuroplasty (not using annuloplasty ring which restricts growth potential). Valve repair has a lower mortality rate (<1%), and anticoagulation is not necessary.

2. Valve replacement is rarely necessary for unrepairable regurgitation. Frequently used low-profile prostheses are the Bjork-Shiley tilting disk and the St. Jude pyrolytic carbon valve. The surgical mortality rate is 2% to 7% for valve replacement. If a prosthetic valve is used, anticoagulation therapy must be continued.

Postoperative Follow-up

1. Valve function (of either the repaired natural valve or the replacement valve) should be checked by echo and Doppler studies every 6 to 12 months.

2. After replacement with a mechanical valve with no risk factors (e.g., atrial fibrillation, previous thromboembolism, LV dysfunction, and hypercoagulable state), warfarin is indicated to achieve an INR of 2.5 to 3.5 along with low-dose aspirin. After replacement with a bioprosthesis with no risk factors, aspirin alone is indicated at the dose of 75 to 100 mg/day; when there are risk factors, warfarin is also indicated.

AORTIC REGURGITATION

Prevalence

Aortic regurgitation is more often congenital than rheumatic in origin in the developed countries. AR of rheumatic origin is almost always associated with mitral valve disease.

Pathology

1. Congenital causes of AR include the following:

   a. Congenital bicuspid aortic valve

   b. Associated with VSD (either subpulmonary or membranous)

   c. Secondary to subaortic stenosis

   d. In association with dilated aortic root (Marfan's syndrome, Ehlers-Danlos syndromes)

2. Acquired type of AR is seen in rheumatic heart disease or after aortic balloon dilatation.

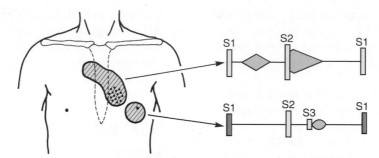

Fig. 21.4 Cardiac findings of aortic regurgitation. The S1 is abnormally soft *(black bar)*. The predominant murmur is a high-pitched, diastolic decrescendo murmur at the third left intercostal space.

Clinical Manifestations
History

1. Patients with mild regurgitation are asymptomatic.
2. Exercise tolerance is reduced with more severe AR or CHF.

Physical Examination (Fig. 21.4)

1. With moderate or severe AR, the precordium may be hyperdynamic with a laterally displaced apical impulse. A diastolic thrill occasionally is present at the third left intercostal space. A wide pulse pressure and a bounding water-hammer pulse may be present with severe AR.
2. The heart sounds are normal with mild AR. The S1 is decreased in intensity with moderate to severe AR. The S2 may be normal or single. A high-pitched diastolic decrescendo murmur, best audible at the third or fourth left intercostal space, is the auscultatory hallmark. This murmur is more easily audible with the patient sitting and leaning forward. The longer the murmur, the more severe the regurgitation (see Fig. 21.4). A systolic murmur of varying intensity may be present at the second right intercostal space because of relative AS caused by an increased stroke volume. The combination of the diastolic and systolic murmurs gives rise to a to-and-fro murmur in patients with severe AR. A mid-diastolic mitral rumble (Austin Flint murmur) may be present at the apex when the AR is severe.

Electrocardiography

The ECG is normal in mild cases. In severe cases, LVH usually is present. LAH may be present in long-standing cases.

Radiography

Cardiomegaly of varying degree involving the LV is present. A dilated ascending aorta and a prominent aortic knob frequently are present. Pulmonary venous congestion develops if LV failure supervenes.

Echocardiography

The LV dimension is increased, but the LA remains normal in size. The LV diastolic dimension is proportional to the severity of AR. Color-flow and Doppler examination can aid in estimating the severity of the regurgitation. LV systolic dysfunction develops at a later stage in severe AR.

Natural History

1. Patients with mild to moderate AR remain asymptomatic for a long time, but when symptoms begin to develop, many patients deteriorate rapidly.
2. Anginal pain, CHF, and multiple premature ventricular contractions are unfavorable signs occurring with severe AR.
3. Infective endocarditis is a rare complication.

Management
Medical

1. In case of rheumatic cause, prophylaxis should be continued against the recurrence of rheumatic fever with penicillin or sulfonamides (see Chapter 20).
2. Activity need not be restricted in mild cases, but varying degrees of restriction are indicated in more severe cases. Aerobic exercise is a better form of exercise; weightlifting exercise should be discouraged.
3. When used on a long-term basis, the angiotensin-converting enzyme (ACE) inhibitors have been shown to reduce (or even reverse) the dilatation and hypertrophy of the LV in children with AR but without CHF.
4. Patients with hypertension should be treated with calcium channel blockers or ACE inhibitors (or angiotensin receptor blockers).
5. If CHF develops, afterload-reducing agents and diuretics may be beneficial, but the benefits are rarely maintained.

Surgical

Indications. A major clinical decision in AR is the timing of aortic valve replacement (AVR). Ideally, it should be performed before irreversible dilatation of the LV develops, but there is no reliable method of detecting that point. According to ACC/AHA 2014 guidelines (Nishimura et al, 2014), the following are surgical indications in adult patients with chronic AR. (Refer to the publication, Nishimura et al, Circulation 2014, for detailed guidelines.) Similar indications may apply for adolescents and younger children.

1. AVR is indicated for symptomatic patient with severe AR regardless of LV systolic function.
2. AVR is indicated for asymptomatic patients with chronic severe AR and LV systolic dysfunction (LVEF <50%).

3. AVR is reasonable for asymptomatic patients with severe AR with normal LV systolic function (LVEF ≥50%) but with severe LV dilatation (LV end-systolic dimension >50 mm or indexed LV end-systolic dimension >25 mm/m^2).

Procedure and Mortality. Aortic valve repair is favored over valve replacement whenever possible. Valve replacement does not incorporate growth potential, except for the Ross procedure. Surgery is performed under cardiopulmonary bypass. The mortality rate for valve repair is near zero and that for valve replacement is about 2% to 5%.

1. Valve repair may include repair of simple tears or valvuloplasty for prolapsed cusps.
2. Valve replacement surgery
   a. The antibiotic-sterilized aortic homograft has been widely used and appears to be the device of choice.
   b. The porcine heterograft has the risk of accelerated degeneration.
   c. The Bjork-Shiley and St. Jude prostheses require anticoagulation therapy and are less suitable for young patients.
3. A pulmonary root autograft (Ross procedure) may be an attractive alternative to the conventional valve replacement surgery (see Fig. 13.9) in selected adolescents and young adults. In this procedure, the patient's own pulmonary valve and the adjacent PA are used to replace the diseased aortic valve and the adjacent aorta. The coronary ostia and buttons of aortic wall around the ostia are detached from the aorta and implanted into the PA. The surgical mortality rate is near zero. This procedure does not require anticoagulant therapy, the autograft may last longer than a porcine bioprosthesis, and there is a growth potential for the autograft pulmonary valve.

Complications. 1. Postoperative acute cardiac failure is the most common cause of death.
2. Thromboembolism, chronic hemolysis, and anticoagulant-induced hemorrhage may occur with prosthetic valves.
3. Porcine valves tend to develop early calcification in children.
4. Prosthetic valve endocarditis is a rare complication.

Postoperative Follow-up. 1. Regular follow-up of valve function should be done every 6 to 12 months by echo and Doppler studies.
2. Anticoagulation is needed after a prosthetic mechanical valve replacement. INR should be maintained between 2.5 and 3.5 for the first 3 months and 2.0 to 3.0 beyond that time. Low-dose aspirin (75–100 mg per day for adolescents) is also indicated in addition to warfarin (ACC/AHA 2006 guidelines).
3. After AVR with bioprosthesis and no risk factors, aspirin (75–100 mg) is indicated, but warfarin is not indicated. When there are risk factors (which include atrial fibrillation, previous thromboembolism, and LA thrombus),

warfarin is indicated to achieve an INR of 2.0 to 3.0 (ACC/AHA 2006 guidelines).
4. After the Ross procedure, anticoagulation is not indicated.
5. The importance of good oral hygiene and antibiotic prophylaxis against subacute bacterial endocarditis (SBE) should be emphasized.

MITRAL VALVE PROLAPSE

Prevalence

The reported incidence of MVP of 2% to 5% in the pediatric population probably is an overestimate. The prevalence of MVP increases with age. This condition usually occurs in older children and adolescents (it is more common in adults) and has a female preponderance (male-to-female ratio of 1 to 2).

Pathology

1. The primary form of MVP is associated with several of the most common heritable disorders of connective tissue disease, such as Marfan's syndrome, Ehlers-Danlos syndrome, osteogenesis imperfecta, and Stickler syndrome as well as polycystic kidney disease in adults. Nearly all patients with Marfan's syndrome have MVP.
2. Secondary cases of MVP can be caused by other conditions, including rupture or dysfunction of the papillary muscles caused by myocardial infarction or ischemia, rupture of chordae tendineae caused by infective endocarditis, or abnormal LV wall motion associated with ischemia or primary myocardial disease. Only primary MVP is discussed in this chapter.
3. In the primary form of MVP, thick and redundant mitral valve leaflets bulge into the mitral annulus (caused by myxomatous degeneration of the valve leaflets, the chordae, or both). The posterior leaflet is more commonly and more severely affected than the anterior leaflet.
4. A CHD is present in one third of patients with MVP. Secundum atrial septal defect is most common; VSD and Ebstein's anomaly are found rarely.

Clinical Manifestations
History

1. MVP usually is asymptomatic, but a history of nonexertional chest pain, palpitation, and, rarely, syncope may be elicited.
2. Chest discomfort may be typical of anginal pain but more atypical in that it is not related to exertion and is often brief attacks or stabbing pain at the apex. Whether the chest pain is actually cardiac in origin (from papillary muscles) has not been fully determined, but the discomfort could be secondary to abnormal tension on papillary muscle.
3. Palpitation may be related to cardiac arrhythmias. Syncope or presyncope may be caused by arrhythmias or a manifestation of an orthostatic phenomenon.
4. The patient occasionally has a family history of MVP.

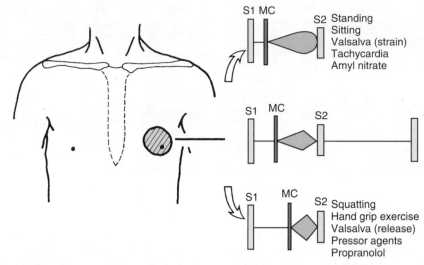

Fig. 21.5 Diagram of auscultatory findings in mitral valve prolapse and the effect of various maneuvers on the timing of the midsystolic click (MC) and the murmur. The maneuvers that reduce ventricular volume enhance leaflet redundancy and move the click and murmur earlier in systole. An increase in left ventricular dimension has the opposite effect.

Physical Examination (Fig. 21.5)

1. An asthenic build with a high incidence of thoracic skeletal anomalies (80%), including pectus excavatum (50%), straight back (20%), and scoliosis (10%), is common. (*Straight-back syndrome* is a condition in which the normal dorsal curvature of the spine is lost, resulting in a shortening of the chest's anteroposterior diameter.)
2. The midsystolic click with or without a late systolic murmur is the auscultatory hallmark of this syndrome and is best audible at the apex (see Fig. 21.5). The presence or absence of the click and murmur, as well as their timing, varies from one examination to the next.
   a. The click and murmur may be brought out by held expiration, left decubitus position, sitting, standing, or leaning forward. They may disappear on inspiration.
   b. Various maneuvers can alter the timing of the click and the murmur:
      1) The click moves toward the S1, and the murmur lengthens with maneuvers that decrease the LV volume, such as standing, sitting, Valsalva's strain phase, tachycardia, and the administration of amyl nitrite.
      2) The click moves toward the S2, and the murmur shortens with maneuvers that increase the LV volume, such as squatting, hand grip exercise, Valsalva's release phase, bradycardia, and the administration of pressor agents or propranolol.

Electrocardiography

1. The ECG is usually normal, but a superiorly directed T vector (with flat or inverted T waves in II, III, and aVF) occurs in 20% to 60% of patients (Fig. 21.6).
2. Arrhythmias are relatively uncommon and include supraventricular tachycardia (SVT), premature atrial contractions, and premature ventricular contractions.

3. First-degree AV block and right bundle branch block are occasionally present.
4. The incidence of Wolff-Parkinson-White preexcitation or prolonged QT interval is higher in patients with MVP than in the general population.
5. LVH or LAH rarely is present.

Chest Radiography

1. Chest radiographs unremarkable except for LA enlargement in patients with severe MR.
2. Thoracoskeletal abnormalities (e.g., straight back, pectus excavatum, scoliosis) may be present.

Echocardiography

Echo findings for adult patients with MVP have been established, but those for pediatric patients are not clearly defined.

1. Two-dimensional echo shows prolapse of the mitral valve leaflet(s) superior to the plane of the mitral valve. The parasternal long-axis view is most reliable. The superior displacement seen only on the apical four-chamber view is not diagnostic because more than 30% of preselected normal children show this finding. The "saddle-shaped" mitral valve ring explains the superior displacement of the mitral valve seen in normal people in the apical four-chamber view.
2. In adults, one or both mitral valve leaflets bulge by at least 2 mm into the LA during systole in the parasternal long-axis view. Thickening of the involved leaflet to more than 5 mm supports the diagnosis. In more severe myxomatous disease, leaflet redundancy, chordal elongation, and dilatation of the mitral annulus may be present.
3. Some pediatric patients with characteristic body build and auscultatory findings of the condition do not show the adult echo criterion of MVP; they may only show thickened mitral leaflets with systolic straightening or

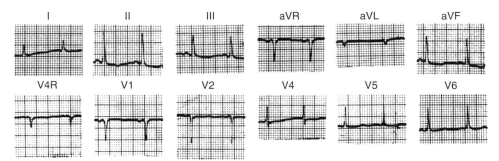

Fig. 21.6 Tracing from a 14-year-old girl with mitral valve prolapse. The T wave in aVF is inverted.

systolic superior doming and some posterosuperior displacement of the coaptation point of the mitral valve, some even with mild MR. This may be because MVP is a progressive disease that shows the full manifestations only in adult life.

4. A large number of first-degree relatives of patients with MVP have echo findings of MVP.

Natural History

1. The majority of patients are asymptomatic, particularly during childhood.
2. Complications that are reported in adult patients, although rare in childhood, include sudden death (probably from ventricular arrhythmias), SBE, spontaneous rupture of chordae tendineae, progressive MR, CHF, arrhythmias, and conduction disturbances.

Management

1. Asymptomatic patients require no treatment or restriction of activity.
2. Antibiotic prophylaxis against bacterial endocarditis is recommended when significant MR is present by auscultation or by echo studies.

3. Beta-adrenergic blockers (propranolol or atenolol) are often used in the following situations.
   a. Patients who are symptomatic (with palpitation, lightheadedness, dizziness, or syncope) secondary to ventricular arrhythmias. Symptomatic patients suspected to have arrhythmias should undergo ambulatory ECG monitoring or treadmill exercise testing. Although beta-blockers are the drugs of choice, other drugs, such as calcium blockers, quinidine, or procainamide, may prove to be effective in some patients.
   b. Patients with self-terminating episodes of SVT may also receive beta-blockers.
   c. Patients with chest discomfort may also be treated with propranolol. (It is not relieved by nitroglycerin but may worsen.)
4. Physical activities that require prolonged periods of straining, such as weightlifting, push-ups, pull-ups, sit-ups, or hanging on a monkey bars, are discouraged; these activities add stress to the mitral apparatus.
5. Reconstructive surgery or mitral valve replacement rarely may be indicated in patients with severe MR. MVP is the most common cause of isolated MR requiring surgical treatment in the United States.

Cardiac Tumors

PREVALENCE

Cardiac tumors in the pediatric age group are extremely rare. A primary cardiac tumor was diagnosed in 0.001% to 0.003% of admissions at large children's referral centers. The male-to-female distribution is equal.

PATHOLOGY

Types and Frequency of Tumors

Table 22.1 shows relative incidence of cardiac tumors in infants and children (Becker, 2000). Becker's data include 55 cases from the Armed Forces Institute of Pathology, Washington, DC, series 3f, and 21 cases from the Cardiovascular Pathology Registry in the Academic Medical Center, Amsterdam, Netherlands. Data in Table 22.1 show the following.

1. A large portion of primary heart tumors in the pediatric age group presents at younger than 1 year of age.
2. The most common cardiac tumor in the pediatric age group is rhabdomyoma. In infants younger than 1 year old, more than 50% of tumors are rhabdomyomas, followed by fibromas (25%). In children 1 to 16 years of age, nearly 40% of benign tumors are fibromas and myxomas (see Table 22.1). Rhabdomyomas accounted for only 8% of benign tumors in this age group.
3. More than 90% of primary tumors are benign in infants. Although primary malignant tumors are extremely rare in infants (~5%), approximately 40% of primary tumors were malignant in children older than 1 year of age. Malignant tumors reported in children include rhabdomyosarcoma, leiomyosarcoma, angiosarcoma, fibrosarcoma, and many others.

Recently, 120 operated cases of cardiac tumors in infants and children were reported by Bielefeld et al (2012). Although the data are not presented according to two age groups, younger than 12 months and older than 12 months, a similar trend exists with earlier reports. Rhabdomyomas were the most frequent, representing 35% of pediatric cardiac tumors (mean age, 7 months). Myxomas were the second most frequent (23%) with a mean age of 9 years. Fibromas represented

20% of the cases with mean age of 3.25 years. These three tumors accounted for three fourths of all surgically treated pediatric cardiac tumors.

Pathology of Individual Cardiac Tumors

Common pediatric cardiac tumors are briefly summarized next.

Rhabdomyoma

1. Rhabdomyomas are by far the most frequent tumors in the pediatric age group, accounting for about half the cases of cardiac tumors.
2. They usually are multiple, ranging in size from several millimeters to several centimeters. The most common location is in the ventricles, either in the ventricular septum or free wall, but they may rarely appear in the atrium.
3. More than half the cases with multiple rhabdomyomas have tuberous sclerosis (e.g., with adenoma of the sebaceous glands, mental retardation, seizures).
4. Tumors regress in size or number or both in most patients younger than 4 years of age (but less so in older patients) (Nir et al, 1995). Spontaneous complete regression may occur.
5. The tumors may produce symptoms of obstruction to blood flow, arrhythmias (usually ventricular tachycardia, occasionally supraventricular tachycardia), or sudden death.
6. Cardiac rhabdomyomas are associated with a higher incidence of Wolff-Parkinson-White (WPW) preexcitation and may increase the risk for arrhythmias.

Fibroma

1. Fibroma is the second most common tumor type encountered in infants and small children.
2. Cardiac fibromas usually occur as a single solid tumor, most commonly in the ventricular septum, although they may occur in the wall of any cardiac chamber. The size of the tumor varies from several millimeters to centimeters. Occasionally, the tumor calcifies.

TABLE 22.1 Relative Incidence of Cardiac Tumors in Infants and Children[a]			
Tumors	Incidence (%)	Tumors	Incidence (%)
Infant (Younger Than 12 mo) (n = 52)		**Children (1–16 yr of Age) (n = 25)**	
Benign Tumors (94%)		**Benign Tumors (58%)**	
Rhabdomyoma	52	Rhabdomyoma	8
Fibroma	25	Fibroma	21
Hemangioma or angioma	6	Myxoma	17
Teratoma	2	Hemangioma or angioma	4
Others	8	Teratoma	0
		Others	8
Malignant Tumors (6%)		**Malignant Tumors (43%)**	
Rhabdomyosarcoma	2	Rhabdomyosarcoma	8
Leiomyosarcoma	4	Leiomyosarcoma	2
Others	0	Others	33

[a]Rearranged data from Becker AE: Primary heart tumors in the pediatric age group: a review of salient pathologic features relevant for clinicians, *Pediatr Cardiol* 21:317–323, 2000.

3. The tumor may obstruct blood flow and disturb atrioventricular (AV) or ventricular conduction.
4. In some cases, the tumor can be removed completely, but in others, the tumor intermingles with myocardial tissue so that complete resection is not possible. The tumors probably represent hamartomatous lesions that may eventually regress. This has led to a tendency for a less aggressive surgical resection to reduce potential risks for complications.

Myxoma

1. Myxomas are the most common type of cardiac tumors in adults, accounting for about 30% of all primary cardiac tumors, but they are very rare in infants and children.
2. The majority of myxomas arise in the left atrium, 25% arise in the right atrium, and very few arise in the ventricles.
3. Myxomas can produce hemodynamic disturbances, commonly interfering with mitral valve function or producing thromboembolic phenomenon in the systemic circulation. With right atrial myxoma, similar effects on the tricuspid valve and thromboembolic phenomenon in the pulmonary circulation may be found. Rarely, patients may have symptoms while sitting and standing, but their symptoms improve when they lie down because of the intermittent protrusion of the tumor through the mitral valve.
4. Surgical removal usually is successful.

Teratoma

1. Teratomas contain elements from all three germ layers.
2. Most of the tumors are intrapericardial and are attached to the root of the aorta and pulmonary trunk, but the heart wall can be involved; occasionally, they may present as an intracardiac mass.
3. Surgical excision is usually possible.

Cardiac Angioma

1. This is a relatively rare tumor in infants and children.

2. They show preference for the epicardium, in which they may produce hemopericardium. Intramyocardial location may cause myocardial dysfunction, AV block, or both.
3. They are not rapid growing, and spontaneous involution has been documented.

Clinical Manifestations

1. Cardiac tumors usually are found on routine echo studies when the diagnosis is not suspected, especially in small infants.
2. Syncope or chest pain may be a presenting complaint in older children. Sudden unexpected death may be the first manifestation. Rarely, symptoms vary with posture in cases of pedunculated tumors (e.g., myxoma).
3. Clinical manifestations of cardiac tumors often are nonspecific and vary primarily with the location and the size of the tumor.
   a. Tumors near cardiac valves may produce heart murmurs of stenosis or regurgitation of valves. So-called tumor plop may occur with a pedunculated and sessile tumor, such as a left atrial myxoma.
   c. Tumors involving the conduction tissue may manifest with arrhythmias or conduction disturbances (such as seen with fibromas).
   d. Intracavitary tumors may produce inflow or outflow obstruction (such as seen with rhabdomyoma), with clinical findings similar to those of mitral or semilunar valve stenosis.
   e. Involvement of the myocardium (mural tumors) may result in heart failure or cardiac arrhythmias.
   f. Pericardial tumors, which may signal malignancy, can produce pericardial effusion and cardiac tamponade or features simulating infective pericarditis.
4. Fragmentation of intracavitary tumors may lead to embolism of the pulmonary or systemic circulations (as seen with myxoma).

5. Occasionally, for unknown reasons, fever and general malaise may manifest, especially with myxomas.

6. The electrocardiogram may show nonspecific ST-T changes, an infarct-like pattern, low-voltage QRS complexes, or WPW preexcitation. Various arrhythmias and conduction disturbances have been reported.

7. Chest radiographs occasionally may reveal altered contour of the heart, with or without changes in pulmonary vascular markings.

Diagnostic Procedures

1. Two-dimensional (2D) Doppler echo is the primary tool for the evaluation of cardiac tumors in pediatric patients. Echo and Doppler studies allow accurate determination of the extent and location of the tumor as well as the hemodynamic significance of the lesion.
   a. Multiple intraventricular tumors in infants and children most likely are rhabdomyomas (Fig. 22.1).
   b. A solitary tumor of varying size, arising from the ventricular septum or the ventricular wall, is likely to be a fibroma (Fig. 22.2).
   c. Left atrial tumors, especially when pedunculated, usually are myxomas (Fig. 22.3).
   d. An intrapericardial tumor arising near the great arteries most likely is a teratoma.
   e. Pericardial effusion suggests a secondary malignant tumor.

2. Transesophageal echo can provide more precise delineation of the tumor preoperatively and intraoperatively.

3. Magnetic resonance imaging (MRI) also provides the same information as the 2D echo study does. MRI techniques have certain advantages over the echo study.
   a. MRI provides high-resolution images of cardiac cavitary, valvular, myocardial, pericardial, and extracardiac masses, in addition to its relationship with mediastinal and other intrathoracic structures.
   b. It can provide spatial relationship of the tumor mass to the coronary arteries, which may help guide surgical management.
   c. MRI allows differentiation of tumors from myocardium and differentiation of the type of tumor (e.g., cardiac hemangiomas from rhabdomyomas and fibromas).
   d. MRI is better than echo in detecting apical tumors.

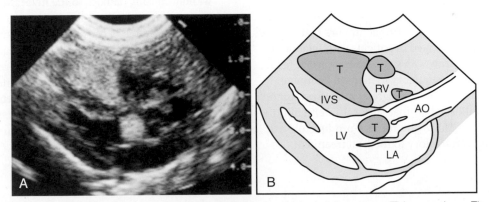

Fig. 22.1 Parasternal long-axis view (A) and diagram (B) of multiple rhabdomyomas (T) in a newborn. There is a round, mobile mass in the left ventricular outflow tract, with resulting obstruction. One large and at least two other smaller tumor masses are imaged in the right ventricle (RV). The tumor in the left ventricular outflow tract was surgically removed because of the obstructive nature of the mass. *AO,* Aorta; *IVS,* interventricular septum; *LA,* left atrium.

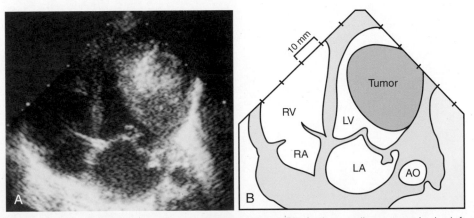

Fig. 22.2 Apical four-chamber view (apex up) (A) and diagram (B) of a large solitary tumor in the left ventricular (LV) cavity in a newborn. The mass is attached to the LV free wall. Because of symptoms, a surgical attempt was made to remove the mass, but the infant died. Pathologic examination revealed the mass to be fibroma. *AO,* Aorta; *LA,* left atrium; *RA,* right atrium; *RV,* right ventricle.

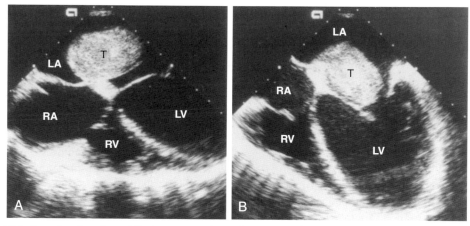

Fig. 22.3 Four-chamber view of the transverse plane of a transesophageal echo from a 54-year-old man with left atrial myxoma (T). **A,** A systolic freeze frame showing a large oval mass in the left atrium (LA). This mass is attached to the atrial septum. The primum atrial septum is also thickened. **B,** During diastole, the myxoma protrudes through the mitral valve. *LV,* Left ventricle; *RA,* right atrium; *RV,* right ventricle.

4. Cardiac catheterization and angiography are usually not necessary. Attempts at tissue diagnosis can be risky because of possible embolization of tumor fragments.

Management

Surgery is the only treatment for cardiac tumors that require intervention. Surgery is indicated in patients with inlet or outlet obstruction and in patients with symptoms of cardiac failure or ventricular arrhythmias refractory to medical treatment.

1. **Rhabdomyomas.** Spontaneous regression of these tumors has been well established so that surgical intervention is no longer indicated unless the tumors produce obstruction or arrhythmias refractory to medical treatment.

2. **Fibromas.** A successful complete resection of a fibroma is possible. In some cases, the tumor intermingles with myocardial tissue so that complete resection is not possible without causing damage to the myocardium or conduction tissues. Currently, there is a tendency for less than radical surgical resection because cardiac fibromas probably represent hamartomatous lesions that may regress spontaneously.

3. Surgical removal is a standard procedure for myxomas and has a favorable outcome. The stalk of the tumor should be removed completely to prevent recurrence.

4. If myocardial involvement is extensive, surgical treatment is not possible. Cardiac transplantation may be an option in such cases.

Cardiovascular Involvement in Systemic Diseases

Many collagen, neuromuscular, endocrine, and other systemic diseases may have important cardiovascular manifestations. The involvement of the cardiovascular system usually becomes evident when the diagnosis of the primary disease is well established, but occasionally cardiac manifestations may precede evidence of the basic disease. Cardiac manifestations of selected systemic diseases are briefly described here.

ACUTE GLOMERULONEPHRITIS

Clinically evident myocardial involvement is found in 30% to 40% of patients with acute poststreptococcal glomerulonephritis. Pulmonary edema, systemic venous congestion, and cardiomegaly also are common, resulting from salt and water retention. Systemic hypertension, sometimes appearing with hypertensive encephalopathy, is a frequent manifestation and may be responsible for signs of congestive heart failure (CHF) in some, but not all, patients. Although hypertension probably reflects fluid expansion (secondary to impaired salt and water excretion), peripheral resistance has been found to be elevated. Increased renin activity may be responsible for the latter. Acute phase generally resolves within 6 to 8 weeks.

Treatment is directed toward lowering blood pressure and inducing diuresis. Sodium restriction; diuresis usually with intravenous Lasix; and antihypertensive therapy with calcium channel antagonists, vasodilators, or angiotensin-converting enzyme (ACE) inhibitors are standard treatment.

DIGEORGE SYNDROME

The same syndrome has been described by different researchers in different areas of expertise. Angelo DiGeorge, an endocrinologist, reported DiGeorge syndrome in 1960s, and Robert Shprintzen, PhD, a speech pathologist, reported velocardiofacial syndrome in the 1970s. A Japanese cardiologist group called it conotruncal anomaly face (CTAF) syndrome in 1978. These syndromes share a common genetic cause, in most cases, a chromosome 22q11 deletion; therefore, currently the term "22q11 deletion syndrome" is used. The great majority of patients with these syndromes have serious congenital heart diseases (CHDs).

DiGeorge syndrome occurs in both males and females. Clinical features in these syndromes include abnormal facies, CHDs, and absence or hypoplasia of the thymus (with congenital immune deficiency and increased susceptibility to infection) or parathyroid gland (with hypocalcemia). Clinical features of the syndrome are collectively grouped under the acronym of CATCH-22 (cardiac, abnormal facies, thymic hypoplasia, cleft palate, and hypocalcemia resulting from 22q11 deletion).

Approximately 90% of patients have a deletion of the long arm of chromosome 22 (22q11.2) detectable with current cytogenetic and florescence in situ hybridization (FISH) technique. In 90% of cases, the disorder occurs as the result of a new mutation, and in 10%, the disorder is inherited from a parent in an autosomal dominant fashion. Rarely, the syndrome may be caused by other chromosomal abnormalities or maternal environmental factors (e.g., alcohol, retinoids).

Clinical Manifestations

1. **Abnormal facies.** Abnormal facies is characterized by hypertelorism, micrognathia, a short philtrum with a fishmouth appearance, an antimongoloid slant, telecanthus with short palpebral fissures, and low-set ears, often with defective pinna.

2. **Cardiac.** Many patients (85%) have cardiac defects. The most common cardiac anomalies include tetralogy of Fallot (TOF; 25%); interrupted aortic arch (15%); ventricular septal defect (VSD), usually perimembranous (15%); persistent truncus arteriosus (9%); and isolated aortic arch anomalies (5%). Less common anomalies include pulmonary stenosis (PS), atrial septal defect (ASD), atrioventricular (AV) canal defect, and transposition of the great arteries.

3. **Cleft.** Anomalies in the palate are common (70-80%), with speech and feeding disorders. The palatal abnormalities may be overt or submucosal cleft. Occasionally, a bilateral cleft lip and palate may be present. Velopharyngeal insufficiency with delayed and hypernasal speech may occur.

4. **Metabolic.** Hypocalcemia (observed in 60%) is caused by hypoparathyroidism.

5. **Immunologic.** Thymic hypoplasia or aplasia leads to mild to moderate decrease in T-cell number. Occasionally, humoral deficits, including IgA deficiency, have been observed (~10%).

6. **Recurrent infections** are common, an important cause of later mortality.

7. **General.** Short statue, mental retardation, and hypotonia in infancy are frequent. Occasionally, psychiatric disorders (e.g., schizophrenia and bipolar disorder) develop.

8. Lateral view of chest radiograph shows a **defective thymic shadow.**

9. Cytogenetics analysis will detect only 20% of the deletion in the region. The deletion is best identified by FISH.

Management

1. Correction of cardiac malformation as discussed in other sections. Cardiac defects are major causes of early death.

2. Irradiated, cytomegalovirus-negative blood products must be administered because of the risk of graft-versus-host disease with nonirradiated products.

3. Monitoring of serum calcium levels and supplementation of calcium and vitamin D are important.
   a. Calcium gluconate (Kalcinate), 500 to 750 mg/kg/day, orally, four times a day, or calcium carbonate (Oscal, Titralac, Oystercal, Caltrate), 112.5 to 162.5 mg/kg/day, given four times a day
   b. Ergocalciferol (vitamin D2), 25,000 to 200,000 U orally four times a day

4. Live vaccines are contraindicated in patients with DiGeorge syndrome and in household members because of the risk of shedding live organism.

5. Usual prophylactic regimen for T- and B-cell deficiency

6. Early thymus transplantation may promote successful immune reconstitution.

Prognosis

The prognosis depends on cardiac and immune systems disorders. The prognosis is poor with complex cyanotic heart defects, if not repaired, with a 1-month mortality rate of 55% and a 6-month mortality rate of 86%.

FRIEDREICH ATAXIA

Friedreich ataxia is inherited as an autosomal recessive trait. The onset of ataxia usually occurs before age 10 years and it progresses slowly involving the lower extremities to a greater extent than the upper extremities. Explosive dysarthric speech and nystagmus are characteristic but their intelligence is preserved.

Echo studies reveal evidence of cardiomyopathy in approximately 30% of the cases. Concentric hypertrophy of the left ventricular (LV) with normal LV systolic function is the most common finding. In advanced stage, the LV enlarges, and the LV wall thickness decreases with decreasing fractional shortening, suggesting the presence of fibrosis in the myocardium (Weidemann et al, 2012). Diastolic dysfunction of the LV may be present. The thickness of the interventricular septum correlates well with LV mass determined by magnetic resonance imaging (MRI). Microscopically, diffuse interstitial fibrosis and fatty degeneration of the myocardium, with compensatory hypertrophy of the remaining cells, frequently are found. CHF is the terminal event with most patients dying before 40 years of age.

Cardiac symptoms (e.g., dyspnea, chest pain) are common. Because of physical disability, cardiac problems may not be recognized until arrhythmias or signs of CHF develop. Importantly, there appears to be no clear correlation between the severity of myocardial involvement and that of neurologic dysfunction. A systolic murmur may be audible at the upper left sternal border. Electrocardiographic (ECG) abnormalities are very common. The most common finding is the T-vector change in the limb leads or left precordial leads. Occasionally, left ventricular hypertrophy (LVH), right ventricular hypertrophy (RVH), abnormal Q waves, or a short PR interval is found. Chest radiographs usually are normal.

Treatments are the same as those described under different types of cardiomyopathy.

HYPERTHYROIDISM: CONGENITAL AND ACQUIRED

The thyroid hormones increase oxygen consumption, stimulate protein synthesis and growth, and affect carbohydrates and lipid metabolism. On the cardiovascular system, the thyroid hormones (1) increase heart rate, cardiac contractility, and cardiac output; (2) increase systolic pressure and decrease diastolic pressure, with mean pressure unchanged; and (3) may increase myocardial sensitivity to catecholamines. Hyperthyroidism results from excess production of triiodothyronine (T_3), thyroxine (T_4), or both.

Congenital hyperthyroidism most often is caused by increased thyroid-stimulating immunoglobulin in infants of mothers who had Graves' disease during pregnancy. A newborn infant with congenital hyperthyroidism often is premature and usually has a goiter. The baby appears anxious, restless, alert, and irritable. The eyes are widely open and appear exophthalmic.

Juvenile hyperthyroidism is believed to be caused by thyroid-stimulating antibodies and often is associated with lymphocytic thyroiditis and other autoimmune disorders. The incidence of juvenile hyperthyroidism peaks during adolescence, with females affected more often than males. These children become hyperactive, irritable, and excitable. The thyroid gland is enlarged.

Both congenital and acquired hyperthyroidisms manifest with tachycardia, full and bounding pulses, and increased systolic and pulse pressures. A nonspecific systolic murmur may be audible. Bruits may be audible over the enlarged thyroid in children but not in newborns. In severely affected patients, cardiac enlargement and cardiac failure may develop, requiring prompt recognition and treatment.

Chest radiographs usually are normal but may show cardiomegaly and increased pulmonary vascularity, especially in the presence of heart failure. ECG abnormalities may include sinus tachycardia, peaked P waves, various arrhythmias (supraventricular tachycardia, junctional rhythm), complete heart block, RVH, LVH, or biventricular hypertrophy (but arrhythmias are rare in acquired [juvenile] hyperthyroidism). Echo studies reveal a hyperkinetic state with increased fractional shortening.

In severely affected patients, a beta-adrenergic blocker, such as propranolol, is indicated to reduce the effect of catecholamines. It is interesting to note that some actions of T_3 on the heart are similar to those of beta-adrenergic stimulation and that essentially all beta-blockers can alleviate many of the symptoms of hyperthyroidism. The mechanism of the similarity between these two is unclear; it may involve increased beta-adrenergic receptor density, or it may occur independently of beta-adrenergic receptor stimulation. Treatment of hyperthyroidism consists of oral administration of antithyroid drugs, propylthiouracil or methimazole (Tapazole). If CHF develops, treatment with anticongestive medications is indicated (see Chapter 27).

HYPOTHYROIDISM: CONGENITAL AND ACQUIRED

Hypothyroidism results from deficient production of thyroid hormone or a defect in its receptor. The disorder may manifest from birth or may be acquired.

Congenital hypothyroidism most often is caused by a developmental defect of the thyroid gland. Hypothyroidism may not be apparent until 3 months of age. The typical picture includes a protuberant tongue, cool and mottled skin, subnormal temperature, carotenemia, and myxedema. Untreated children become mentally retarded and slow in physical development. In the congenital type, patent ductus arteriosus and PS are frequently found.

The patient may have significant bradycardia, a weak arterial pulse, hypotension, and nonpitting facial and peripheral edema. ECG abnormalities occur in more than 90% of cases and consist of some or all of the following: (1) low QRS voltages, especially in the limb leads; (2) low T-wave amplitude, not affecting the T axis; (3) prolongation of PR and QT intervals; and (4) dome-shaped T wave with an absent ST segment ("mosque" sign) (Fig. 23.1). Echo studies may show cardiomegaly, pericardial effusion, hypertrophic cardiomyopathy, or asymmetric septal hypertrophy in addition to CHDs, if present. Sodium-l-thyroxine given orally is the treatment of choice.

Acquired (or juvenile) hypothyroidism most often results from lymphocytic thyroiditis (Hashimoto's disease or autoimmune thyroiditis). Hypothyroidism may result from subtotal or complete thyroidectomy or from protracted ingestion of goitrogens, iodides, or cobalt mediations. Rarely, amiodarone can cause hypothyroidism. Serum levels of T_3 and T_4 are low or borderline.

The heart rate is relatively slow, and the heart sounds may be soft. A weak arterial pulse and hypotension may be present. Myxedema may be present. There is an increased occurrence of hypercholesterolemia. Echo studies frequently show pericardial effusion and asymmetric septal hypertrophy. The ECG, chest radiograph, and echo findings of juvenile hypothyroidism are the same as for congenital hypothyroidism. Treatment of hypothyroidism corrects the lipid abnormalities.

MARFAN SYNDROME

Marfan syndrome is a generalized connective tissue disease with clinical features involving skeletal, cardiovascular, and ocular systems. Mutation in the *FBN1* gene located on chromosome 15 is the cause of Marfan syndrome. It is inherited as an autosomal dominant pattern with variable expressivity. New mutations are the cause of at least 25% of Marfan syndrome cases.

Skeletal features include tall stature with long slim limbs, little subcutaneous fat and muscle hypotonia, arachnodactyly, joint laxity with scoliosis and kyphosis, pectus excavatum or carinatum, and narrow facies. Eye manifestation may include lens subluxation, increased axial global length, myopia, and retinal detachment.

Clinically evident cardiovascular involvement occurs in more than 50% of patients by the age of 21 years. Microscopic changes probably are present in almost all patients, even during infancy and childhood. A wide spectrum of cardiovascular abnormalities is seen in Marfan syndrome.

1. The common abnormalities include dilatation of the sinus of Valsalva, dilatation of the ascending aorta (with or without dissection or rupture), and aortic regurgitation (AR). Microscopic examination of the proximal aorta (and the proximal coronary arteries) reveals disruption of the elastic media, with fragmentation and disorganization of the elastic fibers. Large accumulations of dermatan sulfate, heparan sulfate, and chondroitin sulfate have been reported in the media of the aorta.

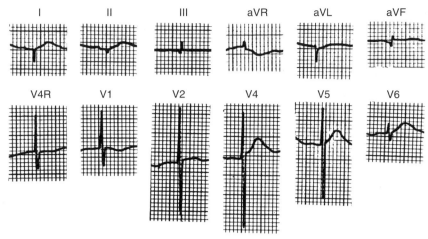

Fig. 23.1 Tracing from a 3-month-old infant with congenital hypothyroidism. Note low QRS voltages in the limb leads, relatively low T-wave amplitude, and dome-shaped T wave with an absent ST segment in V6.

2. Mitral valve abnormalities are more common in children and young adults than aortic lesions. The mitral valve and left atrium (LA) endocardium often undergo a fibromyxoid degeneration, resulting in dilatation of the mitral valve annulus, mitral regurgitation (MR), and mitral valve prolapse (MVP).

3. Aneurysm of the pulmonary artery (PA) is less frequently seen.

4. Rarely, myocardial fibrosis and infarction, rupture of chordae tendineae, aneurysm of the abdominal aorta, and aneurysmal dilatation of the proximal coronary arteries have been reported.

Auscultatory findings of MR and MVP appear in more than 50% of patients (see Chapter 21). Rarely, the murmur of AR is audible. The S2 may be accentuated in many patients, especially in those with thin chest walls or dilated PAs. The ECG findings may include LVH; T-wave inversion in leads II, III, aVF, and left precordial leads; and first-degree AV block. Chest radiographs may show cardiomegaly, either generalized or involving only the LV and LA or a prominence of the ascending aorta, aortic knob, or the main PA segment.

Echo studies show an increased dimension of the aortic root with or without AR and a "redundant" mitral valve or MVP with thickened valve leaflets and MR. Periodic examination of the aortic root dimension and the status of the MR and MVP is important. As to the diagnosis of MVP in children, however, the adult criterion of MVP is met infrequently, probably because MVP is a progressive disease, and a full manifestation of the disease does not occur until the adulthood.

Early death in individuals with this syndrome is most commonly precipitated by aortic dissection, chronic AR, or severe MR. Use of beta-blockers, ACE inhibitors, or angiotensin II receptor blockers (ARBs) has significantly diminished the progression of aortic root dilation, thus delaying surgical intervention. Timely and improved surgery has significantly increased the life expectancy of these patients in recent years.

1. Beta-blockers (atenolol, propranolol) are effective in slowing the rate of aortic dilatation and reducing the development of aortic complications. In addition to traditional beta-blocker treatment, over the past decade, enalapril (an ACE inhibitor) and losartan (an ARB) have been added to the medical regimen to treat dilated aortic root in patients with Marfan syndrome. The role of prophylactic medical treatment in children with Marfan syndrome remains controversial, although some physicians choose to start medications at the time of diagnosis of Marfan syndrome even without aortic root dilation. Nevertheless, the treatment should be started the latest when the aortic root exceeds a Z score of more than 2.

2. Certain physical activities are discouraged to reduce the damage to the aortic root and regurgitant aortic and mitral valves. Exercises such as weightlifting, rowing, push-ups, pull-ups, sit-ups, and hanging on a monkey bar, should be avoided.

3. Cardiac failure caused by severe MR is treated with mitral valve repair or valve replacement.

4. Surgery should be considered when the diameter of the aortic root increases significantly. However, there is controversy as to what is considered significant enlargement of the aortic root to require surgery in children. The current general recommendation for surgery is an aortic root diameter of 50 mm or greater or rapid growth of more than 5 mm/year in patients with Marfan syndrome. Additionally, modifications should be done to these recommendations when there is family history of aortic dissection at a diameter less than 50 mm or significant and progressive aortic valve regurgitation or in children with significant and rapid aortic root dilation (>10 mm/year). Normal two-dimensional (2D) echo dimensions of the aortic root and the aorta are presented in Table D.3 in Appendix D.

5. Valve-sparing aortic root reconstruction appears to be preferable to composite graft surgery.

6. Aortic root dilatation or aortic aneurysm may occur in other connective tissue diseases and similar surgical procedure may become necessary. The conditions may include, in addition to Marfan syndrome, Ehlers-Danlos syndrome, Turner syndrome, Loeys-Dietz syndrome, and

others. Dilatation of the ascending aorta or the aortic root can also occur after surgery for CHDs, such as aortic stenosis, TOF, and truncus arteriosus.

MUCOPOLYSACCHARIDOSES

The mucopolysaccharidoses (MPS) are a diverse group of inherited metabolic disorders in which excessive amounts of glycosaminoglycans (previously called mucopolysaccharides) accumulate in various tissues, including the myocardium and coronary arteries. Stored glycosaminoglycans vary with different types and include dermatan sulfate, heparin sulfate, keratan sulfate, and dermatan sulfate. Hurler (type IH) Hunter (II), Scheie (IS), Sanfilippo (III), and Morquio (IV) are well-known eponyms. A wide variety of clinical manifestations occur, including growth and mental retardation, skeletal abnormalities, clouded cornea, upper airway obstruction, and cardiac abnormalities. In most cases, the cause of death is cardiorespiratory failure secondary to cardiac involvement and upper airway obstruction.

Echo studies show involvement of mitral and aortic valves (most frequently valve regurgitation) in more than 50% of the cases; about 25% of patients show cardiomyopathy. The prevalence of these abnormalities increases as the patient becomes older.

1. MR is present in approximately 30% of the patients. It is more frequent in types IH (38%) than other types (24% in type II and 20% in type III). Thickening of the mitral valve is common.
2. AR is present in about 15% of the cases often with thickening of the valve. It is more common in types II (56%) and IV (24%).
3. Myocardial abnormalities, such as asymmetric septal hypertrophy, hypertrophic cardiomyopathy, dilated cardiomyopathy (DCM), and endocardial thickening, are present in about 25% of patients.
4. Occasionally, systemic hypertension is present.
5. Rarely, myocardial infarction can occur.

Heart murmur may represent cardiac valve involvement. Chest radiographs may show cardiomegaly in severe cases of valve regurgitation. The ECG may show a prolonged QT interval, RVH, LVH, or left atrial hypertrophy (LAH). Management depends on the abnormalities present.

MUSCULAR DYSTROPHY

Duchenne muscular dystrophy is a sex-linked recessive disease. Involvement of the pelvic muscles leads to lordosis, a waddling gait, a protuberant abdomen, and difficulty rising. Becker muscular dystrophy is the same fundamental disease as Duchenne dystrophy, but it follows a milder and more protracted course.

Cardiac enlargement, with occasional endocardial thickening of the LV and LA, is found on gross examination. Fatty degeneration and lymphocytic infiltration are found on microscopic examination. Dystrophic changes in the papillary muscles may be evident with MR or MVP.

Exertional dyspnea and tachypnea are common symptoms. The P2 may be loud if pulmonary hypertension is present. One may hear either a systolic ejection murmur at the base or a regurgitant apical systolic murmur of MR. CHF is an ominous terminal sign.

Electrocardiogram abnormalities occur in 90% of teenagers with the Duchenne type, and RVH and right bundle branch block are the most common abnormalities. Deep Q waves frequently are seen in the left precordial leads. Short PR interval is occasionally seen. T-vector changes may be seen in the limb leads or left precordial leads. Holter monitoring may show atrial tachycardia or frequent ventricular ectopies, especially in patients with low LV ejection fraction.

Echo studies show significant cardiac involvement in the form of DCM in both Duchenne and Becker types of muscular dystrophy and manifests clinically during adolescence. In early stages of the disease, only diastolic dysfunction (of reduced diastolic relaxation pattern) may be present. Systolic dysfunction appears later in the disease process. Echo features of MR or MVP may be seen. Cardiac MRI is used to quantify ventricular function as well as extent of myocardial fibrosis in patients with muscular dystrophy.

Treatment is the same as that described for DCM (see Chapter 18). Recent reports suggest a more aggressive treatment with ACE inhibitors (e.g., perindopril) appears to lead to improved LV function and possible delay of progression of the disease (Duboc et al, 2005). Although prospective treatment may be better, the treatment appears to improve LV function even if started after abnormal echo findings appear. Addition of carvedilol (0.5–1 mg/kg, twice daily) to the standard treatment was shown to prevent dilatation of the ventricle over baseline and to increase fractional shortening (Kajimoto et al, 2006). Recently, Viollet et al (2012) reported that treatment with of an ACE inhibitor (lisinopril) with or without additional beta blockers (metoprolol) in 42 patients significantly improved the myocardial function. Beta-blockers were added to the ACE inhibitor when average heart rate exceeded 100 beats/min on a 24-hour Holter monitoring.

MYOTONIC DYSTROPHY

Myotonic muscular dystrophy is the second most common muscular dystrophy. This disease is characterized by myotonia (increased muscular irritability and contractility with decreased power of relaxation) combined with muscular weakness. This autosomal dominant disease causes dysfunction in multiple organ systems, including musculoskeletal, gastrointestinal, cardiovascular, endocrine, and immunologic systems.

In infancy, myotonic dystrophy presents with feeding difficulties. Later in life, developmental retardation, poor coordination, and muscle weakness are evident. During childhood, the trunk and proximal muscle groups are involved, and in late in life, the distal muscle groups and the facial and neck muscles are involved. "Hatchet" face is characteristic with open mouth, drooling, and expressionless face.

Cardiac abnormalities are frequent with involvement of the AV conduction and structural abnormalities. Fatty infiltration in the myocardium and fibrofatty degeneration in the sinus node and AV conduction system may be responsible for the manifestations.

1. The ECG may show first-degree AV block and intraventricular conduction delay. As disease progresses, second-degree and complete heart block may develop. In addition, atrial fibrillation and flutter, abnormal Q waves, and ventricular arrhythmias may develop. Sudden death is frequent, attributable to conduction abnormalities or arrhythmias.
2. MVP may develop, usually by adulthood.
3. LV systolic dysfunction may appear with advancing age. Rarely, LV hypertrophy or LA dilatation, or regional wall motion abnormality is seen.

Patients with symptoms or evidence of dysrhythmias should be considered for pacemaker treatment. LV dysfunction, if present, should be treated.

NOONAN SYNDROME

Noonan syndrome, once referred to as "male Turner syndrome," is an autosomal dominant genetic disorder occurring in both males and females. Mutations in the *PTPN11* gene located on chromosome 12 have been found in about 50% of the patients with Noonan syndrome. It was first described by Dr. Jacqueline A. Noonan, a pediatric cardiologist, in the early 1960s. Noonan syndrome occurs in about 1 in 1000 to 2500 live births.

The diagnosis of Noonan syndrome is suspected by distinctive facial features, short stature, chest deformity, and CHD (Romano et al, 2010).

1. The facial appearance is most characteristic in infancy and early to middle childhood. It includes a large head, wide-spaced eyes, prominent epicanthal folds, horizontal or down-slanting palpebral fissures, low-set ears, and short and broad nose with depressed root. The neck is short with excess skin (webbed neck) and a low posterior hairline (55%).
2. Cubitus valgus is found in more than half of the patients. Hyperextensibility is common.
3. A characteristic pectus deformity of the chest with pectus carinatum superiorly and pectus excavatum inferiorly is seen in many children with the syndrome. Scoliosis is reported in 10% to 15%.
4. Although some clinical features are similar to those of Turner syndrome, patients with Noonan syndrome are often mentally retarded, and normal sexual maturation usually occurs, although it is delayed.
5. More than 80% of patients with the syndrome have an abnormality of the cardiovascular system.
   a. Pulmonary valve stenosis is the most common one. The valve may be dysplastic in 25% to 35% of the cases.
   b. Secundum ASD is often associated with pulmonary valve stenosis.
   c. Hypertrophic cardiomyopathy is present in approximately 20% of patients. The condition may resolve, become rapidly progressive, or remain stable.

6. Abnormal ECG is present in about 50% of patients with LAD, LVH, and abnormal Q waves.

Management

1. For significant PS, initial treatment is usually pulmonary balloon valvuloplasty, but it may be unsuccessful because the valve is at times extremely dysplastic. With severe dysplasia, a pulmonary valvectomy or pulmonary homograft may be needed in childhood.
2. Patients with hypertrophic cardiomyopathy may require the use of beta-blockers or surgical myomectomy to reduce outflow obstruction.
3. Individuals without heart disease on their initial evaluation should be followed every 5 years because of possible late appearance of cardiac problems.
4. The patients should be followed by endocrinologists for:
   a. Possible growth failure, which may require growth hormone therapy
   b. Thyroid hormone replacement for hypothyroidism
   c. Possible pubertal induction with estrogen (for females) or testosterone (for males) for absence of breast development in girls by the age of 13 years or no testicular enlargement in boys by 14 years of age

RHEUMATOID ARTHRITIS

Rheumatoid arthritis represents an autoimmune disease in which the synovium is the principal target of inappropriate immune attack. Autopsy cases may exhibit multiple hemorrhages on parietal and visceral pericardial surfaces with dense fibrous adhesion. The myocardium may be hypertrophied with infiltration of inflammatory cells, and irregular nodular thickening may be seen on cardiac valves.

In clinical settings, the following cardiac manifestations may occur.

1. Pericarditis is the most common finding, occurring in about 50% of cases. Chest pain and friction rub signify pericarditis. It is most frequent in systemic-onset juvenile rheumatoid arthritis (JRA), occasionally in patients with polyarticular-onset JRA, and very rarely in pauciarticular-onset JRA. Small pericardial effusion occurs without symptoms, but large effusion may cause symptoms. Cardiac tamponade only rarely occurs.
2. Myocarditis occurs infrequently (1%–10%) in JRA but can lead to life-threatening CHF and arrhythmias.
3. Rarely, MR and AR with thickening of these valves occur.
4. Occasionally, LV systolic dysfunction (decreased ejection fraction and fractional shortening) with dilated LV occurs.
5. ECG abnormalities occur in 20% of cases, with the most common findings being nonspecific ST-T changes. Rarely, involvement of the conduction system with heart block can occur.

Asymptomatic and mild pericarditis may be treated with nonsteroidal antiinflammatory agents (e.g., naproxen 15 mg/kg/day in two divided doses). Symptomatic or severe pericarditis may require treatment with corticosteroids for 8 to 16 weeks. Prednisone 0.5 to 2 mg/kg/day (three or four times a day) for more than 1 week is gradually reduced by approximately 20% each week (later given as a single dose). Tamponade is treated with pericardiocentesis.

SICKLE CELL ANEMIA

In sickle cell anemia, erythrocytes become rigid and "sickle," leading to capillary occlusion and sickle cell "crisis." The increased stroke volume of the heart compensates for anemia, and the heart gradually dilates and hypertrophies. Heart failure may be a late complication.

Most of the clinical manifestations reflect anemia. The arterial pulse is brisk, and the precordium is hyperactive. The diastolic pressure is low with a wide pulse pressure. An ejection systolic murmur usually is audible along the upper right and left sternal borders. Rarely, one may hear an apical rumble and a gallop rhythm. ECG abnormalities may include first-degree AV block, LVH, and nonspecific T-wave changes. Chest radiographs show generalized cardiomegaly in nearly all patients. Echo findings include increased LV dimension and vigorous LV contraction, but the ejection fraction and systolic time intervals are within normal limits.

SYSTEMIC LUPUS ERYTHEMATOSUS

This chronic multisystem autoimmune disease can affect the cardiovascular system. The condition most commonly affects girls older than 8 years of age (78%), with a girl-to-boy ratio of 6.3 to 1.

The most common symptoms of lupus include constitutional complaints (fever, fatigue, anorexia, weight loss), joint pain and stiffness with or without swelling (commonly finger joints), skin rash (typical malar "butterfly" rash, seen only in 50%), and chest pain (from pleuritis or pericarditis). Evidence of renal involvement, hypertension, and Raynaud's phenomenon are also frequent. Chorea may be the sole presenting manifestation, requiring differentiation from acute rheumatic fever.

A positive antinuclear antibody (ANA) result is present in more than 95% of the cases, making it the most helpful initial screening test. However, a positive ANA test result is not diagnostic of the disease, particularly if the titer is low. Positive ANA test is seen in other connective tissue diseases, such as juvenile rheumatoid arthritis (JRA) (but not in systemic-onset type), dermatomyositis, scleroderma, Sjögren's syndrome, and mixed connective tissue disease and in some healthy children and adults. If the ANA test result is positive, further screening by a rheumatologist should be carried out.

Cardiovascular manifestations occur in about 30% to 40% of patients with lupus erythematosus, a higher rate than with other connective tissue diseases. Pathologically, varying degrees of immune-mediated changes occur in all layers of the heart, including the pericardium (patchy infiltration of inflammatory cells, fibrous adhesion), myocardium (mild to moderate acute and chronic inflammatory foci, perivasculitis

of intramural arteries, increased interstitial connective tissue, myocardial cell atrophy), and cardiac valves (classical verrucous Libman-Sacks lesion).

1. Pericarditis with pericardial effusion is the most common manifestation (~25%) and is often asymptomatic. Tamponade is rare, and constrictive pericarditis is extremely rarer.
2. Clinically evident myocarditis occurs in 2% to 25%, with resting tachycardia.
3. The classic verrucous endocarditis (Libman-Sacks) is found most commonly on the mitral valve, less commonly on the aortic valve, and only rarely on the tricuspid and pulmonary valves. Echo studies show irregular vegetations 2 to 4 mm in diameter on the valve or subvalvular apparatus (seen in ~10%). Rarely, embolization of the vegetations can occur to a coronary or cerebral artery. Recent studies indicate that, instead of verrucous lesion, the mitral or aortic valve may exhibit diffuse thickening with or without regurgitation.

Anterior chest pain may occur with pericarditis. Apical systolic murmur of MR frequently is found, but pericardial friction rub rarely is audible. The ECG shows nonspecific ST-T changes, arrhythmias, or conduction disturbances. With pericarditis, T-wave inversion and ST segment elevation may develop.

If active valvulitis is suspected, corticosteroid therapy may be warranted. Anticoagulation therapy should also be considered.

TURNER SYNDROME

Turner syndrome occurs in about 1 out of 2000 live female births. Standard karyotyping shows a missing X chromosome in more than 50% of the patients (45,X), and others have a combination of monosomy X and normal cells (45,X/46,XX), called mosaic Turner syndrome.

Diagnosis of Turner syndrome is suspected at birth by a characteristic edema of the dorsa of the hands and feet and loose skin folds at the nape of the neck. Clinical manifestations in childhood include webbing of the neck, a broad chest with widely spaced nipples, cubitus valgus, and small stature. Cardiac abnormalities are found in about 35% of the patients with Turner syndrome.

Important cardiac abnormalities are as follows:

1. Bicuspid aortic valve (BAV), COA, and aortic wall abnormalities (ascending aortic dilatation, aneurysm formation, and aortic dissection) are more commonly found in patients with webbing of the neck. BAV may lead to clinically significant AS or AR.
2. Less common CV anomalies include the following:
   a. Elongated transverse arch is present, which may be prone to dilatation and perhaps dissection.
   b. Partial anomalous pulmonary venous return (PAPVR) involving the left upper PV is found in 13%.
   c. Persistent left superior vena cava (13%)
3. The ECG may show RAD, T-wave abnormalities, accelerated AV conduction, and QTc prolongation.

4. 2D echo and color Doppler studies usually detect most cardiovascular abnormalities but MRI should also be performed to evaluate other abnormalities when it can be done without sedation.

The following are suggested in the follow-ups according to the organ systems (Bondy, 2007).

1. Cardiac follow-up is required with attention to the following:
   a. Monitoring blood pressure for hypertension. Hypertension is treated with beta-blockers.
   b. Aortic dimension should be determined on a regular basis. If the aorta is enlarged, treat it with beta-blockers.
   c. Also monitor for diabetes and dyslipidemia.
   d. MRI may be advised to evaluate the aortic dimension every 5 to 10 years.
2. They should be followed by pediatric endocrinologists.
   a. Growth hormone is indicated as early as possible and through puberty to attain normal adult height. Optimal age for starting growth hormone is not established, but it may be as early 9 months of age.
   b. Puberty induction is done with estrogen therapy at around 12 years of age if pubertal development is absent (although 30% will have spontaneous pubertal development). Spontaneous pregnancy occurs in 2% to 5% of the patients.
3. Cautions with regard to pregnancy.
   a. Aortic dissection during pregnancy and the postpartum period is possible.
   b. If pregnancy is being considered, cardiology evaluation with MRI of the aorta is indicated.
   c. History of surgically repaired cardiovascular defect, BAV, aortic dilatation, and systemic hypertension are relative contraindications of pregnancy.
4. Exercise. Regular moderate aerobic activity is emphasized. Highly competitive sports and very strenuous or isometric exercise are not recommended for patients with a dilated aortic root.

WILLIAMS SYNDROME

Williams syndrome is a rare genetic condition, occurring in 1 per 7500 to 20,000 births; most cases are sporadic. It occurs with equal prevalence in males and females. A microdeletion in the chromosomal region 7q11.23 near the elastin gene *(ELN)* is identified in virtually all individuals with Williams syndrome. Elastin is protein that allows blood vessels and other tissues in the body to stretch. Elastin arteriopathy is generalized, but it most commonly affects the ascending aorta and the PAs.

Patients with Williams syndrome have multisystem manifestations, including cardiovascular disease, developmental delay, learning disability, mental retardation, hearing loss, severe dental disease, ocular problems, nephrolithiasis, and bowel and bladder diverticula.

1. Many children have history of failure to thrive, poor weight gain, colic, and delayed motor development during early life.

2. Most young children with the syndrome have similar characteristic features. These features include a small upturned nose, a long philtrum (upper lip length), a wide mouth, full lips, a small chin, a stellate pattern in the iris (seen in 50%), and puffiness around the eyes.
3. They have personality traits of being very friendly, trusting strangers, fearing loud sounds, and being interested in music. They are also hyperactive, inattentive, and easily distracted (attention deficit disorder).
4. Other findings include a hoarse voice, joint hyperelasticity, contractures, kyphoscoliosis, and lordosis.

Important cardiovascular pathology includes the following.

1. Supravalvular aortic stenosis and PA stenosis are the two most common defects, occurring singly or together in 55% to 80% of the patients. PA stenosis has been reported in up to 83% of cases (in some reports).
2. Less common defects include coarctation, hypoplastic aortic arch, ASD, VSD, TOF, complete AV canal, and hypertrophic cardiomyopathy.
3. Systemic hypertension may be present or develop in approximately 50% of the patients.
4. High pressure in the sinus of Valsalva may lead to coronary ostial narrowing and coronary artery stenosis and may result in increased risk for sudden death.
5. There may also be renal artery stenosis with resulting hypertension. Renal ultrasonography may find anatomic abnormalities (found in 15%–20%) or nephrolithiasis (caused by hypercalcemia).
6. The ECG may show LVH in severe cases of supravalvular AS. BVH or RVH may be present with severe PA stenosis. Rarely, ST-T wave abnormalities may be present.
7. Echocardiography may show most of the known cardiac abnormalities (as described earlier).
8. Hypercalcemia, which is noted in approximately 15% of infants with Williams syndrome, is frequently asymptomatic and resolves in the first few years of life but can be lifelong.

The diagnosis of the syndrome is suspected by facial characteristics and cardiac abnormalities (supravalvular aortic stenosis or PA stenosis). Most deletions are detected through FISH, not through standard karyotyping.

A less well-recognized fact is an increased chance of sudden death (Bird et al, 1996). It has been estimated that sudden death can occur in patients with Williams syndrome at a rate 25- to 100-fold higher than in age-matched control participants. Deaths have been reported after the use of anesthesia or sedation or during invasive procedures (e.g., cardiac catheterization and heart surgery). Sudden deaths with no apparent instigating event have also been reported. Several factors have been cited as the potential causes of sudden death.

1. Severe supravalvular aortic stenosis or severe PS leading to ventricular hypertrophy and myocardial ischemia
2. Coronary artery stenosis secondary to exposure to a high systolic pressure in the sinus of Valsalva
3. Recently, prolongation of QTc interval has been raised as a possibility. Collins et al (2010) reported a much

higher prevalence of prolonged QTc interval in patients with the syndrome. Prolonged QTc interval ($\geq$460 msec) was found in 13.6% of the patients compared to 2.0% in control participants. Thus, prolonged cardiac repolarization seen in this condition may be a cause of sudden death.

Management of the patients may include the following.

1. Hypercalcemia should be treated, if present. Patients should avoid taking extra calcium and vitamin D.

2. Annual cardiology evaluation is indicated with assessment of the cardiac conditions, measurement of blood pressure, and checking the QTc interval.

3. When planning a procedure, history should be evaluated carefully for syncope, angina, fatigue or dyspnea, and hemodynamic instability during previous anesthesia or sedation.

4. Management of cardiac defects is described under specific defects (supravalvular AS in Chapter 13, and PA stenosis in Chapter 15).

PART 6

Arrhythmias and Atrioventricular Conduction Disturbances

This part discusses cardiac arrhythmias, atrioventricular conduction disturbances, and cardiac pacemakers and implantable cardioverter–defibrillators in children.

Cardiac Arrhythmias

The frequency and clinical significance of arrhythmias are different in children compared with adults. Although arrhythmias are relatively infrequent in infants and children, the common practice of monitoring cardiac rhythm in children requires primary care physicians, emergency department physicians, and intensive care physicians to be able to recognize and manage basic arrhythmias.

TACHYCARDIA VERSUS BRADYCARDIA

The normal heart rate varies with age: the younger the child, the faster the heart rate. Therefore, the definitions of *bradycardia* (<60 beats/min) and *tachycardia* (>100 beats/min) used for adults do not apply to infants and children. *Tachycardia* is defined as a heart rate beyond the upper limit of normal for the patient's age, and *bradycardia* is defined as a heart rate slower than the lower limit of normal. Normal resting heart rates by age are presented in Table 24.1.

This chapter discusses basic arrhythmias according to the origin of their impulse. Each arrhythmia is described along with its causes, significance, and treatment.

RHYTHMS ORIGINATING IN THE SINUS NODE

All rhythms that originate in the sinoatrial (SA) node (sinus rhythm) have two important characteristics (Fig. 24.1). Both are required for a rhythm to be called sinus rhythm.
1. P waves precede each QRS complex with a regular PR interval. (The PR interval may be prolonged, as in first-degree atrioventricular [AV] block; in this case, the rhythm is sinus with first-degree AV block.)
2. The P axis falls between 0 and +90 degrees, an often neglected criterion. This produces upright P waves in lead II and inverted P waves in aVR. (See Chapter 3 for a detailed discussion of sinus rhythm.)

Regular Sinus Rhythm
Description
The rhythm is regular, and the rate is normal for age. The two characteristics of sinus rhythm described previously are present (see Fig. 24.1).

Significance
This rhythm is normal at any age.

Management

No treatment is required.

Sinus Tachycardia

Description

Characteristics of sinus rhythm are present (see previous description). The rate is faster than the upper limit of normal for age (see Table 24.1). A rate above 140 beats/min in children and above 170 beats/min in infants may be significant. The heart rate usually is below 200 beats/min in sinus tachycardia (see Fig. 24.1).

Causes

Anxiety, fever, hypovolemia or circulatory shock, anemia, congestive heart failure (CHF), administration of catecholamines, thyrotoxicosis, and myocardial disease are possible causes.

Significance

Increased cardiac work is well tolerated by healthy myocardium.

TABLE 24.1	Normal Ranges of Resting Heart Rate		
Age	Mean (range)	Age (yr)	Mean (range)
Newborn	145 (90–180)	4	108 (72–135)
6 mo	145 (106–185)	6	100 (65–135)
1 yr	132 (105–170)	10	90 (65–130)
2 yr	120 (90–150)	14	85 (60–120)

From Davignon A, Rautaharju P, Boisselle E, Soumis F, Megelas M, Choquette A: Normal ECG standards for infants and children, *Pediatr Cardiol* 1:123–131, 1979/1980.

Management

The underlying cause is treated.

Sinus Bradycardia

Description

The characteristics of sinus rhythm are present (see previous description), but the heart rate is slower than the lower limit of normal for the age (see Table 24.1). A rate slower than 80 beats/min in newborn infants and slower than 60 beats/min in older children may be significant (see Fig. 24.1).

Causes

Sinus bradycardia may occur in normal individuals and trained athletes. It may occur with vagal stimulation, increased intracranial pressure, hypothyroidism, hypothermia, hypoxia, hyperkalemia, and administration of drugs such as beta-adrenergic blockers.

Significance

In some patients, marked bradycardia may not maintain normal cardiac output.

Management

The underlying cause is treated.

Sinus Arrhythmia

Description

There is a phasic variation in the heart rate caused by respiratory influences on the autonomic nervous system, increasing during inspiration and decreasing during expiration. The arrhythmia occurs, with maintenance of characteristics of sinus rhythm (see Fig. 24.1).

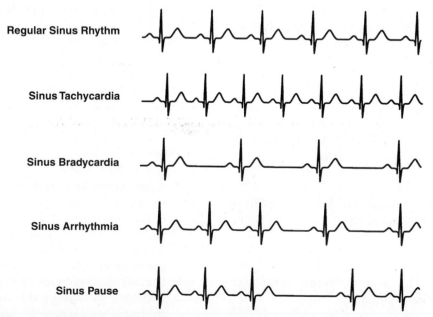

Fig. 24.1 Normal and abnormal rhythms originating in the sinoatrial node. Two characteristics of sinus rhythm are (1) P waves in front of each QRS complex with a regular PR interval and (2) normal P-axis (between 0 and +90 degrees). (From Park MK, Guntheroth WG: *How to Read Pediatric ECGs*, ed 4, Philadelphia, 2006, Mosby.)

Causes

This is a normal phenomenon and is caused by phasic variation in the firing rate of cardiac autonomic nerves with the phases of respiration.

Significance

Sinus arrhythmia has no significance because it is a normal finding in children and a sign of good cardiac reserve.

Management

No treatment is indicated.

Sinus Pause

Description

In sinus pause, the sinus node pacemaker momentarily ceases activity, resulting in absence of the P wave and QRS complex for a relatively short time (see Fig. 24.1). *Sinus arrest* is of longer duration and usually results in an escape beat (see later discussion) by other pacemakers, such as the AV junctional or nodal tissue (junctional or nodal escape beat).

Causes

Increased vagal tone, hypoxia, sick sinus syndrome, and digitalis toxicity are possible causes. Well-conditioned athletes may have bradycardia and sinus pause of greater than 2 seconds because of prominent vagal influence.

Significance

Sinus pause of less than 2 seconds is normal in young children and adolescents. It usually has no hemodynamic significance but may reduce cardiac output in patients with frequent and long periods of sinus pause.

Management

Treatment is rarely indicated except in sinus node dysfunction (or sick sinus syndrome; see later discussion).

Sinoatrial Exit Block

Description

A P wave is absent from the normally expected P wave, resulting in a long RR interval. The duration of the pause is a multiple of the basic PP interval. An impulse formed within the sinus node fails to propagate normally to the atrium.

Causes

Causes include excessive vagal stimulation; myocarditis or fibrosis involving the atrium; and drugs such as quinidine, procainamide, or digitalis.

Significance

It is usually transient and has no hemodynamic significance. Rarely, the patient may have syncope.

Management

The underlying cause is treated.

Sinus Node Dysfunction (Sick Sinus Syndrome)

Description

In sinus node dysfunction, the sinus node fails to function because the dominant pacemaker of the heart or performs abnormally slowly, resulting in a variety of arrhythmias. These arrhythmias may include profound sinus bradycardia, sinus pause or arrest, sinus node exit block, slow junctional escape beats, and ectopic atrial or nodal rhythm. Clear documentation is not always possible. Long-term recording with Holter is better in documenting overall heart rate variation and the prevalence of abnormally slow and fast rhythm.

Bradytachyarrhythmia occurs when bradycardia and tachycardia alternate. Whereas bradycardia may originate in the sinus node, atria, AV junction, or ventricle, tachycardia is usually caused by atrial flutter or fibrillation and less commonly by reentrant supraventricular tachycardia (SVT). When these arrhythmias are accompanied by symptoms such as dizziness or syncope, sinus node dysfunction is referred to as sick sinus syndrome.

Causes

1. Injury to the sinus node caused by extensive cardiac surgery, particularly involving the atria (e.g., the Senning operation, Fontan procedure, or surgery for partial or total anomalous pulmonary venous return or endocardial cushion defect) are possible causes.
2. Some cases of sick sinus syndrome are idiopathic, involving an otherwise normal heart without structural defect.
3. Rarely, myocarditis, pericarditis, or rheumatic fever is a cause.
4. Congenital heart diseases (CHDs) (e.g., sinus venosus atrial septal defect [ASD], Ebstein's anomaly, left atrial [LA] isomerism [polysplenia syndrome])
5. Secondary to antiarrhythmic drugs (e.g., digitalis, propranolol, verapamil, quinidine)
6. Hypothyroidism

Significance

Bradytachyarrhythmia is the most worrisome. Profound bradycardia after a period of tachycardia (overdrive suppression) can cause presyncope, syncope, and even death.

Management

1. For severe bradycardia:
   a. Acute symptomatic bradycardia is treated with intravenous (IV) atropine (0.04 mg/kg IV every 2–4 hours) or isoproterenol (0.05–2 mcg/kg IV) or transcutaneous pacing. Temporary transvenous or transesophageal pacing can be used until a permanent pacing system can be implanted.
   b. Chronic medical treatment using drugs has not been uniformly successful and is not accepted as standard treatment of sinus node dysfunction.
   c. Symptomatic bradycardia is treated with permanent pacing. Asymptomatic patients with heart rate under

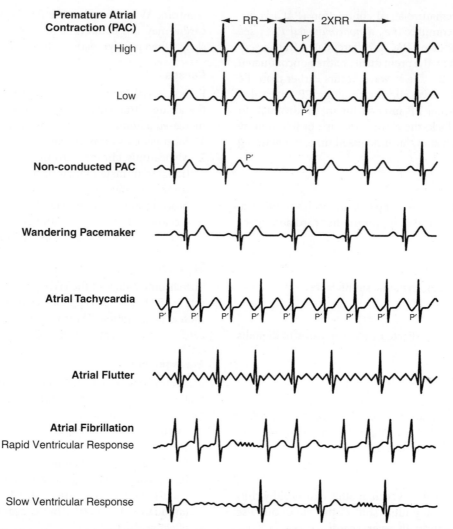

Fig. 24.2 Arrhythmias originating in the atrium. Characteristics of atrial arrhythmias are (1) abnormal P axis and/or an abnormal number of P waves per QRS complex and (2) normal duration of QRS complexes. *PAC,* Premature atrial contraction. (From Park MK, Guntheroth WG: *How to Read Pediatric ECGs,* ed 4, Philadelphia, 2006, Mosby.)

40 beats/min or pauses longer than 3 seconds are less clear indications for permanent pacing.

   d. Permanent implantation of a pacemaker is the treatment of choice in symptomatic patients, especially those with syncope. Most patients receive atrial demand pacing. Patients with any degree of AV nodal dysfunction receive dual-chamber pacemakers. Ventricular demand pacemakers may be used.

2. For symptomatic tachycardia:

   a. Antiarrhythmic drugs, such as propranolol or quinidine, may be given to suppress tachycardia, but they are often unsuccessful.

   b. Digoxin or amiodarone may help to decrease AV conduction of rapid tachycardia.

   c. Catheter ablation of arrhythmia substrates (often requiring concomitant surgical revision of previous surgeries) may be indicated.

   d. Patients with tachycardia–bradycardia syndrome may benefit from antitachycardia pacemakers.

RHYTHMS ORIGINATING IN THE ATRIUM

Rhythms that originate in the atrium (ectopic atrial rhythm) are characterized by the following (Fig. 24.2):

1. P waves have an unusual contour, which is caused by an abnormal P axis or an abnormal number of P waves per QRS complex.

2. QRS complexes are usually of normal configuration, but occasional bizarre QRS complexes caused by aberrancy may occur (see later discussion).

Premature Atrial Contraction
Description

The QRS complex appears prematurely. The P wave may be upright in lead II when the ectopic focus is high in the atrium. The P wave is inverted when the ectopic focus is low in the atrium (so-called coronary sinus rhythm). The compensatory pause is incomplete; that is, the length of two cycles, including one premature beat, is less than the length of two normal cycles (see Fig. 24.2).

An occasional premature atrial contraction (PAC) is not followed by a QRS complex (i.e., a *nonconducted PAC*; see Fig. 24.2). A nonconducted PAC is differentiated from a second-degree AV block by the prematurity of the nonconducted P wave (P′ in Fig. 24.2). The P′ wave occurs earlier than the anticipated normal P wave, and the resulting PP′ interval is shorter than the normal PP interval for that individual. In second-degree AV block, the P wave that is not followed by the QRS complex occurs at the anticipated time, maintaining a regular PP interval.

Causes

Premature atrial contraction appears in healthy children, including newborns. It also may appear after cardiac surgery and with digitalis toxicity.

Significance

Isolated PAC has no hemodynamic significance.

Management

Usually no treatment is indicated except in cases of digitalis toxicity.

Wandering Atrial Pacemaker
Description

Wandering atrial pacemaker is characterized by *gradual* changes in the shape of P waves and PR intervals (see Fig. 24.2). The QRS complex is normal.

Causes

Wandering atrial pacemaker is seen in otherwise healthy children. It is the result of a gradual shift of the site of impulse formation in the atria through several cardiac cycles.

Significance

Wandering atrial pacemaker is a benign arrhythmia and has no clinical significance.

Management

No treatment is indicated.

Ectopic (or Autonomic) Atrial Tachycardia
Description

There is a narrow QRS complex tachycardia (in the absence of aberrancy or preexisting bundle branch block) with visible P waves at an inappropriately rapid rate. The P axis is different from that of sinus rhythm. When the ectopic focus is near the sinus node, the P axis may be the same as in sinus rhythm. The usual heart rate in older children is between 110 and 160 beats/min, but the tachycardia rate varies substantially during the course of a day, reaching 200 beats/min with sympathetic stimuli. This arrhythmia is sometimes difficult to distinguish from the reentrant AV tachycardia, and thus it is included under SVT. It represented 18% of SVT in one study.

Holter monitoring may demonstrate a characteristic gradual acceleration of the heart rate, the so-called warming up period, rather than abrupt onset and termination seen with reentrant AV tachycardia. The P waves of ectopic atrial tachycardia may not conduct to the ventricle, especially during sleep, when parasympathetic tone is heightened.

Causes

Ectopic atrial tachycardia originates from a single focus in the atrium. This arrhythmia is believed to be secondary to increased automaticity of nonsinus atrial focus.
1. Most patients have structurally normal heart (idiopathic).
2. Myocarditis, chronic cardiomyopathy, AV valve regurgitation, atrial dilatation, atrial tumors, and previous cardiac surgery involving atria (e.g., Senning operation, Fontan procedure) may be the cause.
3. Occasionally, respiratory infections caused by mycoplasma or viruses may trigger the arrhythmia.

Significance

The chronic nature of the arrhythmia at a relatively low heart rate (<150 beats/min) can escape detection, and CHF is common at presentation. There is a high association of this tachycardia with tachycardia-induced cardiomyopathy.

Management

It is refractory to medical therapy and cardioversion. Drugs that are effective in reentrant atrial tachycardia (e.g., adenosine) do not terminate the tachycardia. Cardioversion is ineffective because the ectopic rhythm resumes immediately.
1. Drugs to slow the ventricular rate are not usually successful. There are conflicting reports regarding the efficacy of digoxin and beta-blockers in slowing down the ventricular rate. Class IC (e.g., flecainide) and class III (e.g., amiodarone) antiarrhythmic agents are generally most effective (up to 75%).
2. Radiofrequency ablation may prove to be effective in 95% to 100%. In children, a majority of the foci are found in the LA near the pulmonary veins and the atrial appendage in contrast to the right atrium found in adults.

Chaotic (or Multifocal) Atrial Tachycardia
Description

This is an uncommon tachycardia characterized by three or more distinct P-wave morphologies. The PP and RR intervals are irregular with variable PR intervals. The arrhythmia may be misdiagnosed as atrial fibrillation (AF).

Causes

Most patients with the condition are infants; it is very rare after 5 years of age. About 30% to 50% have respiratory illness. Myocarditis and birth asphyxia have been described. Structural heart disease may or may not be present.

Significance

The mechanism of this arrhythmia has been poorly defined. Cardiac enlargement or reduced left ventricular (LV) systolic function may be present at the diagnosis. Sudden death has been reported in up to 17% while on therapy. Spontaneous resolution frequently occurs.

Management

This arrhythmia is refractory to cardiac pacing, cardioversion, and adenosine.

1. When there is no evidence of cardiac dysfunction, observation on a regular basis may be reasonable.
2. Drugs that slow AV conduction (propranolol or digoxin) and those that decrease automaticity (such as class IA or IC or class III) have not been very effective, but they may control the heart rate.
3. Concurrent illness should be treated.
4. If the patient has cardiac dysfunction, medical therapy with amiodarone should be begun. Amiodarone appears to be the current treatment of choice.

Atrial Flutter

Description

The pacemaker lies in an ectopic focus, and "circus movement" in the atrium is the mechanism of this arrhythmia.

1. Typical atrial flutter is characterized by an atrial rate (F wave with "sawtooth" configuration) of about 300 (ranges, 240–360) beats/min, a ventricular response with varying degrees of block (e.g., 2:1, 3:1, 4:1), and normal QRS complexes (see Fig. 24.2).
2. Another form of atrial flutter may be seen in children who have undergone atrial surgery with multiple suture lines. Atrial flutter is secondary to a reentry mechanism within the scarred atrial muscle (called *incisional intraatrial reentrant tachycardia*). In this situation, the atrial rates are commonly 250 beats/min or slower, the P-wave morphology is variable without the usual sawtooth F waves, and the P wave is often difficult to detect. Either 2:1 or 1:1 AV conduction is present.

Causes

Atrial flutter usually suggests a significant cardiac pathology, although most fetuses and neonates with atrial flutter have normal hearts, and spontaneous conversion is common. Structural heart disease with dilated atria, acute infectious illness, myocarditis or pericarditis, digitalis toxicity, and thyrotoxicosis are possible causes. Previous surgical procedures involving atria (e.g., Senning operation for transposition, Fontan operation, and other CHDs) may cause incisional intraatrial reentrant tachycardia.

Significance

The ventricular rate determines eventual cardiac output. With a reasonable ventricular rate, the arrhythmia is well tolerated for a long time. A too-rapid ventricular rate may decrease cardiac output and result in heart failure. Uncontrolled atrial flutter may precipitate heart failure. Thrombus formation may lead to embolic events. The flutter may be associated with syncope, presyncope, or chest pain.

Management

Management of atrial flutter is divided into acute conversion, chronic suppression of the arrhythmia, control of ventricular rate, prevention of recurrences, and for refractory cases.

1. Acute situation
   a. Adenosine does not convert the arrythmia to sinus rhythm, although it may be helpful in confirming the diagnosis of atrial flutter by temporarily blocking AV conduction (as shown in Fig. 24.4).
   b. Immediate synchronized DC cardioversion is the treatment of choice for atrial flutter of short duration if the infant or child is in severe CHF.
   c. Transesophageal atrial overdrive pacing may be used for the same purpose. Pacing stimuli are delivered at rates 20% to 25% faster than the flutter rate until the flutter circuit is captured.
   d. In children, IV amiodarone (class III) or IV procainamide (class IA) may be effective.
2. For chronic cases
   For long-standing atrial flutter or fibrillation (of 24 to 48 hours' duration) or those with unknown duration, thrombus formation may lead to cerebral embolic events, especially when the atrial arrhythmia is terminated.
   a. It is essential to rule out atrial thrombi, preferably by echocardiography. Transesophageal echo (TEE) may define atrial thrombi better than transthoracic echo.
   b. If a thrombus is found or its absence uncertain, anticoagulation with warfarin (with an international normalized ratio between 2.0 and 3.0) is started and cardioversion delayed for 2 to 3 weeks. After conversion to sinus rhythm, anticoagulation is continued for an additional 3 to 4 weeks.
3. For rate control
   For control of ventricular rate, calcium channel blockers appear to be the drug of choice. Propranolol may be equally effective. In the past, digoxin was popular for this purpose.
4. For prevention of recurrences
   Class I and class III antiarrhythmic drugs have been shown to be successful in preventing recurrences in some cases. However, class IA drugs (procainamide, quinidine, disopyramide) also have anticholinergic effects that may produce a faster conduction through the AV node, worsening the situation. Therefore, they should be used with drugs that offset the anticholinergic effect, such as digoxin, beta-blockers, or diltiazem. Amiodarone and ibutilide (class III) have also been shown to be effective in treating atrial flutter. For a quick review of antiarrhythmic drugs, readers are recommended to see Tables A.4 and A.5 in Appendix A.
5. For refractory cases
   For incisional intraatrial reentry tachycardia, radiofrequency ablation to interrupt the flutter circuit may be indicated. The success rate for this condition is not as high as in typical atrial flutter (with acute success rate of 75% with recurrence as high as 50%).

Atrial Fibrillation

Description

Atrial fibrillation is the most common arrhythmia seen in adults, but it is rare in children and is less common than atrial flutter in children. The mechanism of this arrhythmia is "circus movement," as in atrial flutter. AF is characterized by an extremely fast atrial rate (f wave at a rate of 350–600 beats/min) and an "irregularly irregular" ventricular response with narrow QRS complexes (see Fig. 24.2).

Causes

Atrial fibrillation usually is associated with structural heart diseases with dilated atria, such as seen with mitral stenosis and regurgitation, Ebstein's anomaly, tricuspid atresia, ASD, or previous intraatrial surgery. Thyrotoxicosis, pulmonary emboli, and pericarditis should be suspected in a previously normal child who develops AF.

Significance

The rapid ventricular rate, in addition to the loss of coordinated contraction of the atria and ventricles, decreases the cardiac output, as occurs in atrial tachycardia. AF usually suggests a significant cardiac pathology.

Management

Some part of medical management for AF is similar to that described under atrial flutter (see previous discussion).

1. If AF has been present for more than 48 hours, anticoagulation with warfarin for 2 to 3 weeks is recommended to prevent systemic embolization of atrial thrombus if the conversion can be delayed. Anticoagulation is continued for 3 to 4 weeks after the restoration of sinus rhythm. If cardioversion cannot be delayed, IV heparin should be started and cardioversion performed when the activated partial thromboplastin time (aPTT) reaches 1.5 to 2.5 times control levels (in 5–10 days), with subsequent oral anticoagulation with warfarin. An alternative to anticoagulation is TEE to rule out atrial thrombus.
2. Propranolol, verapamil, or digoxin may be used to slow the ventricular rate.
3. Class I antiarrhythmic agents (e.g., quinidine, procainamide, flecainide) and the class III agent amiodarone may be used, but the success rate in rhythm conversion is disappointingly low. Tables A.4 and A.5 in Appendix A provide a quick review of antiarrhythmic drugs.
4. In patients with chronic AF, anticoagulation with warfarin should be considered to reduce the incidence of thromboembolism. In chronic cases, rate control, rather than conversion, is increasingly used.
5. In the Cox maze procedure (or the "cut-and-sewmaze"), multiple surgical incisions are made in the right and left atria that are then repaired in an attempt to minimize the formation of reentrant loop. The procedure showed greater than a 96% cure rate 10 years after the surgery in adult patients. Freedom from stroke has generally been reported as exceeding 99% for Cox maze procedures.
6. Radiofrequency ablation to electrically isolate the pulmonary veins from the LA or directly ablating the ectopic focus within the pulmonary veins has shown better results than pharmacologic agents in rhythm control in adults.

Supraventricular Tachycardia

Description

Supraventricular tachycardia is a general term that refers to any rapid heart rhythm originating above the ventricular tissue. In general, SVTs are caused by two separate mechanisms. The first mechanism is reentry, and the second is automaticity. The majority of SVTs are caused by reentrant (or reciprocating) AV tachycardia rather than rapid firing of a single focus in the atria. Examples of the reentry (reciprocating) SVT include atrioventricular reentry tachycardia (AVRT) and atrioventricular nodal reentry tachycardia (AVNRT). Examples of automatic types of SVT are atrial ectopic tachycardia and junctional ectopic tachycardia (JET). These arrhythmias share a number of clinical, electrocardiographic, and therapeutic similarities. Most of the discussion will focus on the reentry type of SVTs; others are discussed under specific headings.

Reentry (Reciprocating) Type of Supraventricular Tachycardia

In the reentry type of SVT, the heart rate is extremely rapid and regular (usually 240 ± 40 beats/min). The P wave usually is invisible. When visible, the P wave has an abnormal P axis and either precedes or follows the QRS complex (see Fig. 24.3). The QRS complex is usually normal (narrow), but occasionally, aberrancy increases the QRS duration, making differentiation from ventricular tachycardia (VT) difficult (see later discussion).

Atrioventricular reentry (or reciprocating) tachycardia is not only the most common mechanism of SVT but also the most common tachyarrhythmia seen in the pediatric age group. This arrhythmia was formerly called *paroxysmal atrial tachycardia (PAT)* because the onset and termination of this arrhythmia were characteristically abrupt.

In SVT caused by reentry, two pathways are involved; at least one of these is the AV node, and the other is an accessory pathway. The accessory pathway may be an anatomically separate bypass tract, such as the bundle of Kent (which produces AVRT; Fig. 24.3A and B), or only a functionally separate bypass tract, such as in a dual AV node pathway (which produces AVNRT; see Fig. 24.3C and D). Patients with accessory pathways frequently have Wolff-Parkinson-White (WPW) preexcitation.

Fig. 24.3 shows the mechanism of reentry AV tachycardia in relation to electrocardiographic (ECG) findings. If a PAC occurs, the prematurity of the extrasystole may find the accessory bundle refractory, but the AV node may conduct, producing a normal QRS complex; when the impulse reaches the bundle of Kent from the ventricular side, the bundle will have recovered and allows reentry into the atrium, producing a superiorly directed P wave that is difficult to detect. In turn, the cycle is maintained by reentry into the AV node, with a very fast heart rate. When there is an antegrade conduction through the AV node (slow pathway), the rhythm is called orthodromic AVRT (see Fig. 24.3A).

Less common is a widened QRS complex with antegrade conduction into the ventricle via the accessory (fast) pathway

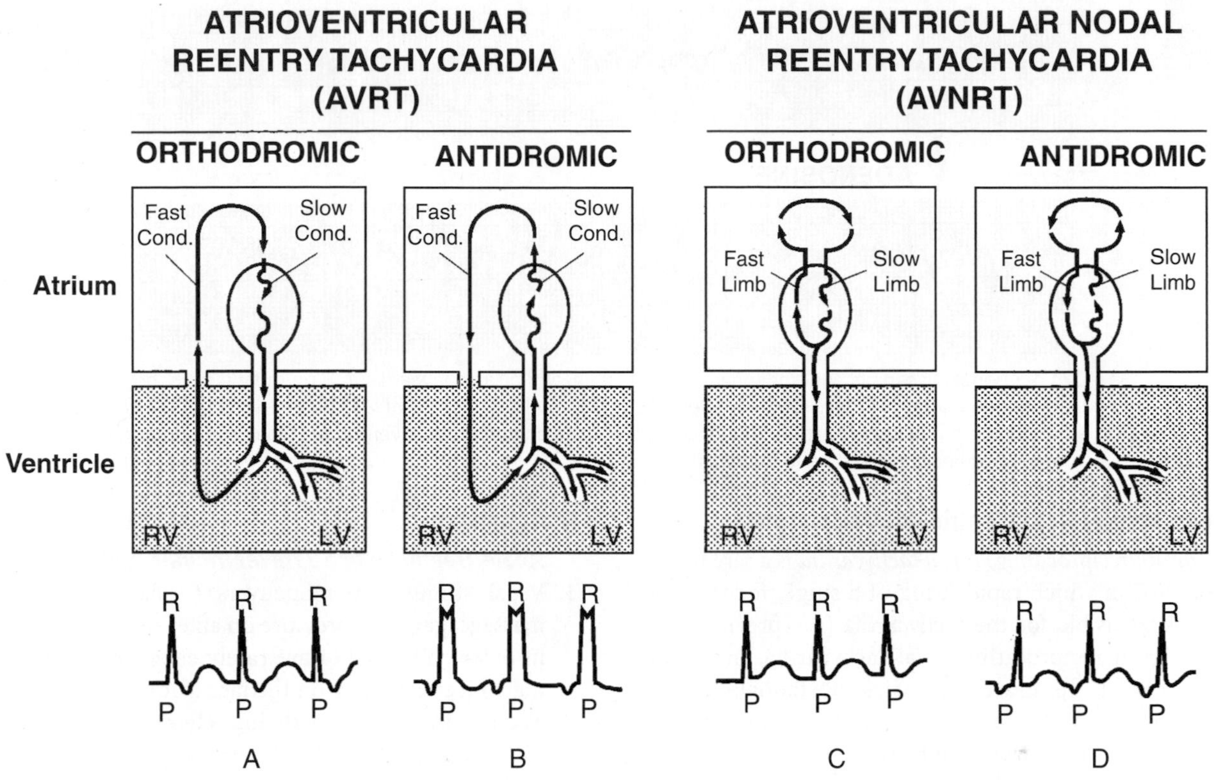

ATRIOVENTRICULAR REENTRY TACHYCARDIA (AVRT)

ORTHODROMIC   ANTIDROMIC

ATRIOVENTRICULAR NODAL REENTRY TACHYCARDIA (AVNRT)

ORTHODROMIC   ANTIDROMIC

Fig. 24.3 Diagram showing the mechanism of reentry type of supraventricular tachycardia (SVT) in relation to electrocardiographic (ECG) findings. **A,** Orthodromic atrioventricular reentry tachycardia (AVRT) is the most common mechanism of SVT in patients with Wolff-Parkinson-White preexcitation. Antegrade conduction through the normal, slow atrioventricular (AV) node produces a normal QRS complex, and the retrograde conduction through the bypass tract creates inverted P waves after the QRS complex (with a short RP interval). **B,** In antidromic AVRT, the antegrade conduction through the bypass tract produces a wide QRS complex. Retrograde P waves precede the wide QRS complex with a short PR interval (and a long RP interval). **C,** In orthodromic atrioventricular nodal reentry tachycardia (AVNRT) (common form), the retrograde P waves are usually concealed in the QRS complex of normal duration. The ECG is similar to that of orthodromic AVRT, and differentiation between these two is possible only when the tachyarrhythmia terminates by the presence of preexcitation in the AVRT. **D,** In antidromic AVNRT, narrow QRS complexes are preceded by retrograde P waves, with a short PR interval. The ECG is similar to that of ectopic atrial tachycardia. *Cond,* conduction; *LV,* left ventricle; *RV,* right ventricle. (From Park MK, Guntheroth WG: *How to Read Pediatric ECGs,* ed 4, Philadelphia, 2006, Mosby.)

and retrograde conduction through the (slower) AV node (antidromic AVRT; see Fig. 24.3B). A premature ventricular contraction (PVC) could initiate this arrhythmia if the recovery time of the two limbs is ideal for the initiation of the reentry.

Dual pathways in the AV node are more common than accessory bundles, at least as functional entities. For SVT to occur, the two pathways would have to have, at least temporarily, different conduction and recovery rates, creating the substrate for a reentry tachycardia. When the normal, slow pathway through the AV node is used in antegrade conduction to the bundle of His (orthodromic), the resulting QRS complex is normal with an abnormal P vector, but the latter is unrecognizable because it is superimposed on the QRS complex (see Fig. 24.3C). The resulting tachycardia could be the same as that seen with SVT associated with WPW syndrome. The two can be differentiated only after conversion from the SVT; after conversion, the patient with accessory bundle would have WPW preexcitation. In antidromic AVNRT (see

Fig. 24.3D), which is uncommon, the fast tract of the AV node transmits the antegrade impulse to the bundle of His, and the normal, slow pathway of the AV node transmits the impulse retrogradely. The resulting SVT demonstrates normal QRS duration, a short PR interval, and an inverted P wave.

In general, AVNRT is more influenced by increased sympathetic tone than AVRT. AVNRT is more likely triggered by physical activity, emotional stress, and abrupt changes in body position. In addition, AVNRT is less likely to be incessant (and therefore rarely causing tachycardia-induced cardiomyopathy). SVT, seen in the first year of life but few afterward, is more likely to have accessory AVRT, and an adolescent who has first SVT is more likely to have AVNRT.

Any type of AV block is incompatible with reentrant tachycardia; AV block would abruptly terminate the tachycardia, at least temporarily. This is the reason that adenosine, which transiently blocks AV conduction, works well for this type of arrhythmia.

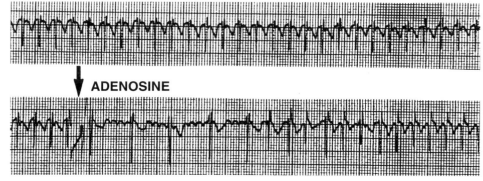

Fig. 24.4 Adenosine can uncover the mechanism of supraventricular tachycardia. A 3-month-old infant developed an extremely fast, narrow QRS complex tachycardia and a heart rate of 220 beats/min after insertion of a central line through a jugular vein. Adenosine produced a transient atrioventricular block and unmasked very rapid atrial fibrillation waves (570 beats/min).

Automatic Type of Supraventricular Tachycardia

Ectopic (or nonreciprocating) atrial tachycardia is a rare mechanism of SVT in which rapid firing of a single focus in the atrium is responsible for the tachycardia (see previous section). Unlike in reciprocating atrial tachycardia, in ectopic atrial tachycardia, the heart rate varies substantially during the course of a day, and second-degree AV block may develop. In contrast, in reentrant tachycardia, second-degree AV block terminates the SVT. *Nodal ectopic tachycardia* may superficially resemble atrial tachycardia because the P wave is buried in the T waves of the preceding beat and becomes invisible but the rate of nodal tachycardia is relatively slower (120 to 200 beats/min) than the rate of ectopic atrial tachycardia. These two arrhythmias are further discussed under separate headings.

Causes

1. WPW preexcitation is present in 10% to 20% of cases, which is evident only after conversion to sinus rhythm. Approximately 10% of WPW patients have multiple (two to four) accessory pathways.
2. No heart disease is found in about half of patients. This idiopathic type of SVT occurs more commonly in young infants than in older children.
3. Some congenital heart defects (e.g., Ebstein's anomaly, single ventricle, congenitally corrected transposition of the great arteries) are more prone to this arrhythmia.
4. SVT may occur after cardiac surgeries.

Significance

1. Many infants tolerate SVT well. If the tachycardia is sustained for 6 to 12 hours, signs of CHF usually develop in infants. Clinical manifestations of CHF include irritability, tachypnea, poor feeding, and pallor. When CHF develops, the infant's condition can deteriorate rapidly.
2. Older children may complain of chest pain, palpitation, shortness of breath, lightheadedness, and fatigue. A pounding sensation in the neck (i.e., neck pulsation) is fairly unique to the reentrant type SVT and considered to be the result of cannon waves when the atrium contracts against a simultaneously contracting ventricle.

Management

Acute Treatment of Supraventricular Tachycardia.

1. Vagal stimulatory maneuvers (unilateral carotid sinus massage, gagging, pressure on an eyeball) may be effective in older children but are rarely effective in infants. Placing an ice-water bag on the face (for ≤10 seconds) is often effective in infants (by diving reflex). In children, a headstand often successfully interrupts the SVT.
2. If the vagal maneuver is ineffective, adenosine is considered the drug of choice. It has negative chronotropic, dromotropic, and inotropic actions with a very short duration of action (half-life <10 seconds) and minimal hemodynamic consequences. Adenosine is effective for almost all reciprocating SVT (in which the AV node forms part of the reentry circuit) of both narrow- and wide-complex *regular* tachycardia. It is not effective for irregular tachycardia. It is not effective for nonreciprocating atrial tachycardia, atrial flutter or fibrillation, and VT, but it has differential diagnostic ability. Its transient AV block may unmask atrial activities by slowing the ventricular rate and thus help clarify the mechanism of certain supraventricular arrhythmias (see Fig. 24.4).

   Adenosine is given by rapid IV bolus followed by a saline flush, starting at 50 μg/kg and increasing in increments of 50 μg/kg every 1 to 2 minutes. The usual effective dose is 100 to 150 μg/kg with maximum dose of 250 μg/kg. Adenosine is 90% to 100% effective.
3. If the infant is in severe CHF and adenosine is not readily available, emergency treatment is directed at immediate cardioversion. The initial dose of 0.5 joule/kg is increased in steps up to 2 joule/kg.
4. IV administration of propranolol may be used to treat SVT in the presence of WPW syndrome. IV verapamil should be avoided in infants younger than 12 months of age because it may produce extreme bradycardia and hypotension in infants. Esmolol, other beta-adrenergic blockers, verapamil, and digoxin also have been used with some success.
5. Overdrive suppression (by transesophageal pacing or by atrial pacing) may be effective in children who have been digitalized.

Prevention of Recurrence of Supraventricular Tachycardia.

1. In infants without WPW preexcitation, oral propranolol for 12 months is effective.
2. Children with breakthrough SVT while taking a beta-blocker or not responsive to beta-blockers benefit from amiodarone orally.
3. Verapamil can also be used, but it should be used with caution in patients with poor LV function and in young infants.
4. In infants or children with or without WPW preexcitation on the ECG, beta-blockers such as atenolol or nadolol are often the medication of choice in the long-term management. In the presence of WPW preexcitation, digoxin or verapamil may increase the rate of antegrade conduction of the impulse through the accessory pathway and therefore should be avoided.
5. For children who have infrequent episodes of SVT that result in little hemodynamic compromise, observation is indicated. They should be taught how to apply vagal maneuvers (e.g., gagging, headstands). If not effective, adenosine is used to correct the rhythm. Alternatively, the use of a beta-blocker or calcium channel blocker can be effective in slowing and terminating the SVT.
6. Recently, intranasal etripamil, a short-acting L-type calcium channel blocker, was successfully used to terminate in the used SVT in adult patients. This new approach may be a promising option for out-of-hospital management of patients with breakthrough SVTs (Stambler et al, 2018).
7. Radiofrequency catheter ablation or surgical interruption of accessory pathways should be considered if medical management fails or frequent recurrences occur. Ablation therapy is controversial for asymptomatic patients with WPW pre-excitation. Ablation is not recommended in infants 1 to 2 years of age because of a possibility of spontaneous resolution of SVT.

Radiofrequency ablation can be carried out with a high degree of success and a low complication rate. The success rate of the procedure for accessory pathway ablation is between 90% and 95%; the highest success rates are found in patients with left-sided accessory pathways. Patients with para-Hisian pathways have the lowest success rate because of more cautious applications (fearing risk of AV block). A risk of heart block is 1.2% with risk as high as 10.4% for patients with midseptal ablation site. The overall risk of complication is 3% to 4%.

RHYTHMS ORIGINATING IN THE ATRIOVENTRICULAR NODE

Rhythms that originate in the AV node are characterized by the following findings (Fig. 24.5):

1. The P wave may be absent, or inverted P waves may follow the QRS complex.
2. The QRS complex usually is normal in duration and configuration.

Only the lower part (NH region) of the AV node has pacemaker ability. The upper (AN region) and middle (N region) parts do not function as pacemakers but delay the conduction of an impulse, either antegrade or retrograde.

Junctional (or Nodal) Premature Beats
Description
A normal QRS complex occurs prematurely. P waves usually are absent, but inverted P waves may follow QRS complexes (see Fig. 24.5). The compensatory pause may be complete or incomplete.

Causes
Nodal premature beats usually are idiopathic in an otherwise normal heart; they may result from cardiac surgery and digitalis toxicity.

Significance
Nodal premature beats usually have no hemodynamic significance.

Management
Treatment is not indicated unless the cause is digitalis toxicity.

Junctional (or Nodal) Escape Beats
Description
When the SA node impulse fails to reach the AV node, the NH region of the AV node initiates an impulse (junctional or nodal escape beat). The resulting QRS complex occurs later than the anticipated normal beat. The P wave may be absent, or an inverted P wave follows the QRS complex (see Fig. 24.5). The duration and configuration of QRS complexes are normal.

Causes
Nodal escape beats may occur after cardiac surgery involving the atria (the Senning procedure or Fontan operation) or in otherwise healthy children.

Significance
Nodal escape beats have little hemodynamic significance.

Management
Generally, no specific treatment is required.

Nodal (or Junctional) Rhythm
Description
If the SA node consistently fails, the AV node may function as the main pacemaker of the heart, producing a relatively slow rate (40–60 beats/min). Nodal rhythm is characterized by no P waves or inverted P waves after QRS complexes and normal (narrow) QRS complexes with a rate of 40 to 60 beats/min (see Fig. 24.5).

Causes
Nodal or junctional rhythm may occur in an otherwise normal heart, increased vagal tone (increased intracranial

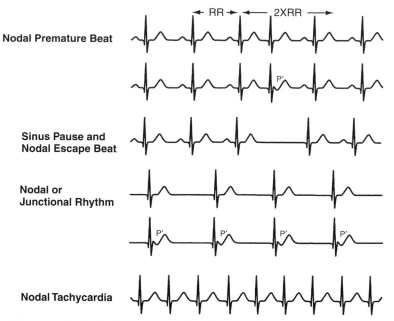

Fig. 24.5 Arrhythmias originating in the atrioventricular (AV) node. Characteristics of arrhythmias of the AV node origin are (1) absent P wave or inverted P wave following the QRS complex and (2) normal duration of QRS complex. (From Park MK, Guntheroth WG: *How to Read Pediatric ECGs*, ed 4, Philadelphia, 2006, Mosby.)

pressure, pharyngeal stimulation), and digitalis toxicity or as a result of cardiac surgery. Rarely, it may be seen in children with polysplenia syndrome (LA isomerism).

Significance

The slow heart rate may significantly decrease cardiac output and produce symptoms.

Management

No treatment is indicated if the patient is asymptomatic. Known causes such as digitalis toxicity should be treated. Atropine or electric pacing is indicated if the patient is symptomatic from bradycardia.

Accelerated Nodal Rhythm

Description

When the patient has a normal sinus rate and AV conduction and the AV node (NH region) has enhanced automaticity and captures the pacemaker function at a faster rate (60–120 beats/min) than the normal junctional rate (40–60 beats/min), the rhythm is called *accelerated nodal* (*or AV junctional*) *rhythm*. P waves are either absent or inverted P waves follow the normal QRS complexes.

Causes

Accelerated nodal rhythm may be idiopathic, may result from digitalis toxicity or myocarditis, or may follow cardiac surgery.

Significance

Accelerated nodal rhythm has little hemodynamic significance.

Management

No treatment is necessary unless caused by digitalis toxicity.

Junctional Ectopic Tachycardia (Nodal Tachycardia)

Description

Either the P waves are absent or inverted P waves follow QRS complexes (see Fig. 24.5). The ventricular rate varies from 140 to 240 beats/min. The QRS complex is usually normal, but *aberration* may occur on rare occasions, as in atrial tachycardia. JET is sometimes difficult to separate from other types of SVT.

Causes

Enhanced automaticity of the junctional area is the suspected mechanism of the arrhythmia. There are two types: postoperative and congenital.

Postoperative type is the most common form of junctional autonomic rhythm in children. It is a transient disorder seen immediately after open heart surgery lasting 24 to 48 hours. Trauma, stretch, or ischemia to the AV node and electrolyte imbalances resulting from surgical procedures may be responsible for the rhythm abnormality.

Rare congenital form may occur without heart defect or may be associated with a cardiac malformation (≤50%). Developmental abnormalities of the AV node and superimposed fibrosis, inflammation, and focal degeneration may be the underlying causes.

Significance

In the postoperative type, there is a loss of AV synchrony in the presence of a fast rate (nearly 200 beats/min), which compromises cardiac output, leading to a fall in blood pressure. Increased endogenous catecholamine levels and administered inotropic support (to maintain adequate blood pressure and renal perfusion) may result in peripheral vasoconstriction, leading to a raise in the core temperature. The rising core temperature exacerbates the tachycardia, worsening ventricular performance.

In the congenital form, most patients present before 6 months of age, usually with congestive heart failure. The overall mortality rate is about 35% for this form of tachycardia.

Management

A number of complementary measures are used to treat postoperative JET. They are aimed at correcting pathophysiology of the postoperative tachycardia.

1. Heart rate less than 170 beats/min is well tolerated, but a rate faster than 170 to 190 beats/min needs to be slowed. Atrial overdrive pacing (typically 10 beats/min higher than the rate) often restores AV synchrony.
2. Mild systemic hypothermia is induced, usually a core temperature of 34°C to 35°C. At a core temperature below 32°C, ventricular function may be impaired.
3. Maximize cardiac output by carefully titrating fluid and electrolyte balance, inotropic support, and pain management.
4. IV amiodarone appears to be the drug of choice as antiarrhythmic therapy. Digoxin, used in the past, has little place in treatment.
5. As an alternative, extracorporeal membrane oxygenation can be used for this arrhythmia.

For the congenital type, amiodarone appears to be the drug of choice. Amiodarone in high dose was effective in 85% of the patients with an almost 75% survival rate. If amiodarone is not effective, ablation therapy may be tried.

RHYTHMS ORIGINATING IN THE VENTRICLE

Rhythms that originate in the ventricle (ventricular arrhythmias) are characterized by the following (Fig. 24.6):
1. Bizarre and wide QRS complexes
2. T waves pointing in directions opposite of QRS complexes
3. QRS complexes randomly related to P waves, if visible

Premature Ventricular Contraction
Description

A bizarre, wide QRS complex appears earlier than anticipated, and the T wave points in the opposite direction. A full compensatory pause usually appears; that is, the length of two cycles, including the premature beat, is the same as that of two normal cycles (see Fig. 24.6). The presence of a full compensatory pause indicates that the sinus node is not prematurely discharged by the PVC. If the retrograde impulse discharges and resets the sinus node prematurely, it produces a pause that is not fully compensatory.

Premature ventricular contractions may be classified into several types, depending on their interrelationship, similarities, timing, and coupling intervals.

Interrelationship.
1. **Ventricular bigeminy or coupling.** Each abnormal QRS complex regularly alternates with a normal QRS complex.
2. **Ventricular trigeminy.** Each abnormal QRS complex regularly follows two normal QRS complexes.
3. **Couplets.** Two abnormal QRS complexes appear in sequence.
4. **Triplets.** Three abnormal QRS complexes appear in sequence. Three or more successive PVCs arbitrarily are termed *ventricular tachycardia.*

Similarities among PVCs. Depending on the similarities of the bizarre QRS complex, PVCs may be classified into the following types:
1. **Uniform (monomorphic or unifocal) PVCs.** Abnormal QRS complexes have the same configuration in a single lead. They are assumed to originate from a single focus.
2. **Multiform (polymorphic or multifocal) PVCs.** Abnormal QRS complexes have different configurations in a single lead. They are assumed to originate from different foci.

Timing in the cardiac cycle. Depending on their timing in the cardiac cycle, PVCs may be classified into several types (Fig. 24.7):
1. **Interpolated PVC.** The PVC appears between two conducted sinus beats. Sinus rhythm is not interrupted, and there is no compensatory pause after the PVC. The PR interval after the PVC is slightly increased (see Fig. 24.7B).

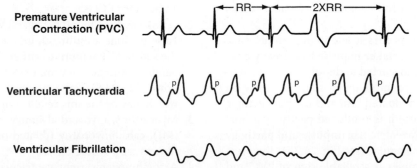

Fig. 24.6 Ventricular arrhythmias. Ventricular rhythms are characterized by bizarre and wide QRS complexes with the T wave, when visible, pointing in opposite directions. *PVC,* Premature ventricular contraction; *VF,* ventricular fibrillation; *VT,* ventricular tachycardia. (From Park MK, Guntheroth WG: *How to Read Pediatric ECGs,* ed 4, Philadelphia, 2006, Mosby.)

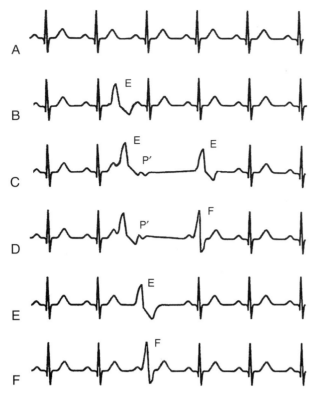

Fig. 24.7 Types of premature ventricular contractions (PVCs) according to timing in the cardiac cycle. **A,** Regular sinus rhythm. **B,** Interpolated PVC followed by a slightly prolonged PR interval. **C,** Early PVC, which results in a retrogradely conducted P wave (P′) with a less than full compensatory pause. The first postectopic beat is a ventricular escape beat (E). **D,** Early PVC with a retrogradely conducted P wave (P′) with a less than full compensatory pause. A ventricular fusion beat (F) resumes the cardiac cycle. **E,** Late PVC, which results in a full compensatory pause; presumably, retrograde discharge of the sinus node did not occur. **F,** Ventricular fusion beat with a full compensatory pause.

2. **Early PVC.** The PVC appears shortly after the normal T wave of the preceding beat. A compensatory pause may appear. If the sinus rate is slow and a retrograde atrial conduction prematurely discharges the sinus node, a noncompensatory pause results. Either a ventricular escape beat or a fusion beat resumes the cardiac cycle (see Fig. 24.7C and D).

3. **Late PVC.** The PVC appears slightly before the normal P wave of the next beat. A full compensatory pause results (see Fig. 24.7E).

4. **Fusion beats.** The PVC occurs so late in the cardiac cycle that a normal sinus pacemaker impulse has already penetrated the AV node and started to depolarize the ventricle. The resulting QRS complex appears midway between the patient's normal conducted beat and the pure ectopic ventricular beat because it is produced partly by a normally conducted supraventricular impulse and partly by an ectopic ventricular impulse (see Fig. 24.7F). The presence of a "fusion" complex is a reliable sign of PVC and helps differentiate VT from a supraventricular arrhythmia with aberrant ventricular conduction (see later discussion).

Coupling Interval

1. **Fixed coupling.** PVCs appear at a constant interval after the QRS complex of the previous cardiac cycle. This suggests ventricular *reentry* within the Purkinje system as the underlying mechanism. Most PVCs in children have a fixed coupling interval and a uniform left bundle branch block (LBBB) morphology.

2. **Varying coupling.** When coupling intervals vary by more than 80 msec, the PVCs may result from parasystole. If the intervals between ectopic beats can be factored so that each interval is a multiple of a single basic interval (within 0.08 second), ventricular parasystole is diagnosed. Ventricular parasystole consists of an impulse-forming focus in the ventricle that is independent of the sinus node–generated impulse and is protected from depolarization (entrance block) by sinus impulses.

Aberration

Occasionally, aberrantly conducted atrial impulse resulted in a wide QRS complex that resembles a PVC. This may occur in patients with atrial arrhythmias, including atrial premature contraction. When an atrial impulse prematurely reaches the AV node or bundle of His, it may find one bundle branch excitable and the other still refractory. Therefore, the resulting QRS complex resembles a bundle branch block pattern. The right bundle branch usually has a longer refractory period than the left bundle branch, producing QRS complexes similar to those of right bundle branch block (RBBB).

The following features help in differentiating aberrant ventricular conduction from ectopic ventricular impulses:

1. An rsR′ pattern in V1 that resembles QRS complexes of RBBB suggests aberration. In ventricular ectopic beats, the QRS morphology is bizarre and does not resemble the classic form of RBBB or LBBB.

2. Occasional wide QRS complexes after visible P waves with regular PR intervals suggest an aberration.

3. The presence of a ventricular "fusion" complex (see previous discussion) is a reliable sign of ventricular ectopic rhythm.

Causes

1. PVC may appear in otherwise healthy children. Up to 50% to 70% of normal children may show PVCs on 24-hour ambulatory ECGs.

2. A link has been found between LV false tendon and PVCs. False tendons are thin, chordal strands that extend from the ventricular septum to either the LV free wall or an LV papillary muscle; they are detectable by two-dimensional echo (Fig. 24.8). False tendons contain Purkinje fibers, which may be the source of the arrhythmia.

3. Myocarditis, myocardial injury or myocardial infarction (MI), cardiomyopathy (dilated or hypertrophic), cardiac tumors are possible causes.

4. Arrhythmogenic right ventricular dysplasia (RV cardiomyopathy) may be the cause in children with symptomatic tachycardia (see the section on primary myocardial disease in Chapter 18).

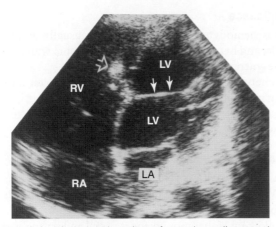

Fig. 24.8 Apical four-chamber view of an echocardiogram showing a false tendon *(solid arrows)* in the left ventricle (LV) in a 13-year-old boy who had surgical repair of a ventricular septal defect *(open arrow)*. This patient had a "twanging string" type of systolic murmur and occasional uniform premature ventricular contractions. *LA,* Left atrium; *RA,* right atrium; *RV,* right ventricle.

5. Long QT syndrome (LQTS; see later section)
6. Congenital or acquired heart disease, preoperative or postoperative
7. Drugs such as catecholamines, theophylline, caffeine, amphetamines, digitalis toxicity, and some anesthetic agents are possible causes.
8. Mitral valve prolapse (MVP) is a possible cause.

Significance

1. Occasional PVCs are benign in children, particularly if they are uniform and disappear or become less frequent with exercise.
2. PVCs are more significant if the following are true:
   a. They are associated with underlying heart disease (preoperative or postoperative status, MVP, cardiomyopathy).
   b. There is a history of syncope or a family history of sudden death.
   c. They are precipitated by, or become more frequent with, activity.
   d. They are multiform, particularly couplets.
   e. There are runs of PVCs with symptoms.
   f. There are incessant or frequent episodes of paroxysmal VT (more likely myocardial tumors).
3. Ventricular parasystole does not appear to have any consequences in children.

Management

1. In children with otherwise normal hearts, occasional isolated uniform PVCs that are suppressed by exercise do not require extensive investigation or treatment. ECG, echo studies, and 24-hour Holter monitoring suffice.
   a. ECGs are used to detect QTc prolongation, ST-T changes, and other abnormalities.
   b. Echo studies detect structural heart disease or functional abnormalities.
   c. 24-hour ambulatory ECG (Holter monitoring) or event recorder detects the frequency and severity of the arrhythmia.
2. Children with uniform PVCs, including ventricular bigeminy and trigeminy, do not need to be treated if the echo and exercise stress test results are normal. Arrhythmias that are potentially related to exercise are significant and require documentation of the relationship. The induction or exacerbation of arrhythmia with exercise may be an indication of underlying heart disease. In children, PVCs characteristically are reduced or eliminated by exercise.
3. Asymptomatic children with multiform PVCs and ventricular couplets should have 24-hour Holter monitoring, even if they have structurally normal hearts, to detect the severity and extent of ventricular arrhythmias.
4. All children with symptomatic ventricular arrhythmias and those with complex PVCs (multiform PVCs, ventricular couplets, unsustained VT) should be treated. Tables A.4 and A.5 in Appendix A provide a quick review of antiarrhythmic drugs.
   a. Beta-blockers (e.g., atenolol, 1–2 mg/kg orally in a single daily dose) are effective for cardiomyopathy and occasionally for RV dysplasia.
   b. Other antiarrhythmic drugs, such as phenytoin sodium (Dilantin) and mexiletine, may be effective. Antiarrhythmic agents that prolong the QT interval, such as those of class IA (quinidine, procainamide), class IC (encainide, flecainide), and class III (amiodarone, bretylium), should be avoided (Box 24.1).
   c. Frequent PVCs occasionally require treatment with an IV bolus of lidocaine (1 mg/kg per dose) followed by an IV drip of lidocaine (20–50 µg/kg/min).
5. For patients with symptomatic ventricular arrhythmias or sustained VT and seemingly normal hearts, magnetic resonance imaging (MRI) may be indicated to investigate for RV dysplasia.
6. Children with multiform PVCs and runs of PVCs (VT) with or without symptoms need to be evaluated by an electrophysiologist. Invasive electrophysiologic studies with RV endomyocardial biopsy may be indicated.

Accelerated Ventricular Rhythm
Description

1. Accelerated ventricular rhythm (AVR) is also known by many other names, such as slow VT, idioventricular tachycardia, slow ventricular rhythm, and nonparoxysmal ventricular tachycardia.
2. Wide QRS complex rhythm of short duration is present (usually several beats but can be longer than 120 beats).
3. The ventricular rate approximates the patient's sinus rate, within ±10% to 15% of the sinus rate (*isochronicity*). The *isochronicity* with sinus rhythm is more important than the rate per minute. The ventricular rate is usually 120 beats/min or less in children (and 140–180 beats/min in newborns). The rate helps differentiate AVR from VT (with rate >120 beats/min).

BOX 24.1 Acquired Causes of QT Prolongation[a]

Drugs

Antibiotics: erythromycin, clarithromycin, telithromycin, azithromycin, trimethoprim–sulfamethoxazole

Antifungal agents: fluconazole, itraconazole, ketoconazole

Antiprotozoal agents: pentamidine isethionate

Antihistamines: astemizole, terfenadine (Seldane; Seldane has been removed from the market for this reason)

Antidepressants: tricyclics such as imipramine (Tofranil), amitriptyline (Elavil), desipramine (Norpramin), and doxepin (Sinequan)

Antipsychotics: haloperidol, risperidone, phenothiazines such as thioridazine (Mellaril) and chlorpromazine (Thorazine)

Antiarrhythmic agents
- Class IA (sodium channel blockers): quinidine, procainamide, disopyramide
- Class III (prolong depolarization): amiodarone (rare), bretylium, dofetilide, N-acetyl-procainamide, sotalol

Lipid-lowering agent: probucol

Antianginal: bepridil

Diuretics (through K loss): furosemide (Lasix), ethacrynic acid (Edecrin)

Oral hypoglycemic agents: glibenclamide, glyburide

Organophosphate insecticides

Promotility agent: cisapride

Vasodilator: prenylamine

Electrolyte Disturbances

Hypokalemia: diuretics, hyperventilation

Hypocalcemia

Hypomagnesemia

Underlying Medical Conditions

Bradycardia: complete atrioventricular block, severe bradycardia, sick sinus syndrome

Myocardial dysfunction: anthracycline cardiotoxicity, congestive heart failure, myocarditis, cardiac tumors

Endocrinopathy: hyperparathyroidism, hypothyroidism, pheochromocytoma

Neurologic: encephalitis, head trauma, stroke, subarachnoid hemorrhage

Nutritional: alcoholism, anorexia nervosa, starvation

[a]A more exhaustive updated list of medications that can prolong the QTc interval is available at the University of Arizona Center for Education and Research on Therapeutics' website (www.qtdrugs.org).

4. The QRS morphology is LBBB pattern in the great majority.

Causes

1. In the majority of the patients, AVR is usually an isolated finding. Rarely, it may be associated with underlying heart disease, such as CHD, myocarditis, digitalis toxicity, hypertension, cardiomyopathy, metabolic abnormalities, postoperative state, or MI (in adults).
2. The mechanism of AVR is unknown; ectopic ventricular focus may accelerate its rate enough to overcome sinus rate.

Significance

1. It is hemodynamically insignificant, usually asymptomatic, and benign. It is rarely seen in patients with syncope, presyncope, or palpitation.
2. Sometimes it is found by routine ECG or Holter monitoring in asymptomatic patients.
3. Exertional sinus tachycardia usually converts it to sinus rhythm.

Management

1. In children, AVR is generally considered benign.
2. AVR is notably resistant to antiarrhythmic agents (no treatment is required).
3. Follow-up Holter monitoring is useful and it usually shows resolution of AVR.

Ventricular Tachycardia

Description

1. VT is a series of three or more PVCs with a heart rate of 120 to 200 beats/min. QRS complexes are wide and bizarre, with T waves pointing in opposite directions (see Fig. 24.6).
2. VT may be classified in various ways by its onset, duration, and morphology.
   a. The onset may be paroxysmal (sudden) or nonparoxysmal.
   b. By duration, VT may be (1) a salvo of VT–a few beats in a row; (2) nonsustained VT—duration of less than 30 seconds; (3) sustained VT—longer than 30 seconds; and (4) incessant VT, referring to lengthy sustained VT that dominates the cardiac rhythm.
   c. By morphology, it may be (1) monomorphic, referring to one dominant QRS form; (2) polymorphic, referring to a beat-to-beat change in the QRS shape; or (3) "bidirectional VT," a specific from of polymorphic VT in which the QRS axis shifts across the baseline.
3. Torsades de pointes (meaning "twisting of the points") is characterized by a paroxysm of VT during which there are progressive changes in the amplitude and polarity of QRS complexes separated by a narrow transition QRS complex. It is a distinct form of polymorphic VT, occurring in patients with marked QT prolongation.
4. Differentiating VT from SVT with aberrant conduction (see later discussion) is sometimes difficult. However, in children, almost all wide QRS tachycardias are VT. They should be treated as such until proved otherwise.

Causes

1. VT may occur in patients with structural heart diseases such as TOF, AS, hypertrophic or dilated cardiomyopathy, or mitral valve prolapse.
2. Postoperative CHDs (such as TOF, D-TGA, or double-outlet right ventricle)
3. Myocarditis, cardiomyopathies, Chagas disease (trypanosomiasis, in South America), myocardial tumors, myocardial ischemia and MI
4. Pulmonary hypertension

5 Arrhythmogenic RV dysplasia (in patients of southern European ancestry), Brugada syndrome (young men from Southeast Asia), and LQTS

6. Metabolic causes include hypoxia, acidosis, hyperkalemia, hypokalemia, and hypomagnesemia.

7. Mechanical irritation (intraventricular catheter)

8. Pharmacologic or chemical causes include catecholamine infusion, digitalis toxicity, cocaine, and organophosphate insecticides. Most antiarrhythmic drugs (especially classes IA, IC, and III) are also proarrhythmic.

9. Certain drugs that prolong the QT interval may cause VT, including:
   a. Antiarrhythmic drugs, especially class IA (quinidine, procainamide), class IC (encainide, flecainide), and class III (amiodarone, bretylium)
   b. Antipsychotic agents (phenothiazines such as chlorpromazine or thioridazine)
   c. Tricyclic antidepressants (imipramine, desipramine)
   d. Certain antibiotics (erythromycin, trimethoprim–sulfamethoxazole) (see Box 24.1)

   Class II and IV antiarrhythmic agents do not prolong the QT interval. For a quick review of antiarrhythmic drugs, readers are recommended to see Tables A.4 and A.5 in Appendix A.

10. VT may occur in healthy children who have structurally and functionally normal heart. This group is discussed under a separate heading (see later).

Significance

1. VT may signify a serious myocardial pathology or dysfunction and can be a cause of sudden cardiac death. These events are, however, unusual in patients with structurally normal hearts.

2. Presenting symptoms may be dizziness, syncope, palpitation, or chest pain. Family history may be positive for ventricular arrhythmia or sudden death.

3. With a fast heart rate, cardiac output may decrease notably, and the rhythm may deteriorate to ventricular fibrillation (VF), in which effective cardiac output does not occur.

4. Chronic low-rate VT may lead to a tachycardia-mediated cardiomyopathy.

5. A condition called *accelerated ventricular rhythm* is similar to VT but the heart rate is slower (< 120 beats/min) and occurs in patients with structurally normal hearts. It is discussed under a separate heading.

4. Polymorphic VTs are more significant than monomorphic ones.

5. Those associated with abnormal cardiac structure (pre- and postoperative) or function are more significant than those seen with structurally and functionally normal hearts.

6. Some VTs are provoked by exercise, but others are suppressed by exercise. The former is usually more significant than the latter.

7. VTs associated with certain forms of cardiomyopathy (arrhythmogenic RV dysplasia, hypertrophic or dilated cardiomyopathy) and genetic electrical heart diseases (LQTS; Brugada syndrome) can be a cause of sudden death.

Management

1. The following investigations may be indicated.
   a. History of congenital or acquired heart disease or substance abuse and family history of syncope, seizure, sudden cardiac death, or familial arrhythmia are important.
   b. Echo and Doppler studies identify most conditions that may cause sudden cardiac death, such as cardiomyopathies (hypertrophic, dilated, noncompaction), myocarditis, coronary artery anomalies (congenital, Kawasaki's disease), primary pulmonary hypertension, and various CHDs (pre- and postoperative).

   Structurally and functionally normal hearts on echo studies may include a group of benign conditions as well as some potentially lethal conditions, including the following:
      1) Right ventricular outflow tract (RVOT) VT, RBBB VT (Belhassen's), and AVR are generally benign conditions. These conditions are discussed further under separate headings.
      2) Electrical myopathies: LQTS, Brugada syndrome, and RV dysplasias and potentially fatal conditions. The ECG usually suggests these conditions.
   c. Holter monitoring may be useful for assessing the frequency of PVCs or VTs.
   d. Exercise stress test is useful for detecting exercise-induced VT and for assessing the effectiveness of therapy (either medical or ablation).
   e. MRI is useful to rule out arrhythmogenic RV dysplasia.
   f. Electrophysiologic investigation may be indicated for:
      1) Those with high-density PVCs and symptoms suspicious for tachyarrhythmia
      2) Those with underlying heart disease, especially those in postoperative status, with potentially life-threatening inducible sustained VT
      3) To target the VT focus or reentry circuit for ablation
      4) To check for the effectiveness of orally administered antiarrhythmic therapy

2. Acute therapy
   a. Symptomatic VT must be treated promptly with synchronized DC cardioversion (0.5–1 joule/kg) if the patient is unconscious or has cardiovascular instability with clinical evidence of low cardiac output.
   b. Rarely, if the patient is conscious, an IV bolus of lidocaine (1 mg/kg per dose over 1 to 2 minutes) followed by an IV drip of lidocaine (20–50 μg/kg/min) may be effective. Lidocaine or procainamide is often initiated after cardioversion in an attempt to suppress reinitiation of the tachycardia.
   c. IV amiodarone is used in patients with drug-refractory VT, particularly those seen in postoperative patients. The mechanism of action of amiodarone appears to be by reducing transmural heterogeneity of repolarization in the ventricular muscle.
   d. IV injection of magnesium sulfate is reportedly an effective and safe treatment for torsade de pointes in adults (2 g in an IV bolus).

e. A trial of adenosine may be helpful in some patients with structurally normal hearts. VT with RBBB and superior axis (LV septal origin) may be calcium channel dependent and respond to slow IV push of verapamil.

3. The physician should research for reversible conditions contributing to the initiation of VT (e.g., hypokalemia, hypoxemia, postoperative TOF with severe PR) and correct the conditions, if possible.

4. Chronic therapy
   a. Conservative management may be safe for asymptomatic patients with repetitive nonsustained VT in the absence of any evidence of ventricular dysfunction.
   b. Antiarrhythmic drug treatment

Complete pharmacologic suppression may not be achieved without serious complications. Therefore, controlling the rate to an asymptomatic level may be adequate. A combination of 24-hour Holter monitoring and treadmill exercise testing is the best noninvasive means of evaluating drug effectiveness.

   1) Virtually all classes of antiarrhythmic agents have been used for various types of VT, including all class I and III drugs, with varying levels of success. Tables A.4 and A.5 in Appendix A provide a quick review of antiarrhythmic drugs.
   2) Beta-blockers may be very effective for patients who have no underlying heart disease and those who have exercise-provokable monomorphic VT from the RVOT left ventricular outflow tract (LVOT). Beta-blockers have fewer side effects than most other antiarrhythmic agents.
   3) In patients with reduced LV function, digitalis and afterload reducer may be beneficial (to improve LV function).
   c. Patients with LQTS are treated with beta-blockers, which alleviate symptoms in 75% to 80%. An implantable cardioverter–defibrillator (ICD) is sometimes recommended as initial therapy.
   d. Catheter ablation. Ablation is most successful in patients with structurally normal hearts with focal origin of the tachycardia. Patients with underlying heart disease are more likely to have reentry circuits, and they have lower effectiveness than those with focal origin of VT.
   e. ICD has become the established standard for treating many, if not most, forms of VT, which are potentially lethal. ICDs that can be used without thoracotomy are gaining experience in the young.

Ventricular Arrhythmias in Children with Normal Hearts

Although recurrent sustained VT usually signals organic cause of the arrhythmia, some VTs are seen in healthy adolescents and young adults with structurally and functionally normal hearts. The prognosis is good. So-called RVOT VT and RBBB VT are examples of this group of VT.

1. **RVOT VT.** This special form of VT seen in children with structurally and functionally normal hearts originates from the RV conal septum and thus has inferior QRS axis

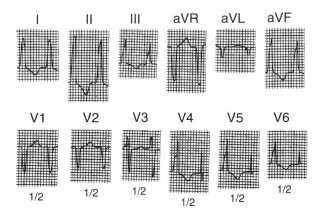

Fig. 24.9 Tracing from a 4-year-old girl who is asymptomatic even while having ventricular tachycardia (VT). The child is on atenolol. In this figure, P waves are not identifiable in front of each QRS complex. The QRS duration is wide (0.10 sec), and ventricular tachycardia is present with the ventricular rate of 160 beats/min. The QRS complexes have left bundle branch block morphology, indicating the right ventricle (RV) as the ectopic focus, and the axis of VT is directed inferiorly. Spontaneous temporary interruption of VT occurred while recording the V4, V5, and V6 leads.

and LBBB morphology (Fig. 24.9). This is usually benign tachycardia. It may manifest as PVCs or short runs or salvos of VT, but many children are asymptomatic or minimally symptomatic. Exercise stress may not completely abolish the tachycardia. Beta-blockers are sufficient for treatment. Verapamil and other agents may also prove to be effective. Radiofrequency ablation can be curative.

2. **RBBB VT (Belhassen's tachycardia).** It appears to arise from the septal surface of the LV and is less common than RVOT VT. It is characterized by RBBB morphology and superior QRS axis. They may be calcium channel dependent and respond to slow IV push of verapamil or adenosine. Long-term treatment with verapamil can prevent recurrences. When refractory to medical therapy, radiofrequency ablation or surgery is effective. The long-term outcome is excellent.

Ventricular Fibrillation
Description

Ventricular fibrillation is rare in the pediatric population. It is characterized by bizarre QRS complexes of varying sizes and configurations. The rate is rapid and irregular (see Fig. 24.6). The arrhythmia is maintained by multiple reentrant circuits because portions of the myocardium are depolarizing constantly.

Causes

All the causes listed for VT can cause VF. Predisposing factors include electrolyte abnormalities, proarrhythmic medications, increased sympathetic activities or catecholamine infusion, hypoxia, or ischemia. Certain CHD (pre- and postoperative) and hereditary conditions are possible causes.

Abrupt VF after blunt chest wall trauma that typically occurs in young participants in sports (notably, ice hockey, lacrosse, baseball, and softball) can cause the arrhythmia (called commotio cordis).

Significance

Ventricular fibrillation usually is a degeneration of VT and is terminal arrhythmia because it results in ineffective circulation. Immediate resuscitation must be provided.

Management

Resuscitation from VF is successful if performed in a timely fashion; the longer the myocardium is allowed to fibrillate, the more difficult is conversion to a sinus rhythm. Electric shocks (delivered in an asynchronous fashion) are aimed at depolarizing the myocardium to terminate fibrillating rhythm and allow an intrinsic cardiac pacemaker to resume control.

1. Acute care
   a. In a witnessed cardiac arrest, immediate cardiac and pulmonary resuscitation (CPR); providing CAB (compressions, airway and breathing); airway management with 100% oxygen; and rhythm monitoring is essential.
   b. Defibrillation with 2, 4, 6, and 8 joule/kg if needed
   c. Administration of epinephrine via the IV or intraosseous (IO) route, 0.01 mg/kg (1:10,000 solution, 0.1 mL/kg) or via endotracheal tube 0.1 mg/kg (1:1000 solution, 0.1 mL/kg)
   d. One should identify and treat causes, including metabolic environment (hypoxia, acidosis).
   e. One of the following antiarrhythmic agents may be used:
      1) Amiodarone 5 mg/kg bolus, IV/IO
      2) Lidocaine 1 mg/kg, IV, IO, or endotracheal
      3) Magnesium sulfate 25 to 50 mg/kg, IV/IO (not to exceed 2 g) for torsade de pointes or hypomagnesemia
2. A child with susceptibility to VF and those resuscitated from the arrhythmia should have a comprehensive pediatric electrophysiology evaluation.

3. An ICD is often indicated in patients who survive VF. This device can be deployed through epicardial patch or transvenous lead placement.

Long QT Syndrome

Long QT syndrome is a genetic disorder of myocardial repolarization characterized by a prolonged QT interval on the ECG and ventricular arrhythmias, usually torsade de pointes, that may result in sudden death. There are four groups of patients with congenital types of LQTS.

1. Jervell and Lange-Nielsen (1957) first described families in Norway in which a long QT interval on the ECG was associated with congenital deafness, syncopal spells, and a family history of sudden death. This syndrome is transmitted in an autosomal recessive manner.
2. Romano-Ward (RW) syndrome, reported independently by Romano and colleagues in Italy (1963) and Ward in Ireland (1964), has all the features of Jervell and Lange-Nielsen (JLN) syndrome but without deafness. It is much more common than JLN syndrome.
3. Unlike JLN syndrome, which is inherited in an autosomal recessive pattern, RW syndrome transmits in an autosomal dominant mode, but a significant number of individuals with this syndrome appear to represent sporadic cases, with a negative family history of the syndrome.
4. Two new syndromes, Anderson-Tawil syndrome and Timothy syndrome, have been added recently (Table 24.2). Anderson-Tawil syndrome is sometimes designated as LQT7, in which the QU interval, rather than QT interval, is prolonged, along with muscle weakness (periodic paralysis), ventricular arrhythmias, and developmental abnormalities. Timothy syndrome is associated with webbed fingers and toes and long QT measurement.

TABLE 24.2   Congenital Causes of Long QT Syndrome

Molecular Genotype	Frequency (%)	Chromosomes Involved	Mutant Genes	Defective Ionic Channel
Romano-Ward Syndrome (Autosomal Dominant) with Normal Hearing				
LQT1	42	11p15.5	KCNQ1/KVLQT1	Potassium channel (I_{Ks})
LQT2	45	7q35-36	KCNH2/HERG	Potassium channel (I_{Kr})
LQT3	8	3p21-24	SCN5A	Sodium channel (I_{Na})
LQT4	?	4q25-27	AKNB	Na/Ca exchanger (I_{Na-Ca})
LQT5	3	21q22.2-22.2	KCNE1/mink	Potassium channel (I_{Ks})
LQT6	2	21q22.2-22.2	KCNE2/MiRP1	Potassium channel (I_{Ks})
Jervell and Lange-Nielsen Syndrome (Autosomal Recessive) with Deafness				
JLN1	80	11p15.5	KCNQ1/KVLQT1	Potassium channel (I_{Ks})
JLN2	20	21q22.1-22.2	KCNE1/mink	Potassium channel (I_{Ks})
Anderson-Tawil Syndrome (Autosomal Dominant)				
ATS1	50	17q23	KCNJ2	Inward rectifier potassium channel (I_{K1})
Timothy Syndrome (Sporadic)				
TS1	?	1q42-q43	CACNA1C	Cardiac L-type calcium channel ($I_{ca.L}$)

Modified from Collins KK, van Hare GF: Advances in congenital long QT syndrome, *Curr Opin Pediatr* 18:497–502, 2006.

Causes

The QT prolongation may be congenital or acquired.

1. Congenital LQTS is a heterogeneous disorder. LQTS is caused by mutations of cardiac ion channel genes. Recent advances in molecular biology have revealed that ion channels that govern the electrical activity of the heart are defective in congenital LQTS. Meanwhile, 15 genetic mutations have been identified responsible for LQTS; some of them are presented in Table 24.2. Because there is rapid progression in identifying genetic abnormalities and evolving understanding of various genetic defects, Table 24.2 will be an incomplete list of molecular genotypes, frequency, chromosomes involved, mutant genes, and defective ionic channels according to subtypes of congenital LQTS. Readers may refer to the publication by Schwartz et al (2012) for additional information on the genetics of LQTS. In the remainder of the discussion, emphasis is placed on the congenital form of LQTS.

2. Acquired prolongation of the QT interval can be caused by a number of drugs, electrolyte disturbances, and other underlying medical conditions (see Box 24.1). In the acquired type of LQTS, a similar ionic mechanism may be involved as is observed in congenital LQTS. Individuals who manifest acquired LQTS are believed to be genetically predisposed to the condition.

Pathophysiology

A prolonged QT interval on the ECG represents prolonged recovery from electrical excitation, which contributes to an increased likelihood of dispersion of refractoriness with some parts of myocardium remaining refractory to subsequent depolarization. Consequently, the wave of excitation may pursue a distinctive pathway around a focal point in the myocardium (circus reentry rhythm), leading to VT.

Clinical Manifestations

1. The family history is positive in about 60% of patients, and deafness is present in 5% of patients with the syndrome.

2. Presenting symptoms may be syncope (26%), seizure (10%), cardiac arrest (9%), presyncope, or palpitation (6%). The majority of these symptoms occur during exercise or with emotion. Symptoms of LQTS are related to ventricular arrhythmias. The first symptom of the syndrome appears usually in the first decade or by the end of the second decade of life. The first manifestation may be cardiac arrest.

3. Syncope occurs in the setting of intense adrenergic arousal, intense emotion, and during or after rigorous exercise. Swimming appears to be a particular trigger among exercises. Abrupt auditory signals such as a loud doorbell, alarm clock, telephone, or security alarm can trigger symptoms.

4. The ECG shows the following:
   a. A prolonged QT interval with a corrected QT interval (QTc) usually longer than 0.46 second (Fig. 24.10). The upper limit of normal is 0.44 second.
   b. Abnormal T-wave morphology (bifid, diphasic, or notched) is frequent.
   c. Bradycardia (20%), second-degree AV block, multiform PVCs, and monomorphic or polymorphic VT (10% to 20%) may be present.

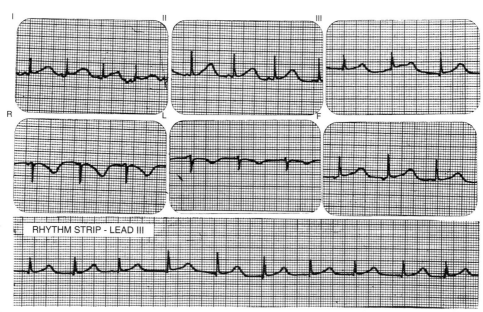

Fig. 24.10 Electrocardiogram from a patient with Romano-Ward syndrome at age 6 years demonstrates the longest QTc interval (0.56 sec). The precordial leads are not shown. Two negative P waves in aVF suggest a junctional mechanism. This child received 10 mg of propranolol four times a day until the age of 13 years, with complete cessation of syncopal attacks. There were seven cases of sudden death associated with syncopal attacks on the maternal side of the family. His mother (age 27 years) and sister (age 5 years) had moderate prolongation of QTc interval but experienced no syncopal attacks.

5. Echocardiographic studies usually show a structurally and functionally normal heart.

Diagnosis

Correct diagnosis and treatment are important to prevent sudden death. However, the diagnosis of this disease, which has a poor prognosis, should not be made lightly because it implies a lifelong commitment to treatment.

Any child who has a prolonged QTc 0.46 second or longer or a compelling borderline QTc interval with symptoms, family history, or unusual T waves (T wave alternans or notched T waves) should be carefully evaluated.

1. Accurate measurement of the QTc interval is necessary for the diagnosis of LQTS. A 12-lead ECG is the current screening tool for identification of LQTS.
   a. Lead II is the preferred lead to measure the QT interval because a q wave is usually present in this lead, but precordial leads (V1, V3, or V5) may also be used because they provide better definition of T waves.
   b. The QTc interval is calculated by using Bazett's formula (see Chapter 3). The QTc interval represents the QT interval normalized for a heart rate of 60 beats/min.
   c. The presence of sinus arrhythmia creates problems in measuring accurate and reliable QTc interval because the QTc interval varies with the R-R interval. It has been recommended that the longest QTc interval following the shortest R-R interval be used. By this method, it is rare to have LQTS with a QTc less than 0.46 ms (Martin et al, 1995). This recommendation is still controversial. Bazett's formula is reliable only for the steady state, but sinus arrhythmia is not steady state. In addition, there is a phenomenon called QT hysteresis in which the QT interval adapts slowly to changing heart rate, and certainly not in one beat. Therefore, it may be worthwhile repeating the measurement of the QTc interval in a tracing that does not have marked sinus arrhythmia.
   d. In patients with a prolonged QRS duration (as seen in bundle branch block), the QT interval may be prolonged secondary to the lengthening of the QRS duration. In such cases, the JT interval may be a more sensitive predictor of repolarization abnormalities than the QTc interval. The JT interval is measured from the J point (the junction of the S wave and the ST segment) to the end of the T wave. Rate correction is accomplished by the use of Bazett's formula (Berul et al, 1994). Normal JTc interval (mean ± standard deviation) is 0.32 ± 0.02 second with the upper limit of normal 0.34 second in children and adolescents.
2. The diagnosis of LQTS is clear-cut when there is a marked prolongation of the QTc interval with positive family history of the syndrome. However, many cases are at borderline, making it difficult to make or reject the diagnosis. Schwartz et al refined the diagnostic criteria in 1993 and re-refined them recently in 2011. A point system is used to distinguish the likelihood of a patient having disease. The criteria take into account the ECG findings, clinical history, and family history and rank the findings by points based on the "importance" of the findings (Table 24.3). According to these criteria, the scoring of the probability of LQTS is done as follows.
   ≤1 point = low probability of LQTS
   1.5 to 3 points = intermediate probability of LQTS
   ≥3.5 points = high probability of LQTS
3. Initial diagnostic strategy. Initially, the following five steps are considered in making the diagnosis of LQTS.
   a. History of presyncope, syncope, seizure, or palpitation and family history are carefully examined.
   b. Causes of acquired LQTS are excluded (see Box 24.1).
   c. ECGs are examined for the QTc interval and morphology of the T waves. ECGs are also obtained from immediate family members.
   d. Exercise testing. Some centers routinely perform exercise testing. In most normal children and young adults, the QT interval shortens with exercise with increasing heart rate. However, in patients with LQTS, the QT interval may fail to shorten or may lengthen at higher heart rates and with exertion. A lack of appropriate shortening of the QTc duration as well as abnormal T-wave morphology are most often seen in patients with LQTS. The QTc of 480 msec or greater at 4 minutes of recovery after the exercise stress may be significant.
   e. The LQTS score is calculated (see Table 24.3), and the diagnostic possibility is graded as described earlier.

TABLE 24.3 Schwartz's Updated Diagnostic Criteria for Long QT Syndrome

ECG Findings[a]	
A. QTc interval (msec)	
>480	3
460–470	2
450–459	1
B. QTc ≥4809 ms at 4 min of recovery from exercise stress test	1
C. Torsades de pointes	2
D. T-wave alternans	1
E. Notched T waves in three leads	1
F. Low heart rate for age (<second percentile)	0.5
Clinical History	
A. Syncope	
With stress	2
Without stress	1
B. Congenital deafness	0.5
Family History	
A. Family members with definite LQTS	1
B. Unexplained sudden cardiac death younger than 30 among immediate family members	0.5

[a]In the absence of medications or disorders known to prolong the QTc interval.

ECG, Electrocardiogram; *LQTS*, long QT syndrome.
Modified from Schwartz PJ, Crotti L, Insolia R: Long QT syndrome: from genetics to management, *Circ Arrhythm Electrophysiol* 5:868–877, 2012.

e. Patients with an LQTS score of 3.5 are considered to have LQTS, but an LQTS score of 1 or less is excluded from the diagnosis. Patients with an LQTS score of 2 or 3 are followed up for possible LQTS.

4. For borderline cases, some centers carry out additional testing, such as Holter monitoring, pharmacologic test, or electrophysiology study. However, the interpretation and significance of these tests are controversial.

5. Because a large number of patients may be incorrectly given the clinical diagnosis of LQTS by their cardiologists, it appears to be the smart approach to recommend molecular screening for those patients with 1.5 to 3 points on the Schwartz score. The commercially available genetic testing can identify the most common gene mutations. The genetic testing has limitations, though. It is important to realize that the testing can identify a particular mutation, but it cannot rule out LQTS; a negative genetic test result does not rule out LQTS.

Management

1. The known risk factors should be considered when making a treatment plan for the congenital type of LQTS.
   a. Known risk factors for sudden death include:
      1) Bradycardia for age (from sinus bradycardia, junctional escape rhythm, or second-degree AV block)
      2) An extremely long QTc interval (>0.55 sec)
      3) Symptoms at presentation (syncope, seizure, cardiac arrest)
      4) Young age at presentation (< 1 month)
      5) Documented torsades de pointes or VF
   b. T-wave alternation (major changes in T-wave morphology) is a relative risk factor.
   c. Noncompliance with medication is an important risk factor for sudden death.

2. General measures
   a. Physicians should be aware of the conditions and medications that prolong the QT interval (see Box 24.1). Physicians should avoid prescribing QT prolonging medications (and discontinue the medications if possible). A list of drugs that are known to prolong the QT interval (see Box 24.1) along with the websites for it (www.qtdrugs.org) should be given to the parents.
   b. Catecholamines and sympathomimetic drugs should also be avoided if possible because they can potentially trigger torsade de pointes in patients with LQTS.
   c. No competitive sports policy applies. This is particularly important in patients with LQT1. Physicians should also advise against swimming without supervision.
   d. Alarm clocks and bedside telephones should be removed because they are known triggers of VT in patients with LQTS.
   e. The patients and the parents should be educated about the importance of being compliant with their medication because noncompliance can result in sudden death.

3. Treatment of congenital LQTS

For congenital LQTS, the initial treatment is aimed at interrupting sympathetic input to the myocardium with beta-blockers. An ICD may be needed in some patients who continue to have symptoms while taking beta-blockers. Left cardiac sympathetic denervation is less popular because of the availability of other options, such as pacing and ICD.

   a. **Beta-blockers.** The present therapy of choice is treatment with beta-blockers. The protective effect of beta-blockers is related to their ability to reduce both syncope and sudden cardiac death. Two most effective beta-blockers are propranolol and nadolol. Propranolol (at 2–3 mg/kg/day) is the most widely used drug. Sometimes the dose is reached 4 mg/kg and even higher in the more malignant cases. Nadolol (1–1.5 mg/kg/day) is also used often because its longer half-life allows twice-a-day administration. Atenolol and metoprolol appear to be less effective than nadolol. Patients with severe JLN or Timothy syndrome are often not adequately protected by beta-blockers and require additional protection.

Whether to start beta-blockers on asymptomatic children with QTc prolongation has been controversial. Any patients who score 3.5 or greater on the Schwartz diagnostic criteria should be treated regardless of symptoms. However, it may be prudent to follow asymptomatic children with the borderline scores. In addition, beta-blocker treatment may be dangerous to some patients with the syndrome because treatment tends to produce bradycardia, a known risk factor for sudden death.

Definitive treatment of asymptomatic patients with congenital LQTS has been suggested by Schwartz (1997) in the following circumstances: (1) newborns and infants, (2) patients with sensorineural hearing loss, (3) affected siblings with LQTS and sudden cardiac death, (4) extremely long QTc (>0.60 sec) or T-wave alternans, and (5) to prevent family or patient anxiety.

   b. **Left cardiac sympathetic denervation (LCSD).** LCSD is another method to reduce cardiac events in patients who continue to have symptoms by reducing sympathetic discharge. LCSD requires removal of the first 3 to 4 thoracic ganglia. The cephalic portion of the left stellate ganglion is left intact to avoid the Horner syndrome. Whenever syncopal episodes recur despite full-dose beta-blockers therapy, LCSD should be considered and implemented without hesitation. However, physicians should also provide the pros and cons of LCSD versus ICD implant; it may carry medico legal consequences.

   c. **ICD.** Implantation of an ICD appears to be the most effective therapy for high-risk patients. The Schwartz group recommend ICD implantation in the following situations: (1) all those who survived a cardiac arrest on therapy; (2) most of those who survived a cardiac arrest off therapy, except those with a reversible or preventable cause; (3) those with syncope despite a full dose of beta-blockers therapy, whenever the option of LCSD is either not available or discarded after discussion with the patients; (4) all patients with syncope, despite a full dose of beta-blockers and LCSD; and (5) exceptionally, rare asymptomatic patients with QTc greater than 550 msec who also manifest signs of high electric instability (e.g., T-wave alternans) or other evidence of being at high risk (e.g., long sinus pauses followed by abnormal T-wave morphologies) despite beta-blockers and LCSD.

   d. Targeted pharmacologic therapy has reported some success. The sodium channel blocker mexiletine was used in patients with mutation in the sodium channel gene *SCN5A (LQT3)* with significant shortening of the QTc. In patients with LQT2 (with potassium channel abnormalities), potassium supplementation in combination with spironolactone was associated with a significant reduction in QTc and some improvement in T-wave morphology.

   f. "Gene-specific" approach. Gene or gene-specific therapy, or more accurately, mutation specific therapy has been of special interest over the recent years.

Prognosis

Long QT syndrome is a serious disease, and treatment is at best only partially effective. The prognosis is very poor in untreated patients, with an annual mortality rate as high as 20% and 10-year mortality rate of 50%. Beta-blockers may reduce mortality to some extent, but they do not completely protect patients from sudden death. ICDs appear promising in improving prognosis.

Short QT Syndrome

Short QT syndrome (SQTS) is a cardiac channelopathy associated with a predisposition to AF and sudden cardiac death, first described by Gassak et al in 2000. Mutations in the *KCNH2, KCNJ2, and KCNQ1* genes appear to be the cause of SQTS. It is transmitted in an autosomal dominant manner. It is characterized by a short QTc (usually ≤360 ms) with tall, symmetric, peaked T waves on the ECG. These patients present with sudden death; symptoms of palpitation, dizziness, or syncope; and sometimes, paroxysmal AF. Most patients have easily inducible VF. Most patients have a family history of sudden death. The cause of death is believed to be VF. Although it usually occurs in the adult (median age, 30 years), a sudden cardiac death was also observed in early infancy. Some infants and neonates present with AF and a slow ventricular response; it may present in utero as persistent bradycardia.

Recently, diagnostic criteria for SQTS were proposed by Gollob et al (2011) (Table 24.4). It is based on a point system similar to Schwartz's criteria for LQTS. According to these criteria, the scoring of the probability of SQTS is done as follows.

≤2 point = low probability of SQTS

3 points = intermediate probability of SQTS

≥4 points = high probability of SQTS

The therapy of choice is an ICD. Recent studies suggest that use of certain antiarrhythmic agents, such as quinidine,

TABLE 24.4 Short QT Syndrome Diagnostic Criteria

ECG Findings	
A. QTc interval (msec)	
<370	1
<350	2
<330	3
B. J point to T peak interval <120 msec	1
Clinical History	
Sudden cardiac arrest	2
Polymorphic VT or VF	2
Unexplained syncope	1
Atrial fibrillation	1
Family History	
First- and second-degree relative with SQTSC	2
First- and second-degree relative with sudden death	1
Sudden infant death syndrome	1
Genotype	
Genotype positive	2
Mutation of undetermined significance in a culprit gene	1

ECG, Electrocardiogram; *SQTS,* short QT syndrome; *VF,* ventricular fibrillation; *VT,* ventricular tachycardia.
Modified from Gollob M, Redpath C, Roberts J: The short QT syndrome: proposed diagnostic criteria, *J Am Coll Cardiol* 57(7):802–812, 2011.

propafenone, or sotalol, may be of benefit, may help prolong the QT interval, and may decrease the potential for VF.

Brugada Syndrome

This inherited arrhythmogenic disorder with a high risk of sudden cardiac death occurring during sleep, resulting from ventricular tachyarrhythmias, appears to be inherited as an autosomal dominant pattern. Mutations in the sodium channel (SCN5A) appear to be the cause of the condition, at least in 20% of affected patients. It is primarily a disease of men, seen most commonly in Southeast Asian men with a reported mean age at sudden death of 40 years. However, this syndrome has been demonstrated in children and infants. No male preponderance is observed in children, raising a possibility of high levels of androgens in the occurrence of the fatal event.

The ECG is abnormal but without demonstrable structural abnormalities of the heart. The ECG typically shows cove-type ST-segment elevation (type 1 Brugada ECG pattern) or saddle-back ST segment elevation (type 2 Brugada ECG pattern) with J-point elevation followed by a negative T wave in the right precordial leads (V1–V3) with or without an RBBB appearance. Only a type 1 ECG pattern can be used to confirm the diagnosis of Brugada syndrome because type 2 is frequently seen in persons without the disease. This so-called type-1 ECG pattern may be present either spontaneously or after provocation with ajmaline or flecainide. The

PR interval is frequently prolonged. An estimated 10% to 20% of the patients also have AF. SVT is also frequent. Fever is an important precipitating factor of syncope, including one that develops after vaccination. The patient may present with complaints of syncope or palpitations. Most syncope takes place at rest (90%). There may be a family history of sudden death. Cardiac examination is usually normal.

Diagnosis is suspected based on the ECG appearance, which may not always be present. It can be provoked with ajmaline, flecainide, or procainamide (class 1 sodium channel blockers). The condition can carry a poor prognosis, particularly in those who are symptomatic (i.e., at least a 10% death rate per year). ICDs are standard practice for all symptomatic patients (either aborted cardiac arrest or arrhythmic syncope) to prevent sudden cardiac death. Beta-blockers do not appear to reduce the risk of death in these patients. Hydroquinidine has been shown to be a good alternative to ICD implantation in adult patients and appears to be effective in preventing syncope in children as well (Probst et al, 2007).

Disturbances of Atrioventricular Conduction

Atrioventricular (AV) block is a disturbance in conduction between the normal sinus impulse and the eventual ventricular response. The block is assigned to one of three classes, depending on the severity of the conduction disturbance. First-degree AV block is a simple prolongation of the PR interval, but all P waves are conducted to the ventricle. In second-degree AV block, some atrial impulses are not conducted into the ventricle. In third-degree AV block (or complete heart block), none of the atrial impulses is conducted into the ventricle (Fig. 25.1). Holter monitoring often reveals patterns not apparent in the relatively short electrocardiogram.

FIRST-DEGREE ATRIOVENTRICULAR BLOCK

Description

The PR interval is prolonged beyond the upper limits of normal for the patient's age and heart rate (see Table 3.2 and Fig. 25.1). The PR interval includes the time required for depolarization of the atrial myocardium (PA interval), the delay of conduction in the AV node (AH interval), conduction through the bundle of His, and the time of onset of ventricular depolarization (HV interval).

Causes

First-degree AV block can appear in otherwise healthy children and young adults, particularly in athletes, mediated through excessive parasympathetic tone. Other causes include congenital heart diseases (CHDs) (e.g., endocardial cushion defect, atrial septal defect [ASD], Ebstein's anomaly), infectious disease, inflammatory conditions (rheumatic fever), cardiac surgery, and certain drugs (e.g., digitalis, calcium channel blockers).

Significance

Slow intraatrial or AV nodal conjunction is almost always the mechanism for first-degree AV block. First-degree AV block

does not produce hemodynamic disturbance. Exercise, both recreational and during stress testing, induces parasympathetic withdrawal, resulting in normalization of AV conduction and the PR interval. The PR interval can be very long, but in the absence of heart disease, it usually does not progress.

Management

No treatment is indicated except when the block is caused by drugs.

SECOND-DEGREE ATRIOVENTRICULAR BLOCK

Some, but not all, P waves are followed by QRS complex (dropped beats). There are three types: Mobitz type I (Wenckebach phenomenon), Mobitz type II, and high-grade (or advanced) second-degree AV block.

Mobitz Type I (Wenckebach)
Description

The PR interval becomes progressively prolonged until one QRS complex is dropped completely (see Fig. 25.1).

Causes

Mobitz type I AV block appears in otherwise healthy children. Other causes include myocarditis, cardiomyopathy, myocardial infarction, CHD, cardiac surgery, and digitalis toxicity.

Significance

The block is at the level of the AV node (with prolonged AH interval). It usually does not progress to complete heart block. It occurs in individuals with vagal dominance.

Management

The underlying causes are treated.

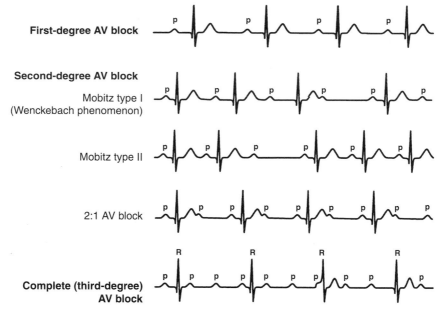

Fig. 25.1 Atrioventricular (AV) block. (From Park MK, Guntheroth WG: *How to Read Pediatric ECGs*, ed 4, Philadelphia, 2006, Mosby.)

Mobitz Type II

Description

The AV conduction is "all or none." AV conduction is either normal or completely blocked (see Fig. 25.1).

Causes

Causes are the same as for Mobitz type I.

Significance

The block usually occurs below the AV node (at the level of the bundle of His). It is more serious than type I block because it may progress to complete heart block, resulting in Stokes-Adams attack.

Management

The underlying causes are treated. Prophylactic pacemaker therapy may be indicated.

Two-to-One (or Higher) Atrioventricular Block

Description

A QRS complex follows every second, third, or fourth P wave, resulting in two-to-one, three-to-one, or four-to-one AV block (see Fig. 25.1). When two or more consecutive P waves are nonconducted, the rhythm is called advanced or high-grade second-degree AV block. In contrast to third-degree complete AV block, some P waves continue to be conducted to the ventricle, and the PR interval of conducted beats is constant.

Causes

Causes are similar to those of other second-degree AV blocks.

Significance

The block is usually at the bundle of His, alone or in combination with the AV nodal block. It may progress to complete heart block. Higher grade second-degree AV block should always be regarded as abnormal. The implications of high-grade AV block appear to be similar to those of complete AV block.

Management

The underlying causes are treated. Electrophysiologic studies may be necessary to determine the level of the block. Symptomatic second-degree AV block, although uncommon, can be acutely treated with atropine, isoproterenol, and temporary pacing. Pacemaker therapy is indicated for symptomatic advanced second-degree AV block.

THIRD-DEGREE ATRIOVENTRICULAR BLOCK (COMPLETE HEART BLOCK)

Description

In third-degree AV block, atrial and ventricular activities are entirely independent of each other (see Fig. 25.1).

1. The P waves are regular (regular PP interval), with a rate comparable to the normal heart rate for the patient's age. The QRS complexes also are regular (regular R-R interval), with a rate much slower than the P rate.
2. In congenital complete heart block (and some acquired types), the duration of the QRS complex is normal because the pacemaker for the ventricular complex is at a level higher than the bifurcation of the bundle of His. The ventricular rate is faster (50–80 beats/min) than that in the acquired type, and the ventricular rate is somewhat variable in response to varying physiologic conditions.
3. In surgically induced (and in some acquired) complete heart block, the QRS duration is prolonged because the pacemaker for the ventricular complex is at a level below

the bifurcation of the bundle of His. The ventricular rate is in the range of 40 to 50 beats/min (idioventricular rhythm), and the ventricular rate is relatively fixed.

Causes

Congenital Type. In the absence of CHD, 60% to 90% of cases of congenital heart block are caused by neonatal lupus erythematosus. Maternal antibodies to the intracellular ribonucleoproteins Ro (SS-A) and La (SS-B) for autoimmune connective diseases cross the placenta to the fetus, causing the heart block. These maternal IgG antibodies may persist in the newborn until 9 months of age (Zuppa et al, 2017). This has the potential of late development of complete heart block at several months of age. In 25% to 33%, it is associated with CHDs, most commonly with L-transposition of the great arteries, single ventricle, or polysplenia syndrome. Neonatal myocarditis and several genetic disorders such as familial ASD and Kearns-Sayre syndrome have been identified.

Acquired Type. Cardiac surgery is the most common cause of acquired complete heart block in children. Other rare causes include severe myocarditis, Lyme carditis, acute rheumatic fever, mumps, diphtheria, cardiomyopathies, tumors in the conduction system, myocardial infarction, and overdoses of certain drugs. These causes produce either temporary or permanent heart block.

Significance

1. Complete heart block can be diagnosed by fetal bradycardia during fetal echocardiographic study between 18 and 28 weeks of gestation. Complications in utero may include hydrops fetalis, myocarditis, and fetal death.
2. Congestive heart failure (CHF) may develop in infancy, particularly when there are associated CHDs.
3. About 40% of congenital heart blocks do not present until childhood (mean age, 5–6 years). Those who survive infancy are usually asymptomatic and achieve normal growth and development for 5 to 10 years. Presenting symptoms may include reduced exercise tolerance, presyncope, syncope, or slow pulse detected during routine examination. Chest radiography may show cardiomegaly (from large stroke volume needed to compensate for the slow heart rate).
4. Syncopal attacks (Stokes-Adams attacks) may occur with a heart rate below 40 to 45 beats/min. A sudden onset of acquired heart block may result in death unless treatment maintains the heart rate in the acceptable range.

Management

1. When detected in utero, steroid therapy may be applied if associated with anti-Ro/SSA and anti-La/SSB.
2. Atropine or isoproterenol is indicated in symptomatic children and adults until temporary ventricular pacing is secured.
3. A temporary transvenous or epicardial ventricular pacemaker is indicated in patients with heart block, or it may be given prophylactically in patients who might develop heart block.
4. No treatment is required for children with asymptomatic congenital complete heart block with acceptable rate, narrow QRS complex, and normal ventricular function. Most of these patients will ultimately require pacemaker placement.
5. Permanent pacemaker therapy is indicated under the following situations:
   a. If the patient is symptomatic or develops CHF. Dizziness or lightheadedness may be an early warning sign of the need for a pacemaker.
   b. If an infant has a ventricular rate below 50 to 55 beats/min or if an infant has a CHD with a ventricular rate below 70 beats/min
   c. If the patient has a wide QRS escape rhythm, complex ventricular ectopy, or ventricular dysfunction
   d. In patients with surgically induced heart block that is not expected to resolve or persists at least 7 days after cardiac surgery
6. A variety of problems may arise after a pacemaker is placed in children. Stress placed on the lead system by the linear growth of the child, fracture of the lead system in a physically active child, electrode malfunction (scarring of the myocardium around the electrode, especially in infants), and the limited life span of the pulse generator require follow-up of children with artificial pacemakers

ATRIOVENTRICULAR DISSOCIATION

Atrioventricular dissociation should not be confused with third-degree AV block. AV dissociation results from a marked slowing of the sinus node or atrial bradycardia or acceleration of the AV node. Whereas in AV dissociation, the atrial rate is slower than the ventricular rate, in complete heart block, the ventricular rate is usually slower than the atrial rate. In AV dissociation, an atrial impulse may conduct to the AV node if it comes at the right time (Fig. 25.2). The conducted beat can be recognized by its relative prematurity.

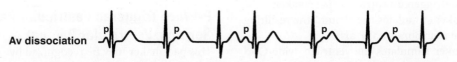

Av dissociation

Fig. 25.2 Diagram of atrioventricular (AV) dissociation owing to either marked slowing of the sinus node or acceleration of the AV node. The fourth complex is conducted, changing the rhythm (called "interference"). All of the other complexes originate in the AV node, where there is higher automaticity than usual.

Cardiac Pacemakers and Implantable Cardioverter–Defibrillators in Children

A pacemaker is a device that delivers battery-supplied electrical stimuli over leads to electrodes that are in contact with the heart. It primarily treats bradycardia. An implantable cardioverter–defibrillator (ICD) is a multiprogrammable antiarrhythmic device for treating ventricular tachycardia (VT) and ventricular fibrillation (VF). ICDs also possess pacemaking capability to treat bradycardia. The electrical leads are placed either directly over the epicardium or inserted transvenously into the cardiac chambers. Electronic circuitry regulates the timing and characteristics of the stimuli. The power source is usually a lithium–iodine battery.

Physicians encounter an increasing number of children with either temporary or permanent pacemakers. Basic knowledge about the pacemaker and the pacemaker rhythm strip is essential in taking care of these children. This chapter presents examples of electrocardiography (ECG) rhythm strips from children with various types of pacemakers and elementary information regarding pacemaker and ICD therapy in children.

ELECTROCARDIOGRAMS OF ARTIFICIAL CARDIAC PACEMAKERS

The need to recognize the rhythm strips of artificial pacemakers has increased in recent years, especially in intensive care and emergency department settings. The position and number of the pacemaker spikes on the ECG rhythm strip are used to recognize different types of pacemakers. Thus, a pacemaker may be classified as a ventricular pacemaker, atrial pacemaker, or P wave–triggered ventricular pacemaker.

1. When the pacemaker stimulates the atrium, the resulting P wave demonstrates an abnormal P axis.
2. When the pacemaker stimulates the ventricle, wide QRS complexes result.
3. The ventricle that is stimulated (or the ventricle on which the pacemaker electrode is placed) can be identified by the

morphology of the QRS complexes. With the pacing electrode on the right ventricle, the QRS complex resembles a left bundle branch block (LBBB) pattern; with the pacemaker placed on the left ventricle, a right bundle branch block (RBBB) pattern results.

Ventricular Pacemaker (Ventricular Sensing and Pacing)

This mode of pacing is recognized by vertical pacemaker spikes that initiate ventricular depolarization with wide QRS complexes (Fig. 26.1A). The electronic spike has no fixed relationship with atrial activity (P wave). The pacemaker rate may be fixed (as in Fig. 26.1A), or it may be on a demand (or standby) mode in which the pacemaker fires only after a long pause between the patient's own ventricular beats.

Atrial Pacemaker (Atrial Sensing and Pacing)

The atrial pacemaker is recognized by a pacemaker spike followed by an atrial complex; when atrioventricular (AV) conduction is normal, a QRS complex of normal duration follows (see Fig. 26.1B). This type of pacemaker is indicated in patients with sinus node dysfunction with bradycardia. When the patient has high-degree or complete AV block in addition to sinus node dysfunction, an additional ventricular pacemaker may be required (AV sequential pacemaker, not illustrated in Fig. 26.1). The AV sequential pacemaker is recognized by two sets of electronic spikes—one before the P wave, and another before the wide QRS complex.

P-Wave Triggered Ventricular Pacemaker (Atrial Sensing, Ventricular Pacing)

This pacemaker may be recognized by pacemaker spikes that follow the patient's own P waves at regular PR intervals and with wide QRS complexes (see Fig. 26.1C). The patient's own P waves are sensed and trigger a ventricular pacemaker after

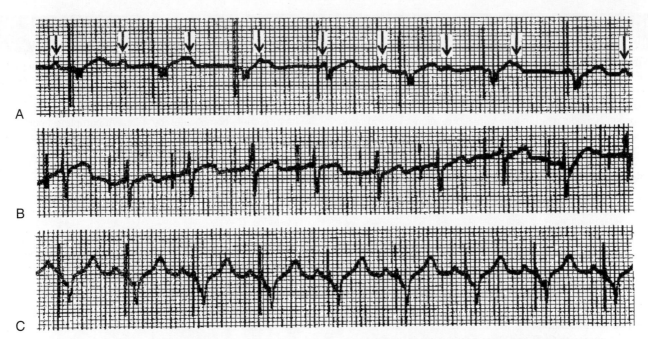

Fig. 26.1 Examples of some artificial pacemakers. **A,** Fixed-rate ventricular pacemaker. The tall spikes (~20 mm) are pacemaker firings and they are followed by low-voltage, wide QRS complexes with predominantly S wave (as seen in a bundle branch block electrocardiogram). Note the regular rate of the electronic spikes with no relationship to the P waves, which are indicated by *arrows.* **B,** Atrial pacemaker. This tracing is from a 2-year-old child in whom extreme symptomatic bradycardia developed after the Mustard operation. Pacemaker spikes (~10 mm) are followed by nearly flat atrial activities and by QRS complexes of normal duration. **C,** P wave–triggered pacemaker. This tracing is from a child in whom surgically induced complete heart block developed after repair of tetralogy of Fallot. (From Park MK, Guntheroth WG: *How to Read Pediatric ECGs,* ed 4, Philadelphia, 2006, Mosby.)

an electronically preset PR interval. This type of pacemaker is the most physiologic and is indicated when the patient has advanced AV block but a normal sinus mechanism. Advantages of this type of pacemaker are that the heart rate varies with physiologic need, and the atrial contraction contributes to ventricular filling and improves cardiac output.

PACEMAKER THERAPY IN CHILDREN

Remarkable technologic advances have been made in pacemaker design and function. Surgical corrections of cardiac defects and their late sequelae have increased the need for pacemaker therapy in children. New permanent pacemakers (physiologic pacemakers) are capable of closely mimicking normal cardiac rhythm, and most of them are small enough to be implanted in an infant.

Indications

The indications for permanent pacemaker implantation in children are continually evolving as the reliability of pacing systems improves and clinical experience increases. Box 26.1 lists conditions for which pacemaker therapy is or is not indicated, based on the 2012 American College of Cardiology/American Heart Association/Heart Rhythm Society (ACCF/AHA/HRS) focused update incorporated into the ACCF/AHA/HRS 2008 guidelines for device-based therapy of cardiac rhythm abnormalities (Epstein et al, 2013). In the guidelines, class I conditions are those for which there is general

agreement that the device will be beneficial, and class II conditions are those for which there is ambivalence regarding whether the device will be beneficial. Class IIa conditions are those for which the weight of evidence or opinion is in favor of usefulness or efficacy, and class IIb conditions are those for which usefulness or efficacy is less well established. Class III conditions are those for which there is agreement that the device will not be useful. Each recommendation is accompanied by the weight of evidence as follows: level A if the data were derived from multiple randomized clinical trials, level B when data were derived either from a limited number of trials or nonrandomized studies, and level C when the consensus of experts was the primary source of the recommendation.

In general, the most common indications for permanent pacemaker implantation in children, adolescents, and patients with heart disease (CHD) fit into one of three categories: (1) symptomatic sinus bradycardia (with symptoms of syncope, dizziness, exercise intolerance, or congestive heart failure), (2) the bradycardia–tachycardia syndrome (caused by overdrive suppression after a period of tachycardia), and (3) advanced second- or third-degree AV block, either congenital or postsurgical.

Bradycardia is the most common and noncontroversial indication for permanent pacemaker therapy in both children and adults. The primary criterion for pacemaker implantation for bradycardia is the concurrent observation of a symptom (e.g., syncope) with bradycardia (e.g., heart rate less than 40 beats/min or asystole longer than 3 seconds). In children,

---

BOX 26.1 Recommendations for Permanent Pacing in Children, Adolescents, and Patients with Congenital Heart Disease

Class I (is indicated)

1. For advanced second- or third-degree AV block associated with symptomatic bradycardia, ventricular dysfunction, or low cardiac output *(level of evidence: C)*
2. For sinus node dysfunction with correlation of symptoms during age-inappropriate bradycardia; the definition of bradycardia varies with the patient's age and expected heart rate *(level of evidence: B)*
3. For postoperative advanced second- or third-degree AV block that is not expected to resolve or that persists at least 7 days after cardiac surgery *(level of evidence: B)*
4. For congenital third-degree AV block with a wide QRS escape rhythm, complex ventricular ectopy, or ventricular dysfunction *(level of evidence: B)*
5. For congenital third-degree AV block in the infant with a ventricular rate <55 beats/min or with congenital heart disease and a ventricular rate <70 beats/min *(level of evidence: C)*

Class IIa (is reasonable)

1. For patients with CHD and sinus bradycardia for the prevention of recurrent episodes of intraatrial reentrant tachycardia; sinus node dysfunction may be intrinsic or secondary to antiarrhythmic treatment *(level of evidence: C)*
2. For congenital third-degree AV block beyond the first year of life with an average heart rate <50 beats/min, abrupt pauses in ventricular rate that are two or three times the basic cycle length, or associated with symptoms due to chronotropic incompetence *(level of evidence: B)*
3. For sinus bradycardia with complex congenital heart disease with a resting heart rate <40 beats/min or pauses in ventricular rate >3 seconds *(level of evidence: C)*

4. For patients with CHD and impaired hemodynamics caused by sinus bradycardia or loss of AV synchrony *(level of evidence: C)*
5. For unexplained syncope in the patient with prior congenital heart surgery complicated by transient complete heart block with residual fascicular block after a careful evaluation to exclude other causes of syncope *(level of evidence: B)*

Class IIb (may be reasonable)

1. For transient postoperative third-degree AV block that reverts to sinus rhythm with residual bifascicular block *(level of evidence: C)*
2. For congenital third-degree AV block in asymptomatic children or adolescents with an acceptable rate, a narrow QRS complex, and normal ventricular function *(level of evidence: B)*
3. For asymptomatic sinus bradycardia after biventricular repair of CHD with a resting heart rate <40 beats/min or pauses in ventricular rate >3 seconds *(level of evidence: C)*

Class III (is not indicated)

1. For transient postoperative AV block with return of normal AV conduction in the otherwise asymptomatic patient *(level of evidence: B)*
2. For asymptomatic bifascicular block with or without first-degree AV block after surgery for CHD in the absence of prior transient complete AV block *(level of evidence: C)*
3. For asymptomatic type I second-degree AV block *(level of evidence: C)*
4. For asymptomatic sinus bradycardia with the longest relative risk interval <3 seconds and a minimum heart rate >40 beats/min *(level of evidence: C)*

AV, Atrioventricular; *CHD,* congenital heart disease.
Adapted from Epstein AE, DiMario JP, Ellenbogen KA, et al: 2012 ACCF/AHA/HRS focused update incorporated into the ACCF/AHA/HRS 2008 guidelines for device-based therapy of cardiac rhythm abnormalities: a report of the American College of Cardiology Foundation/American Heart Association Task Force on Practice Guidelines and the Heart Rhythm Society, *J Am Coll Cardiol* 61(3):e6–75, 2013.

---

significant bradycardia with syncope or near syncope results most commonly from extensive surgery involving the atria (e.g., the Senning operation, the Fontan operation, and surgery for atrial septal defect or total anomalous pulmonary venous return). Another noncontroversial indication is surgically acquired heart block that lasts more than 2 weeks after surgery. The risk of death from surgically acquired heart block is as high as 35% in unpaced patients. Most children with congenital heart block eventually require pacemaker implantation. Patients with additional CHDs require pacemaker therapy at an earlier age than those without heart defects.

Temporary pacing is indicated for (1) patients with advanced second-degree or complete heart block secondary to overdose of certain drugs, myocarditis, or myocardial infarction and (2) certain patients immediately after cardiac surgery.

Types of Pacing Devices

The North American Society of Pacing and Electrophysiology and the British Pacing and Electrophysiology Group devised a generic letter code to describe the types and functions of

pacemakers, and it was updated in 2002 (Table 26.1). The first three letters are used exclusively for antibradyarrhythmia functions.

1. The letter in the first position identifies the chamber paced (O, none; A, atrium; V, ventricle; D, dual chamber; or both A and V).
2. The second is the chamber sensed (O, none; A, atrium; V, ventricle; or D, dual).
3. The third letter corresponds to the response of the pacemaker to an intrinsic cardiac event (O, none; I, inhibited; T, triggered; or D, dual [I + T]).
4. The fourth letter indicates both programmability and rate modulation.
5. The fifth position of the code is used to indicate whether multisite pacing is present.

Some examples of the first three letters (and their indications) are shown below.

1. A VOO device provides ventricular pacing, no sensing, and no response to an intrinsic cardiac event. This type of pacemaker is commonly used as emergency pacing.

TABLE 26.1	**Revised NASPE/BPEG Generic Code for Antibradycardia Pacing**			
I: Chamber(s) Paced	**II: Chamber(s) Sensed**	**III: Response to Sensing**	**IV: Programmability, Rate Modulation**	**V: Antiarrhythmia Function**
O, None	O, None	O, None	O, None	O, None
A, Atrium	A, Atrium	T, Triggered	R, Rate modulation	A, Atrium
V, Ventricle	V, Ventricle	I, Inhibited		V, Ventricle
D, Dual (A + V)	D, Dual (A + V)	D, Dual (T + I)		D, Dual (A + V)

BPEG, British Pacing and Electrophysiology Group; *NASPE,* North American Society of Pacing and Electrophysiology.
Adapted from Bernstein AD, Daubert AC, Fletcher RD, et al: The revised NASPE/BPEG generic code for antibradycardia, adaptive-rate, and multisite pacing. North American Society of Pacing and Electrophysiology/British Pacing and Electrophysiology Group, *Pacing Clin Electrophysiol* 25:260–264, 2002.

2. An AOO device provides atrial pacing with no sensing.
3. A VVI device is ventricle stimulated and ventricle sensed; it inhibits paced output if endogenous ventricular activity occurs (thus preventing competition with native QRS activity). This type is commonly used for episodic AV block or bradycardia in small infants.
4. An AAI device paces and senses the atrium and is inhibited by the patient's own atrial activity. This type is commonly used in sinus node dysfunction with intact AV conduction.
5. A DDD device is a dual-chamber pacemaker that is capable of pacing either chamber, sensing activity in either chamber, and either triggering or inhibiting paced output (with resulting AV synchrony). This type is used in AV block where AV synchrony is important.
6. A DVI device paces the ventricle, senses the ventricle and inhibits ventricular pacing. This type allows AV synchrony and is commonly used in patients with atrial arrhythmias.

Selection of Pacing Mode

The pacemaker choice is based on several factors, including the presence or absence of underlying cardiac disease, the size of the patient, and the relevant hemodynamic factors (including the need for atrial contribution in cardiac output).
1. A patient who has sinus node dysfunction but an intact AV node function may receive a single-chamber atrial pacemaker or ventricular pacemaker if AV synchrony is not necessary.
2. In patients with AV block, if AV synchrony is not necessary, a single-chamber ventricular pacing may be implanted.
3. If the sinus node and AV node are both dysfunctional, a dual-chamber device is implanted.

Rate-adaptive pacemakers have the ability to increase the pacing rate through sensors that monitor physiological processes such as activity (activity sensing with vibration detection by piezoelectric crystal or accelerometer) and minute ventilation.

Battery, Leads, and Route

Lithium anode batteries are used almost exclusively. The most widely used type of lithium battery is the lithium iodide. Battery longevity depends on several factors, such as battery size, stimulation frequency, and output per stimulation. Battery life varies from 3 years for a dual-chamber pacemaker used in a small child to 15 years for a large single-chamber device needed infrequently.

There are two types of leads, unipolar and bipolar. The unipolar lead (in which the tip of the lead is the negative pole and the pacemaker itself is the positive pole) has the advantages of a smaller size and a larger sensing circuit, which amplifies low-voltage P waves. The bipolar lead (which possesses a tip electrode [–] and a ring electrode [+] near the end of the pacing catheter) can screen pectoral muscle "noise," has a lower likelihood of external muscle stimulation, and can function even if the pacemaker is out of contact with the body.

Historically, epicardial pacing was more common in children, but transvenous implantation is the method of choice. With improved technology, generators and leads have become smaller and more advanced, allowing transvenous pacing systems in small children. In general, the transvenous route is a reasonable approach for children weighing at least 10 kg, although others have reported successful transvenous pacing in neonates without complications. Transvenous implantation is performed on the side contralateral to the dominant hand. Transvenous implantation has several advantages over epicardial implantation: both atrial and ventricular capture thresholds generally are lower, and pacing problems are significantly fewer than with epicardial implantation. Epicardial implantation is performed through a xyphoid approach and is chosen when a transvenous implantation is precluded, when the patient is a neonate or a small infant (<10 kg), and when the transvenous approach is not possible (after the Fontan operation or superior vena cava obstruction).

IMPLANTABLE CARDIOVERTER–DEFIBRILLATOR THERAPY

An ICD is used in patients at risk for recurrent, sustained VT or VF. The efficacy of ICD therapy in saving the lives of patients at high risk of sudden death has been shown convincingly. Multiple studies have shown ICDs to be superior to antiarrhythmic drug therapy in patients with a history of life-threatening ventricular tachyarrhythmias (i.e., VT or VF).

All ICDs also have a built-in pacemaker. Pacing may be necessary for bradycardia, which may follow an electrical shock delivered by the ICD. The pacemaker also corrects certain tachycardia by overdrive suppression.

The ICD automatically detects, recognizes, and treats tachyarrhythmias and bradyarrhythmias using tiered therapy (i.e., bradycardia pacing, overdrive tachycardia pacing, low-energy cardioversion, high-energy shock defibrillation).

BOX 26.2 Recommendations for Implantable Cardioverter–Defibrillators in Pediatric Patients and Patients with Congenital Heart Disease

Class I (is indicated)

1. In the survivors of cardiac arrest after evaluation to define the cause of the event and to exclude any reversible causes *(level of evidence: B)*
2. For patients with symptomatic sustained VT in association with CHD who have undergone hemodynamic and electrophysiological evaluation; catheter ablation or surgical repair may offer possible alternatives in carefully selected patients *(level of evidence: C)*

Class IIa (is reasonable)

1. For patients with CHD with recurrent syncope of undetermined origin in the presence of either ventricular dysfunction or inducible ventricular arrhythmias at electrophysiological study *(level of evidence: B)*

Class IIb (may be considered)

1. For patients with recurrent syncope associated with complex CHD and advanced systemic ventricular dysfunction when thorough invasive and noninvasive investigations have failed to define a cause *(level of evidence: C)*

Class III (is not indicated)

1. For patients who do not have a reasonable expectation of survival with an acceptable functional status for at least 1 year even if they meet ICD implantation criteria specific in class I, IIa, and IIb recommendation above *(level of evidence: C)*
2. For patients with incessant VT or VF *(level of evidence: C)*
3. In patients with significant psychiatric illness that may be aggravated by device implantation or that may preclude systemic follow-up *(level of evidence: C)*
4. For NYHA class IV patients with drug-refractory CHF who are not candidates for cardiac transplantation or CTR-D *(level of evidence: C)*
5. For syncope of undetermined cause in a patient without inducible VTs and without structural heart disease *(level of evidence: C)*
6. When VF or VT is amenable to surgical or catheter ablation (e.g., atrial arrhythmias associated with WPW syndrome, RVOT or LVOT VT, idiopathic VT, or fascicular VT) in the absence of structural heart disease *(level of evidence: C)*
7. For patients with ventricular tachyarrhythmias caused by a completely reversible disorder in the absence of structural heart disease (e.g., electrolyte imbalance, drugs, trauma) *(level of evidence: B)*

CHD, Congenital heart disease; *CHF,* congestive heart failure; *CRT-D,* cardiac resynchronization therapy device incorporating both pacing and defibrillation capabilities; *LVOT,* left ventricular outflow tract; *NYHA,* New York Heart Association; *RVOT,* right ventricular outflow tract; *VF,* ventricular fibrillation; *VT,* ventricular tachycardia; *WPW,* Wolff-Parkinson-White.
Adapted from Epstein AE, DiMario JP, Ellenbogen KA, et al: 2012 ACCF/AHA/HRS focused update incorporated into the ACCF/AHA/HRS 2008 guidelines for device-based therapy of cardiac rhythm abnormalities: a report of the American College of Cardiology Foundation/American Heart Association Task Force on Practice Guidelines and the Heart Rhythm Society, *J Am Coll Cardiol* 61(3):e6–75, 2013.

They also offer a host of other sophisticated functions (e.g., storage of detected arrhythmic events and the ability to do "noninvasive" electrophysiologic testing). ICDs can discharge voltages ranging from less than 1 V for pacing to 750 V for defibrillation.

The ICD is implanted beneath the skin over the left chest (for right-handed persons) pectoralis muscle and is then connected to the leads. Virtually all ICD systems are implanted transvenously. The longevity of the ICD depends on the frequency of shock delivery, the degree of pacemaker dependency, and other programmable options, but most are expected to last from 5 to 10 years.

The most common problem with ICDs is inappropriate shocks, which are usually the result of detection of a supraventricular tachycardia, most commonly atrial fibrillation. In adult patients, inappropriate shock has been reported in up to 20% of patients within the first year and 40% by 2 years after implantation, causing pain and anxiety generated by this complication.

Indications

Indications for ICD implantation include patients with life-threatening arrhythmias; aborted sudden death; family history of the same disease that can cause sudden death; those with dilated and hypertrophic cardiomyopathy, especially when unexplained fainting episodes have occurred; and other conditions that may increase sudden arrhythmic death risk. The ICD usually is recommended as initial therapy in patients who present with sustained VT or resuscitated cardiac arrest. Box 26.2 lists recommendations for ICD therapy according to the 2012 revised guidelines by the ACC, AHA, and HRS (Epstein et al, 2013).

Fewer than 1% of all ICD implantations are performed in pediatric patients.

1. Two most common indications for ICD implantation in children are hypertrophic cardiomyopathy and long QT syndrome.
2. Other potential indications include idiopathic dilated cardiomyopathy, Brugada syndrome, and arrhythmogenic right ventricular (RV) dysplasia.
3. A family history of sudden death may influence the decision to use an ICD in a pediatric patient.
4. Some postoperative CHDs with VT, such as tetralogy of Fallot and transposition of the great arteries are rare indications for ICD implantation.

Living with a Pacemaker or Implantable Cardioverter–Defibrillator

Electromagnetic interference (EMI) can cause malfunction of the pacemaker or ICD by rate alteration, sensing abnormalities, reprogramming, and other functions, which may result in malfunction of the device or even damage to the pulse generator. EMI is defined as any signal—biological or nonbiological—that is within a frequency spectrum detectable by the sensing circuitry of the pacemaker or ICD.

Patients should be well educated to avoid situations that may cause malfunction or damage to the device. EMI can occur within or outside the hospital. Patients with pacemakers or ICDs should wear a medical identification bracelet or necklace to show that they have a pacemaker or ICD in case of emergency. The following lists some common situations that may or may not affect pacemakers or ICDs.

1. Most home appliances will *not* interfere with the pacemaker signal. The following home appliances are safe to use.
   a. Kitchen appliances (microwave ovens, blenders, toaster ovens, electric knives)
   b. Televisions, stereos, FM and AM radios, ham radios, and CB radios
   c. Electric blankets, heating pads
   d. Electric shavers, hair dryers, curling irons
   e. Garage door openers, gardening electric trimmers
   f. Computers, copying and fax machines
   g. Properly grounded shop tools (except power generator or arc welding equipment)
2. The patient must use caution in the following situations.
   a. Security detectors at airport and government buildings such as courthouses. The patient should not stay near the electronic article surveillance system longer than is necessary and should not lean against the system.
   b. Cellular phones: one should not carry a cell phone in the breast pocket when the ICD is implanted in the left upper chest. Keep the cell phone at least 6 inches away from the ICD. When talking on the cell phone, hold it on the opposite side of the body from the ICD.
   c. Avoid working with, holding, or carrying magnets near the pacemaker.
   d. Turn off large motors such as cars or boats when working on them. Do not use a chainsaw.
   e. Avoid industrial welding equipment. Most welding equipment used for hobby welding should not cause any significant problem.
   f. Avoid high-tension wires, radar installations, smelting furnaces, electric steel furnaces, and other high-current industrial equipment.
   g. Abstain from diathermy (the use of heat to treat muscles).
   h. Contact sports are not recommended for children with pacemakers or ICDs.
3. Hospital sources of potentially significant EMI are as follows.
   a. Electrocautery during surgical procedures: Notify the surgeon or dentist so that electrocautery will not be used to control bleeding. ICD therapy should be deactivated before surgery and reinitiated after surgery by a qualified professional. Alternatively, a magnet can be placed over the pacemaker throughout the procedure.
   b. For cardioversion or defibrillation: Paddles should be placed in the anteroposterior position, keeping the paddles at least 4 inches from the pulse generator. A qualified pacemaker programmer should be available.
   c. Magnetic resonance imaging is considered a relative contraindication in patients with a pacemaker or ICD.

Follow-up for Pacemaker and Implantable Cardioverter–Defibrillator

Patients with pacemakers and ICDs must be followed up on a regular schedule. Many of the same considerations are relevant to both pacemaker and ICD follow-up. The follow-up schedule varies from institution to institution, but one popular approach is to see the child 2 weeks after cardiac pacemaker implantation to make sure that the incisions are healing well and there is no electrode dislodgement. A repeat follow-up appointment is scheduled at 6 weeks. Subsequent visits are scheduled at 3 months, 6 months, and 1 year. Thereafter, visits are usually done once every 12 months for single-chamber pacemakers and once every 6 months for dual-chamber pacemakers.

After the initial pacemaker follow-ups, some physicians prefer regular office assessment, others prefer transtelephonic follow-up, and still others prefer a combination of the two techniques. Monthly transtelephonic pacing system evaluation is simple, convenient, and relatively inexpensive, allowing follow-up with fewer cardiology office visits. Transtelephonic assessment includes a collection of (1) a nonmagnet ECG strip, (2) an ECG strip with magnet applied to the pacemaker, and (3) measurement of magnet rate (see the next paragraph for a discussion of an ECG with magnet application) and pulse duration. (Pulse duration is measured on both atrial and ventricular channels for dual-chamber pacemaker.) During an office visit, the clinical status of the patient is assessed, and the same information as described for transtelephonic assessment should be collected.

ECG and magnet application. The 12-lead ECG with and without a magnet (placed over a pacemaker generator) is a useful tool in pacemaker follow-up assessment.

1. The integrity of atrial and ventricular pacing can be quickly identified with magnet placement. Without the magnet, the patient's intrinsic rhythm inhibits pacer firing.
2. With the magnet on, it begins to pace at a fixed rate in an asynchronous mode (or "magnet mode"). It does not sense the patient's own rhythm (i.e., it paces at a fixed rate regardless of what the patient's own heart rhythm is).
3. The fixed rate that a pacemaker paces at after magnet placement is termed the *magnet rate*. A decrease in the magnet rate (e.g., from the fixed pacing rate of 85 beats/min to 75 beats/min) over time is indicative of a pacemaker battery that is beginning to wear down.
4. It will help locate the side of the ventricle paced (i.e., RBBB pattern with left ventricular pacing and LBBB pattern with RB pacing). Whereas a superior QRS axis suggests leads in the RV apex, an intermediate or inferiorly directed QRS axis suggests leads high on the septum or in the outflow tract.

In many institutions, ICD follow-up is similar to pacemaker follow-up. For an ICD follow-up, the following specific information is collected and assessed. Many cardiologists follow up every 3 to 6 months for the first 3 to 4 years, after which follow-up frequency increases.

1. History: specific emphasis on awareness of delivered therapy and any tachycardia events
2. Device interrogation
3. Assessment of battery status and charge time
4. Retrieval and assessment of stored diagnostic data, such as the cycle length or rate of the detected tachyarrhythmias and ECGs of detected arrhythmias
5. Periodic radiographic assessment
6. Periodic arrhythmia induction in the electrophysiology laboratory to assess defibrillation threshold and efficacy

PART 7

Special Problems

This part explores common pediatric cardiac problems not discussed in previous chapters. The topics include congestive heart failure, systemic hypertension, pulmonary hypertension, child with chest pain, syncope, palpitation, dyslipidemia and other cardiovascular risk factors, athletes with cardiac problems, and cardiac transplantation.

Congestive Heart Failure

Congestive heart failure (CHF) is a clinical syndrome in which the heart is unable to pump enough blood to the body to meet its needs, to dispose of systemic or pulmonary venous return adequately, or a combination of the two.

CAUSES

The heart failure syndrome may arise from diverse causes. Common causes of CHF are volume or pressure overload (or both) caused by congenital or acquired heart disease and myocardial diseases. Tachyarrhythmias and heart block can also cause heart failure at any age. By far the most common causes of CHF in infancy result from congenital heart defects (CHDs). Beyond infancy, myocardial dysfunctions of various etiologies are important causes of CHF. Among the rare causes of CHF are metabolic and endocrine disorders, anemia, pulmonary diseases, collagen vascular diseases, systemic or pulmonary hypertension, neuromuscular disorders, and drugs such as anthracyclines.

Congenital Heart Disease

Volume overload lesions, such as ventricular septal defect (VSD), patent ductus arteriosus (PDA), and endocardial cushion defect (ECD), are the most common causes of CHF in the first 6 months of life. In infancy, the time of the onset of CHF varies predictably with the type of defect. Table 27.1 lists common CHDs according to the age at which CHF develops. When looking at the table, the following should also be noted.
1. Children with tetralogy of Fallot (TOF) do not develop CHF unless they have received a large systemic-to-pulmonary

artery shunt procedure (e.g., too large a Gore-Tex interposition shunt).
2. Atrial septal defect (ASD) rarely causes CHF in the pediatric age group, although it causes CHF in adulthood.
3. Large left-to-right shunt lesions, such as VSD and PDA, do not cause CHF before 6 to 8 weeks of age because the pulmonary vascular resistance does not fall low enough to cause a large left-to-right shunt until this age. The onset of CHF resulting from these left-to-right shunt lesions may be earlier in premature infants (within the first month) because of an earlier fall in the pulmonary vascular resistance in these infants.

Acquired Heart Disease

Acquired heart disease of various causes can lead to CHF. With acquired heart disease, the age at onset of CHF is not as predictable as with CHD, but the following generalities apply:
1. Dilated cardiomyopathy (DCM) is probably the most common cause of CHF beyond infancy. It may cause CHF at any age during childhood and adolescence. The cause of the majority of DCM is idiopathic, but it may be caused by infectious, endocrine, or metabolic disorders; autoimmune diseases; or after antineoplastic treatment (e.g., anthracycline).
2. Doxorubicin cardiomyopathy may manifest months to years after the completion of chemotherapy for malignancies in children.
3. Cardiomyopathies associated with muscular dystrophy and Friedreich's ataxia may cause CHF in older children and adolescents.

TABLE 27.1 Causes of Congestive Heart Failure Resulting from Congenital Heart Disease

Age of Onset	Cause
At birth	HLHS Volume overload lesions: • Severe tricuspid or pulmonary insufficiency • Large systemic arteriovenous fistula
First wk	TGA PDA in small premature infants HLHS (with more favorable anatomy) TAPVR, particularly those with pulmonary venous obstruction Others: • Systemic arteriovenous fistula • Critical AS or PS
1–4 wk	COA with associated anomalies Critical AS Large left-to-right shunt lesions (VSD, PDA) in premature infants All other lesions previously listed
4–6 wk	Some left-to-right shunt lesions such as ECD
6 wk–4 mo	Large VSD Large PDA Others such as anomalous left coronary artery from the PA

AS, Aortic stenosis; *COA,* coarctation of the aorta; *ECD,* endocardial cushion defect; *HLHS,* hypoplastic left heart syndrome; *PA,* pulmonary artery; *PDA,* patent ductus arteriosus; *PS,* pulmonary stenosis; *TAPVR,* total anomalous pulmonary venous return; *TGA,* transposition of the great arteries; *VSD,* ventricular septal defect.

4. Myocarditis associated with Kawasaki's disease is seen in children 1 to 4 years of age.
5. Patients who received surgery for some types of CHDs (e.g., Fontan operation, surgery for TOF, transposition of the great arteries and other cyanotic defects) may remain in or develop CHF after varying period of time.
6. Viral myocarditis tends to be more common in small children older than 1 year. It occurs occasionally in the newborn period, with a fulminating clinical course with a poor prognosis.
7. Acute rheumatic carditis is an occasional cause of CHF that occurs primarily in school-age children.
8. Rheumatic valvular heart diseases, usually volume overload lesions such as mitral regurgitation (MR) or aortic regurgitation (AR), cause CHF in older children and adults. These diseases are uncommon in industrialized countries.
9. Endocardial fibroelastosis, a rare primary myocardial disease, causes CHF in infancy; 90% of cases occur in the first 8 months of life.

Miscellaneous Causes

Miscellaneous causes of CHF include the following:
1. Metabolic abnormalities (severe hypoxia and acidosis, as well as hypoglycemia and hypocalcemia) can cause CHF in newborns.
2. Endocrinopathy such as hyperthyroidism
3. Supraventricular tachycardia (SVT) causes CHF in early infancy.
4. Complete heart block associated with structural heart defects causes CHF in the newborn period or early infancy.
5. Severe anemia may be a cause of CHF at any age. Hydrops fetalis may be a cause of CHF in the newborn period and severe sicklemia at a later age.

6. Bronchopulmonary dysplasia seen in premature infants causes predominantly right-sided heart failure in the first few months of life.
7. Primary carnitine deficiency (plasma membrane carnitine transport defect) causes progressive cardiomyopathy with or without skeletal muscle weakness that begins at 2 to 4 years of age.
8. Acute coronary pulmonale caused by acute airway obstruction (such as seen with large tonsils) can cause CHF at any age but most commonly during early childhood.
9. Acute systemic hypertension, as seen in acute postinfectious glomerulonephritis, causes CHF in school-age children. Fluid retention with poor renal function is important as a cause of hypertension in this condition.

PATHOPHYSIOLOGY

A quick review of physiology of cardiac output is described. Cardiac output is determined by preload, afterload, myocardial contractility, and heart rate. Cardiac output is proportional to filling pressure (preload) and inversely proportional to the resistance against which the heart pumps (afterload).

Preload

According to the Frank-Starling law, as the ventricular end-diastolic volume (or preload) increases, the healthy heart increases cardiac output until a maximum is reached and cardiac output can no longer be augmented (see Fig. 27.1). This is a built-in property of the heart that normally allows it to pump out automatically whatever amount of blood flows into the heart. When the left ventricular (LV) end-diastolic pressure reaches a certain point, however, pulmonary congestion develops with congestive symptoms (tachypnea and dyspnea)

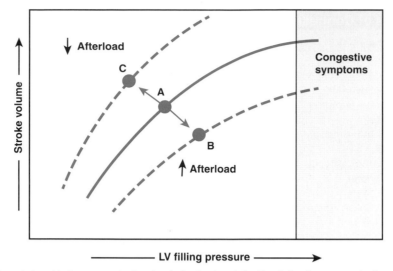

Fig. 27.1 The relationship between the levels of afterload and the Frank-Starling curve. An increase in afterload shifts the Frank-Starling curve down and to the right (from point *A* to *B*), which decreases stroke volume and at the same time increases left ventricular (LV) end-diastolic pressure (preload). In contrast, a decrease in afterload shifts the Frank-Starling curve up and to the left (from point *A* to *C*) and increases stroke volume and at the same time reduces LV end-diastolic pressure. The relationship between afterload and preload is used in the treatment of heart failure; vasodilator drugs augment stroke volume by decreasing arterial pressure (afterload) and at the same time reduce the LV preload (moving point *A* to *C*).

(see Fig. 27.2, which appear in the Management section in this chapter). Congestive symptoms occur even with normally functioning myocardium if the LV end-diastolic pressure is greatly increased, such as seen with infusion of a large amount of fluid or blood. An increase in the stroke volume is also achieved in failing heart when the preload is increased but the failing heart does not achieve the same level of maximal cardiac output as seen in normal heart.

Afterload

Afterload can be thought of as the "load" that the heart must eject blood against. It is the force that resists myofibril shortening during systole, which contributes to total myocardial wall stress (or tension). A decrease in afterload increases cardiac output, and an acute increase in afterload results in decreases in stroke volume and ejection fraction.

According to the law of LaPlace, the tension on the wall of a sphere is the product of pressure and radius and the tension is inversely related to the thickness of the wall.

LV wall stress =
(LV pressure × radius) / (2 × LV wall thickness)

The LaPlace law emphasizes the following three points. (1) The bigger the LV (the radius), the greater the wall stress; (2) at any given radius (LV size), the greater the pressure developed in the LV, the greater the wall stress; and (3) hypertrophied ventricle (increased wall thickness) has less wall stress.

The increased wall tension in the dilated ventricle leads to ventricular hypertrophy that tends to keep the wall tension (stress) low. Well-trained athletes develop cardiac hypertrophy, which helps reduce wall stress. These are examples of how healthy myocardium will adapt to keep wall stress low.

A failing heart will also hypertrophy to reduce the increase in wall stress, but the hypertrophy in the failing heart is abnormal because it occurs as part of ventricular remodeling secondary to neurohormonal compensatory mechanisms. Although hypertrophy may tend to lower wall tension, abnormally hypertrophied ventricle may interfere with synthesis of some of the contractile proteins and leads to collagen damage, including fibrosis.

Compensatory Mechanisms

In the early stages of heart failure, various compensatory mechanisms are evoked to maintain normal metabolic function (i.e., sympathetic nervous system, renin–angiotensin–aldosterone system [RAAS], and natriuretic peptides). After initial beneficial effects, however, some of these mechanisms may eventually prove to be maladaptive.

1. **Sympathetic nervous system.** The initial beneficial effects of an increase in sympathetic tone (by increased adrenal secretion of circulating epinephrine and increased neural release of norepinephrine) include increased heart rate and myocardial contractility with a resulting increase in cardiac output. However, chronic adrenergic stimulation eventually leads to adverse myocardial effects, including increased afterload, arrhythmogenesis, and direct myocardial toxicity (possibly by inhibiting synthesis of contractile protein or by decreasing the density of beta-adrenergic receptors on the surface of the myocardial cell). In clinical settings, the use of beta-adrenergic blockers has resulted in clinical improvement in patients with DCM, in whom increased levels of catecholamines have been shown to be present.

2. **RAAS:** The reduced blood flow to the kidneys in patients with CHF causes marked increase in renin output, and

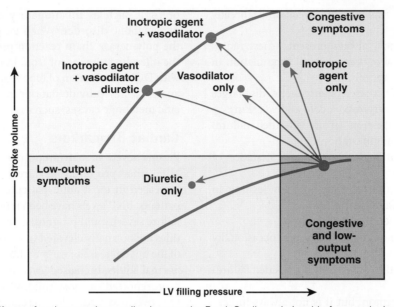

Fig. 27.2 Effects of anticongestive medications on the Frank-Starling relationship for ventricular function. In persons with normal heart, cardiac output increases as left ventricular (LV) filling pressure (preload) increases (*upper curve*). Even in normal heart, congestive symptoms (dyspnea, tachypnea) may appear if the LV filling pressure reaches a certain point (reaching the *top right quadrangle* of the figure). In patients with heart failure, the normal relationship between cardiac output (stroke volume) and filling pressure (preload) is shifted lower and to the right such that a low-output state and congestive symptoms may coincide (the *lower curve* seen in two quadrangles in the lower part of the figure). The effects of various medications, alone and in combination, are shown in the figure. At one extreme, the addition of a pure inotropic agent, such as digoxin, primarily increases the stroke volume with minimal impact on LV filling pressure (so that the patient may still have congestive symptoms). Conversely, the addition of a diuretic primarily decreases the LV filling pressure (with improved congestive symptoms) but without improving cardiac output. Addition of vasodilators reduces afterload and moves the curve up and to the left, thus relieving congestive symptoms and increasing stroke volume. Clinically, it is common to use multiple classes of agents (usually a combination of inotropic agents, diuretics, and vasodilators) to produce both increased cardiac output and decreased LV filling pressure. (Adapted from Cohn JN, Franciosa JS: Vasodilator therapy of cardiac failure [first of two parts], *N Engl J Med* 297:27–31, 1977.)

this in turn causes the formation of angiotensin II. Angiotensin II (a) leads to a further increase in reabsorption of both water and salt from the renal tubules, (b) may cause constriction of vascular smooth muscle (vasoconstriction) and myocardial hypertrophy, and (c) promotes myocardial fibrosis. Thus, angiotensin II plays a maladaptive role in CHF by initiating fibrosis and altering ventricular compliance. In addition, aldosterone tends to retain water. Angiotensin-converting enzyme (ACE) inhibitors used in the treatment of patients with CHF block the maladaptive role of the RAAS.

3. **Natriuretic peptides** (e.g., atrial natriuretic peptide [ANP] and B-type (brain) natriuretic peptide [BNP]): ANP is stored mainly in the RA and is released when the atrial distending pressure increases. BNP is stored in ventricular myocardium and appears to be released when the ventricular filling pressure increases. Both peptides exhibit vasodilating effects and natriuretic effects on the kidneys and counteract the water-retaining effects of the RAAS.

DIAGNOSIS

The diagnosis of CHF relies on several sources of clinical findings, including history, physical examination, chest radiography, and echocardiographic studies. No single test is specific for CHF. In addition to physical findings discussed later, cardiomegaly on a chest radiograph (or echo study) is nearly a prerequisite sign of CHF. An echocardiographic study is the most helpful noninvasive study that confirms the diagnosis of heart failure and estimates the severity of heart failure. It may also help identify the cause of heart failure.

History

1. Poor feeding of recent onset, tachypnea that worsens during feeding, poor weight gain, and cold sweat on the forehead suggest CHF in infants.
2. Older children may complain of shortness of breath, especially with activities; early fatigability; puffy eyelids; or swollen feet.

Physical Examination

Physical findings of CHF may be classified according to their pathophysiologic consequences: impaired cardiac function, pulmonary venous congestion, and systemic venous congestion. The more common findings are in italics.

1. The following are found as compensatory responses to impaired cardiac function:

a. *Tachycardia*, *gallop rhythm*, and weak and thready pulses are common.
b. *Cardiomegaly* is almost always present. Chest radiographs are more reliable than physical examination in demonstrating cardiomegaly.
c. There are signs of increased sympathetic discharges (e.g., *growth failure*; *perspiration*, cold and wet skin).
2. Pulmonary venous congestion (from left-sided failure) results in the following manifestations:
   a. *Tachypnea* is common and is an early manifestation of CHF in infants.
   b. Dyspnea on exertion (equivalent to poor feeding in small infants) is common in children.
   c. Orthopnea may be seen in older children.
   d. Wheezing and pulmonary crackles are occasionally audible.
3. Systemic venous congestion (caused by right-sided failure) results in the following:
   a. Hepatomegaly is common, but it is not always indicative of CHF. A large liver may be palpable in conditions that cause hyperinflated lungs (asthma, bronchiolitis, during hypoxic spells) and in infiltrative liver disease. Conversely, the absence of hepatomegaly does not rule out CHF: hepatomegaly may be absent in (early) left-sided failure.
   b. Puffy eyelids are common in infants.
   c. Distended neck veins and ankle edema, which are common in adults, are not seen in infants.
   d. Splenomegaly is not indicative of CHF; it usually indicates infection.

Radiography

The presence of cardiomegaly should be demonstrated by chest radiographic films. The absence of cardiomegaly almost rules out the diagnosis of CHF. The only exception to this rule is when the pulmonary venous return is obstructed; in such cases, the lung parenchyma will show pulmonary edema or venous congestions.

Electrocardiography

Electrocardiography (ECG) helps determine the type of heart defect causing heart failure but is not helpful in deciding whether CHF is present.

Echocardiography

Echo studies may confirm enlargement of ventricular chambers and impaired LV systolic function (decreased fractional shortening or ejection fraction) as well as impaired diastolic function by the use of Doppler techniques. A more important role of echo may be its ability to determine the cause of CHF. Echo is also helpful in serial evaluation of the efficacy of therapy. Normal echo values for LV diastolic and systolic dimensions are found in Table D.1 in Appendix D.

Tissue Diagnosis

Endomyocardial biopsy obtained during cardiac catheterization offers a new approach to specific diagnosis of the cause of CHF, such as inflammatory disease, infectious process, or metabolic disorder. When viral myocarditis is suspected, the polymerase chain reaction provides a means of isolating the offending viral agent from biopsy specimens. In a patient with DCM, evaluation of biopsy specimens, including genetic analysis, may provide data permitting the diagnosis of specific metabolic causes, such as carnitine deficiency.

Cardiac Biomarkers

Plasma levels of natriuretic peptides (e.g., ANP, BNP, and N-terminal pro-brain natriuretic peptide [NT-proBNP]) are increased in most adult patients with heart failure. In adult patients, BNP levels have been reported to correlate with heart failure severity and prognosis. The plasma levels of these peptides are normally elevated in newborns and in the first weeks of life but decrease in early childhood to the levels observed in normal adults. Increased levels of BNT and NT-ProBNT have been reported in most children with either pressure or volume overload cardiac lesions compared with the levels seen in normal children (Nir et al, 2005). BNP levels of 140 pg/mL or greater identified heart failure patients at a higher risk of poor outcome (Auerbach et al, 2010). The levels of these peptides are different depending on the commercial testing kits used.

MANAGEMENT

The treatment of patients with CHF consists of (1) elimination of the underlying causes, (2) treatment of the precipitating or contributing causes (e.g., infection, anemia, arrhythmias, fever), and (3) control of heart failure state. Eliminating the underlying causes is the most desirable approach whenever possible. Surgical correction of CHDs is such an approach. The heart failure state is controlled by the use of multiple drugs, including inotropic agents, diuretics, and afterload-reducing agents, along with general supportive measures.

Treatment of Underlying Causes or Contributing Factors

1. When surgically feasible, surgical correction of underlying CHDs and valvular heart disease is the best approach for complete cure.
2. If hypertension is the underlying cause of CHF, antihypertensive treatment should be given.
3. If arrhythmias or advanced heart block is the cause of or a contributing factor to heart failure, antiarrhythmic agents or cardiac pacemaker therapy is indicated.
4. If hyperthyroidism is the cause of heart failure, this condition should be treated.
5. Fever should be controlled with antipyretics.
6. When there is a concomitant infection, it should be treated with appropriate antibiotics.
7. For anemia, packed cell transfusion is given to raise the hematocrit to 35% or higher.

General Measures

General support to improve congestive symptoms and nutritional support are important.

TABLE 27.2 Increasing Caloric Density of Feedings

1. Human milk fortifier (Enfamil, Mead Johnson), 1 packet per 25 mL of breast milk = 24 kcal/oz
2. Formula concentration to 24 kcal/oz by:
   a. 1 cup powdered formula + 3 cups water or
   b. 4 oz ready-to-feed + ½ scoop powdered formula
3. Supplementation of formula to 26–30 kcal/oz is accomplished in the following manner.
   a. Fat modular products
      1) MCT oil (Mead Johnson), 8 kcal/mL
      2) Microlipid (safflower oil emulsion, Mead Johnson), 4.5 kcal/mL
   b. Low-osmolality polymers
      1) Polycose (Ross), 23 kcal/Tbsp
      2) Moducal (Mead Johnson), 30 kcal/Tbsp
4. Pediasure (Ross), 30 kcal/oz ready-to-feed (for children older than 1 year of age)

MCT, Medium-chain triglyceride.
From Wright GE, Rochini AP: Primary and general care of the child with congenital heart disease, *ACC Curr J Rev* Mar/Apr:89–93, 2002.

---

1. A "cardiac chair" or "infant seat" is used to keep infants in semi-upright position to relieve respiratory distress.
2. Oxygen (40%–50%) with humidity is administered to infants with respiratory distress if pulse oximetry indicates compromise of blood oxygenation.
3. For infants with CHF, adequate calories and fluid should be provided to permit appropriate weight gain. Infants in CHF need significantly higher caloric intakes than recommended for average infants. The required calorie intake may be as high as 150 to 160 kcal/kg/day for infants in CHF. Compounding this problem is that these infants typically cannot take in needed calories even for normal growth owing to tachypnea, increased work of breathing, and diminished strength of sucking, and difficulty with coordination of sucking and swallowing.
   a. Increasing caloric density of feeding may be required and it may be accomplished with fortification of feeding (Table 27.2).
   b. Frequent small feedings are better tolerated than large feeding in infants.
   c. If oral feedings are not well tolerated, intermittent or continuous nasogastric (NG) feeding is indicated. To promote normal development of oral-motor function, infants may be allowed to take calorie-dense oral feeds throughout the day and then be given continuous NG feeds overnight.
   d. Salt restriction in the form of a low-salt formula and severe fluid restriction are not indicated in infants. Use of diuretics has replaced these measures.
   e. Parents should be taught proper feeding techniques.
4. In older children, salt restriction (<0.5 g/day) and avoidance of salty snacks (chips, pretzels) and table salt are recommended. Bed rest remains an important component of management. The availability of a television screen and computer games for entertainment assures bed rest in older children.
5. If respiratory failure accompanies cardiac failure, intubation and positive-pressure ventilation are occasionally required. Respiratory failure usually signifies that surgical intervention will be needed for CHDs when the patient is stabilized.
6. Daily weight measurement is essential in hospitalized patients.

Drug Therapy

Three major classes of drugs are commonly used in the treatment of CHF in children: diuretics, inotropic agents, and afterload-reducing agents. Rapid acting inotropic agents (dopamine, dobutamine) are used in critically or acutely ill infants and children. Digoxin is the only safe and effective oral inotropic agent. Diuretics are usually used with inotropic agents. Afterload-reducing agents, such as ACE inhibitors, have gained popularity because they can increase cardiac output without increasing myocardial oxygen consumption. Recently, low-dose beta-adrenergic blockade has been added to the treatment of DCM with encouraging results. Effects of various anticongestive medications, alone or in combination, on the Frank-Starling curve are schematically illustrated in Fig. 27.2.

Diuretics

Diuretics remain the principal therapeutic agent to control pulmonary and systemic venous congestion. Diuretics only reduce preload and improve congestive symptoms but do not improve cardiac output or myocardial contractility (see Fig. 27.2). Patients with mild CHF may improve rapidly after a dose of fast-acting diuretics, such as ethacrynic acid or furosemide, even without inotropic agents. Table 27.3 shows dosages of commonly available diuretic preparations.

Three main classes of diuretics are commercially available.
1. Thiazide diuretics (e.g., chlorothiazide, hydrochlorothiazide), which act at the proximal and distal tubules, are no longer popular.
2. Rapid-acting diuretics, such as furosemide and ethacrynic acid, are the drugs of choice. They act primarily at the loop of Henle ("loop diuretics").
3. Aldosterone antagonists (e.g., spironolactone) act on the distal tubule to inhibit sodium–potassium exchange. The serum aldosterone level is significantly increased in

TABLE 27.3 Diuretic Agents and Dosages

Preparation	Route	Dosage
Thiazide Diuretics		
Chlorothiazide (Diuril)	PO	20–40 mg/kg/day in 2 divided doses
Hydrochlorothiazide (HydroDIURIL)	PO	2–4 mg/kg/day in 2 divided doses
Loop Diuretics		
Furosemide (Lasix)	IV	1 mg/kg/dose
	PO	2–3 mg/kg/day in 2–3 divided doses
Ethacrynic acid (Edecrin)	IV	1 mg/kg/dose
	PO	2–3 mg/kg/day in 2–3 divided doses
Aldosterone Antagonist		
Spironolactone (Aldactone)	PO	1–3 mg/kg/day in 2–3 divided doses

IV, Intravenous; *PO,* oral.

patients with persistent CHF, contributing to fluid and salt retention. Patients with increased levels of circulating aldosterone have a diminished response to diuretic agents because aldosterone increases tubular reabsorption of sodium and water at a site distal to the sites of action of other diuretic agents (thiazides or furosemide). Aldosterone antagonists have value in preventing hypokalemia produced by other diuretics and thus are used in conjunction with a loop diuretic. However, when ACE inhibitors are used, spironolactone should be discontinued to avoid hyperkalemia.

Side Effects of Diuretic Therapy. Diuretic therapy alters the serum electrolytes and acid–base equilibrium.

1. Hypokalemia is a common problem with diuretic therapy, except when used with spironolactone. It is more profound with potent loop diuretics. Hypokalemia may increase the likelihood of digitalis toxicity.
2. Hypochloremic alkalosis may result because the loss of chloride ions is greater than the loss of sodium ions through the kidneys, with a resultant increase in bicarbonate levels. Alkalosis also predisposes to digitalis toxicity.

Rapidly Acting Inotropic Agents

In critically ill infants with CHF, in those with renal dysfunction (e.g., infants with coarctation of the aorta), and in postoperative cardiac patients with heart failure, rapidly acting catecholamines with a short duration of action are preferable to digoxin. This class of agents includes dopamine, dobutamine, isoproterenol, and epinephrine. These agents possess inotropic and vasodilator actions and thus are useful in acute situations. Dobutamine has fewer chronotropic effects than dopamine. Dopamine in high doses causes α-receptor stimulation with vasoconstriction and reduction of renal blood flow. There is an added beneficial effect when an inotropic agent has vasodilating action as in dopamine. Inotropic agents in general increase the contractile property of the myocardium toward the normal curve (see Fig. 27.2). Dosages for intravenous drip of these catecholamines are suggested in Table 27.4.

Milrinone is a phosphodiesterase-3 (PDE-3) inhibitor with lusitropic (myocardial relaxation) and vasodilatory as well as some mild inotropic effects. It improves the cardiac output by augmenting the contractility as well as decreasing the afterload with less chronotropy compared with other acute inotropic agents. Amrinone is another PDE-3 inhibitor and noncatecholamine agent that exerts its inotropic and vasodilator effects by inhibiting phosphodiesterase. Thrombocytopenia is a side effect; the drug should be discontinued if the platelet count falls below 150,000/mm^3. Amrinone is useful in patients with severe CHF (DCM) who have received prolonged treatment with beta-stimulants (see Appendix E, Table E.1 for dosage).

Digitalis Glycosides

Use of Digoxin. The popularity of digoxin in the treatment of heart failure has waxed and waned. Until the early 1980s, there were only two classes of drugs available to treat patients with CHF: cardiac glycosides and diuretics. During that period of time, open-heart surgeries carried a high mortality rate in small infants with CHDs, so maximum pharmacologic efforts were made using digoxin and diuretics to delay the surgeries in small infants with heart failure from CHDs.

Afterload-reducing agents, mainly ACE inhibitors, became available in the 1980s. At that time, it became apparent that many infants with large left-to-right shunt lesions had congestive symptoms, but their LV systolic function remained normal, the so-called pulmonary overcirculation state. With the increasing popularity of ACE inhibitors and new understanding of pathophysiology of congestive symptoms (with normal LV systolic function) in infants with large left-to-right shunt lesions, the benefits of digoxin in these infants were questioned, and the use of digoxin became controversial. Salutary effects of combined use of diuretics and afterload-reducing agents, without digoxin, were reported. Thereafter, the use of digoxin in small infants with congestive symptoms from large left-to-right shunt lesions gradually lost popularity.

However, studies have shown that digoxin improves symptoms in these infants with pulmonary overcirculation, perhaps because of other actions of digoxin (Berman et al,

TABLE 27.4 Suggested Starting Dosages of Catecholamines

Drug	Dosage and Route (μg/kg/min IV)	Side Effects
Epinephrine (Adrenalin)	0.1–1	Hypertension, arrhythmias
Isoproterenol (Isuprel)	0.1–0.5	Peripheral and pulmonary vasodilatation
Dobutamine (Dobutrex)	2–8	Little tachycardia and vasodilatation, arrhythmias
Dopamine (Intropin)	5–10	Tachycardia, arrhythmias, hypertension or hypotension
		Dose-related cardiovascular effects (mcg/kg/min):
		Renal vasodilatation: 2–5
		Inotropic: 5–8
		Tachycardia: >8
		Mild vasoconstriction: >10
		Vasoconstriction: 15–20

IV, Intravenous.

1983). In addition to inotropic action, digoxin also has parasympathomimetic action with slowing of heart rate, reducing sinoatrial firing, and slowing the atrioventricular (AV) conduction. Several earlier studies showed that digoxin reduces circulating norepinephrine, renin, and aldosterone levels. Digoxin is a diuretic agent as well. Digoxin can increase inotropy without increasing myocardial oxygen consumption. Research has shown that myocardial oxygen consumption is increased in normal hearts by the positive inotropic action of glycosides, and oxygen consumption is actually reduced or remains constant in failing hearts (Braunwald, 1985). Therefore, some cardiologists still favor the use of digoxin in infants with CHF from large-shunt lesions. A usual approach may be that a diuretic and an afterload-reducing agent are initially started, and digoxin is added later if further improvement is needed.

With regards to patients with dilated LV with decreased systolic function, such as those with DCM, digoxin, the only safe and effective positive inotropic agent, clearly increases the cardiac output (or contractile state of the myocardium), thereby resulting in an upward and leftward shift of the Frank-Starling curve (see Fig. 27.1). When inotropic agents are used with a vasodilator or a diuretic, a much greater improvement is seen both in the contractile state and in congestive symptoms than when a single class of agent was used (see Fig. 27.2). Thus, the use of a combination of inotropic agents, diuretics, and vasodilators has become popular.

Dosage of Digoxin. The total digitalizing dose and maintenance dosage of digoxin in treating CHF by oral and intravenous routes are shown in Table 27.5. The maintenance dose is more closely related to the serum digoxin level than is the digitalizing dose, which is given to build a sufficient body store of the drug and to shorten the time required to reach the pharmacokinetic steady state.

The pediatric dosage of digoxin is much larger than the adult dosage on the basis of body weight. Pharmacokinetic studies indicate that infants and children require larger doses of digoxin than adults to attain comparable serum levels, primarily because of a larger volume of distribution and, less important, a more rapid renal clearance, including tubular secretion. The volumes of distribution of digoxin are 7.5 L/kg

in neonates, 16 L/kg in infants and children, and 4 L/kg in adults. Much higher concentrations of digoxin are found in the myocardium and skeletal muscles from young patients.

How to Digitalize. Loading doses of the total digitalizing dose are given over 12 to 18 hours followed by maintenance doses. This results in a pharmacokinetic steady state in 3 to 5 days. The intravenous route is preferred over the oral route, particularly when dealing with infants in severe heart failure. The intramuscular route is not recommended because absorption of the drug from the injection site is unreliable. When an infant is in mild heart failure, the maintenance dose may be administered orally without loading doses; this results in a steady state in 5 to 8 days.

The following is a suggested step-by-step method of digitalization:

1. Obtain a baseline ECG (rhythm and PR interval) and baseline levels of serum electrolytes. Changes in ECG rhythm and PR interval are important signs of digitalis toxicity (see later discussion). Hypokalemia and hypercalcemia predispose to digitalis toxicity.
2. Calculate the total digitalizing dose (see Table 27.5).
3. Give half the total digitalizing dose immediately followed by one fourth and then the final one fourth of the total digitalizing dose at 6- to 8-hour intervals.
4. Start the maintenance dose 12 hours after the final total digitalizing dose. Obtaining an ECG strip before starting the maintenance dose is advised.

Monitoring for Digitalis Toxicity by Electrocardiography. Digitalis toxicity is best detected by monitoring with ECGs, not serum digoxin levels, during the first 3 to 5 days after digitalization (when the pharmacokinetic steady state is not reached). Box 27.1 lists signs of digitalis effects and toxicity. In general, whereas the digitalis effect is confined to ventricular repolarization, toxicity involves disturbances in the formation and conduction of the impulse. One should assume that any arrhythmia or conduction disturbance occurring *with* digitalis is *caused by* digitalis until proved otherwise.

Serum Digoxin Levels. Therapeutic ranges of serum digoxin levels for treating patients with CHF are 0.8 to 2 ng/mL. Levels obtained during the first 3 to 5 days after digitalization tend to be higher than those obtained when the

TABLE 27.5 Oral Digoxin Dosages for Congestive Heart Failure

Age	Total Digitalizing Dose (mcg/kg)	Maintenance Dose[a] (mcg/kg/day)
Premature infants	20	5
Newborn infants	30	8
<2 yr	40–50	10–12
>2 yr	30–40	8–10

[a]The maintenance dose is 25% of the total digitalizing dose in two divided doses. The intravenous dose is 75% of the oral dose.
Adapted from Park MK: The use of digoxin in infants and children with specific emphasis on dosage, *J Pediatr* 108:871–877, 1986.

BOX 27.1 Electrocardiogram Changes Associated with Digitalis

Effects
Shortening of QTc, the earliest sign of digitalis effect
Sagging ST segment and diminished amplitude of T wave (the T vector does not change)
Slowing of heart rate

Toxicity
Prolongation of PR interval: sometimes a prolonged PR interval is seen in children without digitalis, making a baseline ECG mandatory; the prolongation may progress to second-degree AV block
Profound sinus bradycardia or SA block
Supraventricular arrhythmias, such as atrial or nodal ectopic beats and tachycardias (particularly if accompanied by AV block), which are more common than ventricular arrhythmias in children
Ventricular arrhythmias such as ventricular bigeminy and trigeminy, which are extremely rare in children, although they are common in adults with digitalis toxicity; isolated PVCs, which are common in children, are a sign of toxicity
AV, Atrioventricular; *ECG,* electrocardiogram; *PVC,* premature ventricular contraction; *SA,* sinoatrial.

BOX 27.2 Factors That May Predispose to Digitalis Toxicity

High Serum Digoxin Level
High-dose requirement, as in treatment of certain arrhythmias (e.g., SVT)
Decreased renal excretion
• Premature infants
• Renal disease
Hypothyroidism
Drug interaction (e.g., quinidine, verapamil, amiodarone)

Increased Sensitivity of Myocardium (without high serum digoxin level)
Status of myocardium
• Myocardial ischemia
• Myocarditis (rheumatic, viral)
Systemic changes
• Electrolyte imbalance (hypokalemia, hypercalcemia)
• Hypoxia
• Alkalosis
Adrenergic stimuli or catecholamines
Immediate postoperative period after heart surgery under cardiopulmonary bypass

SVT, Supraventricular tachycardia.

Digitalis Toxicity. Digitalis toxicity may result during treatment with digoxin or from an accidental overdose of digoxin. With the relatively low dosage recommended in Table 27.5, digitalis toxicity is unlikely to develop. However, one should beware of possible digitalis toxicity in every child receiving digitalis preparations. Patients with conditions listed in Box 27.2 are more likely to develop toxicity. The diagnosis of digitalis toxicity is a clinical decision and usually is based on the following clinical and laboratory findings.

1. The patient has a history of accidental ingestion.
2. Noncardiac symptoms appear in digitalized children: anorexia, nausea, vomiting, diarrhea, restlessness, drowsiness, fatigue, and visual disturbances in older children.
3. Heart failure worsens.
4. ECG signs of toxicity probably are more reliable and appear early (see Box 27.1).
5. An elevated serum level of digoxin (>2 mg/mL) is likely to be associated with toxicity in a child if the clinical findings suggest digitalis toxicity.

Afterload-Reducing Agents

Vasoconstriction which occurs as a compensatory response to reduced cardiac output seen in CHF may be deleterious to the failing ventricle. Vasoconstriction is produced by a rise in sympathetic tone and circulating catecholamines and by an increase in the activity of the renin–angiotensin system. Reducing afterload tends to augment the stroke volume without a great change in the contractile state of the heart and therefore without increasing myocardial oxygen consumption (see Fig. 27.2). When a vasodilator is used with an inotropic agent, the degree of improvement in the inotropic state as well as in congestive symptoms is much greater than

pharmacokinetic steady state is reached. Blood for serum digoxin levels should be drawn at least 6 hours after the last dose or just before a scheduled dose; samples obtained earlier than 6 hours after the last dose will give a falsely elevated level.

Determining serum digoxin levels frequently and using those levels for therapeutic goals are neither justified nor practical; occasional determination of the levels is adequate. Determination of the serum digoxin levels is useful in evaluating possible toxicity (see later section), determining the patient's compliance, and detecting abnormalities in absorption and excretion and is mandatory in managing accidental overdoses.

Serum digoxin levels may be elevated when administered concomitantly with other drugs such as quinidine, verapamil, amiodarone, beta-blockers, tetracycline, and erythromycin. Lower serum levels have been noted with rifampin, kaolin-pectin, neomycin, and cholestyramine.

TABLE 27.6 Dosages of Vasodilators

Drug	Route and Dosage	Comments
Arteriolar Vasodilator		
Hydralazine (Apresoline)	IV: 0.15–0.2 mg/kg/dose every 4–6 hr (maximum, 20 mg/dose)	May cause tachycardia; may be used with propranolol
	Oral: 0.75–3 mg/kg/day, in 2–4 doses (maximum, 200 mg/day)	May cause GI symptoms, neutropenia, and lupus-like syndrome
Venodilators		
Nitroglycerin	IV: 0.5–1 mcg/kg/min (maximum, 6 mcg/kg/min)	Start with small dose and titrate based on effects
Mixed Vasodilators		
Captopril (Capoten)	PO:	May cause hypotension, dizziness, neutropenia, and proteinuria
	Newborn: 0.1–0.4 mg/kg, TID–QID	
	Infants: initially 0.15–0.3 mg/kg QD–QID; titrate upward if needed; maximum dose, 6 mg/kg/24 hr	Dose should be reduced in patients with impaired renal function
	Children: initially 0.3—0.5 mg/kg BID–TID; titrate upward if needed; maximum, 6 mg/kg/24 hr	
	Adolescents and adults: initially 12.5–25 mg, BID–TID; increase weekly if needed by 25 mg/dose to maximum dose of 450 mg/24 hr	
Enalapril (Vasotec)	PO: 0.1 mg/kg QD or BID	Patient may develop hypotension, dizziness, or syncope
Nitroprusside (Nipride)	IV: 0.3–0.5 mcg/kg/min; titrate to effect; maximum dose, 10 mcg/kg/min	May cause thiocyanate or cyanide toxicity (e.g., fatigue, nausea, disorientation), hepatic dysfunction, or light sensitivity

BID, Twice a day; *GI,* gastrointestinal; *IV,* intravenous; *PO,* oral; *QD,* once a day; *QID,* four times a day; *TID,* three times a day.

when a vasodilator alone is used. Combined use of an inotropic agent, a vasodilator, and a diuretic produces the most improvement in both inotropic state and congestive symptoms (see Fig. 27.2).

Afterload-reducing agents now occupy a prominent role in the treatment of infants with CHF secondary to a large left-to-right shunt lesions (e.g., VSD, AV canal, PDA). Infants with large left-to-right shunts have been shown to benefit from captopril and hydralazine. Beneficial effects of afterload-reducing agents are also seen in DCM, adriamycin-induced cardiomyopathy, myocardial ischemia, postoperative cardiac status, severe MR or AR, and systemic hypertension. These agents usually are used in conjunction with diuretics and often with digitalis glycosides for a maximal benefit.

Afterload-reducing agents may be divided into three groups based on the site of action: arteriolar vasodilators, venodilators, and mixed vasodilators. Dosages of these agents are presented in Table 27.6.

1. Arteriolar vasodilators (hydralazine) augment cardiac output by acting primarily on the arteriolar bed, with resulting reduction of the afterload. Hydralazine often is administered with propranolol because it activates the baroreceptor reflex, with resulting tachycardia.
2. Venodilators (nitroglycerin, isosorbide dinitrate) act primarily by dilating systemic veins and redistributing blood from the pulmonary to the systemic circuit (with a resulting decrease in pulmonary symptoms). Venodilators are most beneficial in patients with pulmonary congestion but may have adverse effects when preload has been restored to normal by diuretics or sodium restriction.
3. Mixed vasodilators include ACE inhibitors (captopril, enalapril), nitroprusside, and prazosin. These agents act on both arteriolar and venous beds. ACE inhibitors are popular in children with chronic severe CHF, but sodium nitroprusside is used primarily in acute situation such as after cardiac surgery under cardiopulmonary bypass, especially in patients who had pulmonary hypertension and those with postoperative rises in PA pressure. When nitroprusside is used, blood pressure must be monitored continuously. ACE inhibitors reduce systemic vascular resistance by inhibiting angiotensin II generation and augmenting production of bradykinin.

Other Drugs

β-Adrenergic Blockers. Beneficial effects of beta-adrenergic blockers were reported in adult patients with DCM. Studies have suggested that adrenergic overstimulation often seen in patients with chronic CHF may have detrimental effects on the hemodynamics of heart failure by inducing myocyte injury and necrosis rather than being a compensatory mechanism, as traditionally thought.

Although some earlier small-scale noncontrolled pediatric studies have reported beneficial effects of beta blockers (metoprolol and carvedilol) in the treatment of patients with DCM, a 26 multicenter large-scale, prospective, randomized trials on 150 patients did not reach the same conclusion

(Shaddy et al, 2007). In that study, the patients were divided into three groups: placebo group and low and high doses of carvedilol groups (0.4 mg and 0.8 mg/kg/day, respectively). All patients were on standard treatment with ACE inhibitors and diuretics. They found no significant differences among the three groups in terms of symptoms and echo indices over 6-month period of follow-up. However, they found a surprising number of patients showing spontaneous improvement in all three groups. They also found a trend to better outcome in patients who have morphologic LV (as seen in patients with tricuspid atresia). Another more recent study on 89 children with heart failure who were treated with carvedilol showed no significant clinical improvement; however improved serum BNP levels as well as echocardiographic parameters were noted (Huong et al, 2013).

Although, at this time, no randomized control trials are available, however, most authorities and centers advocate the use of beta-blockers in children with CHF when they are hemodynamically stable. Contraindication to the use of beta-adrenergic blockers also includes symptomatic bradycardia or heart block, significant hypotension, active asthma, or severe bronchial disease.

Carnitine. Carnitine, which is an essential cofactor for transport of long-chain fatty acids into mitochondria for oxidation, has been shown to be beneficial in some cases of cardiomyopathy, especially those with suggestive evidence of disorders of metabolism (Helton et al, 2000). Most of these patients had DCM. The dosage of L-carnitine was 50 to 100 mg/kg/day, given twice or thrice orally (maximum daily dose, 3 g). It improved myocardial function, reduced cardiomegaly, and improved muscle weakness. Animal studies suggest potential protective and therapeutic effects on doxorubicin-induced cardiomyopathy in rats.

SURGICAL MANAGEMENT

If medical treatment with the previously mentioned regimens does not improve CHF caused by CHDs within a few weeks to months, one should consider either palliative or corrective cardiac surgery for the underlying cardiac defect when technically feasible. Cardiac transplantation is an option for a patient with progressively deteriorating cardiomyopathy despite maximal medical treatment.

Systemic Hypertension

DEFINITION

For adults, 2017 Guidelines by the American College of Cardiology, American Heart Association, and several other organizations jointly revised the earlier definition and classification of hypertension (HTN) by the 2003 Joint National Committee on Prevention, Detection, Evaluation, and Treatment of High Blood Pressure. According to the new classification (Whelton et al, 2018), normal blood pressure (BP) is defined as less than 120 mm Hg systolic blood pressure (SBP) and less than 80 mm Hg diastolic blood pressure (DBP) in adults. SBP between 120 and 129 mm Hg and DBP less than 80 mm Hg are now called "elevated blood pressure," formerly called "prehypertension." HTN is classified as stage 1 and stage 2, depending on the level of abnormalities. Stage 1 HTN is defined as SBP 130 to 139 systolic *or* DBP of 80 to 89 mm Hg. Stage 2 HTN is defined as SBP 140 mm Hg or greater *or* DBP 90 mm Hg or greater. Table 28.1 shows different levels of BP readings by the new definition of elevated BP.

In children, HTN is defined statistically because BP levels vary with age and gender, and outcome-based data are not available for children. Following the new definition of HTN in adults (Whelton et al, 2017), the American Academy of Pediatrics (AAP) updated the earlier guidelines of 2004 (The Fourth Report, 2004), which was endorsed by the American Heart Association (Flynn et al, 2017). In the new guidelines, the term "prehypertension" has been replaced with "elevated blood pressure" for children as in adults.

1. *Normal BP* is defined as SBP and DPB less than 90th percentile.
2. *Elevated BP* is defined as an average SBP and DPB between the 90th and 95th percentiles for age and gender.

3. *HTN* is defined as SBP or DPB levels that are greater than the 95th percentile for age and gender. As in adults, adolescents with BP levels 120/80 mm Hg or greater by auscultatory method are considered hypertensive even if they are below the 95th percentile. HTN is further classified into stage 1 and stage 2.
   a. Stage 1 HTN is present when BP readings are between the 95th and 99th percentiles + 12 mm Hg.
   b. Stage 2 HTN is present when BP readings are higher than the 95th percentile + 12 mm Hg.
4. *White-coat HTN* is present when BP readings in health care facilities are greater than the 95th percentile but are normotensive outside a clinical setting. This condition may not be as benign as once thought to be, and regular follow-up is now recommended. This topic is discussed further later in this chapter.

WHICH NORMATIVE BLOOD PRESSURE STANDARDS?

A prerequisite to the use of the above definition for pediatric HTN is the availability of reliable normative BP standards. An unfortunate part of the problem is that there are no reliable evidence based BP standards for children. The BP tables recommended by the Working Group of the National High Blood Pressure Education Program (NHBPEP) are not as good as it was made to believe because (1) the BP data are not derived by the methodology currently recommended by the Working Group, (2) expressing BP levels by age and height percentiles is statistically unsound and unjustified, and (3) additional computation of BP levels by height percentile on such highly variable office BP readings is unscientific and impractical for busy practitioners. NHBPEP's statistical processing on

TABLE 28-1   Classification of Blood Pressure for Adults and Children

	ADULTS[a]* AND ADOLESCENT >13 YEARS[b]			
	Systolic P		Diastolic P	Children and Adolescents <13 years[b]
Normal BP	<120	and	<80	<90th %
Elevated BP	120–129	and	<80	≥90th%–<95th% or >120/80 mm Hg
Stage 1 HTN	130–139	or	80–89	≥95th%–95th% + 12 or 130/80 to 139/89 mm Hg (whichever is lower)
Stage 2 HTN	≥140	or	≥90	Higher than 95th% + 12 or ≥140/90 mm Hg (whichever is lower)

Blood pressrue levels are based on an average of ≥2 careful readings or ≥2 occasions.

Individuals with systolic and diastolic pressure in two different categories should be designaed to the higher BP category.

BP, blood pressure; *HTN*, hypertension; *%*, percentile.

Adapted from

[a]Whelton PK, Carey RM, Aronow WS, et al: 2017 ACC/AHA/AAPA/ABC/ACPM/AGS/APhA/ASH/ASPC/NMA/PCNA guidelines for the prevention, dectection, evaluation, and management of high blood pressure in adults. J Am Coll Cardiol 71:e127-e247, 2018.

[b]Flynn JT, Kaelber DC, Barker-Smith CM, et al: Clinical practice guideline for screening and management of high blood pressure in children and adolescents, 140(3):e20171904, 2017.

unscientifically obtained data does not improve their validity (this part has been discussed in depth in the section on blood pressure measurement, in Chapter 2.)

In addition, it is important to know that the BP standards of the NHBPEP cannot be used when BP is measured by an oscillometric device. This conclusion is based on a single study that specifically lookcd at BP readings obtained by the two different methods, alternating the order of device used (Park et al, 2001). In the San Antonio Children's Blood Pressure Study (SACBPS) using both the auscultatory and a popular oscillometric device (Dinamap Model 8100), BP levels obtained by Dinamap were on average 10 mm Hg higher for SP and 5 mm Hg higher for DP than those obtained by the auscultatory method (Park et al, 2001). Therefore, BPs obtained by the auscultatory method are not interchangeable with those obtained by the oscillometric method, which is being used in increasing frequency. Therefore, when BPs are obtained by an oscillometric device, one should not use the BP standards derived from the auscultatory method. Only normative BP standards by Dinamap Monitor are thosc from the SACBPS (Park et al, 2005), and they are presented in Appendix B (Tables B.6 and B.7).

Kaelber et al (2009) have recommended a simplified table of BP levels according to age and gender (without height percentiles), above which further evaluation should be carried out for possible HTN. This approach is well justified and more practical because one does not need to use the unscientific normative standards of the NHBPEP and because height is not measured at some BP screening sites (as discussed in Chapter 2). Table 28.2 shows the 90th percentile BP values by both methods side by side. The values in Table 28.2 are the same as those presented in Table 2.4. It is interesting to note that the Kaelber's auscultatory BP levels are almost the same as the 90th percentile of BP levels by the SACBPS (Park et al, 2005).

WHAT ABOUT OTHER MEANS OF BLOOD PRESSURE MEASUREMENT?

The above classification of BP is based on the auscultatory BP method measured on the upper arm.

Wrist BP should not be used in the detection of patients with possible HTN. The radial artery SBP is expected to be higher than the arm SBP, more so in children than adults, because of a physiologic phenomenon known as "peripheral amplification of systolic blood pressure." This topic is discussed in depth in the section on BP measurement in Chapter 2.

Ambulatory BP measurement (ABPM) has been recommended by the US Preventive Services Task Force for the confirmation of HTN in adults before starting treatment. Although the issue of ABPM is gaining popularity in pediatrics, there are still gaps regarding its usefulness in pediatric patients. There is evidence that ABPM is more accurate for the diagnosis of HTN than clinic-measured BP and that left ventricular hypertrophy (LVH) correlated more strongly with ABPM parameters than casual BP measurement. In addition, ABPM is more reproducible than casual or home BP measurement. Therefore, it has been recommended to use for the confirmation of HTN in children older than 5 years of age (for technical reasons). Normative ambulatory BP standards are presented in Tables B.8 and B.9 in Appendix B.

Home or school BP measurement. Home BP measurement (or self-monitoring), using an automated device with memory capacity, has certain advantages over both office BP and ABMP. A problem with this approach is that there are no reliable normative BP standards for this approach, and the accuracy of some such devices is uncertain. Therefore, home BP measurement should not be used to diagnose HTN; it may be a useful tool for follow-up after HTN has been diagnosed. School BP measurement may have a similar role to home BP measurement. It should not be used to make the diagnosis of HTN, but it can be a useful tool to identify children who require formal evaluation and children with possible white-coat HTN. It can be a helpful adjunct in the monitoring of children with diagnosed HTN.

Cause

Hypertension is classified into two general types, essential (or primary) HTN, in which a specific cause cannot be identified, and secondary HTN, in which a cause can be (Box 28.1).

TABLE 28.2 90th Percentiles of Blood Pressure by Auscultatory and Oscillometric Methods from the San Antonio Study

Age (yr)	AUSCULTATORY[A,C]				Age (yr)	OSCILLOMETRIC[B]			
	MALE		FEMALE			MALE		FEMALE	
	SBP	DBP	SBP	DBP		SBP	DBP	SBP	DBP
5	103	60	102	60	5	115	68	114	68
6	105	64	103	63	6	117	68	115	68
7	107	66	104	65	7	118	69	116	69
8	108	68	106	67	8	119	70	118	70
9	109	68	108	67	9	121	70	119	70
10	111	68	110	68	10	122	71	121	71
11	113	68	112	68	11	124	71	122	71
12	116	68	113	68	12	126	71	123	71
13	118	68	115	68	13	129	71	125	71
14	120	68	116	68	14	131	72	125	72
15	120	69	117	69	15	133	72	126	72
16	120	71	117	69	16	134	72	126	72
17	120	73	118	70	17	134	72	126	72
≥18	120	73	120	70					

[a]Data from Park MK, Menard SW, Yuan C: Comparison of blood pressure in children from three ethnic groups, *Am J Cardiol* 87:1305–1308, 2001.
[b]Data from Park MK, Menard SW, Schoolfield J: Oscillometric blood pressure standards for children, *Pediatr Cardiol* 26:601–607, 2005. These values were obtained by Dinamap model 8100 and in general fall between the 90th and 95th percentiles of blood pressure (prehypertension range).
[c]The 90th percentiles of systolic blood pressure (SBP) for males 14 years and older are higher than 120 mm Hg, but 120 mm Hg is listed in the table to be consistent with the definition of "elevated blood pressure" in adults.
DBP, Diastolic blood pressure.

1. The exact prevalence of primary HTN in children and adolescents is not known. It is estimated that about 60% of pediatric patients with HTN have essential HTN. Among the patients with essential HTN, 75% of them are obese. Thus, the most common cause of pediatric HTN appears to be obesity; about 10% to 30% of obese children are reported to have HTN.

2. Among patients with secondary HTN, more than 90% of the cases are caused by three conditions: renal parenchymal disease, renovascular diseases (both accounting for 70%), and coarctation of the aorta (COA) (20%). Fewer than 10% of secondary HTN cases are caused by endocrine and other disorders.

3. In newborns, the causes of HTN may include renal artery thrombosis, congenital renal malformation, and COA. Transient HTN may be found in neonates with bronchopulmonary dysplasias, which resolves when oxygenation improves.

Table 28.3 lists the common causes of sustained HTN by age group in children. Box 28.1 lists causes of secondary HTN.

Diagnosis and Workup
Steps to Confirm the Diagnosis

1. The diagnosis of HTN relies on accurate BP measurement and comparing the reading with reliable BP standards. In evaluating for possible diagnosis of HTN, it is important to remember that (a) the most common cause of high BP readings, especially of a single BP reading, in a health care facility is anxiety, called the white-coat phenomenon, and (b) BPs measured by the auscultatory and oscillometric methods are significantly different, and thus they are not interchangeable (as mentioned earlier). The following is one way of handling a case of high BP reading in the office setting.

   a. If an abnormal reading is the result of a single reading, two additional measurements should be made to help reduce the effects of anxiety associated with a visit to the doctor's office.

   b. If BP is still high, a repeat set of three readings at the end of the office visit may help identify some of the children with the white-coat phenomenon.

   c. Even if these BP readings are still high, a possibility of white-coat HTN still exists. The diagnosis of HTN should not be made until one confirms persistently elevated BP levels greater than the 95th percentile on three or more separate office visits over a period of time.

   d. One should consider ways to identify cases of white-coat HTN by measuring BPs outside the health care facility.

      1) Having reliable school nurses to take daily BP for 3 to 4 weeks may be a cost-effective way to get the same information.

      2) Home BP monitoring can be an option. For adult patients, new position papers from the United States and Europe recommend home BP monitoring as a routine part of diagnosis and management of HTN. They recommend recording an average of 2 (or 3) BP readings taken in the morning and at night for 1 week, with a total of at least 12 readings being averaged to make clinical decisions. It is reasonable to try home BP measurement in children under certain circumstances using protocol similar to the one described for adults.

Box 28.1 Causes of Secondary Hypertension

Renal

Renal parenchymal disease (34%–79% of secondary HTN)
  Glomerulonephritis, acute and chronic
  Pyelonephritis, acute and chronic
  Congenital anomalies (polycystic or dysplastic kidneys)
  Obstructive uropathies (hydronephrosis)
  Hemolytic-uremic syndrome
  Collagen disease (periarteritis, lupus)
  Renal damage from nephrotoxic medications, trauma, or radiation
Renovascular (12%–13% of secondary HTN)
  Renal artery disorders (e.g., stenosis, polyarteritis, thrombosis)
  Renal vein thrombosis

Cardiovascular

Coarctation of the aorta
Conditions with large stroke volume (PDA), aortic insufficiency, systemic AV fistula, complete heart block (these conditions cause only systolic hypertension)

Endocrine

Hyperthyroidism (systolic hypertension)
Excessive catecholamine levels
  Pheochromocytoma
  Neuroblastoma
Adrenal dysfunction
  Congenital adrenal hyperplasia
    11-β-Hydroxylase deficiency
    17-Hydroxylase deficiency
  Cushing's syndrome
  Hyperaldosteronism
    Primary
      Conn's syndrome
      Idiopathic nodular hyperplasia
      Dexamethasone-suppressible hyperaldosteronism

Secondary
  Renovascular hypertension
  Renin-producing tumor (juxtaglomerular cell tumor)
Hyperparathyroidism (and hypercalcemia)

Neurogenic

Increased intracranial pressure (any cause, especially tumors, infections, trauma)
Poliomyelitis
Guillain-Barré syndrome
Dysautonomia (Riley-Day syndrome)

Drugs and Chemicals

Sympathomimetic drugs (nose drops, cough medications, cold preparations, theophylline)
Amphetamines
Corticosteroids
NSAIDs
Oral contraceptives
Heavy-metal poisoning (mercury, lead)
Cocaine, acute or chronic use
Cyclosporine
Thyroxine
Tacrolimus

Miscellaneous

Hypervolemia and hypernatremia
Stevens-Johnson syndrome
Bronchopulmonary dysplasia (newborns)

AV, Atrioventricular; *HTN,* hypertension; *NSAID,* nonsteroidal antiinflammatory drug; *PDA,* patent ductus arteriosus.

TABLE 28.3 Common Causes of Chronic Sustained Hypertension

Age Group	Causes
Newborns	Renal artery thrombosis, renal artery stenosis, congenital renal malformation, COA, bronchopulmonary dysplasia
<6 yr	Renal parenchymal disease, COA, renal artery stenosis
6–10 yr	Renal artery stenosis, renal parenchymal disease, primary hypertension
>10 yr	Primary hypertension, renal parenchymal disease

COA, Coarctation of the aorta.
Adapted from Report of the Second Task Force on Blood Pressure Control in Children—1987. Task Force on Blood Pressure Control in Children. National Heart, Lung, and Blood Institute, Bethesda, Maryland, *Pediatrics* 79:1-25, 1987.

For home BP monitoring, the monitor should be checked for its accuracy, and the patient should be taught correct measurement technique and correct BP cuff size. Wrist monitors are not acceptable because the reading will reflect peripheral amplification of SBP. In evaluating home BP readings, one should not use BP standards by NHBPEP, which are based on the auscultatory method. One may use the oscillometric BP data from the SACBPS. Appendix B provides normative oscillometric BP values (Table B.6 for boys; Table B.7 for girls).

2. If multiple BP readings obtained outside the health care facility show persistently elevated BP levels above the 95th percentile most of the time, one could make a tentative diagnosis of HTN and proceed with initial investigation for HTN (as described later). The AAP guidelines (Flynn et al, 2017) recommend routine use of ABPM to confirm the diagnosis of HTN in children and adolescents older than 5 years of age for technical reasons. It is recommended (a) in patients with office BP measurements

TABLE 28.4 Screening Tests and Relevant Populations

Patient Population	Screening Tests
All patients	Urinalysis Chemistry panel (electrolytes, BUN, creatinine) Lipid profile, fasting or non-fasting (total cholesterol, HDL) Renal ultrasonography in those <6 yr of age or those with abnormal urinalysis or renal function
Obese (BMI >95th percentile) children and adolescents	Hemoglobin A1c AST and ALT (screen for fatty liver) Fasting lipid panel (dyslipidemia)
Optional tests to be obtained on the basis of history, physical examination, and initial studies	Fasting glucose for those at high risk for diabetes mellitus TSH Drug screen Sleep study (if found snoring, daytime sleepiness, or reported history of apnea) CBC (those with growth delay or abnormal renal function)

AST, Aspartate transaminase (formerly SGOT); ALT, alanine transaminase (formerly SGPT); BMI, body mass index; BUN, blood urea nitrogen; CBC, complete blood count; HDL, high density lipoprotein; TSH, thyroid-stimulating hormone.
From Flynn JT, Kaelber DC, Barker-Smith CM, et al: Clinical practice guideline for screening and management of high blood pressure in children and adolescents, *Pediatrics* 140(3):e20171904, 2017.

in the elevated BP category for 1 year or more or (b) in patients with stage 1 HTN over three clinic visits, and (c) in patients suspected to have "white-coat HTN." Normative ABPM data are available in Appendix B, Tables B.8 and B.9.

3. If the repeated BP measurements fall between the 90th and 95th percentiles (elevated BP), the patient should be followed on a regular basis (every 3–6 months) with repeat BP measurements.

4. When the diagnosis of HTN is established or strongly suspected:
   a. One should evaluate the history (present, past, and family), perform careful physical findings, and proceed with initial investigation to look for the cause of HTN.
   b. The initial investigation should include urinalysis, serum electrolytes, renal function tests (blood urea nitrogen [BUN], creatinine), and lipid profile (total cholesterol, high-density lipoprotein cholesterol) (Table 28.4).
   c. In overweight children, additional laboratory tests such as hemoglobin A1c, alanine transaminase, aspartate transaminase, and fasting lipid panel should be ordered.
   d. When COA is suspected, electrocardiography (ECG), chest radiography, and echocardiography are indicated.
   e. Renal ultrasonography is recommended in children younger than 6 years of age or those with abnormal urinalysis or renal function test results.

History
Past and Present History

1. Present history
   a. Most children with mild HTN are asymptomatic, and HTN is diagnosed as the result of routine BP measurement, highlighting the importance of accurate measurement of BP.
   b. Children with acute severe HTN may be symptomatic, such as that seen with acute glomerulonephritis (with headache, dizziness, nausea and vomiting, irritability, or personality changes). Occasionally, neurologic manifestations, congestive heart failure, renal dysfunction, and stroke may be the presenting symptoms.
   c. Weakness and muscle cramp from hypokalemia may be seen with primary aldosteronism.
   d. A history of palpitation, headache, and excessive sweating may suggest increased catecholamine levels.
   e. Tachycardia with systolic HTN may suggest hyperthyroidism or catecholamine excess.

2. Neonatal: use of umbilical artery catheters (a possible cause of renovascular HTN)

3. Cardiovascular: history of COA or surgery for it

4. Renal: history of obstructive uropathies; urinary tract infection; and radiation, trauma, or surgery to the kidney area

5. Medications: corticosteroids, amphetamines, antiasthmatic drugs, cold medications, oral contraceptives, nephrotoxic antibiotics (e.g., aminoglycosides, sulfonamides, amphotericin B, trimethoprim, and others), cyclosporin, cocaine use, excessive dose of thyroxin, ingestion of large quantity of licorice. (Licorice inhibits 11β-hydroxysteroid dehydrogenase with a resulting increase in cortisol levels and producing hypokalemia.)

6. Habits: smoking or consumption of excessive amount of coffee or tea

Family History

1. Essential HTN, atherosclerotic heart disease, and stroke

2. Familial or hereditary renal disease (polycystic kidney, cystinuria, familial nephritis)

Physical Examination

1. Accurate measurement of BP is essential (as described in Chapter 2).

2. Complete physical examination also is essential, with emphasis on the following.

a. Delayed growth (renal disease)

b. Bounding peripheral pulse (patent ductus arteriosus or aortic regurgitation)

c. Weak or absent femoral pulses or BP differential between the arms and legs (COA). In normal children, SBP in the lower limbs is more than 5 to 10 mm Hg higher than that in the upper limbs.

d. Abdominal bruits (renovascular)

e. Tenderness over the kidney (renal infection)

f. Children's weight status, including body mass index percentile, should be obtained because obesity is a common cause of primary HTN. Children with secondary HTN from renal diseases are rarely obese, although those with HTN from adrenocortical disorders may be obese.

Initial Investigation

1. The initial investigations should be directed toward detecting renal parenchymal disease and COA and therefore include the following (see Table 28.4).

   a. **Urinalysis.** Abnormal urinalysis with red blood cells or white blood cells suggests nephritis or infectious processes. Urine culture is indicated if urinalysis suggests infectious processes. Urinalysis is normal in essential HTN, renovascular HTN, and endocrine HTN.

   b. **Serum electrolytes.** Low potassium levels suggest aldosterone excess, either from primary aldosteronism or secondary hyperaldosteronism (including renovascular HTN). Serum electrolyte changes also occur in endocrine disorders causing HTN; hypokalemia may be seen with Cushing's syndrome or certain (not all) types of congenital adrenal hyperplasias (11-β hydroxylase deficiency and 17-hydroxylase deficiency). Hypercalcemia suggests hyperparathyroidism.

   c. **BUN and creatinine.** Abnormal values suggest renal parenchymal or renovascular disease, although renal function is usually not affected in renovascular HTN. Normal BUN and creatinine do not rule out renovascular HTN.

   d. **Uric acid level:** Uric acid level above 5.5 mg/dL was found in 89% of subjects with primary HTN, 30% of children with secondary HTN, and 0% of children with white-coat HTN and normal control participants. This finding suggests that uric acid level might have a role in the pathogenesis of primary HTN (Feig et al, 2003). Furthermore, there is independent association between uric acid level and the severity of HTN.

2. When obesity is the likely cause of HTN, metabolic aspects of risk factors should be evaluated (including fasting lipid profile, liver function test, blood glucose, and so on). Renal Doppler ultrasound adds very little in obese children. The presence of metabolic abnormalities may help in convincing patients to adopt a healthy lifestyle.

3. In a nonobese child younger than 10 years of age who has moderate to severe HTN, one should consider the possibility of renovascular HTN. History of umbilical catheterization and abdominal radiation are important clues to renovascular HTN. The following preliminary screening tests may be indicated.

   a. Renal ultrasonography and renal Doppler sonography

   b. Plasma renin activity (PRA)

4. Thyroid function test (TSH, thyroxine) may be indicated when a rapid heart rate and HTN coexist.

5. When COA is suspected, ECG, chest radiography, and echo study are indicated.

Depending on the results of the initial laboratory tests, more specialized tests have been used in the diagnosis of secondary HTN (see Specialized Studies). The decision to undertake special tests and procedures depends on the availability of and familiarity with the procedure, severity of HTN, age of the patient, and history and physical findings suggestive of a certain cause. For example:

1. Nonobese children younger than 10 years of age with sustained HTN require extensive evaluation because identifiable and potentially curable causes are more likely to be found.

2. Adolescents with mild HTN and a positive family history of essential HTN are more likely to have essential HTN, and extensive studies are not cost effective.

3. In obese children with mild HTN, renal Doppler ultrasound study does not add any clinical value.

When renovascular or renoparenchymal HTN is a possibility, nephrology consultation is indicated because most of the specialized tests belong to the domain of nephrology. Consultation with endocrinology should be obtained when endocrine disorders are suspected to be the cause of HTN.

Specialized Studies
Echocardiography

In addition to be essential in the diagnosis of COA, echocardiography is a tool to measure and follow LV target organ injury related to HTN in children.

1. The following three measurements are checked to assess LV target organ injury:

   a. LVH is defined as left ventricular (LV) mass greater than 51 g/m$^{2.7}$ (for boys or girls) or LV mass greater than 115 g per body surface area (BSA) for boys and LV mass greater than 95 g/BSA for girls.

   b. LV relative wall thickness of 0.42 cm indicates concentric geometry; LV wall thickness greater than 1.4 cm is abnormal.

   c. Decreased LV ejection fraction is a value less than 53%.

2. Repeat echo study is done to monitor improvement or progression of target organ damage at 6- to 12-month intervals.

3. In patients with no LV target organ injury at initial echo assessment, repeat echo at yearly intervals may be considered in those with suspected to have HTN.

4. Echo study may be indicated in patients with stage 2 HTN, secondary HTN, or chronic stage 1 HTN to assess for the development of worsening LV target organ injury.

Images for Renovascular Disease

The following specialized studies may be indicated for the detection of renal artery stenosis as a cause of secondary HTN.

1. Doppler renal ultrasonography may be used as a noninvasive screening study for the evaluation of possible renal

artery stenosis in normal-weight children and adolescents 8 years of age or older who are suspected of having renovascular HTN.

2. In addition, computed tomography angiography (CTA) or magnetic resonance angiography (MRA) may be used to investigate renal artery stenosis.

Specialized Chemistries

1. Peripheral PRA is a useful screening test for renal cause of HTN. Whereas elevated value (high-renin HTN) suggests renal parenchymal or renovascular diseases, a suppressed value (low-renin HTN) suggests excess mineralocorticoid effects such as seen with hyperaldosteronism. The usefulness of captopril-stimulated PRA is controversial at best.

2. PRA in blood collected from both renal veins and the inferior vena cava at the time of angiography is helpful in diagnosing unilateral or bilateral kidney disease.

3. Aldosterone levels in serum and urine is indicated in patients with hypokalemia for possible hyperaldosteronism.
    a. High plasma aldosterone levels seen in primary aldosteronism are caused by a benign adrenal adenoma (Conn's syndrome) or bilateral idiopathic adrenal hyperplasia.
    b. Secondary hyperaldosteronism is caused by overactivity of the renin–angiotensin system. Examples of secondary hyperaldosteronism include juxtaglomerular cell tumor and renal artery stenosis (which increases renin levels). Other conditions, such as liver cirrhosis, heart failure, nephrotic syndrome, or a very low-sodium diet, may also increase aldosterone levels.

4. Twenty-four-hour urine collection for catecholamine levels and their metabolites (metanephrine, normetanephrine, and vanillylmandelic acid [VMA]) is indicated when a catecholamine-secreting tumor (e.g., pheochromocytoma, neuroblastoma) is suspected. Collection of urine for 24 hours is preferable to plasma for detection of increased levels of catecholamines or their metabolites because plasma levels of these fluctuate throughout the day.

5. Twenty-four-hour urine collection for free cortisol and 17-ketosteroid. The former is elevated in Cushing syndrome, and the latter is elevated in congenital adrenal hyperplasia (adrenogenital syndrome).

MANAGEMENT OF ESSENTIAL HYPERTENSION

Nonpharmacologic Intervention

Nonpharmacologic intervention should be started as an initial treatment. Counseling should encourage weight reduction if the patient is overweight or obese, healthful diets, low-salt (and potassium-rich) foods, regular aerobic exercise, and avoidance of smoking and oral contraceptives.

Pharmacologic Intervention

Drug therapy is not recommended initially. Drugs are used when nonpharmacologic approaches have not been found to be effective because the possible adverse effects of long-term drug therapy on growing children have not been evaluated adequately and because many antihypertensive agents have side effects.

Indications for Drug Therapy

There are no clear guidelines for identifying those who should be treated with antihypertensive drugs. However, based on the recent AAP guidelines (Flynn et al, 2017) and other recommendations, the following are generally considered indications for initiating antihypertensive drug therapy in children.

1. Severe symptomatic HTN (should be treated with intravenous antihypertensive medications initially)
2. Persistent HTN despite a trial of lifestyle modification
3. Symptomatic HTN
4. Stage 2 HTN without clearly modifiable factor (e.g., obesity)
5. Any stage of HTN associated with renovascular and renoparenchymal disease or diabetes
6. Hypertensive target-organ damage: LVH, increased LV mass, and so on
7. Family history of early complications of HTN
8. Child who has dyslipidemia and other coronary artery risk factors

End-Organ Damage

The most reliable evidence of end-organ damage at this time appears to be the presence of LVH evidenced by echocardiographic studies.

1. Increased LV mass by echocardiography may be an indication of LVH, but the values are not very reproducible, and controversies exist as to how to express LV mass (i.e., by 2.7 power of height or by BSA). Normal M-mode–derived LV mass data indexed by 2.7 power of height are available in Table D.7 in Appendix D. Normal two-dimensional echo-derived LV mass data indexed by BSA are shown in Table D.8.
2. Other valuable markers of end-organ damage include carotid intima-media thickening and urinary albumin excretion. Although these are frequently used in evaluation of adult HTN, they are infrequently used in the evaluation of pediatric HTN. Carotid intima-media thickening is nonspecific and is also seen in children with familial hypercholesterolemia and obesity. Urinary albumin excretion is a sign of HTN-related renal damage.

The Choice of Drug

Recent studies in adults suggest that beta-blockers are not as effective as other classes of antihypertensive agents. European studies have shown superiority of calcium channel blockers (CCBs) over beta-blockers in lowering BP. Other studies have found that angiotensin-converting enzyme (ACE) inhibitors or angiotensin receptor blockers (ARBs) are definitely better than diuretics and are as effective as CCBs. Currently, many adult cardiologists strongly favor using ACE inhibitors (or ARBs) or CCBs as the choice of initial therapy in adult patients with HTN.

Most pediatric cardiologists now recommend ACE inhibitors (or ARBs), CCBs, and possibly thiazide diuretics as the initial drugs for treatment of HTN in children and adolescents. Beta-blockers are not recommended as initial treatment in children. Besides, diuretics and beta-blockers tend to raise blood glucose levels. Because ACE inhibitors and ARBs are contraindicated in pregnancy, CCBs may be a better choice for female adolescents with HTN.

1. For children and adolescents with HTN and chronic renal disease, proteinuria, or diabetes mellitus, an ACE inhibitor or ARB is recommended as the initial therapeutic agent because they also have renoprotective effects.
2. For overweight patients at risk of developing diabetes, ACE inhibitors, ARBs, and CCBs are preferable to beta-blockers and diuretics. Besides, diuretics and beta-blockers tend to raise blood glucose levels.
3. African American children do not show as robust a response to ACE inhibitors, so CCBs appear to be a better choice for African Americans.
4. Adolescent males with primary HTN
   a. ACE inhibitors or ARBs. These agents alone or in combination with a CCB (e.g., Lotrel, the combination of amlodipine and benazepril) are a good choice in obese children with high glucose and triglyceride levels.
   b. CCBs are equally good as ACE inhibitors as the initial antihypertensive agent.
   c. ACE inhibitors + diuretic are a good combination because diuretics enhance ACE inhibitors' effects. However, this combination is not recommended in

obese patients with acanthosis nigricans because it could cause diabetes.

5. Female adolescents or childbearing age women with primary HTN
   a. CCBs (e.g., amlodipine [Norvasc] or extended-release nifedipine) are good choices in women because they lack teratogenic effects. ACE inhibitors and ARBs are known teratogens in pregnancy.
   b. Diuretics or beta-blockers are probably safe. However, blood glucose level should be checked regularly because they raise glucose levels.
   c. ACE inhibitors or ARBs should not be used in female adolescents because they are known teratogens. If a patient becomes pregnant, the drug should be discontinued; it may be resumed at the end of the third trimester if needed.
6. Coexisting conditions. The choice of initial therapy has been influenced by other conditions that frequently coexist with HTN. Preferences, contraindications, and side effects of different classes of antihypertensive agents are summarized in Table 28.5, which may help in choosing the drug for initial therapy. Most of the information has been derived from adult experiences.
   a. Migraine patients: Beta-blockers or CCBs are preferred. Beta-blockers appear to be more effective in prevention of migraines than CCBs.

TABLE 28.5 Classes of Antihypertensive Agents: Preferences, Contraindications, and Side Effects

Drug Classes	Preferred In	Contraindicated In (Not to Use In)	Adverse Effects
Thiazide diuretics	Asthma (±)	*Do not use in:* Diabetic or prediabetic (increases glucose level)	Hypokalemia, hyponatremia (±) May increase glucose May increase uric acid
Beta-blockers	Migraine Hyperthyroidism Hyperdynamic hypertension Coarctation of the aorta	*Contraindicated in:* Asthma and diabetes *Not to use in:* Prediabetic patients	Increases glucose Increases triglycerides Rarely hypoglycemia
Angiotensin-converting inhibitors	Male adolescents Diabetic or prediabetic Obese males (may be used in combination with the CCB Lotrel) Renal failure	*Contraindicated in:* Pregnancy (because of teratogenic effects) *Do not use in:* Childbearing aged women Patients with asthma (can cause cough)	Hyperkalemia Azotemia Angioedema Dry cough Rash, loss of taste, and leukopenia
Angiotensin receptor blockers	Male adolescents Diabetic or prediabetic Renal failure	*Contraindicated in:* Pregnancy (because of teratogenic effects) *Do not use in:* Childbearing aged women	Angioedema rarely (but no cough)
Calcium channel blockers	Female adolescents Male adolescents African Americans Migraine Asthma Renal failure	*Contraindicated in:* Heart block	Occasional headache, flushing, ankle edema

CCB, Calcium channel blocker.

b. Patients with asthma: CCBs may be the drug of first choice. ARBs and diuretics may work well. ACE inhibitors may cause persistent dry cough in 10% of 20% of patients with asthma, and this may possibly cause bronchospasm. Beta-blockers are contraindicated in patients with asthma because they may cause bronchospasm.

c. Hyperthyroidism or hyperdynamic HTN with fast heart rates: Beta-blockers are preferred. Beta-blockers are used as treatment adjuncts in hyperthyroidism.

d. Patients with diabetes: ACE inhibitors or ARBs are preferred. Thiazide diuretics or beta blockers should not be used because they increase blood glucose levels.

e. Renal failure: CCBs or ACE inhibitors are preferred.

The goal of the treatment is to lower BP levels to below the 90th percentile. Lifestyle modification should be continued while the patient is on pharmacologic therapy. After the most appropriate agent for initial therapy has been selected, a relatively small dose of a single drug should be started. The dose of the initial medication can be increased every 2 to 4 weeks until BP is controlled (e.g., <90th percentile), the maximal dose is reached, or adverse effects occur. If the first drug is not effective, a second drug may be added to, or substituted for, the first drug, starting with a small dose and proceeding to a full dose. In many situations, however, more than one drug is needed to control severely elevated BPs like those seen in patients with renal disease, and thus starting with a combination of two drugs from classes with complementary mechanism of action may be acceptable. A single daily dose of a long-acting agent improves adherence to the medication. Long-acting preparations are available within each class of antihypertensive drugs. Table 28.6 shows the dosage of antihypertensive drugs for children.

Classes of Antihypertensive Drugs
Diuretics

Diuretics are the oldest class of antihypertensive drugs.

1. The thiazide diuretics (hydrochlorothiazide and chlorthalidone) have the longest history of being used in the treatment of HTN, sometimes in combination with a potassium-sparing diuretic. The action of thiazide diuretics is related to a decrease in extracellular and plasma

TABLE 28.6 Oral Dosages of Selected Antihypertensive Drugs for Children

Drugs	Initial Dose	Times/Day
Angiotensin-Converting Enzyme Inhibitors		
Captopril (Capoten)	0.3–0.5 mg/kg/dose (maximum, 6 mg/kg/day)	3
Enalapril (Vasotec)	0.08 mg/kg/day up to 5 mg/day (maximum, 0.6 mg/kg/day up to 40 mg/day)	1–2
	Adults: 2.5–5 mg (maximum, 40 mg/day)	
Lisinopril (Zestril, Prinivil)	0.07 mg/kg/day up to 5 mg/day (maximum, 0.6 mg/kg/day up to 40 mg/day)	1
	Adults: 10 mg (maximum, 80 mg/day)	
Angiotensin Receptor Blocker		
Losartan (Cozaar)	0.7 mg/kg/day up to 50 mg/day (maximum, 1.4 mg/kg/day up to 100 mg/day)	1
	Adults: 50 mg (maximum, 100 mg/day)	
Calcium Channel Blockers		
Amlodipine (Norvasc)	6–17 yr: 2.5–5 mg/day	1
	Adults: 5–10 mg (maximum, 10 mg/24 hr)	
Isradipine (DynaCirc)	0.15–0.2 mg/kg/day (maximum, 0.8 mg/kg/day up to 20 mg/day	3–4
Diuretics		
Hydrochlorothiazide (HydroDIURIL)	1 mg/kg/day (maximum, 3 mg/kg/day up to 50 mg/day)	1
	Adults: 25-100mg	
Chlorthalidone	0.3 mg/kg/day (maximum, 2 mg/kg/day up to 50 mg/day)	1
	Adults: 12.5–25 mg	
Furosemide (Lasix)	0.5–2 mg/kg/dose (maximum, 6 mg/kg/day)	1–2
Spironolactone (Aldactone)	1 mg/kg/day (maximum, 3.3 mg/kg/day up to 100 mg/day)	1–2
Triamterene (Dyrenium)	1–2 mg/kg/day (maximum, 3-4 mg/kg/day up to 300 mg/day)	2
Adrenergic Inhibitors		
Propranolol (Inderal)	1–2 mg/kg/day (maximum, 4 mg/kg/day up to 640 mg/day)	2–3
Metoprolol (Lopressor)	1–2 mg/kg/day (maximum, 6 mg/kg/day up to 200 mg/day)	2
Atenolol (Tenormin)	0.5–1 mg/kg/day (maximum, 2 mg/kg/day up to 100 mg/day)	1–2
Direct-Acting Vasodilators		
Hydralazine (Apresoline)	0.75 mg/kg/day (maximum, 7.5 mg/kg/day up to 200 mg/day)	4
Minoxidil (Loniten)	>12 yr: 5 mg/day (maximum, 100 mg/day)	1–3

Modified from The fourth Report on the Diagnosis, Evaluation, and Treatment of High Blood Pressure in Children and Adolescents, *Pediatrics* 114:555–576, 2004.

volume initially, and later the action is related to a decline in peripheral resistance. An important side effect of thiazide diuretics in children is hypokalemia, occasionally requiring potassium supplementation in the diet or as potassium salt. They may also increase glucose, insulin, and cholesterol levels. One should check serum electrolytes and glucose levels initially and periodically.

2. Aldosterone antagonists (or aldosterone receptor blockers), such as spironolactone, are weak potassium-sparing diuretics. Spironolactone antagonizes the action of aldosterone at mineralocorticoid receptors, with resulting inhibition of sodium resorption in the collecting duct of the nephron in the kidneys (by interfering with Na/K exchange with reduction of urinary potassium loss). This group of drugs is often used as adjunctive therapy, in combination with other drugs, for the management of chronic heart failure. They are also used in the management of hyperaldosteronism (including Conn's syndrome).

3. Sodium channel blockers, such as triamterene (Dyrenium) and amiloride, are potassium-sparing diuretics used in combination with thiazide diuretics for the treatment of HTN and edema. They directly block the epithelial sodium channel on the lumen side of the collecting tubule. Potassium-sparing diuretics (spironolactone, triamterene) may cause hyperkalemia, especially if given with ACE inhibitors or ARBs.

Adrenergic Inhibitors

The mechanism of action of beta-blockers is not fully understood. It may involve suppressing cardiac contractility, decreasing systemic vascular resistance, or suppressing the renin–angiotensin system. Beta-blockers appear to be less effective than other classes of antihypertensives. β-Adrenergic blockers are contraindicated in patients with asthma (because of bronchospasm) and diabetes mellitus (because of hyperglycemic effects). Propranolol (Inderal) is a short-acting form requiring dosing three times a day. Atenolol (Tenormin) has the advantage of being a longer acting beta-blocker requiring only a single daily dose.

Angiotensin-Converting Enzyme Inhibitors

Captopril is a short-acting ACE inhibitor widely used in the treatment of pediatric HTN. Enalapril and lisinopril are long-acting ACE inhibitors that have also been shown to be effective in children with HTN. A diuretic clearly enhances the effectiveness of ACE inhibitors. Side effects of ACE inhibitors include rash, loss of taste, and leukopenia. Occasional side effects include cough, angioedema, hyperkalemia, and azotemia. If cough appears, an ARB may be used. ACE inhibitors are contraindicated in pregnancy because of their known teratogenic effects. Serum electrolytes and creatinine should be checked for hyperkalemia and azotemia.

Angiotensin Receptor Blockers

Angiotensin receptor blockers are a new class of antihypertensive agents that act by displacing angiotensin II from its receptor, antagonizing all of angiotensin's known effects with

a resulting decrease in peripheral resistance. Cough is not a side effect, although angioedema can occur.

Calcium Channel Blockers

Calcium channel blockers are being used increasingly in the treatment of adult HTN. Nifedipine has the greatest peripheral vasodilatory action, with little effect on cardiac automaticity, conduction, or contractility. Concomitant dietary sodium restriction or the use of a diuretic agent may not be necessary because calcium antagonists cause natriuresis by producing renal vasodilatation. Recently, the safety and efficacy of amlodipine (Norvasc) have been reported for children with various forms of HTN (Flynn et al, 2004). Occasional side effects include headache, flushing, and local ankle edema.

Vasodilators

Hydralazine (Apresoline), a direct-acting vasodilator, is popular in the treatment of acute HTN in children. When used alone, it produces side effects related to increased cardiac output (flushing, headache, tachycardia, palpitation) and salt retention. Therefore, the concomitant use of a β-adrenergic blocker and a diuretic is recommended. Hydralazine can cause lupus-like syndrome. Minoxidil, a less commonly used vasodilator, can cause hypertrichosis when used on a chronic basis.

Follow-up Evaluation of Patients with Chronic Hypertension

1. Follow-up examinations should include ongoing monitoring of BP levels, target-organ damage, periodic serum electrolyte determination in children treated with ACE inhibitors or diuretics, counseling regarding other cardiovascular risk factors, and adherence with a newly adopted healthy lifestyle.
2. Goals of treatment
   a. For children with uncomplicated primary HTN without hypertensive end-organ damage, the goal of the treatment is reduction of BP to below the 95th percentile.
   b. For children with chronic renal disease, diabetes, or hypertensive target organ damage, the goal is reduction of BP to below the 90th percentile.
3. A "step-down" therapy or cessation of therapy may be considered in selected patients with uncomplicated primary HTN that is well under control, especially overweight children who successfully lose weight. Such patients require ongoing follow-up of their BP levels and their weight status.

White-Coat Hypertension

White-coat HTN is defined as persistent HTN in a health care facility with concomitant normal BP during usual daily life. The prevalence of white-coat HTN in children and adolescents is estimated to be about 30% to 50%.

White-coat HTN may not be as benign as it was once thought to be. Several recent studies in adults and children suggest that about 30% to 40% of patients with white-coat HTN spontaneously evolve into having HTN with accompanying end-organ damage (e.g., increase in LV mass or increase in carotid intima-media thickness). Thus, white-coat

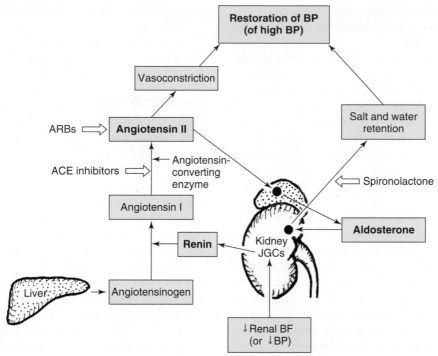

Fig. 28.1 The renin–angiotensin–aldosterone system. When the system is activated, high levels of angiotensin II and aldosterone result. Angiotensin II constricts vascular structure with resulting increase in blood pressure. Aldosterone retains sodium and water, thereby helping to maintain elevated blood pressure. The sites of action of antihypertensive agents used in this condition are shown with *open arrows. ARB,* Angiotensin receptor blockers; *ACE,* angiotensin-converting enzyme; *BF,* blood flow; *BP,* blood pressure; *JGCs,* juxtaglomerular cells.

HTN can be considered a prehypertension. Therefore, it is important to identify individuals with white-coat HTN before labeling them as hypertensive or dismissing them as normotensive. Patients with white-coat HTN should be followed up on a regular basis.

How are individuals with white-coat HTN identified, and how should they be followed? One needs a reliable way of accurately measuring BP outside of health care facilities. There are a few ways of identifying patients with white-coat HTN.

1. Twenty-four-hour ambulatory BP measurements provide reliable BP readings outside the doctor's office. The ambulatory BP values can then be compared with available ABP standards, such as those reported by Wühl and colleagues (2002), which provide both the 90th and 95th percentiles (see Table B.8 and B.9). It is noteworthy that the left ventricular mass index (LVMI) correlates well with ambulatory SBPs only but not well with ambulatory diastolic pressures or clinic BPs (Sorof et al, 2002). Ambulatory diastolic BP does not change much with increasing age. Drawbacks of ambulatory BP are that it is costly and reflects BP changes for only 1 day, but there are day-to-day variations in BP readings.

2. Another way of getting BP readings outside the doctor's office is by having reliable outside persons, such as school nurses, take daily BP measurements for 3 to 4 weeks. One then examines the overall distribution of BP readings and compares them with clinic BP readings as well as with normative BP standards to see if the readings are in the hypertensive range.

3. Home BP monitoring with an oscillometric device is controversial because the accuracy of many commercially available BP measuring devices is questionable. Besides, those that take BP on the wrist are more likely to cause confusion than solving the problem because of the well-known peripheral amplification of SBP (discussed in depth in Chapter 2). Physicians should never recommend or use the wrist device.

Secondary Hypertension

Among patients with secondary HTN, more than 90% of the cases of secondary HTN are caused by chronic renal disease, renovascular diseases, and COA. The remaining 10% of cases are caused by other diseases and conditions listed in Box 28.1. In this section, renovascular HTN and pheochromocytoma are discussed in some detail. Management of HTN caused by COA is discussed in Chapter 13.

Renovascular Hypertension

Renovascular HTN results from a lesion that impairs blood flow to a part or all of one or both kidneys. It is the second most common cause of correctable secondary HTN, second only to COA. It accounts for 3% to 10% of children with HTN.

Pathogenesis of Renovascular Hypertension. The renin–angiotensin–aldosterone system (RAAS) is involved in the pathogenesis of renovascular HTN. Angiotensin and aldosterone together influence arterial pressure and sodium and the water content of the body. Therefore, knowledge of the RAAS is essential in the management of patients with renovascular HTN by using such drugs as ACE inhibitors, ARBs, and aldosterone antagonists (Fig. 28.1).

Renin is stored and released from juxtaglomerular cells associated with the afferent arteriole entering the glomerulus. Renin release from the juxtaglomerular cells of the kidney is stimulated by a reduction in BP in the afferent arteriole, such as seen with renal artery stenosis or systemic hypotension, whereas its release is inhibited by increased BP. Renin causes the cleavage of angiotensinogen in circulation to form angiotensin I, which has no known biological activity. Angiotensin I is further broken down to angiotensin II by ACE. Angiotensin II is a potent vasoconstrictor, constricting arteries and veins and increasing BP. Angiotensin II acts on the adrenal cortex to stimulate the secretion of aldosterone. Aldosterone in turn acts on the kidneys to increase the reabsorption of sodium and fluid retention, which may help sustain BP and lead to secondary suppression of renin release. Aldosterone also stimulates the excretion of potassium in the distal tubule with resulting hypokalemia. Thus, the end results of the activation of the RAAS are an increase in BP (primarily by angiotensin II) and retention of sodium and water (by aldosterone); the latter helps sustain elevated BP. This is the pathogenesis of HTN seen in patients with renal artery stenosis. Aldosterone retains Na but increases K excretion, with resulting hypokalemia.

Causes

1. Fibromuscular dysplasia is the most common cause of renovascular HTN, accounting for up to 70% of the patients, in whom the media of the arterial wall is primarily affected. If the intima is most affected, the term *intimal hyperplasia* is used, which shows a "string of beads" appearance on angiography.
2. Rarely, renal artery stenosis is also seen in other systemic or inherited conditions, including Williams' syndrome, Marfan's syndrome, Kawasaki's disease, and Takayasu's disease; after neonatal renal artery thrombosis; as a sequela to abdominal radiation; and after renal transplantation.

Clinical Manifestations

Many children with renovascular HTN are asymptomatic, and when symptoms are present, they are frequently nonspecific. However, when any or some of the following are found on workup, one should consider a possibility of renovascular HTN.

1. Young age, usually younger than 10 years of age
2. History of umbilical catheterization in the newborn period or history of abdominal irradiation
3. Serum electrolyte abnormalities, notably hypokalemia, but occasionally hyponatremia may also be found. However, an absence of electrolyte abnormalities does not preclude the possibility of severe renovascular HTN.
4. Some normal children may have abdominal bruit.
5. Severe HTN or worsening of HTN refractory to medical treatment. However, HTN is not always severe in renovascular HTN.

6. Unexplained impaired renal function in the presence of HTN
7. Unequal kidney size on renal ultrasonography or any other clinical study. The affected kidney is usually is smaller.
8. Rarely, polyuria and polydipsia may be present.

Diagnostic Workup

When renovascular HTN is a possible cause, one generally needs most of the investigations listed earlier (see Table 28.4) except for endocrine tests.

1. BUN and creatinine are usually normal in renovascular HTN unless there is severe renal artery involvement or accelerated HTN.
2. There may be some hypokalemia caused by secondary hyperaldosteronism.
3. It is common to find a normal size and shape of the kidneys in renal ultrasonography.
4. PRA is increased in most (but not all) cases of patients with renovascular disease or pyelonephritic scarring. ACE inhibitors stimulate PRA selectively in patients with renovascular HTN ("captopril-stimulated PRA test"), but the specificity of the test is controversial. Low PRA in a hypertensive child suggests mineralocorticoid excess or a salt and water overload for other reasons.
5. Renal vein renin measurement is an important diagnostic procedure and helps in identifying surgically curable forms of renal HTN.
6. Doppler ultrasonography, CTA, and MRA are safe tests with high sensitivity and specificity for renovascular HTN. However, renal arteriography is still considered the gold standard for the diagnosis of renovascular HTN. The procedure is mandatory if surgical or transluminal angioplasty is being considered.

Management

1. While waiting for intervention, antihypertensive medication should be started to lower the BP.
   a. ACE inhibitors are most effective, which minimizes the ischemia-induced rise in the angiotensin production. One needs to closely monitor renal function because ACE inhibitors can cause a drop in the glomerular filtration rate. ARBs may be equally effective.
   b. CCBs provide control of HTN in patients with less impaired function of the ischemic kidney. They may have beneficial long-term effects, but this remains uncertain.
2. Restoration of adequate renal blood flow can be accomplished by percutaneous transluminal angioplasty with or without stenting. This is a relatively safe procedure with a success rate up to 90%.
3. Surgical revascularization by using bypass graft may be performed. However, the widespread nature of the disease in children will not offer a benefit to many children. In adults, surgical revascularization was found to offer better long-term results than endovascular revascularization (Ham et al, 2010).

TABLE 28.7	Curable Forms of Systemic Hypertension
Organ or System	**Diseases or Conditions**
Renal	Unilateral kidney disease (pyelonephritis, hydronephrosis, traumatic damage, radiation nephritis, hypoplastic kidney)
	Wilms' and other kidney tumors
Cardiovascular	Coarctation of the aorta
	Renal artery abnormalities (e.g., stenosis, aneurysm, fibromuscular dysplasia, thrombosis)
Adrenal	Pheochromocytoma and neuroblastoma
	Cushing's syndrome (caused by adrenocortical or pituitary tumor)
	Primary aldosteronism
Miscellaneous	Glucocorticoid therapy
	Oral contraceptives
	Hyperthyroidism

Pheochromocytoma

Pheochromocytoma is a catecholamine-secreting tumor that arises from chromaffin cells. The most common site of the tumor is the adrenal medulla, but it can occur anywhere along the abdominal sympathetic chain. It may be inherited as an autosomal dominant trait.

Hypertension results from excess secretion of norepinephrine and epinephrine. Paroxysmal HTN typically suggests the disease, but HTN in children is usually more sustained than paroxysmal. During attacks, the patient complains of headache, palpitation, abdominal pain, dizziness, vomiting, pallor, and sweating. Convulsion and other manifestations of hypertensive emergency may occur. Because of hypermetabolism, growth failure is striking, with frequent polydipsia and polyuria. BP may rise to 180 to 220 mm Hg.

The diagnosis is made by demonstration of increased levels of blood and urine catecholamines and their metabolites. Urinary excretion of VMA and metanephrine is increased. Adrenal tumors are easily detected by sonography, computed tomography scan, or magnetic resonance imaging, and they are often bilateral. However, in children, it often occurs in extraadrenal sites and in multiple sites; thus, it may be difficult to detect and remove all tumors. Removal of these tumors results in cure, but the operation is very high risk. Preoperative α- and β-adrenergic blockade and fluid loading are required.

Management of Other Forms of Secondary Hypertension

Treatment of secondary HTN should be aimed at removing the cause of HTN whenever possible. Table 28.7 lists curable causes of systemic HTN.

Cardiovascular Causes. Hypertension caused by mild coarctation is treated with beta-blockers. Surgical or catheter interventional correction may be indicated for COA.

Renal Parenchymal Disease. In nephritis, medical management should be instituted to lower BP in the same manner as has been discussed for essential HTN. Salt restriction, avoidance of excessive fluid intake, and antihypertensive drug therapy can control HTN caused by most renal parenchymal diseases. Concomitant antibiotic therapy for infectious processes and general supportive measures may be indicated, depending on the nature of the renal disease. If HTN is difficult to control and the disease is unilateral, unilateral nephrectomy may be considered.

Renovascular Disease. Renovascular disease may be cured by successful renal artery balloon angioplasty or surgery, such as reconstruction of a stenotic renal artery, autotransplantation, or unilateral nephrectomy (as discussed earlier). Further discussion of this topic follows.

Adrenal Glands. Hyperaldosteronism caused by bilateral adrenal hyperplasia is treated with a mineralocorticoid antagonist, such as spironolactone or eplerenone. HTN caused by tumors that secrete vasoactive substances, such as pheochromocytoma and neuroblastoma, is treated primarily by surgery.

29

Pulmonary Hypertension

DEFINITION

When measured directly in the cardiac catheterization laboratory, the normal pulmonary artery (PA) systolic pressure of children and adults is 30 mm Hg or less, and the mean PA pressure is 25 mm Hg or less. A diagnosis of pulmonary hypertension can be made when the mean PA pressure is 25 mm Hg or greater in a resting individual older than 3 months of age at sea level. The PA pressure is higher at high elevations. There is a wide range of severity in pulmonary hypertension (PH); in some, it reaches or surpasses the systemic pressure. The status of PH also varies; in some, it is static, and in others, it is dynamic.

CAUSES

Pulmonary hypertension is a group of conditions with multiple causes rather than a single one. Pathogenesis and management differ among entities. Box. 29.1 lists, according to pathogenesis, conditions that cause PH of a temporary or permanent, acute or chronic nature.

The causes of PH can be grouped into the following five. Some oversimplification is inevitable in dividing this diverse group into five categories.
1. Increased pulmonary blood flow (PBF) seen in congenital heart diseases (CHDs) with large left-to-right shunts (hyperkinetic PH)
2. Alveolar hypoxia
3. Increased pulmonary venous pressure

4. Primary pulmonary vascular disease
5. Other diseases that involves pulmonary parenchyma or pulmonary vasculature, directly or indirectly

PHYSIOLOGY OF THE PULMONARY CIRCULATION

The basics of physiology of pulmonary circulation and pulmonary vascular responses are summarized below for a quick review.
1. Vascular endothelium
Normally, balanced release of vasodilators and vasoconstrictors by endothelial cells is a key factor in the regulation of the pulmonary vascular tone. Three endothelium signaling cascades are known: (1) the nitric oxide–cyclic guanosine monophosphate (NO–cGMP) cascade, (2) prostanoids, and (3) endothelin-1 (ET-1). The most widely used drug therapy of PH works by altering one of these signaling cascades (see Management).
  a. **The NO-cGMP cascade.** NO, a vasodilator, is produced in the vascular endothelium by the enzyme endothelial NO synthase from the precursor L-arginine. Once formed, NO diffuses into the adjacent smooth muscle cell and produces cGMP (by activation of guanylate cyclase), which results in smooth muscle relaxation. cGMP is broken down by a family of phosphodiesterases (PDEs), which is prominent in the pulmonary circulation. Blocking breakdown of cGMP (by PDE type 5 [PDE-5] inhibitors) helps maintain vasodilation.

BOX. 29.1 Causes of Pulmonary Hypertension

1. Large left-to-right shunt lesions (hyperkinetic pulmonary hypertension): ventricular septal defect, patent ductus arteriosus, endocardial cushion defect
2. Alveolar hypoxia
   a. Pulmonary parenchymal disease
      (1) Extensive pneumonia
      (2) Hypoplasia of the lungs (primary or secondary, such as that seen in diaphragmatic hernia)
      (3) Bronchopulmonary dysplasia
      (4) Interstitial lung disease (Hamman-Rich syndrome)
      (5) Wilson-Mikity syndrome
   b. Airway obstruction
      (1) Upper airway obstruction (large tonsils, macroglossia, micrognathia, laryngotracheomalacia, sleep-disordered breathing)
      (2) Lower airway obstruction (bronchial asthma, cystic fibrosis)
   c. Inadequate ventilatory drive (central nervous system diseases, obesity hypoventilation syndrome)
   d. Disorders of chest wall or respiratory muscles
      (1) Kyphoscoliosis
      (2) Weakening or paralysis of skeletal muscle
   e. High altitude (in certain hyperreactors)
3. Pulmonary venous hypertension: mitral stenosis, cor triatriatum, total anomalous pulmonary venous return with obstruction, chronic left heart failure, left-sided obstructive lesions (aortic stenosis, coarctation of the aorta); rarely, congenital pulmonary vein stenosis causes incurable pulmonary hypertension.
4. Primary pulmonary vascular disease
   a. Persistent pulmonary hypertension of the newborn
   b. Primary pulmonary hypertension (rare, fatal form of pulmonary hypertension with obscure cause)
5. Other diseases that involve pulmonary parenchyma or pulmonary vasculature, directly or indirectly
   a. Thromboembolism: ventriculoatrial shunt for hydrocephalus, sickle cell anemia, thrombophlebitis
   b. Connective tissue disease: scleroderma, systemic lupus erythematosus, mixed connective tissue disease, dermatomyositis, rheumatoid arthritis
   c. Disorders directly affecting the pulmonary vasculature: schistosomiasis, sarcoidosis, histiocytosis X
   d. Portal hypertension (hepatopulmonary syndrome)
   e. HIV infection

---

b. **Prostanoids.** Arachidonic acid metabolism within vascular endothelial cells results in the production of prostaglandin I_2 (PGI_2 or prostacyclin) and thromboxane (TXA_2). PGI_2 is a vasodilator, and TXA_2 is a vasoconstrictor.

c. **ET-1**, the dominant isoform of endothelin (ET), is produced by vascular endothelial cells. ET-1 is a potent vasoconstrictor. (ET receptor antagonists produce vasodilation.)

2. The lung is unique in its response to hypoxia. Alveolar oxygen tension in the alveolar capillary region is the major physiologic determinant of pulmonary arteriolar tone.

Alveolar hypoxia causes vasoconstriction in the lungs. In all other tissues, hypoxia causes vasodilation. In hypoxia-induced vasoconstriction, NO production is reduced, and ET production is increased. High altitude (with low alveolar oxygen tension) is associated with pulmonary vasoconstriction (and PH) of varying degrees. There is a large species and individual variation in the reactivity of the PAs to low alveolar oxygen tension.

3. Pulmonary vascular resistance (PVR) is primarily determined by the cross-sectional area of small muscular arteries and arterioles. With stenosis or thrombosis of the pulmonary arteries, PVR will increase. Other determinants of PVR include blood viscosity, total mass of the lungs (pneumonectomy or hypoplasia), and extramural compression on the vessels. Normal PVR is 1 Wood unit (or 67 ± 23 standard deviation dyne x sec x cm^{-5}), which is one 10th of systemic vascular resistance.

4. With exercise, a large increase in PBF is accomplished by only a small increase in PA pressure because of recruitment of near collapsed capillaries. The increase in the left atrial (LA) pressure appears to account for most of the increase in PA pressure.

PATHOGENESIS OF PULMONARY HYPERTENSION

Pressure (P) is related to both flow (F) and vascular resistance (R), as shown in the following formula:

$$P = F \times R$$

An increase in flow, vascular resistance, or both can result in PH. Regardless of its cause, PH eventually involves constriction of the pulmonary arterioles, resulting in an increase in PVR and hypertrophy of the right ventricle (RV).

The pathogenesis of PH is discussed according to the (first four) general categories of causes because they are distinctly different from each other.

Hyperkinetic Pulmonary Hypertension

Pulmonary hypertension associated with large left-to-right shunt lesions, such as ventricular septal defect (VSD), patent ductus arteriosus (PDA), is called *hyperkinetic pulmonary hypertension*. It is the result of an increase in PBF, a direct transmission of the systemic pressure to the PA, and an increase in PVR by compensatory pulmonary vasoconstriction. If no vasoconstriction occurs, the increase in PBF will be much larger, and an intractable congestive heart failure (CHF) will result. Defects in the vasodilation machinery of the endothelial cell, such as overproduction of vasoconstrictor elements, have been implicated in this form of PH. Hyperkinetic PH is usually reversible if the cause is eliminated before permanent changes occur in the pulmonary arterioles (see later section).

If large left-to-right shunt lesions (e.g., VSD, PDA, complete atrioventricular [AV] canal) are left untreated, irreversible changes take place in the pulmonary vascular bed, with severe PH and cyanosis caused by a reversal of the left-to-right shunt. This stage is called Eisenmenger's syndrome or pulmonary vascular obstructive disease (PVOD). Surgical correction is not possible at this stage. The time of onset of PVOD varies, ranging from infancy to adulthood, but the majority of patients develop PVOD during late childhood or early adolescence. It develops even later in patients with atrial septal defect. Many patients with uncorrected transposition of the great arteries begin to develop PVOD within the first year of life for reasons not entirely clear. Children with Down syndrome with large left-to-right shunt lesions tend to develop PVOD much earlier than normal children with similar lesions.

Alveolar Hypoxia

An acute or chronic reduction in the oxygen tension (Po_2) in the alveolar capillary region (alveolar hypoxia) elicits a strong pulmonary vasoconstrictor response, which may be augmented by acidosis. The mechanisms of the pulmonary vasoconstrictor response to alveolar hypoxia is not completely understood, but our current understanding is that the vascular endothelium releases two important vasoactive substances, ET and NO. ET is a vasoconstrictor, and NO is a vasodilator. Normally, balanced release of NO and ET by endothelial cells regulates the pulmonary circulation.

Whereas a reduction in NO production occurs in chronically hypoxic animals, prolonged inhalation of NO attenuates hypoxic pulmonary vasoconstriction and vascular remodeling (proliferation) in animals. Conversely, plasma levels of ET-1 arc increased in association with hypoxia in humans. ET receptor antagonists have been demonstrated to reduce hypoxic pulmonary vasoconstriction and vascular remodeling in animals. A number of other growth factors (including platelet-derived growth factors and vascular endothelial growth factor) also mediate pulmonary vascular remodeling in response to hypoxia.

Alveolar hypoxia may be an important basic mechanism of many forms of PH, including that seen in pulmonary parenchymal disease, airway obstruction, inadequate ventilatory drive (central nervous system diseases), disorders of chest wall or respiratory muscles, and high altitude. Even a small area of affected lung may produce vasoconstriction throughout the lungs, possibly through a circulating humoral agent. PH caused by alveolar hypoxia is usually reversible when the cause is eliminated.

Pulmonary Venous Hypertension

Increased pressures in the pulmonary veins produce reflex vasoconstriction of the pulmonary arterioles, raising PA pressure to maintain a high enough pressure gradient between the PA and the pulmonary vein. This pressure gradient maintains a constant forward flow in the pulmonary circulation. There is a marked individual variation in the degree of reactive pulmonary arteriolar vasoconstriction. For example, when the pulmonary venous pressure is elevated in excess of 25 mm Hg from mitral stenosis, marked reactive PH occurs only in less than one third of patients. The mechanism for the vasoconstriction is not entirely clear, but a neuronal component may

be present. Moreover, an elevated pulmonary venous pressure may also narrow or close small airways, resulting in alveolar hypoxia, which may contribute to the vasoconstriction. Mitral stenosis, total anomalous pulmonary venous return (TAPVR) with obstruction (of pulmonary venous return to the LA), and chronic left-sided heart failure are examples of this entity. PH with increased pulmonary venous pressure is usually reversible when the cause is eliminated.

Primary Pulmonary Hypertension

Primary pulmonary hypertension (PPH) is characterized by progressive, irreversible vascular changes similar to those seen in Eisenmenger's syndrome but without intracardiac lesions. There is a decrease in the cross-sectional area of the pulmonary vascular bed caused by the intimal proliferation with partial or complete occlusion of the vessel, thromboembolism, platelet aggregation, or a combination of these. This condition is extremely rare in pediatric patients; it is a condition of adulthood and is more prevalent in women. A familial form of the disease has been reported worldwide in approximately 6% of the cases with PPH. It has a poor prognosis.

The pathogenesis of PPH is not fully understood, but endothelial dysfunction of the pulmonary vascular bed and enhanced platelet activities may be important factors. In normal pulmonary vascular bed, the endothelial cells (1) modulate the tone of vascular smooth muscles (by synthesizing prostacyclin, NO, and ET), (2) control the potential proliferation of smooth muscle cells, and (3) interact with platelets to release anticlotting factors (prostacyclin) in the blood to maintain a nonthrombotic state. These delicate functions are themselves influenced by factors such as shear stress, hypoxia, and tissue metabolism. ET is overproduced in PH, and this excess ET is associated with not only vasoconstriction but also with cell proliferation, inflammation, medial hypertrophy, and fibrosis. ET receptor antagonists (e.g., bosentan) produce vasodilation.

Other Disease States

Pulmonary hypertension associated with other disease states has similar pathophysiologies described in the four categories described, singly or in combination.

PATHOLOGY OF PULMONARY HYPERTENSION

Regardless of the initial events that lead to PH, elevated PA pressure eventually induces varying severity of anatomic changes in the pulmonary vessels. The triad of well-established PH includes vasoconstriction, cell proliferation, and thrombosis through the action of ET, serotonin, and thromboxane A_2.

1. Hyperkinetic PH is the result of CHDs with left-to-right shunts. Heath and Edwards classified the changes into six grades (Fig. 29.1). Grade 1 consists of hypertrophy of the media of the small muscular arteries; grade 2, hyperplasia of the intima; and grade 3, hyperplasia and fibrosis of the intima with narrowing of the vascular lumen. Changes up to grade 3 are considered reversible if the cause is

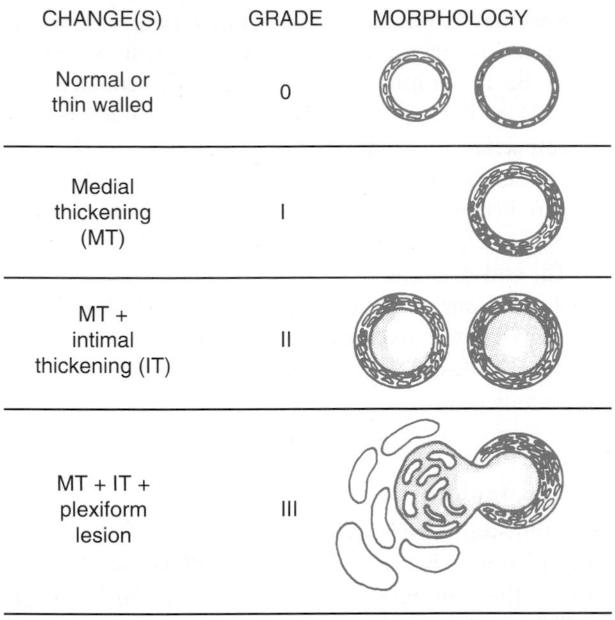

CHANGE(S)	GRADE	MORPHOLOGY
Normal or thin walled	0	
Medial thickening (MT)	I	
MT + intimal thickening (IT)	II	
MT + IT + plexiform lesion	III	

Fig. 29.1 Heath-Edwards grading of the morphologic changes in the pulmonary arteries of patients with pulmonary hypertension (see text). (From Roberts WC: *Congenital heart disease in adults*, Philadelphia, 1979, FA Davis.)

eliminated. In grade 4, dilatation and so-called plexiform lesion of the muscular pulmonary arteries and arterioles are present. Grade 5 changes include complex plexiform, angiomatous, and cavernous lesions and hyalinization of intimal fibrosis. Grade 6 is characterized by the presence of necrotizing arteritis. These advanced changes seen in grades 4 through 6 are considered "irreversible," and they augment the hypertension and sustain it even when the original stimulus is removed. Thus, the presence of irreversible pulmonary vascular changes precludes surgical repair of CHDs.

2. The progressive vascular changes that occur in primary PH are identical to those that occur with CHDs.
3. With pulmonary venous hypertension, the pulmonary arteries may show severe medial hypertrophy and intimal fibrosis. However, the changes are limited to grades I through III of Heath and Edwards classification, and they are often reversible when the cause is eliminated.

PATHOPHYSIOLOGY

1. The normally thin RV cannot sustain sudden pressure loads over 40 to 50 mm Hg. If severe PH develops suddenly in the presence of an unprepared (nonhypertrophied) RV, right-sided heart failure develops. Examples of this include infants who develop acute upper airway obstruction and adult patients who develop massive pulmonary thromboembolism.
2. However, if PH develops slowly, the RV hypertrophies, and it can tolerate mild PH (with a systolic pressure of ~50 mm Hg) without producing clinical problems. The RV pressure rises gradually with accompanying RV hypertrophy, and the PA pressure may eventually exceed the systemic pressure.

3. In patients with PH, a decrease in cardiac output may result from at least two mechanisms:
   a. A volume and pressure overload of the RV impairs cardiac function, primarily by impaired coronary perfusion of the hypertrophied and dilated RV and decreased LV function. The LV dysfunction results from the dramatic leftward shift of the interventricular septum caused by the increasing RV volume. The dilated RV also alters LV structures and decreases the compliance of the LV, resulting in an increase in both LV end-diastolic pressure and LA pressure and thus worsening pulmonary vasoconstriction.
   b. A sudden increase in PVR may decrease pulmonary venous return to the LA, with resulting hypotension in the absence of a right-to-left intracardiac shunt.
4. Pulmonary edema can occur without elevation of LA pressure. Direct disruption of the walls of the small arterioles proximal to the hypoxically constricted arterioles may be responsible (a mechanism similar to that proposed for high-altitude pulmonary edema). The disruption is more likely if there is no hypertrophy of the smooth muscles in the media of these vessels.
5. Deterioration of arterial blood gas levels may occur. Hypoxemia, acidosis, and occasionally hypercapnia may result from pulmonary venous congestion or edema, compression of small airways, or intracardiac shunts, which may worsen PH.

CLINICAL MANIFESTATIONS

Regardless of the cause, clinical manifestations of PH are similar when significant hypertension exists in the PA.

History

1. Exertional dyspnea and fatigue are the earliest and most frequent complaints. Some patients may have a history of headache.
2. Syncope, presyncope, or chest pain also occur on exertion, which generally represent more advanced disease with a fixed cardiac output.
3. History of a heart defect or CHF in infancy is present in most cases of Eisenmenger's syndrome.
4. Patients with underlying lung disease may also complain of frequent episodes of cough or wheezing.
5. Hemoptysis (associated with pulmonary infarction secondary to thrombosis) is a late and sometimes fatal development.

Physical Examination

1. Cyanosis with or without clubbing may be present. The neck veins are distended, with a prominent *a* wave.
2. An RV lift or tap (on the left parasternal area) is present on palpation.
3. There is a single S2, or it splits narrowly with a loud P2. An ejection click and an early diastolic decrescendo murmur of pulmonary regurgitation (PR) are usually present along the mid-left sternal border. A holosystolic murmur

of tricuspid regurgitation (TR) may be audible at the lower left sternal border.

4. Signs of right-sided heart failure (e.g., hepatomegaly, ankle edema) may be present.
5. Arrhythmias occur in the late stage.
6. Patients with associated illness often have clinical findings of that disease.

Electrocardiography

1. Right axis deviation (RAD) and RVH with or without "strain" are seen with severe PH.
2. Right atrial hypertrophy (RAH) is frequently seen late.

Radiographic Studies

1. The heart size is normal or only slightly enlarged with or without right atrial (RA) enlargement. Cardiomegaly appears when CHF supervenes.
2. A prominent PA segment and dilated hilar vessels with clear lung fields are characteristic.
3. With acute exacerbation, pulmonary edema may be seen.

Echocardiography

Echocardiography is the most useful noninvasive screening tool to evaluate patients with clinical suspicion of PH.

1. Associated cardiac defect such as VSD may be imaged.
2. Enlargement of the RA and RV, with normal or small LV dimensions
3. Two-dimensional echo may show thickened interventricular septum that is shifted toward the LV and appears flattened at the end of systole. An inspection of the septal curvature at the end of systole provides an estimate of the RV systolic pressure.
4. Doppler echo study provides semiquantitative estimate of PA pressure.
   a. Peak TR velocity (TR_{max}) determined by continuous-wave Doppler is used to estimate the *systolic* pressure in the PA. The simplified Bernoulli equation ($\Delta P = 4V^2$) is used to estimate a systolic pressure drop across the tricuspid valve; an estimated mean RA pressure (RAP) is added to the result to estimate PA *systolic* pressure. In the absence of pulmonary stenosis (PS), the systolic pressure in the RV equals that in the PA.

$$\text{RV systolic pressure} = 4V^2 + RAP$$

Traditionally, RA pressure is estimated in adult patients by the size and distensibility of inferior vena cava during inspiration at rest and during forced inhalation, but this approach is error prone. Therefore, recently the European Society of Echocardiography guidelines (2015) suggested just using the TR_{max} without adding RAP and suggested the following probabilities (Galie et al 2016):

TR_{max} ≤2.8 m/sec suggests low probability.
TR_{max} 2.9–3.4 m/sec indicates intermediate probability.
TR_{max} >3.4 m/sec suggests a high probability of PH.

   b. With a shunt lesion, such as VSD, PDA, or systemic-to-PA shunt, the peak systolic velocity across the shunt can be used to estimate systolic pressure in the RV or PA. The systolic pressure in the LV (which is equal to the aortic pressure) is estimated by systolic pressure in the arm minus the systolic pressure drop across the VSD or PDA estimates RV and PA systolic pressures, respectively. Note that the systolic pressure in the arm is a little higher (5–10 mm Hg) than the LV systolic pressure because of the peripheral amplification of systolic pressure (see Chapter 2).
   c. The end-diastolic velocity of PR can be used to estimate the *diastolic* pressure in the PA. The end-diastolic (not early diastolic) velocity is measured and entered into the modified Bernoulli equation, and a normal central venous pressure (in lieu of RV end-diastolic pressure) of 5 or 10 mm Hg is added.

Exercise Testing

A symptom-limited exercise, such as the 6-minute walk test, has been found to be useful in the evaluation of adult patients with PH. The 6-minute walk test may be useful in children as well for following disease progression or measuring the response to medical interventions. Figure A.2 in Appendix A shows reference values for healthy children from Switzerland (Ulrich et al, 2013).

DIAGNOSIS

1. Cardiac catheterization is necessary to confirm the diagnosis, to assess the severity of the disease, and to assess the responses to pulmonary vasodilators (acute vasoreactive test [AVT]) before starting therapy and at intervals. It may also assist in the determination of suitability for heart or heart–lung transplantation.
2. After the diagnosis of PH is confirmed, AVT is undertaken to assess the response of the pulmonary vascular bed to pulmonary-specific vasodilators. The test result shows whether the elevated PVR is due to active vasoconstriction ("acute responders") or to permanent changes in the pulmonary arterioles ("nonresponders"). The protocol for vasodilator testing varies from center to center. NO inhalation (20–80 ppm) with or without increased oxygen concentration for 10 minutes is commonly used. One may also use 100% oxygen, inhaled or intravenous (IV) prostacyclin, or IV adenosine.

   "Acute responders" should show (1) a decrease of at least 10 mm Hg in the mean PA to less than 40 mm Hg (with a normal or increase in cardiac output) or (2) a decrease of 20% or more in the mean PA pressure or PVR with an unchanged or increased cardiac output.

   For children with CHD with large left-to-right shunts, AVR is to assess whether the PVR will decrease sufficiently for surgical repair to be undertaken in borderline cases. A decrease in PVR index to less than 6 to 8 WU/m² or PVR-to-SVR ratio less than 0.3 is considered a favorable result.
3. Characteristic angiographic findings of advanced PH secondary to CHD include sparseness of arborization, abrupt tapering of small arteries, and reduced background capillary filling.

4. Lung biopsies have been used in an attempt to evaluate the "operability" of patients with PH and associated CHDs. Unfortunately, pulmonary vascular changes are not uniformly distributed, and the biopsy findings correlate poorly with the natural history of the disease or the operability. Hemodynamic data appear to predict the survival better than biopsy findings.

NATURAL HISTORY

1. PH secondary to the upper airway obstruction is usually reversible when the cause is eliminated.
2. Chronic conditions that produce alveolar hypoxia have a relatively poor prognosis. Superimposed pulmonary infection may be an aggravating factor.
3. PH with large left-to-right shunt lesions (hyperkinetic type) or associated with pulmonary venous hypertension improves or disappears after surgical repair of the cause if treatment of the condition is possible and performed early.
4. PPH is progressive and has a fatal outcome without treatment, usually 2 to 3 years after the onset of symptoms.
5. PH associated with Eisenmenger's syndrome, collagen disease, and chronic thromboembolism is usually irreversible and has a poor prognosis but may be stable for 2 to 3 decades.
6. Two most frequent causes of death are progressive RV failure and sudden death (probably secondary to arrhythmias).
7. Cerebrovascular accident from paradoxical embolization is a rare complication.

MANAGEMENT

Most cases of PH are difficult to treat and impossible to reverse unless the cause can be eliminated. The primary emphasis must be on the prevention and elimination of causes whenever possible.

Treating Underlying Causes

Measures to remove or treat the underlying cause include the following.
1. Timely corrective surgery for CHDs, such as large-shunt VSD, ECD, or PDA, before obstructive anatomic changes occur in the pulmonary vessels
2. Tonsillectomy and adenoidectomy when the cause of PH is the upper airway obstruction
3. Treatment of underlying diseases, such as cystic fibrosis, asthma, pneumonia, obstructive sleep apnea, or bronchopulmonary dysplasia

General Measures

General measures are aimed at preventing further elevation of PA pressure or treating its complications.
1. Avoidance or limitation of strenuous exertion, isometric activities (weightlifting), trips to high altitudes, and possibly flights on commercial aircraft

2. Oxygen supplementation as needed.
3. Avoidance of vasoconstrictor drugs, including decongestants with α-adrenergic properties
4. Patients should be strongly advised to avoid pregnancy. Pregnancy increases circulating blood volume and oxygen consumption, may increase the risk of pulmonary embolism from deep vein thrombosis or amniotic fluid, and may cause syncope and cardiac arrest. Oral contraceptives worsen PH (surgical contraception is preferred).
5. Patients with CHF are treated with chronic administration of digoxin and diuretics and a low-salt diet. Digoxin may improve RV contractility against the elevated afterload and is also useful if there is coexisting LV dysfunction. Diuretics provide marked benefit in symptom relief by reducing intravascular volume, hepatic congestion, and pulmonary congestion.
6. Patients with cardiac arrhythmias are treated with antiarrhythmic drugs.
7. Partial erythropheresis is performed for polycythemia and headache.
8. Annual flu shots are recommended.
9. The use of nitroglycerine for anginal pain is avoided because it may worsen the pain.

Anticoagulation

1. Anticoagulation with warfarin (Coumadin) is widely recommended in patients with thromboembolic disease and may be beneficial in patients with PH from other causes. The international normalized ratio of 2.0 to 2.5 is the goal of therapy.
2. Some recommend antiplatelet drugs (aspirin) instead of warfarin to prevent microembolism in the pulmonary circulation. Unlike in patients with prosthetic mechanical heart valve, concomitant use of aspirin is not recommended because it may increase effects of warfarin.

Pharmacologic Treatment of Chronic Pulmonary Hypertension

The main determinant of treatment of chronic PH is the response to vasodilator testing at AVT during cardiac catheterization (see Diagnosis). The pulmonary vasodilators are used in "responders." For nonresponders, vasodilators have limited success. Vasodilators should not be used without first testing AVT in the catheterization laboratory.

Drugs that are used to relieve pulmonary vasoconstriction can be divided into endothelial-based and smooth muscle-based drugs (Oishi et al, 2011).
- Endothelial-based drugs act on endothelial mechanisms that cause vasoconstriction or induce vasodilatation (see Physiology of Pulmonary Circulation in this chapter for review).
  - NO inhalation
  - PDE-5 inhibitors (sildenafil, tadalafil)
  - Prostacyclin analogues (epoprostenol, treprostinil, iloprost, beraprost)
  - ET receptor antagonists (bosentan, sitaxsentan, ambrisentan)

- Smooth muscle–based drugs act directly on the smooth muscle.
  - Calcium channel blockers (CCBs)

For "Acute Responders"

1. **Nifedipine.** Nifedipine, a CCB, is one of the oldest drugs used with beneficial effects. For "acute responders" with primary PH treated with CCB, the survival rates were 97% and 81% at 1 and 10 years, respectively. Children who were not "acute responders" but were still treated with CCBs had survival rates of 45% and 29% at 1 and 4 years, respectively. CCBs are contraindicated in children who have not undergone AVT, are nonresponders, or have RV failure regardless of acute response. Unfortunately, the majority of children with severe PAH are nonresponders to AVT, and therapy other than CCB is usually required. The oral dose of nifedipine is 0.25 - 0.50 mg/kg/day in three divided doses. The major side effect is systemic hypotension. CCBs should not be used in AVT because these drugs do not act through the pulmonary endothelial mechanism but act on any vascular smooth muscles. Therefore, they can cause a dangerous decrease in cardiac output or a marked drop in systemic arterial pressure. The dosages of other CCBs are diltiazem 1.5-2 mg/kg/day, and amlodipine 2.5 to 10 mg/day. Diltiazem lowers heart rate, so it is used more frequently in younger children with higher heart rates. Verapamil is contraindicated because of its negative inotropic effects.

2. **Prostacyclin.** Prostacyclin is a potent pulmonary and systemic vasodilator with antiplatelet activity. Prostacyclin analogues have been shown to improve quality of life and survival in patients with PPH, Eisenmenger's syndrome, and chronic lung disease.
   a. Epoprostenol is a synthetic prostacyclin and has a very short half-life (1-2 minutes), necessitating a continuous IV infusion through a central venous line and delivered by an ambulatory infusion system. (The starting dose of epoprostenol was 2 ng/kg/min, with increments of 2 ng/kg/min every 15 minutes, until desired effects appeared; the average final dose was 9 to 11 ng/kg/min.) Barst et al (1999) have shown improved survival rate with a 4-year survival rate of 94% compared with 38% in untreated patients. Thrombosis, pump malfunction (with rebound PH), flushing, headache, nausea, diarrhea, and jaw discomfort are reported complications and side effects.
   b. Several prostacyclin analogs have been approved by the US Food and Drug Administration that can be administered intravenously or subcutaneously (treprostinil), by inhalation (iloprost) at the dose of 5 mcg every 2 to 3 hours, or orally (beraprost).

3. **ET receptor antagonists.** The ET receptor antagonists bosentan and sitaxsentan have been used in both PPH and Eisenmenger's syndrome. Two receptors, ETA and ETB receptors, are known. Both ETA and ETB receptors on vascular smooth muscle mediate vasoconstriction, whereas ETB receptors on endothelial cells cause release of NO and prostacyclin and act as clearance receptors

of circulating ET-1 (Tissot et al, 2010). Side effects of ET antagonists include elevation of hepatic aminotransferase levels, teratogenicity, anemia, peripheral edema, decreased effectiveness oral contraceptive agents, and effects on male fertility.
   a. Bosentan, a dual (nonselective) ET receptor blocker, given orally, in a dose of 125 mg twice a day (BID) for 16 weeks, has resulted in a significant improvement in the level of exercise capability in adult patients. Similar beneficial effects have been reported in pediatric patients. In children with PPH or Eisenmenger's syndrome, oral bosentan in the dose of 31.25 mg BID for children weighing less than 20 kg, 62.5 mg BID for children weighing 20 to 40 kg, and 125 mg BID for children weighing more than 40 kg (with or without concomitant IV prostacyclin therapy) for a media duration of 14 months resulted in a significant functional improvement in about 50% of the cases (Barst et al, 2003; Rosensweig et al, 2005; Maiya et al, 2006). A rare side effect of the drug is increased liver enzymes.
   b. Sitaxsentan is a selective ET-A (ET_A) receptor antagonist. When given orally once daily at a dose of 100 mg (for mostly adult patients and children older than 12 years), it resulted in improved exercise capacity after 18 weeks of treatment (Barst et al, 2006). Elevation of alanine transaminase and aspartate transaminase was a rare side effect. Ambrisentan is another oral selective ET_A receptor antagonist, but little data are available for children. A pediatric retrospective cohort study in 2013 was suggestive of safety and clinical improvement similar to the adult patients with PH (Takatsuki et al, 2013).

4. **Sildenafil.** Sildenafil, a PDE inhibitor, prevents the breakdown of cyclic guanosine monophosphate (cGMP), resulting in pulmonary vasodilatation. Given orally, it has been shown to be a potent and selective pulmonary vasodilator with equal efficacy to that of inhaled NO in adult patients. A small pediatric study with sildenafil for 12 months resulted in improvement in hemodynamics and exercise capacity in children with PPH and secondary PH from CHDs. The dosage used was 0.25 to 1 mg/kg four times daily, starting with the lower dose (Humpl et al, 2005). Adverse effects include headache, flushing, exacerbation of nosebleed, and rare systemic hypotension or erections. Tadalafil is also a selective phosphodiesterase inhibitor, but no data are available in children.

5. **NO.** NO inhalation is effective in lowering PA pressure in patients with adult respiratory distress syndrome, PPH, and persistent PH of the newborn. NO can be administered only by inhalation because it is inactivated by hemoglobin. Rebound PH is problematic.

For "Nonresponders"

The following measures can be used in patients with fixed PVR and severe PH, including PPH.

1. NO inhalation and continuous IV or possibly nebulized prostacyclin (prostaglandin I_2) may provide selective pulmonary vasodilatation.

2. Atrial septostomy or septectomy (either by catheter or surgery) improves survival rates and abolishes syncope or intractable right heart failure by providing a right-to-left atrial shunt and thereby helping to maintain cardiac output but with increased hypoxemia. Surgical or transcatheter creation of "reverse" Potts shunt has shown hemodynamic and clinical improvement in drug-refractory patients.

3. Lung transplantation. Lung or heart–lung transplantation remains the only available treatment for patients unresponsive to vasodilator or interventional treatments. It was believed initially that because of severe RV dysfunction, heart–lung transplantation was the only option. However, bilateral or single lung transplantation has been shown to reduce PVR and improve RV function. Bilateral lung transplantation is preferred at most centers because of a greater pulmonary vascular reserve, but some centers prefer single-lung transplantation because of its simpler surgical technique and shorter waiting time for the organ procurement.

30

The Child with Chest Pain

A complaint of chest pain is frequently encountered in children in the office and emergency department (ED). Although chest pain does not indicate serious disease of the heart or other systems in most pediatric patients, in a society with a high prevalence of atherosclerotic cardiovascular disease, it can be alarming to the child and parents. Physicians should be aware of the differential diagnosis of chest pain in children and should make every effort to find a specific cause before making a referral to a specialist or reassuring the child and the parents of the benign nature of the complaint. Making a routine referral to a cardiologist is not always a good idea; it may increase the family's concern and may result in a prolonged and costly cardiac evaluation.

CAUSE AND PREVALENCE

Chest pain occurs in children of all ages and equally in male and female patients, with an average age of presentation at 13 years. Most of the data on the frequency of causes of chest pain in children come from studies performed in pediatric ED and cardiology clinics. Chest pain accounts for approximately 0.3% to 0.6% of pediatric ED visits. Table 30.1 lists the frequency of the causes of chest pain in children according to the organ systems based on published data from six pediatric EDs or pediatric clinics and data from four pediatric cardiology clinics (Thull-Freedman, 2011). According to the table, trauma or muscle strain of the chest wall, costochondritis, and respiratory illness are the three most frequent causes of the pain. Gastrointestinal (GI) and psychogenic causes are identified in fewer than 10% of cases, and a cardiac cause is found infrequently (≤5%). In another report, chest wall pathology including costochondritis was the cause of the pain in 64% of patients seen in an ED and in 88% of the patients seen in a cardiology clinic (Massin et al, 2004). Whereas children younger than 12 years of age were two times more likely

to have an organic cause, adolescents were 2.5 times more likely to have a psychogenic cause. A study published in 2011 reviewed 3700 patients with no known cardiac pathology or no previous cardiac evaluation who presented to Children's Hospital of Boston with a complaint of chest pain. Cardiac pathology or arrhythmias were found in only 1% of these patients, of whom 38% had supraventricular tachycardia and 27% had pericarditis (Saleeb et al, 2011). Box. 30.1 is a partial list of possible causes of noncardiac and cardiac chest pain in children.

CLINICAL MANIFESTATIONS

Idiopathic Chest Pain

No cause can be found in 12% to 85% of patients, even after a moderately extensive investigation. In many children with chronic chest pain, an organic cause is less likely to be found. In some of these children, chest pain is resolved spontaneously, and some of them are eventually referred for specialty evaluation.

Noncardiac Causes of Chest Pain

Most cases of pediatric chest pain originate in the organ systems other than the cardiovascular system. Identifiable noncardiac causes of chest pain are found in 56% to 86% of reported cases. Causes of chest pain are found most often on the thorax and respiratory system.

Costochondritis

Costochondritis causes chest pain in 9% to 22% of children with such pain. A single study reported rates as high as 79%. It is more common in girls than boys. Pain is generally sharp, anterior chest pain and usually unilateral but occasionally bilateral. Pain is usually exaggerated by physical activity or breathing. A specific position may also cause the pain. The

TABLE 30.1 Frequency of Causes of Chest Pain In Children

Causes	Pediatric Emergency Department or Pediatric Clinic (Data from Six Reports) (%)	Cardiology Clinic (Data from Four Reports) (%)
Idiopathic or cause unknown	12–61	37–54
Musculoskeletal or costochondritis	7–69	1–89
Respiratory or asthma	13–24	1–12
Gastrointestinal or gastroesophageal reflux disease	3–7	3–12
Psychogenic	5–9	4–19
Cardiac	2–5	3–7

From Thull-Freedman J: Evaluation of chest pain in the pediatric patients, *Med Clin North Am* 94:327–347, 2010.

Box 30.1 Selected Causes of Chest Pain

Noncardiac Causes

Musculoskeletal

Costochondritis
Trauma to chest wall (from sports, fights, or accident)
Muscle strains (pectoral, shoulder, or back muscles)
Overused chest wall muscle (from coughing)
Abnormalities of the rib cage or thoracic spine
Tietze's syndrome
Slipping rib syndrome
Precordial catch (Texidor's twinge or stitch in the side)

Respiratory

Reactive airway disease (exercise-induced asthma)
Pneumonia (viral, bacterial, mycobacterium, fungal, or parasitic)
Pleural irritation (pleural effusion)
Pneumothorax or pneumomediastinum
Pleurodynia (devil's grip)
Pulmonary embolism
Foreign bodies in the airway

Gastrointestinal

Gastroesophageal reflux
Peptic ulcer disease
Esophagitis
Gastritis
Esophageal diverticulum
Hiatal hernia
Foreign bodies (e.g., coins)
Cholecystitis
Pancreatitis

Psychogenic

Life stressor (death in family, family discord, divorce, failure in school, nonacceptance from peers, sexual molestation)

Hyperventilation
Conversion symptoms
Somatization disorder
Depression
Bulimia nervosa (esophagitis, esophageal tear)

Miscellaneous

Sickle cell disease (vaso-occlusive crisis)
Mastalgia
Herpes zoster

Cardiac Causes

Ischemic Ventricular Dysfunction

Structural abnormalities of the heart (severe aortic or pulmonary stenosis, hypertrophic obstructive cardiomyopathy, Eisenmenger's syndrome)
Mitral valve prolapse
Coronary artery abnormalities (previous Kawasaki disease, congenital anomaly, coronary heart disease, hypertension, sickle cell disease)
Cocaine abuse
Aortic dissection and aortic aneurysm (Turner's, Marfan's, or Noonan's syndromes)

Inflammatory Conditions

Pericarditis (viral, bacterial, or rheumatic)
Postpericardiotomy syndrome
Myocarditis (acute or chronic)
Kawasaki disease

Arrhythmias (and Palpitations)

Supraventricular tachycardia
Frequent premature ventricular tachycardia or ventricular tachycardia (possible)

---

pain may radiate to the remainder of the chest, back, and abdomen. The pain may be preceded by exercise, an upper respiratory infection, or physical activity. Physical examination is diagnostic; the clinician finds a reproducible tenderness on palpation over the chondrosternal or costochondral junctions. It is a benign condition, but the pain may persist for several months.

Tietze's syndrome is a rare form of costochondritis characterized by a large, tender, fusiform (spindle-shaped), nonsup-

purative swelling at the chondrosternal junction. It usually affects the upper ribs, particularly the second and third costochondral junctions.

Musculoskeletal

Musculoskeletal chest pain is also common in children. The pain is caused by strains of the pectoral, shoulder, or back muscles after exercise, overused chest wall muscle for coughing, or chronic or acute trauma to the chest wall from sports, fights, or accidents as well as continued muscle strain from video gaming. A history of vigorous exercise (push-ups, pull-ups), weightlifting, or direct trauma to the chest (boxing) and the presence of tenderness of the chest wall or muscles clearly indicate muscle strain or trauma. Abnormalities of the rib cage or thoracic spine can cause mild, chronic chest pain in children.

Respiratory

Respiratory problems are responsible for about 10% to 20% of cases of pediatric chest pain, which may result from lung pathology, pleural irritation, or pneumothorax. A history of severe cough, with tenderness of intercostal or abdominal muscles, is usually present. The presence of crackles, wheezing, tachypnea, retraction, or fever on examination suggests a respiratory cause of chest pain. Pleural effusion may cause pain that is worsened by deep inspiration. Radiographic examination may confirm the diagnosis of pleural effusion, pneumonia, or pneumothorax.

Exercise-Induced Asthma

The prevalence of exercise-induced asthma is probably underestimated. Exercise triggers bronchospasm in up to 80% of individuals with asthma. The response of the asthmatic patient to exercise is quite characteristic. Running for 1 to 2 minutes often cause bronchodilatation in patients with asthma, but strenuous exercise for 3 to 8 minutes' duration causes bronchoconstriction in virtually all subjects with asthma, especially when the heart rate rises to 180 beats/min. Symptoms range from mild to severe and may include coughing, wheezing, dyspnea, and chest congestion, constriction, or pain. They also complain of limited endurance during exercise. Environmental factors such as cold temperature, pollens, and air pollution, as well as viral respiratory infection can worsen exercise-induced asthma. Exercise-induced bronchospasm provocation test is diagnostic, which is described under Stress Tests in Chapter 6.

Gastrointestinal

Some GI disorders, including gastroesophageal reflux disease (GERD), may present as chest pain in children. In addition to chest pain, children with GERD may complain of abdominal pain, frequent sore throat, gagging or choking, extreme pickiness about foods, frequent respiratory problems (such as bronchitis, wheezing, asthma), and poor weight gain. The onset and relief of pain in relation to eating and diet may help clarify the diagnosis. The incidence of GERD is higher in patients with Down syndrome, cerebral palsy, and other causes of developmental delay. Esophagitis resulting from gastroesophageal reflux should be suspected in a child who complains of burning substernal pain that worsens with a reclining posture or abdominal pressure or that worsens after certain foods are eaten. Cholecystitis presents with postprandial pain referred to the right upper quadrant of the abdomen and part of the chest.

Young children sometimes ingest foreign bodies, such as coins, which lodge in the upper esophagus, or they may ingest caustic substances that burn the entire esophagus. In such cases, the history makes the diagnosis obvious.

Psychogenic

Psychogenic disturbances account for 5% to 17% of cases and are seen in both boys and girls at equal rates. Often a recent major stressful event parallels the onset of the chest pain: a death, divorce or separation in the family, a serious illness, a disability, a recent move, failure in school, or sexual molestation. However, a psychological cause of chest pain should not be lightly assigned without a thorough history taking and a follow-up evaluation. Psychological or psychiatric consultation may reveal conversion symptoms, a somatization disorder, or even depression.

Miscellaneous

- The precordial catch (Texidor's twinge or stitch in the side), a one-sided chest pain, lasts a few seconds or minutes and is associated with bending or slouching. The cause is unclear, but the pain is relieved by straightening and taking a few shallow breaths or one deep breath. The pain may recur frequently or remain absent for months.
- Slipping rib syndrome results from excess mobility of the 8th to 10th ribs, which do not directly insert into the sternum. In many cases, the ligaments that hold these ribs to the upper ribs are weak, resulting in slippage of the ribs, causing pain.
- Some male and female adolescents complain of chest pain caused by breast masses (mastalgia). These tender masses may be cysts (in postpubertal girls) or may be part of normal breast development in pubertal boys and girls.
- Pleurodynia (devil's grip), an unusual cause of chest pain caused by coxsackievirus infection, is characterized by sudden episodes of sharp pain in the chest or abdomen.
- Herpes zoster is another unusual cause of chest pain.
- Spontaneous pneumothorax and pneumomediastinum are serious but rare respiratory causes of acute chest pain in children; children with asthma, cystic fibrosis, or Marfan's syndrome are at risk. Inhalation of cocaine can provoke pneumomediastinum and pneumothorax with subcutaneous emphysema.
- Pulmonary embolism, although extremely rare in children, has been reported in female adolescents who use oral contraceptives or have had elective abortions. It has also been reported in male adolescents with recent trauma of the lower extremities and in children with shunted hydrocephalus. It may occur in in children with hypercoagulation syndromes. Affected patients usually have dyspnea, pleuritic pain, fever, cough, and hemoptysis.
- Hyperventilation can produce chest discomfort and is often associated with paresthesia and lightheadedness.

Cardiovascular Causes of Chest Pain

Cardiovascular disease is identified as the cause of pediatric chest pain in 0% to 5% of cases. Cardiac chest pain may be caused by ischemic ventricular dysfunction, pericardial or myocardial inflammatory processes, or arrhythmias.

TABLE 30.2 Important Clinical Findings of Cardiac Causes of Chest Pain

Condition	History	Physical Findings	ECG	Chest Radiograph
Severe AS	History of CHD (+)	Loud (>grade 3 of 6 SEM at URSB with radiation to neck)	LVH with or without strain	Prominent ascending aorta and aortic knob
Severe PS	History of CHD (+)	Loud (grade >3 of 6) SEM at ULSB	RVH with or without strain	Prominent PA segment
HOCM	Positive FH in one third of cases	Variable heart murmurs Brisk brachial pulses (±)	LVH Deep Q/small R or QS pattern in LPLs	Mild cardiomegaly with globular-shaped heart
MVP	Positive FH (±)	Midsystolic click with or without late systolic murmur Thin body build Thoracic skeletal anomalies (80%)	Inverted T waves in aVF (±)	Normal heart size Straight back (±) Narrow AP diameter (±)
Eisenmenger syndrome	History of CHD (+)	Cyanosis and clubbing RV impulse Loud and single S2 Soft or no heart murmur	RVH	Markedly prominent PA with normal heart size
Anomalous origin of left coronary artery	Recurrent episodes of distress in early infancy	Soft or no heart murmur	Anterolateral MI pattern	Moderate to marked cardiomegaly
Anomalous origin or intramural course of either coronary artery	Exercise-related anginal pain	No murmur	Normal resting ECG	Normal heart size
Sequelae of Kawasaki's disease	History of Kawasaki's disease (±) Typical exercise-related anginal pain	Usually negative Continuous murmur in coronary fistula	ST-segment elevation (±) Old MI pattern (±)	Normal heart size or mild cardiomegaly
Cocaine abuse	History of substance abuse (±)	Hypertension Nonspecific heart murmur (±)	ST-segment elevation (±)	Normal heart size in acute cases
Pericarditis and myocarditis	History of URI (±) Sharp chest pain	Friction rub Muffled heart sounds Nonspecific heart murmur (±)	Low QRS voltages ST-segment shift Arrhythmias (±)	Cardiomegaly of varying degree
Postpericardiotomy syndrome	History of recent heart surgery, pain, and dyspnea	Muffled heart sounds (±) Friction rub	Persistent ST-segment elevation	Cardiomegaly of varying degree
Arrhythmias (and palpitation)	History of WPW syndrome (±) FH of long QT syndrome (±)	May be negative Irregular rhythm (±)	Arrhythmias (±) WPW preexcitation (±) Long QTc interval (>0.46 sec)	Normal heart size

+, Positive; ±, may be present; *AP*, anteroposterior; *AS*, aortic stenosis; *CHD*, congenital heart disease; *ECG*, electrocardiogram; *FH*, family history; *HOCM*, hypertrophic obstructive cardiomyopathy; *LPLs*, left precordial leads; *LVH*, left ventricular hypertrophy; *MI*, myocardial infarction; *MVP*, mitral valve prolapse; *PA*, pulmonary artery; *PS*, pulmonary stenosis; *RV*, right ventricle; *RVH*, right ventricular hypertrophy; *SEM*, systolic ejection murmur; *ULSB*, upper left sternal border; *URI*, upper respiratory infection; *URSB*, upper right sternal border; *WPW*, Wolff-Parkinson-White.

A typical *anginal pain* in adults is located in the precordial or substernal area and radiates to the neck, jaw, either or both arms, the back, or the abdomen. The patient describes the pain as a deep, heavy pressure; the feeling of choking; or a squeezing sensation. Older adolescents are expected to describe the pain as above, but young children may not. Exercise, cold stress, emotional upset, or a large meal typically precipitate anginal pain. Table 30.2 summarizes clinical findings of cardiac causes of chest pain in children for practitioners.

If a noncardiac cause of chest pain is not found and the nature of the pain is consistent with that of cardiac origin, cardiology consultation should be considered. Children with exertional chest pain, especially if it is associated with dizziness or palpitation, should be considered for possible cardiac cause of chest pain. The electrocardiogram (ECG) and echo study should demonstrate or rule out most of the chest pain of cardiac origin, except for those associated with cardiac arrhythmias or substance abuse.

Ischemic Myocardial Dysfunction
Congenital Heart Defects

Severe obstructive lesions, such as aortic stenosis (AS), subaortic stenosis, severe pulmonary stenosis (PS), and pulmonary vascular obstructive disease (Eisenmenger's syndrome), may cause chest pain. Mild stenotic lesions do not cause ischemic chest pain. Chest pain from severe obstructive lesions results from increased myocardial oxygen demands from tachycardia and increased pressure work by the ventricle. Therefore, the pain is usually associated with exercise and may be a typical anginal pain. Cardiac examination often reveals a loud heart murmur best audible at the upper right or left sternal border, usually with a thrill, except in patients with Eisenmenger's syndrome. The ECG usually shows ventricular hypertrophy with or without "strain" pattern. Chest radiography films may be abnormal in patients with AS or PS with a prominent ascending aorta or main pulmonary artery trunk, respectively. Chest films are definitely abnormal in patients with Eisenmenger's syndrome, with a marked prominence of the main pulmonary artery segment. Echocardiography and Doppler studies permit accurate diagnosis of the type and severity of the obstructive lesion.

Mitral Valve Prolapse

Chest pain associated with mitral valve prolapse (MVP) has been reported in about 20% of patients with the condition. The pain is usually a vague, nonexertional pain of short duration, located at the apex, without a constant relationship to effort or emotion. The pain is presumed to result from abnormal tension on papillary muscles, but the causal relationship between chest pain and MVP remains unclear in children. Occasionally, supraventricular or ventricular arrhythmias may result in cardiac symptoms, including chest discomfort. Thoracoskeletal deformities commonly occur in these children and may cause chest pain. Nearly all patients with Marfan's syndrome have MVP.

Cardiac examination reveals a midsystolic click with or without a late systolic murmur. The midsystolic click becomes more prominent on standing. The ECG may show T-wave inversion in the inferior leads (leads II, III, aVF). Two-dimensional echo findings of MVP in adults are well established, but diagnostic echo findings of MVP have not been established in children (see Chapter 21).

Cardiomyopathy

Hypertrophic and dilated cardiomyopathies can cause chest pain from ischemia, with or without exercise, or from rhythm disturbances. Cardiac examination reveals no diagnostic findings, but the ECG or chest radiographic films are abnormal, leading to further studies. Echo studies are diagnostic of the conditions (see Chapter 18).

Coronary Artery Disease

Coronary artery anomalies rarely cause chest pain. They include rare cases of proximal intramural course of either coronary arteries, anomalous origin of the left coronary artery from the pulmonary artery (usually symptomatic during early infancy), single coronary artery, coronary artery fistula, aneurysm or stenosis of the coronary arteries as a result of Kawasaki's disease, or coronary insufficiency secondary to previous cardiac surgery involving the coronary arteries or the vicinity of these arteries.

The pain caused by coronary artery abnormalities is expected to be typical of anginal pain. Cardiac examination may be normal or may reveal a heart murmur (systolic murmur of mitral regurgitation or continuous murmur of coronary artery fistula). The ECG may show myocardial ischemia (ST-segment elevation) or old myocardial infarction. Chest radiographs may reveal abnormalities suggestive of these conditions. Although echo can be helpful, computed tomography or coronary angiography is usually indicated for the definitive diagnosis.

Cocaine Abuse

Even children with normal hearts are at risk of ischemia and myocardial infarction if cocaine is used. Cocaine blocks the reuptake of norepinephrine in the central nervous system and peripheral sympathetic nerves. An increase in the sympathetic output and circulating level of catecholamines causes coronary vasoconstriction. Cocaine also induces the activation of platelets in some patients and causes increased production of endothelin and decreased production of nitric oxide. The resulting increase in heart rate and blood pressure, increase in myocardial oxygen consumption, possible increase in platelet activation, and myocardial electrical abnormalities may collectively produce anginal pain, infarction, arrhythmias, or sudden death. History and drug screening help physicians in the diagnosis of cocaine-induced chest pain.

Aortic Dissection or Aortic Aneurysm

Aortic dissection or aortic aneurysm rarely causes chest pain. Children with Turner's, Marfan's, and Noonan's syndromes are at risk.

Pericardial or Myocardial Disease
Pericarditis

Irritation of the pericardium may result from inflammatory pericardial disease; pericarditis may have a viral, bacterial, or rheumatic origin. In a child who had recent open-heart surgery, the cause of the pain may be postpericardiotomy syndrome. Older children with pericarditis may complain of a sharp, stabbing precordial pain that worsens when lying down and improves after sitting and leaning forward. Examination may reveal distant heart sounds, neck vein distention, friction rub, and paradoxical pulse. The ECG may reveal low QRS voltages and ST-T changes, and chest radiographs may show varying degrees of cardiac enlargement and changes in the cardiac silhouette. Diagnosis of pericardial effusion with or without tamponade can be accurately made by echo examination.

Myocarditis

Acute myocarditis often involves the pericardium to a certain extent and can cause chest pain. Examination may reveal fever, respiratory distress, distant heart sounds, neck vein distention, and friction rub. Chest radiographic films and the ECG may suggest the correct diagnosis, which can be confirmed by echo examination (see Chapter 19).

Arrhythmias

Chest pain may result from a variety of arrhythmias, especially with sustained tachycardia, resulting in myocardial ischemia. Even without ischemia, children may consider palpitation or forceful heartbeats as chest pain. When chest pain is associated with dizziness and palpitation, a resting ECG and a 24-hour Holter monitor should be obtained. Alternatively, an event recorder with telephone transmission device may be used to record the ECG rhythm while the patient experiences symptoms.

DIAGNOSTIC APPROACH

The first goal of evaluating children with a complaint of chest pain is to rule out cardiac cause of chest pain, which is usually the main concern to the child and parents, and to look for three common noncardiac causes of chest pain—costochondritis, musculoskeletal causes, and respiratory diseases—which account for 45% to 65% of chest pain in children.

A thorough history taking and careful physical examination will suffice to rule out cardiac causes of chest pain and often to find a specific cause of the pain. To rule out cardiac causes of chest pain, physicians will need chest radiographic films and an ECG. (Cardiologists may, in addition, obtain an echocardiogram to accomplish the same.) Cardiac causes of chest pain can be ruled out by nonexertional nature of pain, negative cardiac examination, and normal results of other investigations, with exception of cardiac arrhythmia as the cause of the pain. Even if physicians cannot find a specific cause of chest pain, it is relatively easy to rule out cardiac causes of chest pain by following the steps outlined in this chapter. Most patients and parents will be relieved and satisfied to learn that the heart is not the cause of chest pain. Finding a specific, benign, or noncardiac cause of pain establishes the diagnosis of noncardiac chest pain.

History of Present Illness

The initial history should be directed at determining the nature of the pain, in terms of the duration, intensity, frequency, location, and points of radiation. An important history is whether the chest pain occurred during or after heavy physical but dynamic activities or whether it occurred at rest or while sitting in class. It is important to remember that ischemic cardiac chest pain is described as a pressure or squeezing sensation, not a sharp pain. Associated symptoms, concurrent or precipitating events, and relieving factors may help clarify the origin of the pain.

The following are some examples of questions to ask.
- When did the pain begin?
  - Acute onset of pain (within 48 hours) is more likely to have an organic etiology.
  - In young children, a sudden onset of chest pain should raise the possibility of a foreign body (coin or button battery) in the esophagus.
  - Those with chronic pain are more likely to be idiopathic or psychogenic, although some children with costochondritis may have chronic pain.

- How often have you had similar pain (frequency and chronicity)?
- What is the location (e.g., specific point, localized or diffuse)?
- How severe is the pain?
- What is the pain like (e.g., sharp, pressure sensation, squeezing)?
  - The character of the pain is usually nonspecific in children and does not help much in identifying the cause.
  - Although classic description of cardiac pain in adults is that of pressure, crushing, or squeezing sensation, it is uncertain whether this classic description is typical in pediatric cases.
- How long does the pain last (seconds, minutes, hours)?
- What triggers the pain (e.g., exercise, eating, trauma, emotional stress)?
  - Chest pain precipitated by running or exercise may relate to cardiac disease or more commonly exercise-induced asthma.
  - Midsternal or precordial pain that worsens after eating or when lying down may be esophageal.
  - History of recent workouts, trauma, or fight may point to the musculoskeletal system.
  - A recent stressful event may be important clue to psychogenic etiology of pain (after ruling out organic causes).
- What makes the pain better or worse?
  - Pain that worsens with moving, deep breathing, or cough may suggest chest wall pain, pleural pain, or lung pathology.
  - Pain that improves by sitting up and leaning forward may be caused by pericarditis.
- Are there associated symptoms, such as cough; fever; syncope; dizziness; tingling in the hands, feet, or around the mouth; or palpitation?
  - Pain associated with palpitation or syncope may suggest arrhythmia or other cardiac disease.
  - History of fever suggests an infectious process (e.g., pneumonia, myocarditis, pericarditis).
  - History of tingling could be suggestive of hyperventilation.

Past and Family Histories

After gaining some idea about the nature of the pain, the clinician should focus on important past and family histories. Examples of questions are as follows.
1. Have you been hurt while playing, or have you used your arms excessively for any reason?
2. Does the child have any known medical conditions (e.g., congenital or acquired heart disease, cardiac surgery, infection, asthma)?
3. Is there any important past history, such as surgery, Kawasaki's disease, asthma, sickle cell disease, diabetes, or Marfan's syndrome (or other connective tissue disease)?
4. Does any disease run in the family? Is there a family history of heart disease, other conditions, or sudden death?
5. Has there been a recent heart attack or a cardiac death in the family?

6. Is the child taking medicines, such as asthma medicines or birth control pills?
7. Has the child been exposed to drugs (cocaine) or cigarettes?
8. What treatments for the pain have been tried?
9. What is the patient or family member concerned about?

Physical Examination

1. A careful general physical examination should be performed before the focus turns to the chest. The clinician should note whether the child is in severe distress from pain, is in emotional stress, or is hyperventilating.
2. The skin and extremities should be examined for trauma or chronic disease. Bruising elsewhere on the body may indicate chest trauma that cannot be seen.
3. The abdomen should be carefully examined because it may be the source of pain referred to the chest.
4. The chest should be carefully inspected for trauma or asymmetry. The chest wall should be palpated for signs of tenderness or subcutaneous air. Special attention should be paid to the possibility of costochondritis as the cause of chest pain, which is a quite common identifiable cause of the pain. Physical examination is all that is needed for the diagnosis of costochondritis. Physicians should use the soft part of the terminal phalanx of a middle finger to palpate each costochondral and chondrosternal junction, not with the palm of a hand; using the palm may frequently miss the diagnosis. Pectoralis muscles and shoulder muscles should be examined for tenderness, which may be caused by excessive weightlifting or other work requiring the use of these muscles.
5. The heart and lungs should be auscultated for arrhythmias, heart murmurs, rubs, muffled heart sounds, gallop rhythm, crackles, wheezes, or decreased breath sounds.
6. Finally, the child's psychological state should be assessed.

Other Investigations

If the three common causes or other identifiable causes of chest pain are not found by physical examination, the clinician should obtain chest radiographic films and an ECG and direct his or her attention to the cardiac causes of chest pain listed in Table 30.2, which summarizes important history, physical findings, and abnormalities of chest radiography and ECGs for cardiac causes of chest pain.

1. Cardiac examination is done to detect a pathological heart murmur. One must be careful not to interpret commonly occurring innocent murmurs as pathologic.
2. Chest radiography should be evaluated for pulmonary pathology, cardiac size and silhouette, and pulmonary vascularity.
3. A resting 12-lead ECG should be evaluated for cardiac arrhythmias, hypertrophy, conduction disturbances (including Wolff-Parkinson-White preexcitation), abnormal T and Q waves, and an abnormal QTc interval.

If the pain is nonexertional, the family history is negative for hereditary heart disease (e.g., long QT syndrome, cardiomyopathies, unexpected sudden death), the past history is negative for heart disease or Kawasaki's disease, the cardiac examination is unremarkable, and the ECG and chest radiographs are normal, the chest pain is not likely to be of cardiac origin unless palpitation or dizziness is a prominent accompanying symptom. At this point, the clinician can reassure the patient and family of the probable benign nature of the chest pain. If any of the above aspects is positive, a formal cardiac consultation may be indicated. An echocardiographic examination is usually obtained by cardiologists, and it will most likely rule in or out cardiac causes of chest pain.

If a cardiac cause and the three common noncardiac causes of chest pain are not found, the pain is likely due to a condition in other systems, such as GI or respiratory systems, including psychogenic or idiopathic origin. Simple follow-up may clarify the cause. Drug screening for cocaine may be worthwhile in adolescents who have acute, severe chest pain and distress with an unclear cause.

Referral to Cardiologists

The following are some of the indications for referral to a cardiologist for cardiac evaluation:

1. When history reveals that chest pain is triggered or worsened by physical activities, the pain suggests anginal pain, or chest pain is accompanied by other symptoms such as palpitation, dizziness, or syncope
2. When there are abnormal findings in the cardiac examination or when abnormalities occur in the chest radiographs or ECG, cardiology referral is clearly indicated. The examiner's ability to recognize common innocent heart murmurs minimizes the frequency of such referrals.
3. When there is a positive family history for cardiomyopathy, long QT syndrome, sudden unexpected death, or other hereditary diseases commonly associated with cardiac abnormalities
4. High levels of anxiety in the family and patient and a chronic, recurring nature of the pain are also important reasons for referral to a cardiologist.

MANAGEMENT

When a specific cause of chest pain is identified, treatment is directed at correcting or improving the cause.

1. Costochondritis can be treated by reassurance and occasionally by nonsteroidal antiinflammatory drugs (NSAIDs, e.g., ibuprofen) or acetaminophen. Ibuprofen is better than acetaminophen because the former is an analgesic and antiinflammatory agent, and the latter is only analgesic.
   a. Ibuprofen 10 mg/kg, three to four times a day, for 7 days often improves the pain. The same course may be repeated two to three times with a 1-week period of no medicine in between the courses. Alternatively, for more compliance (because of twice-daily dosing), naproxen could be given for 5 to 7 days.
   b. Weight of backpacks should be reduced to a minimum.
   c. Physical activities requiring the use of shoulder girdle muscles should be avoided, which may include sports using arms, push-ups, pull-ups, certain house chores, and others.

2. Most musculoskeletal and nonorganic causes of chest pain can be treated with rest, acetaminophen, or NSAIDs.

3. If respiratory causes of chest pain are found, treatment is directed at those causes. Referral to a pulmonologist should be considered.

4. Exercise-induced asthma is most effectively prevented by inhalation of a β_2-agonist 10 to 15 minutes before exercise. Inhaled albuterol usually affords protection for 4 hours. Other antiasthmatic agents have also been reported to be effective as well. Use of a muffler or cold weather mask to warm and humidify air before inhalation also is effective.

5. If gastritis, gastroesophageal reflux, or peptic ulcer disease is suspected, trials of antacids, hydrogen ion blockers, or prokinetic agent (e.g., metoclopramide [Reglan]) are helpful therapeutically (as well as diagnostically).

6. If serious cardiac anomalies, arrhythmias, or exercise-induced asthma is diagnosed, a referral is made to the cardiology or pulmonary service. Cardiac evaluation requires further specialized studies such as echo, an exercise stress test, Holter monitoring, event recorder, or even cardiac catheterization or electrophysiologic study. Depending on the cause, treatment may be surgical or medical.

7. If organic causes of chest pain are not found and a psychogenic etiology is suspected, psychological consultation may be considered.

8. When or if cocaine-associated chest pain is suspected, physicians should arrange a referral to appropriate specialists for confirmation of the diagnosis and management of the problem.

Cocaine's pharmacologic action is through inhibition of the reuptake of norepinephrine, dopamine, and serotonin, and thus it produces signs of heightened sympathetic nervous system. Cocaine produces chest pain through powerful coronary vasoconstriction with decreased oxygen supply to the myocardium. Cocaine leads to increased heart rate, high blood pressure, dilated pupils, and reduced skin temperature. Cocaine also increases the possibility of thrombus formation (by inhibition of endogenous fibrinolysis, increasing thrombogenicity, and enhancing platelet aggregation via increased production of thromboxane).

The following are several points recommended by the American Heart Association's guideline on treatment for cocaine abuse patients (McCord et al, 2008).

a. If cocaine intoxication is suspected, benzodiazepines are recommended as the primary treatment for anxiety, tachycardia, and hypertension.

b. Aspirin and nitrates continue to be strongly recommended.

c. However, beta-blockers (including agents with mixed α-adrenergic antagonist effects, such as labetalol) are considered contraindicated because the unopposed α-adrenergic effect leads to worsening coronary vasoconstriction and increasing blood pressure.

d. Calcium channel blockers are not recommended; they might increase mortality rates.

e. Early percutaneous coronary intervention is indicated if myocardial infarction is likely the diagnosis.

Syncope

PREVALENCE

The prevalence of syncope and near syncope in children is unknown, but it is estimated that as many as 15% of children and adolescents will have a syncopal event between the ages of 8 and 18 years. The incidence may be as high as 3% of emergency department visits in some areas. Before age 6 years, syncope is unusual except in the setting of seizure disorders, breath holding, and cardiac arrhythmias.

DEFINITION

- Syncope is a transient loss of consciousness and muscle tone that results from inadequate cerebral perfusion.
- Presyncope is the feeling that one is about to pass out but remains conscious with a transient loss of postural tone. It is usually less serious than syncope and is often a manifestation of a benign condition.
- Dizziness is the most common prodromal symptom to the above. It is a nonspecific symptom that may include vertigo and lightheadedness. Vertigo is a feeling that you or your surroundings are spinning or whirling, a manifestation of vestibular disorder. Lightheadedness is a feeling that you are about to faint, but you do not feel as though you or your surroundings are moving. Lightheadedness often accompanies hyperventilation and is frequently associated with psychological distress, including anxiety, depression, and panic attacks.
  Although most of these complaints are benign in pediatric age group, any of these complaints could represent a serious cardiac condition that could cause sudden death.

CAUSES

The normal function of the brain depends on a constant supply of oxygen and glucose. Significant alterations in the supply of oxygen and glucose may result in a transient loss or near loss of consciousness, with manifestation of syncope, presyncope, or dizziness. The differential diagnosis of syncope is rather broad. It may be from noncardiac causes (usually autonomic dysfunction), cardiac conditions, neuropsychiatric, and metabolic disorders. Box 31.1 lists possible causes of syncope.

In contrast to adults, in whom most cases of syncope are caused by cardiac problems, in children and adolescents, most incidents of syncope are benign, resulting from vasovagal episodes (probably the most common cause), orthostatic intolerance syndromes, dehydration (or inadequate hydration), hyperventilation, and breath holding. However, the primary purpose of the evaluation of patients with syncope is to determine whether the patient is at increased risk for death.

In this chapter, only circulatory causes of syncope are discussed in some detail. Discussion of the metabolic and neuropsychiatric causes of syncope is beyond the scope of this book.

NONCARDIAC CAUSES OF SYNCOPE

Noncardiac causes of syncope may be divided into three groups: orthostatic intolerance group, exercise-related syncope, and other rare types of syncope. Improved understanding of disorders of blood flow, heart rate, and blood pressure

Box 31.1 Causes of Syncope

Autonomic (Noncardiac)
Orthostatic intolerance group
    Vasovagal syncope (also known as simple, neurocardiogenic, or neurally mediated syncope)
    Orthostatic (postural) hypotension (dysautonomia)
    Postural orthostatic tachycardia syndrome
Exercise-related syncope
Situational syncope
    Breath holding
    Cough, micturition, defecation
    Carotid sinus hypersensitivity

Cardiac
Arrhythmia
Tachycardia: SVT, atrial flutter or fibrillation, ventricular tachycardia (seen with long QT syndrome, short QT syndrome, Brugada, arrhythmogenic RV dysplasia)
Bradycardia: sinus bradycardia, asystole, complete heart block, pacemaker malfunction

Obstructive Lesions
Outflow obstruction: AS, PS, HCM, pulmonary hypertension
Inflow obstruction: MS, tamponade, constrictive pericarditis, atrial myxoma

Myocardial
Coronary artery anomalies: HCM, DCM, MVP, arrhythmogenic RV dysplasia

Neuropsychiatric
Anxiety disorders: panic disorders, agoraphobia (fear of open space or uncontrollable social situations)
Hyperventilation
Seizure disorders
Migraine
Brain tumors
Hysterical

Metabolic
Dehydration (or inadequate hydration)
Hypoglycemia
Electrolyte disorders
Anorexia nervosa
Drugs/toxins: anti-seizure drugs, sedatives and tranquilizers, anti-psychotic drugs, anti-hypertensive drugs.

AS, aortic stenosis; *DCM,* dilated cardiomyopathy; *HCM,* hypertrophic cardiomyopathy; *MS,* mitral stenosis; *MVP,* mitral valve prolapse; *PS,* pulmonary stenosis; *RV,* right ventricular; *SVT,* supraventricular tachycardia.

(BP) is the result of the recently popularized "head-up tilt test." Three easily definable entities of orthostatic intolerance group are (1) vasovagal syncope, (2) orthostatic hypotension (or dysautonomia), and (3) postural orthostatic tachycardia syndrome (POTS).

Vasovagal Syncope

Vasovagal syncope (also called simple fainting or neurocardiogenic or neutrally mediated syncope) is the most common type of syncope in otherwise healthy children and adolescents. This syncope is uncommon before 10 to 12 years of age but quite prevalent in adolescent girls. It is characterized by a prodrome (warning symptoms and signs) lasting a few seconds to a minute. The prodrome may include dizziness, nausea, pallor, diaphoresis, palpitation, blurred vision, headache, or hyperventilation. The prodrome is followed by the loss of consciousness and muscle tone. The patient usually falls without injury, the unconsciousness does not last more than 1 minute, and the patient gradually awakens. The syncope may occur after rising in the morning, after taking a morning shower, or in association with prolonged standing, anxiety or fright, pain, blood drawing or the sight of blood, fasting, hot and humid conditions, or crowded places. It may occur after prolonged exercise (if exercise is stopped suddenly).

The pathophysiology of vasovagal syncope is not completely understood. The following is a popular hypothesis (although dismissed by some). In normal individuals, an erect posture without movement shifts blood to the lower extremities and pelvis and causes a decrease in venous return, thus decreasing stroke volume and BP. This reduced filling of the ventricle places less stretch on the mechanoreceptor (i.e., C fibers) and causes a decrease in afferent neural output to the brain stem, reflecting hypotension. This decline in neural traffic from the mechanoreceptors and a decreased arterial pressure elicit an increase in sympathetic output, resulting in an increase in heart rate and peripheral vasoconstriction to restore BP to the normal range. Thus, the normal responses to the assumption of an upright posture are a reduced cardiac output (by 25%), an increase in heart rate, an unchanged or slightly diminished systolic pressure (Fig. 31.1), and an increase in diastolic pressure to ensure coronary artery perfusion. Cerebral blood flow decreases by approximately 6% with cerebrovascular autoregulation functioning near its maximal limit.

In susceptible individuals, however, a sudden decrease in venous return to the ventricle produces a large increase in the force of ventricular contraction; this causes activation of the left ventricular mechanoreceptors, which normally respond only to stretch (Fig. 31.2). The resulting paroxysmal increase in neural traffic to the brain stem somehow mimics the conditions seen in hypertension and thereby produces a paradoxical withdrawal of sympathetic activity and vagal activation. Withdrawal of sympathetic activity leads to a peripheral vasodilatation, hypotension, and bradycardia. Vagal activation results in bradycardia (see Fig. 31.2). Characteristically, the reduction of BP and especially the heart rate are severe enough to decrease cerebral perfusion, resulting in either presyncope or syncope (with loss of consciousness). Vasovagal syncope always occurs while the patient is in standing position. Hypovolemia (or dehydration) is often a predisposing factor.

History is most important in establishing the diagnosis of vasovagal syncope. Tilt testing of various protocol is useful in diagnosing vasovagal syncope, but it has not been well standardized, and its specificity and reproducibility are questionable.

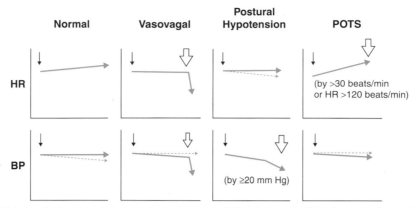

Fig. 31.1 Schematic drawing of changes in heart rate and blood pressure (BP) observed during the head-up tilt test. *Thin arrows* mark the start of orthostatic stress. *Large unfilled arrows* indicate appearance of symptoms with changes seen in heart rate (HR) and BP. In normal individuals, the HR increases slightly with no change or slight reduction in BP. In patients with vasovagal syncope, both the HR and BP drop precipitously with the appearance of symptoms. Postural hypotension is characterized by a drop in systolic BP by 20 mm Hg or more as symptoms appear within 3 minutes of standing. In postural orthostatic tachycardia syndrome (POTS), HR increases significantly by more than 30 beats/min (or the HR is ≥120 beats/min) with development of symptoms within 10 minutes of standing.

Placing the patient in a supine position until the circulatory crisis resolves may be all that is indicated. If the patient feels the prodrome to a faint, he or she should be told to lie down with the feet raised above the chest; this usually aborts the syncope. Success in preventing syncope has been reported with medications, such as α-adrenergic agonists, beta-blockers, pseudoephedrine, fludrocortisone (Florinef), and others. Their points of action are shown in Fig. 31.2 (also see Management section).

Orthostatic Hypotension (Dysautonomia)

The normal response to standing is reflex arterial and venous constriction and a slight increase in heart rate. In orthostatic hypotension, the normal adrenergic vasoconstriction of the arterioles and veins in the upright position is absent or inadequate, resulting in hypotension without a reflex increase in heart rate (see Fig. 31.1). In contrast to the prodrome seen with vasovagal syncope, in orthostatic hypotension, patients experience only lightheadedness. Orthostatic hypotension is usually related to medication (see later) or dehydration, but it can be precipitated by prolonged bed rest, prolonged standing, and conditions that decrease the circulating blood volume (e.g., bleeding, dehydration). Drugs that interfere with the sympathetic vasomotor response (e.g., calcium channel blockers, antihypertensive drugs, vasodilators, phenothiazines) and diuretics may exacerbate orthostatic hypotension.

In patients suspected of having orthostatic hypotension, BPs should be measured in the supine and standing positions. In adults, the American Autonomic Society has defined orthostatic hypotension as a persistent fall in systolic/diastolic pressure of more than 20/10 mm Hg within 3 minutes of assuming the upright position without moving their arms or legs with no increase in the heart rate but without fainting. Orthostatic hypotension may only be demonstrable in the presence of dehydration. In a well-hydrated state when seen in an office setting, orthostatic hypotension may not occur.

The same management as that given for vasovagal syncope is sometimes successful. Elastic stockings, a high-salt diet, sympathomimetic amines, and corticosteroids have been used with varying degrees of success. The patient should be told to move to an upright position slowly.

Postural Orthostatic Tachycardia Syndrome

This is a form of orthostatic intolerance that is most often observed in young women. Venous pooling associated with assuming standing position predominantly affects the lower extremities. This leads to a reduced venous return, a resulting increase in sympathetic discharge, and a significant degree of tachycardia. An increased level of adrenomedullin, a potent vasodilator with natriuretic and diuretic effects, has been observed in some children with the syndrome, possibly as a result of endothelial dysfunction (Zhang et al, 2012).

Children (and adults) with the syndrome often have symptoms of syncope, dizziness, chest discomfort or pain, headache, palpitation, nausea, fatigue, and exercise intolerance. This may be related to "chronic fatigue syndrome" and may be misdiagnosed as having panic attacks or chronic anxiety.

For the diagnosis of POTS, heart rate and BP are measured in the supine, sitting, and standing positions. POTS is defined as the development of orthostatic symptoms that are associated with at least a 30-beat/min increase in heart rate (or a heart rate of ≥120 beats/min) that occurs within the first 10 minutes of standing or upright tilt. An exaggerated increase in heart rate is often accompanied by hypotension in association with the symptoms described (see Fig. 31.1).

The same approaches of management as vasovagal syncope are used with varying level of success. Pharmacologic agents such as fludrocortisone, midodrine (a peripheral vasoconstrictor, at the dosage of 5–10 mg three times a day), and venlafaxine (a selective serotonin reuptake inhibitor) are useful in many patients.

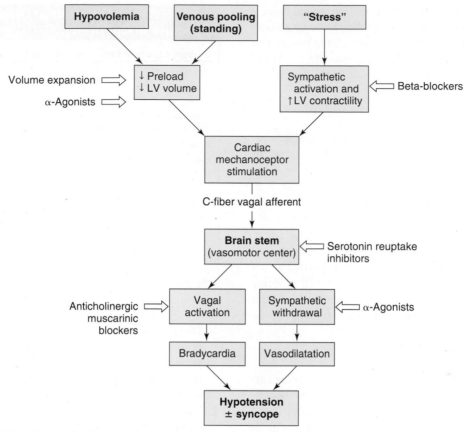

Fig. 31.2 Proposed pathophysiology of vasovagal syncope. Presumed points of action of various pharmacologic agents are also shown by *open arrows*. *LV*, Left ventricular. (Modified from Ross BA, Saul JP: Management of vasovagal syncope: pharmacologic, nonpharmacologic, or pacing. In Walsh EP, Philip Saul J, Triedman JK, eds, *Cardiac Arrhythmias in Children and Young Adults with Congenital Heart Disease*, Philadelphia, 2001, Lippincott Williams & Wilkins.)

Exercise-Related Syncope

Sudden unconsciousness that occurs during or after strenuous physical activities or sports may signal an organic cause such as cardiopulmonary diseases, including cardiac arrhythmia. However, in most cases, exercise-related syncope is not an indicator of serious underlying cardiopulmonary or metabolic disease. It occurs more often because of a combination of venous pooling in vasodilated leg muscles, inadequate hydration, and high ambient temperature. Hyperventilation with hypocapnia (with tingling or numbness of extremities) secondary to strenuous activities may also cause syncope. To prevent venous pooling, athletes should keep moving after running competitions.

Rare Causes of Syncope

Micturition syncope is a rare form of orthostatic hypotension. In this condition, rapid bladder decompression results in decreased total peripheral vascular resistance with splanchnic stasis and reduced venous return to the heart, resulting in postural hypotension.

Cough syncope follows paroxysmal nocturnal coughing in children with asthma. The patient's face becomes plethoric and cyanotic, and the child perspires, becomes agitated, and is frightened. Loss of consciousness is associated with muscle contractions lasting for several seconds. Urinary incontinence is frequent. Consciousness is regained within a few minutes. Paroxysmal coughing produces a marked increase in intrapleural pressure with a reduced venous return and reduced cardiac output, resulting in altered cerebral blood flow and loss of consciousness. Treatment is aimed at preventing bronchoconstriction with aggressive asthma treatment plans.

CARDIAC CAUSES OF SYNCOPE

Cardiac causes of syncope may include obstructive lesions, myocardial dysfunction, and arrhythmias, including long QT syndrome and Brugada syndrome. A cardiac cause of syncope is suggested by the occurrence of syncope even in the recumbent position, syncope provoked by exercise, chest pain associated with syncope, a history of unoperated or operated heart disease, or a family history of sudden death.

Obstructive Lesions

Patients with severe obstructive lesions such as aortic stenosis (AS), pulmonary stenosis (PS), or hypertrophic obstructive cardiomyopathy (HOCM), as well as those with pulmonary hypertension may have syncope. Exercise often precipitates syncope associated with these conditions. Peripheral vasodilatation secondary to exercise is not accompanied by an adequate increase in cardiac output because of the obstructive lesion, which results in diminished perfusion to the brain. Patients may also complain of chest pain, dyspnea, and palpitation.

Myocardial Dysfunction

Although rare, myocardial ischemia or infarction secondary to congenital anomalies of the coronary arteries or acquired disease of the coronary arteries (e.g., Kawasaki's disease or atherosclerotic heart disease) may cause syncope. Patients with dilated cardiomyopathy may have episodes of syncope associated with self-terminating episodes of ventricular tachycardia, which can lead to cardiac arrest. Syncope is a major risk factor for subsequent sudden cardiac death in hypertrophic cardiomyopathy, particularly if it is repetitive and occurs with exertion. Arrhythmogenic right ventricular (RV) dysplasia often develops ventricular tachycardia caused by myocyte replacement by adipose tissue or fibrosis.

Arrhythmias

Either extreme tachycardia or bradycardia can decrease cardiac output and lower the cerebral blood flow below the critical level, causing syncope. The occurrence of syncope in the sitting or recumbent position suggests cardiac arrhythmias (or seizure) as the cause of syncope. Commonly encountered rhythm disturbances include supraventricular tachycardia (SVT), ventricular tachycardia, sick sinus syndrome, and complete heart block. Simple bradycardia is usually well tolerated in children, but the combination of tachycardia followed by bradycardia (overdrive suppression) is more likely to produce syncope. Arrhythmias may or may not be associated with structural heart defects.

No Identifiable Structural Defects

Syncope from arrhythmias in children with structurally normal hearts may be seen in the following conditions.
1. Long QT syndrome
2. Short QT syndrome
3. Wolff-Parkinson-White (WPW) preexcitation may cause SVT.
4. RV dysplasia (RV cardiomyopathy)
5. Brugada syndrome

Structural Heart Defects

The following congenital and acquired heart conditions, unoperated or operated, are associated with arrhythmias that may result in syncope.
1. Preoperative congenital heart diseases (CHDs), such as Ebstein's anomaly, mitral stenosis (MS), or mitral regurgitation (MR), and congenitally corrected transposition of the great arteries (L-TGA), may cause arrhythmias.
2. Postoperative CHDs may cause arrhythmias, especially after repairs of tetralogy of Fallot (TOF) and transposition of the great arteries (TGA) and after the Fontan operation.

TABLE 31.1 Differential Diagnosis of Syncope in Children			
If positive, consider:	**Vasovagal**	**Cardiac**	**Seizure**
Prodrome	✓		✓
Positional	✓		
Chest pain		✓	
Palpitations	±	✓	
Exercise-related	±	✓	
Abnormal movements	±	±[a]	✓
Headache	±		±
Heart murmur		✓	
Neurologic deficits			✓
Prolonged altered mental status			✓
Family history	±	✓	±
Abnormal ECG		✓	

[a]10% of patients with Long QT syndrome present with seizures.
ECG, Electrocardiogram.

These children may have sinus node dysfunction (sick sinus syndrome), SVT or ventricular tachycardia, or complete heart block.
3. Dilated cardiomyopathy can cause sinus bradycardia, SVT, or ventricular tachycardia.
4. Hypertrophic cardiomyopathy is a rare cause of ventricular tachycardia and syncope.
5. Mitral valve prolapse (MVP) is an extremely rare cause of ventricular tachycardia.

EVALUATION OF A CHILD WITH SYNCOPE

Most children who present with presyncope (without loss of consciousness) or even syncope have vasovagal phenomenon or other benign causes of syncope. However, the goal of the evaluation of a patient with syncope (or presyncope) is to identify high-risk patients with underlying heart disease, which may include patients with abnormal electrocardiograms (ECGs) (e.g., long QT syndrome, WPW preexcitation), cardiomyopathy (hypertrophic or dilated), or structural heart diseases. The evaluation of pediatric patients with syncope may extend to other family members when a genetic condition is suspected or identified.

Table 31.1 is a simplified overview of deciding which one of the three major causes of syncope is more likely the cause. Detailed discussion of history, physical examination, and other investigations will follow, which will help in the differential diagnosis of syncope in children and adolescents.

History

Because physical examinations of patients are almost always normal long after the event, accurate history taking is most important in determining a cost-effective diagnostic workup for each patient. Sometimes a complete history cannot be obtained owing to amnesia about the event, but witness accounts are useful. The following are some important aspects of history taking.

1. About the syncopal event
   a. The time of the day
      - Syncope occurring after rising in the morning or after morning shower suggests vasovagal syncope.
      - Hypoglycemia is a very rare cause of syncope, occurring in fasting state in the morning.
   b. The patient's position (supine, standing, or sitting)
      - Syncope while sitting or recumbent suggests arrhythmias or seizures.
      - Syncope after standing for some time suggests orthostatic intolerance group, including vasovagal syncope.
   c. Relationship to exercise
      - Syncope occurring during exercise suggest arrhythmias.
      - Syncope occurring immediately after cessation of physical activities suggests venous pooling in the leg (with reduced venous return and cardiac output).
      - Estimating vigorousness and duration of the activity, relative hydration status, and ambient temperature at the time of syncope is important.
   d. Associated symptoms sometimes are helpful in suspecting the cause of syncope.
      - Palpitation or racing heart rate suggests tachycardia or arrhythmias.
      - Chest pain suggests possible myocardial ischemia (obstructive lesions, cardiomyopathy, carditis).
      - Shortness of breath or tingling or numbness of the extremities suggests hyperventilation.
      - Nausea, epigastric discomfort, and diaphoresis suggest vasovagal syncope.
      - Headache or visual changes suggests vasovagal syncope.
   e. The duration of syncope
      - Syncopal duration less than 1 minute suggests vasovagal syncope, postural hypotension, or hyperventilation.
      - A longer duration of syncope suggests convulsive disorders, migraine, or arrhythmias.
   f. The patient's appearance during and immediately after the episode
      - Pallor indicates hypotension.
      - Abnormal movement or posturing, confusion, focal neurologic signs, amnesia, or muscle soreness suggests the possibility of seizure.
2. Past history of cardiac, endocrine, neurologic, or psychological disorders may suggest a disorder in that system.
3. Medication history, including prescribed, over-the-counter, and recreational drugs, should be checked.
4. Family history should include:
   a. Coronary heart disease risk factors, including history of myocardial infarction in family members younger than 30 years of age
   b. Cardiac arrhythmia, CHD, cardiomyopathies, long QT syndrome, seizures, and metabolic and psychological disorders
   c. Positive family history of fainting is common in patients with vasovagal syncope.

5. Social history is important in assessing whether there is a possibility of substance abuse, pregnancy, or factors leading to a conversion reaction.

Physical Examination

Although the results of the physical examination are usually normal, a complete physical examination should always be performed, focusing on the patient's cardiac and neurologic status.

1. If orthostatic intolerance group is suspected, the heart rate and BP should be measured repeatedly while the patient is supine and after standing without moving for up to 10 minutes. In a well-hydrated state, positive test results for vasovagal syncope or postural hypotension in the office setting are uncommon.
2. Careful auscultation is carried out to detect a heart murmur or an abnormally loud second heart sound.
3. Neurologic examination should include a fundoscopic examination, test for Romberg's sign, gait evaluation, deep tendon reflexes, and cerebellar function.

Diagnostic Studies

History and physical examinations guide practitioners in choosing the diagnostic tests that apply to a given syncopal patient. A complete cardiac evaluation is indicated if there is a heart murmur, a family history of sudden death or cardiomyopathy, or an abnormal ECG finding.

1. Serum glucose and electrolytes is of limited value because the patients are seen hours or days after the episode.
2. In suspected cases of arrhythmia as the cause of syncope, the following may be indicated.
   a. The ECG should be inspected for heart rate (bradycardia), arrhythmias, WPW preexcitation, heart block, and long QTc interval, as well as abnormalities suggestive of cardiomyopathies and myocarditis.
   b. Ambulatory ECG monitoring: A correlation between a patient's symptoms and a diagnostic arrhythmia confirms the arrhythmic cause of syncope. Symptoms without arrhythmia probably exclude an arrhythmic cause of syncope.
      1) Holter monitor usually records ECG for up to 24 hours.
      2) A loop memory event recorder with extended monitoring (usually for a month) may increase the diagnostic yield.
      3) A nonlooping event recorder can be used for symptoms lasting for a few minutes (usually for a month).
      4) An implantable loop recorder (implanted in the left pectoral region) can be used to record ECGs for a period much longer than one month.
   c. Exercise stress test. If the syncopal event is associated with exercise, a treadmill exercise stress test should also be performed, with full ECG and BP monitoring (see Chapter 6).
3. Echocardiographic studies. Echo studies identify structural abnormalities that can cause syncope and chest pain. Identifiable structural causes include severe obstructive

lesions (e.g., AS, PS, HOCM), pulmonary hypertension, certain CHDs (Ebstein's anomaly, MS or MR, L-TGA), and the status of postoperative CHDs (e.g., TOF, TGA, Fontan operation).

4. Head-up tilt table test. If a patient with syncope has autonomic symptoms (e.g., pallor, diaphoresis, or hyperventilation), a tilt table testing will be useful (see subsequent section for full discussion).

5. Cardiac catheterization and electrophysiologic testing may rarely be indicated in some equivocal cases. Because of the low yield of electrophysiologic testing in patients without underlying heart disease, this test is not routinely recommended in such cases.

6. Neurologic consultation. Patients exhibiting prolonged loss of consciousness, seizure activity, and a postictal phase with lethargy or confusion should be referred for neurologic consultation and electroencephalography (EEG). Without the above history, the reported positive yield of EEG or imaging studies is very low.

Head-up Tilt Table Test

The goal of tilt table testing is to provoke the patient's symptoms exactly during an orthostatic stress while being closely monitored, with demonstration of the cardiac rhythm and rate and BP responses associated with symptoms. Orthostatic stress is created by a tilting table with the patient placed in an upright position to obtain the necessary pooling of blood to the lower extremities.

Patients lie supine on an electric tilt table and have an intravenous line established. ECG monitoring and automated BP measurements are performed. Some laboratories perform an autonomic challenge test, which includes deep breathing to accentuate sinus arrhythmia, carotid massage (not done in adults, especially older adults), Valsalva maneuver, and the application of ice to the face to induce the "diving reflex." Patients are then tilted into the 60- to 80-degree head-up position for a period of up to 30 minutes. These patients remain upright, with recording of BP every 1 or 2 minutes and continuous heart rate and rhythm monitoring. If a patient becomes symptomatic or the 30-minute time elapses, the tilt table is immediately returned to the supine position. If result of the tilt test alone is not positive, the procedure is repeated with an infusion of isoproterenol, starting at 0.02 µg/kg/min and increasing to 1 µg/kg/min for 15 minutes; the use of isoproterenol in the evaluation of patients with vasovagal syncope remains somewhat controversial.

Positive responses commonly include lightheadedness, dizziness, nausea, visual changes, and frank syncope. Sinus bradycardia, junctional bradycardia, and asystole for as long as 30 seconds are common. Hypotension generally is manifested by systolic BPs of less than 70 mm Hg, with frequently immeasurable diastolic pressures. Returning these patients to the supine position produces resolution of symptoms rapidly, with a return of normal sinus rhythm, usually with a reactive tachycardia. Patients frequently comment that they "had a spell" and that they feel tired and weak.

Several distinct abnormal patterns have been identified following head-up tilt table tests (see Fig 31.1).

1. Vasovagal: an abrupt decrease in BP usually with bradycardia
2. Dysautonomia (or postural hypotension): a gradual decrease in BP leading to syncope
3. POTS: an excessive heart rate increase to maintain an adequate BP to prevent syncope

After a positive tilt test result, many laboratories begin a therapeutic trial of a short-acting beta-blocker, such as an esmolol infusion, and repeat the tilt test. If these patients do not become symptomatic during this tilt test, an oral beta-blocker is prescribed (see subsequent discussion). If these patients are again symptomatic, they are tested with infusion of an α-agonist (phenylephrine) with a repeat tilt table test. Finally, the patient is tested with a bolus of 1 L normal saline. If the patient remains asymptomatic during the test, these patients are treated with volume expansion therapy using a mineralocorticoid (Florinef) and salt supplementation (see later).

There are, however, serious questions about the sensitivity, specificity, diagnostic yield, and day-to-day reproducibility of the tilt test. In adults, the overall reproducibility of syncope by the tilt test is disappointingly low (62%), which causes doubt about the specificity of the test for diagnosis and the validity of evaluating the effect of oral drug treatment by a repeat tilt test. About 25% of adolescents with no prior fainting history fainted during the tilt test. Moreover, among habitual fainters, 25% to 30% did not faint during the test on a given day.

TREATMENT

The same preventive measures are used for all orthostatic intolerance group of conditions. Beginning the therapy empirically without performing a head-up tilt table test is reasonable. Most patients show spontaneous resolution of syncope in 6 to 12 months, and therefore long-term medical prophylaxis is usually not necessary.

1. Maintaining adequate intravascular volume is the most important element in the prevention of syncope.
   a. The patient is recommended to drink 60 to 90 oz of water a day. Physical activities, especially in a hot environment, require much more fluid intake, preferably electrolyte containing fluids (e.g., Gatorade).
   b. Drinking "soft drinks" with additional sodium is an option.
   c. Liberal use of salt with meals and nonfatty salted snacks (i. e., pretzels, popcorn without butter) are recommended.
   d. Caffeinated beverages should be avoided (because of their renal diuretic effect).
   e. Elastic support hose (waist high) is useful in some patients with postural hypotension.
2. Success in preventing syncope has been reported with the following medications. Their mechanism of action is shown in Fig. 31.2.
   a. Fludrocortisone (Florinef), a mineralocortisone, increases intravascular volume and produces both venous and

arterial vasoconstriction. It can be given in a low dosage (0.1 mg by mouth once or twice a day; adult dose is around 0.2 mg/day) with increased salt intake or a salt tablet (1 g/day). Average preadolescents or adolescents commonly gain 1 kg or 2 kg water weight into their circulating volume within 2 or 3 weeks. The increased vascular volume allows these patients to maintain cerebral BP despite the normal episodic parasympathetic-mediated venodilation.

b. Beta-blocker therapy is used commonly, especially in adolescents and young adults, to modify the feedback loop. Atenolol (1-2 mg/kg/day orally every day) and metoprolol (1.5 mg/kg/day given orally in two or three doses) are most commonly used.

c. α-Agonist therapy using pseudoephedrine or an ephedrine–theophylline combination (Marax) stimulates the heart rate and increases the peripheral vascular tone, preventing reflex bradycardia and vasodilation. Pseudoephedrine, 60 mg given orally twice a day, has been reported to be beneficial in some older children and adolescents. Midodrine, an α_1-agonist, promotes vasoconstriction in the smooth muscle cells of the blood vessels, thus increasing the vascular tone and with that the BP. Midodrine is given at 2.5 to 10 mg orally three times a day. Adverse effects include supine hypertension, urinary retention or urgency, or paresthesia.

d. The efficacy of serotonin agonists (sertraline [Zoloft]) has also been described in the treatment of patients with refractory syncope.

3. Beneficial effects of an implanted pacemaker for vasovagal syncope have been reported by some investigators but not by others. It is generally not indicated in pediatric patients.

Cardiac Arrhythmias

Primary cardiac arrhythmias presenting as syncopal events may require antiarrhythmic medications, pacemakers, or implantable cardioverter–defibrillators as discussed in Chapter 24.

DIFFERENTIAL DIAGNOSIS

A thorough history taking usually directs the physician to the correct diagnosis and thereby reduces the number of unnecessary tests.

Epilepsy

Patients with epilepsy may have incontinence, marked confusion in the postictal state, and abnormal EEGs. Patients are rigid rather than limp and may have sustained injuries. Patients do not experience the prodromal symptoms of syncope (e.g., dizziness, pallor, palpitation, diaphoresis) but may experience mood changes, irritability, or anxiety. The duration of unconsciousness is longer than that typically seen with syncope (<1 minute).

Hypoglycemia

Hypoglycemia has characteristics similar to syncope, such as pallor, perspiration, abdominal discomfort, lightheadedness, confusion, unconsciousness, and possible subsequent occurrence of seizures. However, hypoglycemic attacks differ from syncope in that the onset and recovery occur more gradually, they do not occur during or shortly after meals, and the presyncopal symptoms do not improve in the supine position.

Hyperventilation

Hyperventilation is believed to produce hypocapnia, resulting in intense cerebral vasoconstriction, and causes syncope. A recent study, however, demonstrates that hyperventilation alone is not sufficient to cause syncope, suggesting that it may also have a psychological component. A typical spell usually begins with an apprehensive feeling and "deep sighing respirations" that the patient rarely notices. The patient often experiences air hunger, shortness of breathing, chest tightness, abdominal discomfort, palpitations, dizziness, numbness or tingling of the face and extremities, and rarely loss of consciousness. It often is associated with emotional disturbances. The supine position may help the patient relax and may stop the anxiety–hyperventilation cycle. The syncopal episode can be reproduced in the office when the patient hyperventilates.

Hysteria

Syncope resulting from hysteria is not associated with injury and occurs only in the presence of an audience. A teenager may be able to give an accurate presyncopal history, but during these attacks, he or she does not experience the pallor and hypotension that characterize true syncope. The attacks may last longer (≤1 hour) than a brief syncopal spell. Episodes usually occur in an emotionally charged setting and are rare before 10 years of age. Spells are not consistently related to postural changes and are not improved by the supine position.

Palpitation

DEFINITION

Palpitation is an unpleasant subjective awareness of one's own heartbeats. This usually occurs as a sensation in the chest of rapid, irregular, or unusually strong heartbeats. The patient describes it as pounding, jumping, racing, irregularity of the heartbeat; a "flip flopping" or "rapid fluttering" in the chest; or pounding in the neck. Palpitation can be felt in the chest, throat, or neck. The pulse rate may become faster or rarely slower than normal. The term "palpitation" is used so loosely that specific questions must be asked to determine the exact nature of the symptom.

Causes

Palpitation is one of the most common cardiac symptoms encountered in medical practice, but it poorly corresponds to demonstrable abnormalities. Many palpitations are often not serious. However, palpitation may indicate the possible presence of serious cardiac arrhythmias.

Box 32.1 lists causes of palpitation. The differential diagnosis can range from benign etiologies to life-threatening arrhythmias.

- A high percentage of patients with palpitation have no etiology that can be established.
- Caffeine, a common stimulant, is found in many foods and drinks, such as coffee, tea, hot cocoa, soda, chocolate, and some medicines. Most energy drinks (e.g., Venom, Whoopass, Red Bull, Adrenalin Rush), which are the latest popular fad among youth culture, contain large doses of caffeine and other legal stimulants, including ephedrine, guarana, taurine, and ginseng.
- Certain drugs and substances can be identified as a cause of palpitation.
- Some medical conditions, such as hyperthyroidism, anemia, and hypoglycemia, may be the cause of palpitation.
- Although relatively rare, cardiac arrhythmias and structural heart disease should be looked into as a cause of palpitation. However, most palpitations are not accompanied by arrhythmias, and most arrhythmias are not perceived and reported as palpitations.

- Rarely, slow heart rates may cause palpitation.
- Occasionally, a psychogenic or psychiatric cause for their symptoms can be suspected. Some adult patients and adolescents with palpitations have panic disorder or panic attack. Panic attack and arrhythmias may be difficult to distinguish clinically because both may present as palpitations, shortness of breath, and lightheadedness.

EVALUATION

History

In a child who is old enough to provide a detailed history, careful history taking often suggests possible causes. Palpitation usually occurs without other symptoms. However, the presence of additional symptoms such as dizziness, fainting, nausea, sweating, chest pain, shortness of breath, and so on may be more significant.

1. The nature and onset of palpitation may suggest causes.
   a. Isolated "jumps" or "skips" suggests premature beats.
   b. A sudden start and stop of rapid heartbeat or a pounding of the chest suggests supraventricular tachycardia (SVT). Some children will appear sweaty or pale with SVT.
   c. A gradual onset and cessation of palpitation suggests sinus tachycardia or anxiety state.
   d. When the rate is known to be normal and the rhythm is regular, anxiety state is the cause.
   e. Palpitation characterized by slow heart rate may be caused by atrioventricular (AV) block or sinus node dysfunction.
2. Relationship to exertion:
   a. A history of palpitation during strenuous physical activity may be a normal phenomenon (caused by sinus tachycardia), although it could also be caused by exercise-induced arrhythmias.
   b. Nonexertional palpitation may suggest atrial flutter or fibrillation, febrile state, thyrotoxicosis, hypoglycemia, or anxiety state.

Box 32.1   Causes of Palpitation

Normal Physiologic Events
Exercise, excitement, fever

Psychologic or Psychiatric
Fear, anger, stress, anxiety disorders, panic attack or panic disorder

Certain Drugs and Substances
Stimulants: caffeine (coffee, tea, soda, chocolate), some energy drinks, smoking
Over-the-counter drugs: decongestants, diet pills, and so on
Drugs that cause tachycardia: catecholamines, theophylline, hydralazine, minoxidil, cocaine
Drugs that cause bradycardia: beta-blockers, antihypertensive drugs, calcium channel blockers
Drugs that cause arrhythmias: antiarrhythmics (some of which are proarrhythmic), tricyclic antidepressants, phenothiazines

Certain Medical Conditions
Anemia
Hyperthyroidism
Hypoglycemia
Hyperventilation
Poor physical condition

Heart Diseases
Certain congenital heart defects that are prone to arrhythmias or that result in a poor physical condition
After surgeries for congenital heart disease: Fontan connection, Senning operation
Mitral valve prolapse
Hypertrophic cardiomyopathy
Dilated cardiomyopathy
Valvular disease: aortic stenosis
Cardiac tumors or infiltrative diseases

Cardiac Arrhythmias
Tachycardia
Bradycardia
Premature atrial contractions
Premature ventricular contractions
Supraventricular tachycardias
Ventricular tachycardias
Atrial fibrillation
Wolff-Parkinson-White preexcitation
Sick sinus syndrome

c. A rapidly developing palpitation, although not abrupt, unrelated to exertion or excitement, may occur with hypoglycemia or tumor of adrenal medulla.

d. Palpitation on standing suggests postural hypotension (or orthostatic intolerance).

3. Associated symptoms

a. Symptoms of dizziness or fainting associated with palpitation may indicate ventricular tachycardia.

b. The presence of other symptoms, such as chest pain, sweating, nausea, or shortness of breath, may be more significant and may increase the likelihood of identifiable causes of palpitation.

4. Personal and family history may help identify the cause.

a. Ask about eating and drinking habits, such as sodas, coffee, tea, hot cocoa, and chocolates, which contain caffeine.

b. Ask if the patient is taking energy drinks.

c. Ask about prescription and over-the-counter medications that could cause palpitation.

d. Ask about medical or heart conditions which may cause tachycardia or palpitation (listed in Box 32.1).

e. Ask about family history of syncope, sudden death, or arrhythmias.

Physical Examination

1. Most children with palpitation have normal physical examinations, except for those with hyperthyroidism.

2. Cardiac examination may reveal findings of mitral valve prolapse (MVP), obstructive lesions, or possibly cardiomyopathy.

Recording of Electrocardiogram Rhythm

Recording of electrocardiogram (ECG) rhythm that coincides with the timing of the patient's complaint of palpitation is a certain way of making diagnosis of arrhythmia or ruling it out as the cause of palpitation. A number of different ECG recording techniques are available.

1. Routine ECG during office visit: Check for prolonged QTc interval, delta waves (Wolff-Parkinson-White preexcitation), or AV block.

2. When palpitation occurs almost daily, especially when associated with symptoms, 24-hour Holter monitoring is usually most helpful in making the diagnosis of the rhythm abnormality. This may clarify the diagnosis and secure management plans. Some children actually complain of palpitation during sinus tachycardia.

3. When palpitation occurs infrequently, long-term event monitor recording (≤30 days) is indicated. With infrequent palpitations that are fairly long-lasting, handheld or patient activated event recorders are indicated. However, with infrequent short-lasting palpitation, external loop recorders are indicated.

4. Implantable loop recorder (inserted under the skin at about the second rib on the left front of the chest) can be used to monitor for a period longer than 1 month (may be up to 1 year). This can be worn during swimming or other vigorous exercises.

5. Continuous outpatient telemetry monitoring is a new monitoring modality available at most tertiary care facility. The patient is fitted with a transmitter that sends the ECG data to the area of the hospital where the telemetry monitoring occurs. The patient can move around within the devices transmitting range.

6. If the symptoms occur during exercise, an exercise stress test may be helpful in making the diagnosis.

7. If there is a high suspicion of ventricular tachycardia, sometimes provocative electrophysiologic studies may be indicated.

8. Inappropriate sinus tachycardia (IST) is a condition of exclusion. When all other means have been exhausted and Holter or event monitoring has shown sinus tachycardias

at unexpected times and heart rate is unusually high for the state of activity, IST is suspected. The mechanism of this tachycardia is not clearly understood. Some investigators have postulated an autoimmune mechanism as the cause. Although it is a benign condition, however, it can cause significant disturbance to the patient's daily life. Its diagnosis and management are at times frustrating to the family and to the physician.

Echocardiography

Echo studies help identify possible structural heart disease that may cause arrhythmias, such as hypertrophic cardiomyopathy, dilated cardiomyopathy, cardiac tumors, MVP, and other structural abnormality of the heart.

Laboratory Studies

When other medical conditions are suspected as a cause of palpitation, a full blood count (for anemia), electrolytes, blood glucose, and thyroid function testing may be indicated. When pheochromocytoma is suspected, free metanephrines could be measured in blood plasma.

MANAGEMENT

1. If the rhythm recorded on the 24-hour Holter monitoring shows sinus tachycardia during the complaint of palpitation, all one has to do is to reassure the parent and child of the normal, benign nature of palpitation. Some parents are unaware of the fact that children's heart rate is faster than adults' heart rate and that children's heartbeats are easily palpable when they place their palms over the child's chest.

2. For isolated premature atrial contractions or premature ventricular contractions, nothing needs to be done except avoidance of stimulants such as caffeine, excessive amount of sodas, and energy drinks. If they are so frequent that they are a hindrance to normal daily living, a beta-blocker could be tried.

3. When a significant cardiac arrhythmia or an AV conduction disturbance is the suspected cause of palpitation, further evaluation and therapy are guided by recommendations discussed in Chapters 24 and 25.

4. Examination of all medications that the patient is taking may be helpful in the diagnosis and in modifying the dosage or schedule or changing it to other medications.

5. If palpitation is associated with symptoms, such as fainting, dizziness, chest pain, pallor, or diaphoresis, further evaluation is guided as described in Chapters 30 and 31.

33

Dyslipidemia and Other Cardiovascular Risk Factors

Atherosclerotic cardiovascular disease (CVD) is a major cause of morbidity and mortality in the United States and other Western countries. The pathogenesis of atherosclerosis and death from coronary artery disease (CAD) are importantly related to high levels of total cholesterol and low-density lipoprotein cholesterol (LDL-C) and low levels of high-density lipoprotein cholesterol (HDL-C). Multiple trials in adults have demonstrated that cholesterol reduction results in reduced angiographic progression of CAD and even modest regression in some cases. Recently, a link has been established between increased levels of triglycerides (TGs) and coronary heart disease. It is timely for physicians and other health care providers to review and update their knowledge on dyslipidemia. This chapter begins with a quick review of biochemistry.

REVIEW OF LIPID BIOCHEMISTRY

Lipids and Lipoproteins

Lipids represent an essential constituent of our daily diet. Four major lipids of plasma are cholesterol, TGs, phospholipids, and free fatty acids. TGs form an important energy source for cellular metabolism. Phospholipids are, because of their amphiphilic behavior, excellent emulsifiers of fats and constitute the predominant element of all biological membranes. Free fatty acids are a primary source of energy and play an important role in energy transport within the body. Cholesterol has an ambivalent nature: on the one hand, it is necessary for the stabilization of biological membrane structure and an essential precursor of hormones and bile acids in hepatic metabolism; on the other hand, a surplus of cholesterol is considered to trigger atherosclerosis.

Plasma lipids that are hydrophobic do not circulate freely but rather circulate in the form of lipid–protein macromolecular complexes known as *lipoproteins*. The nonpolar lipids (cholesterol esters and TGs) are present in the lipoprotein core surrounded by a monolayer composed of specific proteins (apolipoproteins [apos]) and the polar lipids (unesterified or free cholesterol and phospholipids). This monolayer allows the lipoprotein to remain miscible in plasma. Lipoproteins function as transport vehicles for water-insoluble lipid fractions and lead them to their sites of metabolism or deposition. Free fatty acids are bound to albumin.

The plasma lipoproteins have been classified into four major groups based on their density: chylomicrons, very-low-density lipoprotein, LDL, and HDL. Most of the cholesterol in plasma is transported by LDL (~65%) with the remainder on HDL (25%) and VLDL (10%). TGs are transported primarily by chylomicron and VLDL.

The lipoproteins can be divided into two by the type of apos in the lipoprotein. Apos serve as enzymatic cofactors and recognition elements in binding to specific receptors.
- The apo B lipoproteins are atherogenic and include chylomicrons, LVDL, LDL, and lipoprotein(a) (Lp[a]).
- The apo A-I–containing lipoproteins are associated with reduced CVD and include HDL and their subfractions.

Small, Dense Low-Density Lipoprotein

Recent studies have shown that it is the size of the LDL particles, not the total concentration of LDL, that is more important in the pathogenesis of CAD. Small, dense LDL particles are expected to be better able to penetrate through the intima of the coronary arteries to deposit in the subendothelial space, where plaque forms. They are also more readily oxidized; only oxidized LDL can enter the macrophages in the lining of the arteries and form

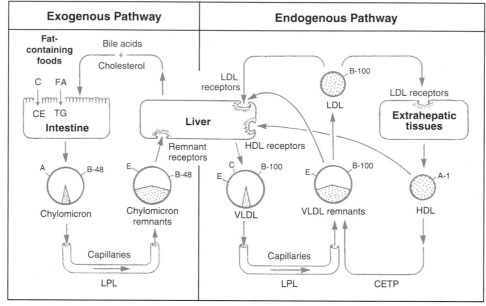

Fig. 33.1 Endogenous and exogenous pathways of plasma lipid and lipoprotein metabolism. Free fatty acid (FA) and cholesterol (C) are esterified in the intestinal mucosa to form triglyceride (TG) and cholesteryl ester (CE), respectively. They combine with apoprotein (apo) A and apo B-48 to form chylomicron and are secreted into the circulation. The *clear portion in the circles* represents TG, and the *shaded portion* represents CE. Chylomicron undergoes lipolysis in the capillary endothelium near adipose tissue and muscle tissue, losing TG via lipoprotein lipase (LPL). The resulting chylomicron remnants are taken up by hepatic apo E receptors for degradation by lysosomes. In the liver, TG and CE are combined with apo B-100, apo C, and apo E and then secreted as very low-density lipoprotein (VLDL). The *clear portion of the circle* represents TG and the *shaded portion* CE. VLDL undergoes lipolysis in the capillary endothelium near adipose tissue and muscle tissue, losing TG via LPL, similar to what happens with chylomicron remnants. The resulting VLDL remnants (or intermediate-density lipoprotein [IDL]) are either converted to low-density lipoprotein (LDL) for transport to peripheral cells via LDL receptor-mediated uptake or are taken up by hepatic receptors. The other major class of lipoprotein, high-density lipoprotein (HDL), participates in the conversion of free cholesterol from peripheral tissues to cholesteryl ester by the action of lecithin–cholesterol acyltransferase (LCAT). Cholesteryl esters are then directly taken up by the HDL receptors in the liver or are transferred to VLDL remnants and LDL by cholesteryl ester transfer protein (CETP), to be ultimately taken up by the liver. This process is known as *reverse cholesterol transport*. (Modified from Goldstein JL, Kita T, Brown MS: Defective lipoprotein receptors and atherosclerosis: lessons from an animal counterpart of familial hypercholesterolemia, *N Engl J Med* 309:288–295, 1983.)

cholesterol-rich plaques. The small, dense LDL phenotype usually occurs associated with elevated TG levels (>140 mg/dL) and decreased HDL levels (<40 mg/dL in men; <50 mg/dL in women). These are typical features of obesity, the metabolic syndrome, insulin resistance, and type 2 diabetes mellitus.

Lipid and Lipoprotein Metabolism

A review of simplified lipid and lipoprotein metabolism is presented in Fig. 33.1 for readers who wish to quickly refresh the metabolism of lipid and lipoproteins before reading clinical aspects of dyslipidemia. The figure legend provides a shorter summary of the topic.

Exogenous Pathway

After ingestion of fat-containing foods, TGs and cholesterol are absorbed into intestinal cells as fatty acids and free cholesterol. Within the intestinal wall, free fatty acids and cholesterol are re-esterified to form TGs and cholesteryl ester, respectively. These lipids are then combined with phospholipids and apos A-I, A-IV, and B-48 to form TG-rich *chylomicron* particles. Apo B-48 is an obligatory protein.

Chylomicrons rapidly enter plasma via the thoracic duct. In the circulation, chylomicrons acquire additional apos (mainly apo E and several forms of apo C). TG-rich chylomicrons are hydrolyzed by the enzyme lipoprotein lipase (LPL) at the capillary endothelium, leaving a smaller and denser remnant particle because they have lost much of their TGs. (The free fatty acid products of this hydrolysis are transferred primarily to adipose tissues for storage as TGs or to muscle for β-oxidation.) This particle is called *chylomicron remnant* and is rich in cholesterol and has gained apo E from HDL (and lost apo A and apo C to HDL).

These remnants are bound and internalized in part via hepatic membrane receptors specific for apo E on the particle. By this mechanism, dietary cholesterol is delivered to the liver, where it plays a role in the regulation of hepatic cholesterol metabolism. In normal persons, chylomicron and chylomicron remnants are very short lived in the circulation, and none of them exists in the plasma after a 12-hour fast. Chylomicron and chylomicron remnants may be atherogenic. Delayed clearance of chylomicron occurs in inherited deficiency of LPL or its activator, apo C-II (type I hypertriglyceridemia).

Endogenous Pathway

Triglycerides synthesized in the liver are packaged with cholesteryl esters and apos B-100, C, and E and then secreted as VLDL. The synthesis of VLDL by the liver is increased by excess carbohydrate, alcohol, or caloric intake and is decreased in the fasting state.

In the capillary beds, TG in the core of the VLDL is hydrolyzed by LPL, with a cofactor apo C-II, to produce a smaller, denser particle called *VLDL remnant* or *intermediate-density lipoprotein* (IDL), which is analogous to chylomicron remnant. (The surface components, except for apos B-100 and E, are transferred to HDL.) Free fatty acids generated by hydrolysis of TG are delivered to adipose tissue and muscle. Compared with VLDL, VLDL remnants have more cholesterol ester and less TG.

Some of these remnant particles (IDLs) are taken up by the hepatic receptors specific for apo E, and some others undergo conversion to LDL by hepatic TG lipase. Elevation of VLDL remnants may predispose the patient to premature CAD and peripheral artery disease (characteristically seen in Frederickson's type III hyperlipoproteinemia).

Low-density lipoprotein is usually formed by means of enhanced conversion of VLDL remnants (see Fig. 33.1) or by direct hepatic production of apo B–containing lipoproteins. LDLs are almost entirely made up of cholesteryl esters and apo B-100.

The content of cholesterol ester in the LDL particle may vary as much as 40%. LDL particles that contain lower amounts of cholesterol ester are known as *small, dense LDL particles*. Patients with increased amounts of small, dense LDL particles are at increased risk for CAD. Small, dense LDL is commonly associated with male gender, diabetes, low HDL-C levels, high TG levels, and familial combined hyperlipidemia (FCH).

Low-density lipoproteins are transported to peripheral cells or liver cells. Apo B-100, the only protein found in LDL, is recognized by a high-affinity LDL receptor on the surfaces of hepatic and certain nonhepatic cells, where LDLs are internalized into the cells. By this mechanism, LDL particles can deliver cholesterol to extrahepatic tissues for use in membrane or steroid hormone synthesis. LDL receptor expression by the liver is a major regulator of plasma LDL-C levels. LDL particles have a half-life of 3 to 4 days.

The liver and small intestine secrete HDL as nascent discoid particles composed primarily of phospholipids and apos (nascent HDL). (Nascent HDL particles secreted by the intestine are rich in apo A-I and apo A-IV, whereas those secreted by the liver contain predominantly apo A-I and apo A-II.) Nascent lipid-poor apo A-I accepts free (unesterified) cholesterol from tissues, and the free cholesterol transferred to the surface of HDL is esterified by the action of the enzyme lecithin–cholesterol acyltransferase (LCAT).

High-density lipoprotein cholesteryl esters may be directly transferred to and selectively taken up by the liver via a hepatic HDL receptor called scavenger receptor class BI (SR-BI). Alternatively, HDL cholesteryl esters may transfer from HDL to VLDL and LDL by the cholesteryl ester transfer protein (CETP), after which it may be taken up by the liver or redistributed to peripheral tissues. Thus, HDLs have two pathways by which they return tissue-derived cholesterol to the liver. The removal of cholesterol from cells by HDL for ultimate disposal in the liver has been termed *reverse cholesterol transport*. These reactions may explain how HDL and apo A-I can protect against the development of atherosclerosis.

Among the several subtypes of HDL particles, HDL_2 and HDL_3 are clinically important. HDL_2 is closely associated with protection against premature atherosclerosis. Alcohol consumption predominantly increases the HDL_3 subfraction. Lower levels of both subfractions are associated with male gender, hypertriglyceridemia, diabetes mellitus, obesity, uremia, smoking, and the use of androgens and progesterones. Estrogen raises HDL levels.

Cholesterol returning to the liver is converted into bile acids by the enzymatic hydroxylation of cholesterol, or cholesterol and phospholipids are excreted directly into the bile. A large portion of secreted bile acid is reabsorbed in the enterohepatic circulation and recycled. Bile acid sequestrants reduce the reabsorption of secreted bile acids, eventually reducing serum cholesterol levels by increasing the conversion of hepatic cholesterol to bile acids, thus reducing the cholesterol content of the hepatocytes. The reduced hepatic cholesterol stimulates the production of surface receptors for LDL-C, clearing more LDL from the serum.

The hepatic and extrahepatic cells can control their own cholesterol content through a feedback control system. In conditions of cellular cholesterol excess, the cell can (1) suppress endogenous cholesterol production by inhibiting the activity of 3-hydroxy-3-methylglutaryl coenzyme A (HMG-CoA) reductase, the rate-limiting enzyme in cholesterol synthesis; (2) decrease its input of cholesterol by suppressing the production of LDL surface receptors through a feedback mechanism; and (3) promote the removal of cholesterol by increasing its movement to the plasma membrane for efflux. The "statins" work through the first mechanism to reduce endogenous cholesterol production.

DIAGNOSIS OF DYSLIPIDEMIA

The diagnosis of dyslipidemia is made by measuring blood lipid, lipoproteins, or apo factors. If any of the measurements are abnormal, the diagnosis of a specific dyslipidemia is made, such as elevated total cholesterol, LDL-C, apo B, non-HDL-C, and TGs or lower than normal level of HDL-C.

Measurement of Lipid and Lipoproteins

A lipoprotein analysis is obtained after an overnight fast of 12 hours. The routine lipid profile typically includes total cholesterol, HDL-C, LDL-C, and TGs. An extended profile may also include VLDL cholesterol (VLDL-C), non-HDL-C, and the ratio of total cholesterol to HDL.

The LDL level is usually estimated by the Friedewald formula:

$$LDL = Total\ cholesterol - HDL - (TG/5)$$

TABLE 33.1   Concentrations of Plasma Lipid, Lipoprotein, and Apolipoprotein in Children and Adolescents (mg/dL): Acceptable, Borderline, and High

Category	Low	Acceptable	Borderline	High
Total cholesterol	—	<170	170–199	≥200
LDL-C	—	<110	110–129	≥130
Non–HDL-C	—	<120	120–144	≥145
Triglycerides: 0–9 yr	—	<75	75–99	≥100
10–19 yr	—	<90	90–129	≥130
HDL-C	<40	>45	40–45	—
Apo A-1	<115	>120	115–120	—
Apo B	—	<90	90–109	≥110

APO, Apolipoprotein; *HDL,* high-density lipoprotein cholesterol; *LDL,* low-density lipoprotein cholesterol.
From Expert Panel on Integrated Guidelines for Cardiovascular Health and Risk Reduction in Children and Adolescents: summary report, *Pediatrics* 128(suppl):S213–S256, 2011.

TABLE 33.2   Recommended Cut Points for Lipid and Lipoprotein Levels in Young Adults (mg/dL)

Category	Low	Borderline Low	Acceptable	Borderline High	High
Total cholesterol	—	—	<190	190–224	≥225
LDL-C	—	—	<120	120–159	≥160
Non–HDL-C	—	—	<150	150–189	≥190
Triglycerides	—	—	<1155	115–149	≥150
HDL-C	<40	40–44	>45	—	—

HDL, High-density lipoprotein cholesterol; *LDL,* low-density lipoprotein cholesterol.
From Expert Panel on Integrated Guidelines for Cardiovascular Health and Risk Reduction in Children and Adolescents: summary report, *Pediatrics* 128(suppl):S213–S256, 2011.

This formula is not accurate if the child is not fasting, if the TG level is above 400 mg/100 mL, or if chylomicrons or dysbetalipoproteinemia (type III hyperlipoproteinemia) is present. Methods are currently available to measure LDL-C directly, which allow LDL-C determination on specimens with the TG level above 400 mg/dL. Direct LDL-C measurement does not require a fasting specimen.

The following derivatives of lipid profile may be useful in the assessment of risks for CVD.

1. **Non–HDL-C.** Serum non–HDL-C (total cholesterol minus HDL-C) is considered a better screening tool than LDL-C for the assessment of CAD risk because it includes all classes of atherogenic (apo B–containing) lipoproteins; it includes VLDL-C, IDLs, LDL-C, and Lp(a). It was found in adults that increased level of non-HDL-C by 1 mg/dL increases the risk of death due to CVD by 5%.

2. **TC to HDL-C ratio.** The total cholesterol to HDL-C (TC to HDL-C) ratio is a useful parameter for assessing risk for CVD. The usual TC to HDL-C ratio in children is approximately 3 (based on TC of 150 mg/dL and an HDL-C of 50 mg/dL). According to the Framingham study, the ratios for average risk were 5.0 for men and 4.2 for women. The higher the ratio, the higher the risk of developing CVD. The ratio of 3.4 halves the risk of developing CVD for both men and women.

3. **Small, dense LDL particles.** In recent years, small, dense LDL particles have been shown to be more important than total LDL levels in CAD. The size of LDL particles is not

routinely measured because the presence of this phenotype is predictable. It occurs in association with elevated TG levels (>140 mg/dL) and a decreased HDL level (<40 mg/dL in men; <50 mg/dL in women). Although not routinely measured, small, dense LDL can be measured directly by various methods in commercial laboratories (including Berkeley HeartLab [www.bhlinc.com], Atherotec [www.thevaptest.com], and LipoScience [www.lipoprofile.com]).

Normal Levels of Lipids and Lipoproteins

Table 33.1 shows normal, borderline, and abnormal levels of lipid and lipoprotein levels in children, and Table 33.2 shows these values for young adults.

CLASSIFICATION OF DYSLIPIDEMIA

Dyslipidemias were traditionally classified by patterns of elevation in lipids and lipoproteins (Fredrickson phenotypes), but a more practical system is to classify them as primary (genetic) or secondary dyslipidemia.

1. Primary dyslipidemia is caused by single or multiple gene mutations that result in either overproduction or defective clearance of TGs and LDL-C or in underproduction or excessive clearance of HDL-C (see later discussion). This entity is much less common than secondary dyslipidemia.

2. Secondary dyslipidemia is caused by associated diseases or conditions and is much more common than primary

BOX 33.1 Causes of Secondary Dyslipidemia

Metabolic	Metabolic syndrome, diabetes, lipodystrophies, glycogen storage disorders
Renal disease	Chronic renal failure, nephrotic syndrome, glomerulonephritis, hemolytic uremic syndrome
Hepatic	Biliary atresia, cirrhosis
Hormonal	Estrogen, progesterone, growth hormone, hypothyroidism, corticosteroids
Lifestyle	Obesity, physical inactivity, diets rich in fat and saturated fat, alcohol intake
Medications	Isotretinoin (Accutane), certain oral contraceptives, anabolic steroids, thiazide diuretics, beta-adrenergic blockers, anticonvulsants, glucocorticoids, estrogen, testosterone, immunosuppressive agents (cyclosporine), antiviral agents (HIV protease inhibitor)
Others	Kawasaki's disease, anorexia nervosa, post–solid organ transplantation, childhood cancer survivor, progeria, idiopathic hypercalcemia, Klinefelter syndrome, Werner syndrome

dyslipidemia (see further discussion later). The majority of the cases found during screening are secondary forms.

Screening of all family members is recommended to determine whether the disorder is a familial one. Family screening is important not only to detect dyslipidemia in other members of the family but also to emphasize the need for all family members to change their eating patterns. Young patients with elevated LDL levels are more likely to have a familial disorder of LDL metabolism. Secondary dyslipidemia can occur in any age group.

Secondary Dyslipidemia

Box 33.1 lists the causes of secondary dyslipidemia. The most common cause of pediatric dyslipidemia is obesity. Medications such as oral contraceptives, isotretinoin (Accutane), anabolic steroids, diuretics, beta-blockers, and estrogens are uncommon causes of dyslipidemia. Medical conditions that include hypothyroidism, renal failure, nephrotic syndrome, and alcohol usage are less common causes of secondary dyslipidemia. Evidence of accelerated atherosclerosis from secondary causes of dyslipidemia is as impressive as that of primary causes.

Most secondary causes of dyslipidemia raise TGs and often lower HDL-C levels, with the exception of estrogen excess, with which HDL-C levels increase.

Each child with dyslipidemia should have certain blood tests to help rule out secondary causes of dyslipidemia. The blood tests should include fasting blood glucose and tests of kidney, liver, and thyroid function. When the diagnosis

of secondary dyslipidemia is made, one should treat the associated disorder producing the dyslipidemia first, such as diabetes, obesity, or nephrotic syndrome, and then treat dyslipidemia using the same guidelines as in primary dyslipidemia.

Selected Primary Dyslipidemias

Primary or inherited dyslipidemia is less commonly found in the screening process. Major primary dyslipidemias found in children include familial hypercholesterolemia (FH), FCH, familial hypertriglyceridemia, and several others. Table 33.3 summarizes changes in the lipid profile seen with primary lipid disorders.

Familial Hypercholesterolemia

Familial hypercholesterolemia is an autosomal dominant condition caused by a lack of or a reduction in LDL receptors. Whereas heterozygotes have about a 50% reduction in LDL receptors, homozygotes have little or no receptor activity. FH results in extreme elevation of LDL-C that may distinguish the condition from other primary and most secondary causes of dyslipidemia. Genetic testing remains the criterion standard for diagnosis of the condition, although it is not widely used.

1. **FH heterozygous disorder** is fairly common, occurring in 1 of every 500 people. It is inherited in an autosomal dominant mode. An evaluation of family members is important in the diagnosis of this condition. In this condition, one of two siblings and one parent have elevated total and LDL-C levels, but unaffected first-degree relatives have completely normal levels.

In heterozygotes, total cholesterol and LDL-C levels are two to three times higher than normal, present at birth or early in life. Their total cholesterol levels are most often above 240 mg/100 mL, with an average of 300 mg/dL, and their LDL-C levels are above 160 mg/100 mL, with an average of 240 mg/dL. HDL-C is reduced, and TG levels are usually normal. The presence of xanthomas of the extensor tendon in the parents of such children almost confirms the diagnosis. A heterozygous child or adolescent has normal physical findings. Tendon xanthomas are rarely found before the age of 10 years; they develop in the second decade, primarily in the Achilles tendons and extensor tendons of the hands, in only 10% to 15% of patients. These patients are likely to develop premature CVD; rarely, angina pectoris develops in the late teenage years.

Treatment of heterozygotes includes a diet low in saturated fat and cholesterol and high in water-soluble fibers. Bile acid sequestrants are safe and moderately effective but difficult to tolerate over the long term because of their gritty texture and gastrointestinal (GI) complaints. Statins are safe, effective, and well tolerated and are considered the drug of choice (see later section). The addition to the statin of a bile acid sequestrant or a cholesterol absorption inhibitor (CAI) is often necessary to achieve LDL-C goals. Niacin is generally not used to treat FH heterozygous children.

TABLE 33.3 Lipid Profile in Major Lipid Disorders in Children and Adolescents

Primary Lipid Disorders	LDL	VLDL	TG	HDL	Others
FH: homozygous	↑↑				
FH: heterozygous	↑				
FCH: type IIa	↑				
FCH: Type IV		↑	↑		
FCH: Type IIb	↑	↑	↑		
FCH: Types IIb and IV				↓	
Familial hypertriglyceridemia (200–1000 mg/dL)		↑	↑		
Severe hypertriglyceridemia (>1000 mg/dL)		↑	↑↑		↑ Chylomicron
Familial hypoalphalipoproteinemia				↓	
Dysbetalipoproteinemia (TC: 250–500 mg/dL; TGL: 50–600 mg/dL)					↑ IDL ↑ Chylomicron remnant

FCH, Familial combined hyperlipidemia; *FH,* familial hypercholesterolemia; *HDL,* high-density lipoprotein; *IDL,* intermediate-density lipoprotein; *LDL,* low-density lipoprotein; *TG,* triglyceride; *VLDL,* very low-density lipoprotein.
From Expert Panel on Integrated Guidelines for Cardiovascular Health and Risk Reduction in Children and Adolescents: summary report, *Pediatrics* 128(suppl):S213–S256, 2011.

2. **Homozygous disorder.** Homozygosity occurs in children who inherit a mutant allele for FH from both parents; it occurs in about 1 in 1 million children. The total cholesterol and LDL-C levels in these children are five to six times greater than normal. Such children have cholesterol levels that average 700 mg/dL but may reach higher than 1000 mg/dL. Clinical signs such as planar xanthomas, which are flat, orange-colored skin lesions, may be present by the age of 5 years in the webbing of the hands and over the elbows and buttocks. Tendon xanthomas, arcus corneae, and clinically significant coronary heart disease are often present by the age of 10 years. The generalized atherosclerosis often affects the aortic valve, with resulting aortic stenosis.

Familial hypercholesterolemia homozygous children respond somewhat to high doses of potent statins and to niacin. CAIs also lower LDL-C in FH homozygotes, especially in combination with a more potent statin. However, most FH homozygotes invariably require LDL apheresis (with extracorporeal affinity LDL absorption column and plasma reinfusion) every 2 weeks to lower LDL to a range that is less atherogenic. The Liposorber system is an example, which selectively binds apo B–containing lipoproteins (LDL, Lp[a], and VLDL).

Familial Combined Hyperlipidemia

Familial combined hyperlipidemia is an autosomal dominant disorder seen three times more frequently than FH. It occurs in 1 of every 200 to 300 people. It is characterized by variable lipid phenotypic expression: elevated LDL level alone, elevated LDL with hypertriglyceridemia, or normal LDL with hypertriglyceridemia. Clinically, it may be difficult to separate this entity from FH. The diagnosis of FCH is suspected when a first-degree family member (often a parent or sibling) has a different lipoprotein phenotype than the proband. Levels of total and LDL-C are somewhat lower than in patients with FH, and LDL-C levels fluctuate from time to time, with TG levels fluctuating in the opposite direction. These children usually have plasma total cholesterol levels between 190 and 220 mg/dL. The LDL-C level is usually normal or only mildly elevated. In FCH, most patients lack tendon xanthomas, and extreme hyperlipidemia is absent in childhood. It may occur in children of survivors of myocardial infarction (MI). Their phenotypes often have other characteristics such as hyperinsulinemia, glucose intolerance, hypertension, and visceral obesity. The combined expression of three or more of these traits constitutes the metabolic syndrome (see earlier section).

A cornerstone of management should be aimed at a fat- and cholesterol-restricted diet and a simple carbohydrate-restricted diet (low glycemic index foods) together with attention to other cardiovascular (CV) lifestyle changes (control of overweight and regular aerobic exercise). Low glycemic index foods are important in reducing carbohydrate-induced hypertriglyceridemia. The statins are the most effective in lowering LDL-C and the total number of atherogenic small, dense LDL particles. Fibric acid and niacin, which are effective in adults, are not ordinarily used in pediatric patients. Drug therapy is reasonable in patients with persistently elevated TGs levels (>350 mg/dL), aimed primarily at preventing an episode of pancreatitis. Metformin has been used to treat obese hyperinsulinemic adolescents with the metabolic syndrome. Metformin may enhance insulin sensitivity and reduce fasting blood glucose, insulin levels, plasma lipids, free fatty acids, and leptin.

Familial Hypertriglyceridemia

In children, this autosomal dominant disorder is caused by LPL deficiency, resulting in hepatic overproduction of VLDL-C. TG levels are typically increased. Cholesterol levels are not increased. Eruptive xanthomas and lipemia retinalis (a creamy appearance of the retinal veins and arteries caused by a high concentration of lipids in the blood) can also be found. Metabolic consequences of hypertriglyceridemia include (1) a lowering of HDL-C; (2) production of smaller, denser LDL particles with more atherogenicity; and (3) a hypercoagulable state.

Treatment is based first on a diet very low in fat and simple sugar and lifestyle modification, including increasing exercise, withdrawing hormones (estrogen, progesterone), and limiting alcohol intake. When the level of TGs is between 200 and 500 mg/dL, the goal of the treatment is to reduce CAD. When TG levels reach 500 to 1000 mg/dL, pancreatitis is a major concern. One may consider using drugs such as fibrate or niacin (see later sections for the use of these antilipidemic agents). If pancreatitis develops, which is usually characterized by severe abdominal pain and elevated plasma levels of amylase and lipase, the patient should be admitted to a hospital for care with intravenous fluid.

Dysbetalipoproteinemia (Type III Hyperlipoproteinemia)

This familial disorder is a rare genetic disorder caused by a defect in apo E, which results in increased accumulation of chylomicron remnants and VLDL remnants. This autosomal recessive disorder is characterized by elevation of both cholesterol and TG equally to greater than 300 mg/dL, but this disorder is not usually seen in childhood. Clinical manifestations may include palmar xanthoma. Patients with this disorder have a moderately increased risk of CVD. A low-fat diet, a low glycemic index diet, and drug treatment (fibric acid or statin) are very effective.

Familial Hypoalphalipoproteinemia (Low High-Density Lipoprotein Syndrome)

This condition is associated with autosomal dominant inheritance. The underlying mechanism is decreased concentration of apo A-I and apo A-II and absent apo C-III. This condition is associated with isolated low HDL-C levels and mild to moderately increased risk of premature CAD. In *Tangiers disease,* HDL-C is nearly absent (with markedly enlarged yellow tonsils).

Although specific drug therapy is not routinely recommended in pediatric age groups, a low-carbohydrate and low-fat diet is indicated in children with inherited disorders of HDL metabolism. Exercise and weight loss are also helpful. The most effective way to reduce CVD risk in these patients is to maintain low LDL-C levels.

MANAGEMENT OF HYPERCHOLESTEROLEMIA

Dietary Management of Hypercholesterolemia

Reduced intake of saturated fat and cholesterol is most basic to the dietary therapy of hypercholesterolemia. The efficacy and safety of dietary therapy have been demonstrated in adults as well as children. Diet therapy is prescribed in two steps that progressively reduce the intake of saturated fats and cholesterol. Physicians should follow the algorithm shown in Fig. 33.2 for managing high LDL-C levels.

1. The Cardiovascular Health Integrated Lifestyle Diet-1 (CHILD-1) diet is the first stage in dietary change for children with dyslipidemia, overweight and obesity, risk-factor clustering, and high-risk medical conditions (Table

33.4). The CHILD-1 diet is also the recommended diet for children with a positive family history of premature CVD, dyslipidemia, obesity, hypertension, diabetes mellitus, or exposure to smoking in the home. This diet is very similar to what has been recommended for the general population of the United States to consume by the Dietary Guidelines for Americans 2010. The use of dietary adjuncts such as plant sterol or stanol esters has shown short-term benefits.

2. If this diet fails to achieve the minimal goal of the dietary therapy for LDL-C (≤130 mg/dL) in 6 months, a more stringent diet with saturated fat at 7% or less of total calories and dietary cholesterol of less than 200 mg/day (CHILD-2-LDL) is used, which has been shown to be safe and effective. A registered dietitian or other qualified nutrition professional should be consulted.

3. If the dietary intervention with CHILD-2-LDL fails, one may proceed with drug therapy.

Indications for Drug Therapy

When dietary management with lifestyle changes of 6 to 12 months duration fails to lower LDL-C levels to the target level (≤130 mg/dL), the use of medication should be considered. Decisions regarding the need for medication therapy should be based on the average of results from at least two fasting lipid profiles (FLPs) obtained at least 2 weeks but no more than 3 months apart, and it should be in consultation with the patient and the family.

1. The following are indications for consideration of drug therapy (Box 33.2; see also Fig. 33.2).
   a. LDL-C of 190 mg/dL or greater after a 6-month trial of lifestyle management (CHILD-1 followed by CHILD-2-LDL) for children 10 years of age or older
   b. LDL-C of 160 to 189 mg/dL after a 6-month trial of lifestyle and diet management (CHILD-2-LDL) in a child 10 years of age or older with a positive family history of premature CVD or events in first-degree relatives or at least one high-level risk factor or risk condition or at least two moderate-level risk factors or risk conditions
   c. LDL-C of 130 to 159 mg/dL in a child 10 years of age or older with a negative family history of premature CVD but with at least two high-level risk factors or risk conditions or at least one high-level risk factor or risk condition together with at least two moderate-level risk factors or risk conditions
   d. LDL-C of 130 to 189 mg/dL in a child 10 years of age or older with a negative family history of premature CVD in first-degree relatives and no high- or moderate-level risk factor or risk condition should continue with lifestyle changes (CHILD-2-LDL), plus weight management if the body mass index is at the 85th percentile or above.
   e. For children age 8 or 9 years with LDL-C persistently 190 mg/dL or above with *multiple* first-degree family members with premature CVD or events or the presence of at least one high-level risk factor or risk conditions or the presence of at least two moderate-level risk factors or risk conditions

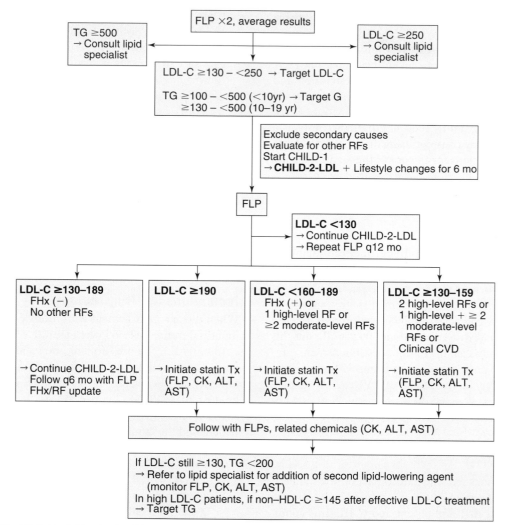

Fig. 33.2 Dyslipidemia algorithm: target low-density lipoprotein cholesterol (LDL-C). Note that the units of milligrams per deciliter (mg/dL) have been omitted. *ALT,* Alanine aminotransferase; *AST,* aspartate aminotransferase; *CHILD,* Cardiovascular Health Integrated Lifestyle Diet; *CK,* creatine kinase; *FHx,* family history; *FLP,* fasting lipid panel; *q,* every; *RF,* risk factor; *TG,* triglyceride; *Tx,* therapy. (Modified from Expert Panel on Integrated Guidelines for Cardiovascular Health and Risk Reduction in Children and Adolescents: Summary report, *Pediatrics* 128[suppl]:S213–S256, 2011.)

TABLE 33.4 Nutrient Composition of CHILD Diets

Nutrients (% total calories)	CHILD-1	CHILD-2-LDL	CHILD-2-TG
Total fat	<30%	25%–30%	25%–30%
Saturated fat	7%–10%	≤7%	≤7%
Cholesterol	300 mg/day	<200 mg/day	<200 mg/day
Mono- and polyunsaturated fatty acids	20%	~10%	~10%
Carbohydrate	50%–55%		
Protein	15%–20%		
Others	Reduce trans-fat intake	Avoid trans-fat as much as possible	Decrease sugar intake
	May add plant sterol, or plant sterol esters, water-soluble fiber psyllium		Increase intake of complex carbohydrates
			Increase dietary fish (omega-3 fatty acids)

CHILD, Cardiovascular Health Integrated Lifestyle Diet; *LDL,* low-density lipoprotein; *TG,* triglyceride.

BOX 33.2 Indications for Drug Therapy for Hypercholesterolemia in Children and Adolescents

- Failure of diet therapy and lifestyle management for 6 to 12 mo *plus*
- Age ≥10 yr with one of the following lipid profiles or risk factors.
  a. LDL-C ≥190 mg/dL
  b. LDL-C 160–189 mg/dL with a positive family history of premature CVD/events in first-degree relatives, at least one high-level risk factor or risk condition, or at least two moderate-level risk factors or risk conditions
  c. LDL-C 130–159 mg/dL with at least two high-level risk factors or risk conditions or at least one high-level risk factor or risk condition together with at least two moderate-level risk factors or risk conditions
  Or
- Children aged 8 or 9 years with LDL-C level persistently ≥190 mg/dL together with *multiple* first-degree family members with premature CVD or events, the presence of at least one high-level risk factor or risk condition, or the presence of at least two moderate-level risk factors or risk conditions

CVD, Cardiovascular disease; *LDL-C*, low-density lipoprotein cholesterol.
From Expert Panel on Integrated Guidelines for Cardiovascular Health and Risk Reduction in Children and Adolescents: summary report, *Pediatrics* 128(suppl):S213–S256, 2011.

f. For children age 8 or 9 years with LDL-C persistently 190 mg/dL or above with *multiple* first-degree family members with premature CVD or events or the presence of at least one high-level risk factor or risk conditions or the presence of at least two moderate-level risk factors or risk conditions

2. Children with homozygous FH and extremely elevated LDL-C levels (>500 mg/dL) have undergone effective LDL-lowering therapy with biweekly LDL apheresis under the care of lipid specialists.

3. In general, pharmacotherapy for children younger than 10 years of age is discouraged. However, there are exceptions to this recommendation. If patient has LDL-C level greater than 500 mg, which occurs with homozygous FH, treatment (apheresis, statin and CAI) is indicated and patient should be referred to a lipid specialist.

Lipid-Lowering Drugs

Five well-known classes of lipid-lowering drugs have been used for adults with dyslipidemia. They are bile acid sequestrants, HMG-CoA reductase inhibitors ("statins"), CAIs, nicotinic acid (niacin, vitamin B$_3$), and fibric acid derivatives. The mechanisms of action, side effects, and ranges of adult dosages of the lipid-lowering agents are presented in Table 33.5.

Experience in children is quite limited, especially with drugs other than the statins, and consensus recommendations are lacking with regard to the use of other lipid-lowering drugs, such as fibrate and niacin.

1. It has been established that the HMG-CoA reductase inhibitors (statins) are the most effective in lowering LDL-C in adults as well as in children and adolescents. A further discussion is presented in the section to follow.

2. The bile acid sequestrants (cholestyramine, colestipol) are other lipid-lowering drugs approved for use in children older than 10 years of age. However, these agents are not used widely because they are associated with a low compliance rate (because of their gritty texture and GI complaints), and they provide only a modest reduction of LDL-C level. No further discussion follows on this topic.

3. Ezetimibe, a CAI, is effective in lowering blood cholesterol levels. Contrary to earlier belief, they are absorbed through the enterohepatic circulation and may have systemic effects, such as rare liver toxicity. Even though ezetimibe decreases cholesterol levels, the results of two major, high-quality clinical trials in adults (in 2008 and 2009) showed a lack of clinically significant improvement in CV events. No further discussion follows on this topic.

4. Nicotinic acid and fibrates have been shown to lower LDL-C and TG levels and increase HDL levels in adults. Although they are frequently used in adults with hypercholesterolemia as a second line of drug, they are not frequently used in adolescents because of limited data available.

The "Statins"

At this time, a statin is recommended as first-line treatment in adolescents with hypercholesterolemia (McCrindle et al, 2007). The statins inhibit HMG-CoA reductase, which is the rate-limiting step in the endogenous production of cholesterol in the hepatic cells.

Adverse Effects of Statins

Adverse effects of statins are infrequent but may include GI upset; elevation of liver transaminases; and myopathy ranging in severity from asymptomatic increases in creatine kinase (CK), muscle aches or weakness, to fatal rhabdomyolysis. Myopathy and elevated liver enzymes are the main concerns.

- More than a 10-time increase in CK levels and more than three times an increase in alanine aminotransferase (ALT) or aspartate aminotransferase (AST) levels above the upper limits of normal are worrisome levels. Therefore, periodic measurements of ALT, AST (preferred because it is also found in muscles), and CK should be done for possible adverse effects of the statins at the same time lipid levels are measured. Box 33.3 provides step-by-step instruction on initiation, titration, and monitoring of statin therapy (McCrindle et al, 2007).

- Patients should be instructed to report immediately any potential signs and symptoms of myopathy (e.g., muscle cramps, weakness, or more diffuse symptoms). Asymptomatic transient increases in CK, although unusual, have been reported. Practitioners should be aware that an increase in CK may be related to vigorous exercise, particularly contact sports or weightlifting. Myopathy is defined as a serum CK level 10 times the upper limit of normal

TABLE 33.5 Summary of Lipid-Lowering Drugs

Daily Dosage Range	Mechanism of Action	Side Effects	Daily Dosage Range
Bile acid sequestrants: cholestyramine (Questran), colestipol (Colestid), colesevelam (WelChol)	Increase excretion of bile acids in stool; increase LDL receptor activity	Constipation, nausea, bloating, flatulence, transient increase in transaminase and alkaline phosphatase levels, increased TG levels (±), possible prevention of absorption of fat-soluble vitamins	Related to levels of cholesterol, not body weight
HMG-CoA reductase inhibitors ("statins"): atorvastatin (Lipitor), fluvastatin (Lescol), lovastatin (Mevacor), pravastatin (Pravachol), rosuvastatin (Crestor), simvastatin (Zocor)	Inhibit HMG-CoA reductase, with a resulting decrease in cholesterol synthesis; increase LDL receptor activity; reduce LDL and VLDL secretion by the liver	Mild GI symptoms, myositis syndrome, elevated hepatic transaminase levels, increased CPK levels. Contraindicated during pregnancy because of potential risk to a developing fetus (Risk of myopathy is higher with a high dose of simvastatin [80 mg] and is lower with atorvastatin or rosuvastatin.)	Children: see text for suggested pediatric dosages. Adult dose ranges (of statins approved for pediatric use): Atorvastatin: 10–80 mg; Fluvastatin: 20–80 mg; Lovastatin: 10–40 mg; Pravastatin: 10–40 mg; Simvastatin: 10–40 mg
Cholesterol absorption inhibitor: ezetimibe (Zetia; Ezetrol)	Selective inhibition of intestinal sterol absorption	Abdominal pain, rhabdomyolysis (±)	Adults: 10 mg/day
Nicotinic acid (niacin, vitamin B₃)	Decreases plasma levels of free fatty acid; possibly inhibits cholesterol synthesis; decreases hepatic VLDL synthesis	Cutaneous flushing, pruritus, GI upset, liver function abnormalities, increased uric acid levels, increased glucose intolerance	Children: only short-term efficacy reported for homozygous FH; not recommended for routine use. Adults: 1–3 g
Fibric acid derivatives: gemfibrozil (Lopid), clofibrate	Decrease hepatic VLDL synthesis; increase LPL activity	Increased incidence of gallstones and perhaps GI cancer, myositis, diarrhea, nausea, rash, altered liver function, increased CPK levels, potentiation of warfarin	Children: not recommended. Adults: gemfibrozil, 600–1200 mg; clofibrate, 1–2 g

CPK, Creatine phosphokinase; *FH,* familial hypercholesterolemia; *GI,* gastrointestinal; *HDL,* high-density lipoprotein; *HMG-CoA,* 3-hydroxy-3-methylglutaryl coenzyme A; *LDL,* low-density lipoprotein; *LPL,* lipoprotein lipase; *VLDL,* very low-density lipoprotein.

with or without muscle weakness or pain. Rhabdomyolysis is defined as unexplained muscle pain or weakness with a serum CK level more than 40 times the upper limit of normal.

- The likelihood of myopathy increases with high doses, especially of simvastatin (80 mg in adults), and when used concomitantly with other medications, such as cyclosporine, erythromycin, gemfibrozil, niacin, azole antifungal agents, or antiretroviral agents (Egan, 2011).
- Increases in liver enzymes up to three times the upper limits of normal have been reported in several patients treated with high doses of simvastatin (40 mg/day) and atorvastatin (20 mg/day). Liver transaminases are not likely to increase in patients taking pravastatin and rosuvastatin.
- The statins are also teratogenic, and female patients should be advised about appropriate contraception if warranted.

Dosages of the "Statins"

Numerous studies have demonstrated the safety and efficacy of the statins in male and female adolescents with FH (Holmes et al, 2005). Five statins—atorvastatin, fluvastatin, lovastatin, pravastatin, and simvastatin—are currently approved by the Food and Drug Administration for use in adolescents. A recent double-blind, placebo-controlled trial with 2 years of pravastatin treatment has shown not only significant reduction of LDL-C but also regression of carotid atherosclerosis in children and adolescents with FH (Wiegman et al, 2004).

Based on published clinical trials in children and adolescents, the following may be a reasonable pediatric dosage of the statins that are approved for pediatric use (Holmes et al, 2005). The Expert Panel has recommended to start with the lowest available dose given once daily at bedtime. The starting doses listed are the lowest available doses for each statin, except for simvastatin (with 5 mg as the lowest available dose).

- Atorvastatin (Lipitor): The starting dose of 10 mg is increased to 20 mg at 3 months and further to a dose of 40 mg/day (maximum adult dose, 80 mg/day).
- Fluvastatin (Lescol): The starting dose is 20 mg. The maintenance dose ranges from 20 to 40 mg.
- Lovastatin (Mevacor): The starting dose is 10 mg with a 10-mg increase every 3 months to a maximum of 40 mg/day.

Box 33.3 Initiation, Titration, and Monitoring of Statin Therapy in Children and Adolescents

- Measure baseline CK, ALT, and AST levels.
- Start with lower dose given once orally (see text for dosage).
- Monitor for potential adverse effects.
  - Instruct the patient to report *immediately* all potential adverse effects, especially myopathy (muscle cramps, weakness, asthenia, and more diffuse symptoms).
  - If myopathy is present, its relationship to recent physical activities should be assessed, the medication stopped, and CK assessed.
  - The patient should be monitored for resolution of myopathy and any associated increases in CK.
  - Consideration can be given to restarting the medication after symptoms and laboratory abnormalities have resolved.
  - Advise female patients about concerns with regard to pregnancy and the need for appropriate contraception if warranted.
- After 4 weeks, measure fasting lipoprotein profile, CK, ALT, and AST.
  - The threshold for worrisome level of CK is 10 times above the upper limit of reported normal; consider the impact of physical activity.
  - The threshold for worrisome level of ALT or AST is three times above the upper limit of reported normal.
  - Target level for LDL: minimal, <130 mg/dL; ideal, 110 mg/dL

- At 4-week follow-up:
  - If target LDL levels are achieved and no laboratory abnormalities are noted:
    - Continue therapy and recheck in 8 wk and then 3 mo.
  - If laboratory abnormalities are noted or symptoms reported:
    - Temporarily withhold the drug and repeat the blood work in ~2 wk.
    - When anomalies return to normal, the drugs may be restarted with close monitoring.
  - If target LDL levels are not achieved:
    - Increase the dose by 10 mg and repeat the blood work in 4 wk.
    - Continue stepped titration up to the maximum recommended dose until target LDL levels are achieved or there is evidence of toxicity.
- Repeat laboratory tests every 3 to 6 mo: fasting lipoprotein profile, CK, ALT, and AST.
- Continue counseling on:
  - Compliance with medications and reduced fat diets
  - Other risk factors, such as weight gain, smoking, and inactivity
  - Counsel female adolescents about statin contraindication in pregnancy and the need for appropriate contraception. Seek referral to an adolescent medicine or gynecologic specialist as appropriate.

ALT, Alanine aminotransferase; *AST,* aspartate aminotransferase; *CK,* creatine kinase; *LDL,* low-density lipoprotein.
Modified from McCrindle BW, Urbina EM, Dennison BA, et al; American Heart Association Atherosclerosis, Hypertension, and Obesity in Youth Committee; American Heart Association Council of Cardiovascular Disease in the Young; American Heart Association Council on Cardiovascular Nursing: Drug therapy of high-risk lipid abnormalities in children and adolescents, *Circulation* 115:1948–1967, 2007.

- Pravastatin (Pravachol): The starting dose of 10 mg is increased to 20 or 40 mg/day.
- Simvastatin (Zocor): The starting dose is 10 mg. It is increased in increments of 10 mg every 3 months to a maximum of 40 mg/day. Note that 80 mg of the drug carries a high risk of myopathy or rhabdomyolysis in adults.

The dose of statin is increased by 10 mg every 3 months to the half or even full dose of the upper range dosage with periodic measurements of cholesterols. The maintenance dosage of the drug is decided by periodic determinations of cholesterol levels. The minimal target level for LDL-C is less than 130 mg/dL, and the ideal target level is 110 mg/dL. If the target level is not reached, a second agent such as a bile acid sequestrant or CAI may be added under the direction of a lipid specialist.

HYPERTRIGLYCERIDEMIA

High TG levels are a marker for atherogenic remnant lipoproteins, such as VLDL-C. Recent studies have found that hypertriglyceridemia is an independent risk factor for major coronary events after controlling for LDL-C and HDL-C. According to the Helsinki Heart Study (1987), people with hypertriglyceridemia alone (without other risk factors for heart disease) had about a 50% increased risk for CAD compared with people with normal TG levels. When high LDL-C coexisted with elevated TG levels, there was a 300% greater risk for CAD.

Management of Hypertriglyceridemia

There are different cutoff points for the treatment of hypertriglyceridemia in children and adults: 100 mg/dL for children younger than 10 years of age, 130 mg/dL for ages 10 to 19 years, and 150 mg/dL for young adults (Tables 33.1 and 33.2). An algorithm for managing hypertriglyceridemia is shown in Fig. 33.3.

1. Diet therapy is the primary tool in treating high TG level using a low-fat diet and low glycemic index foods, such as CHILD-2-TG (see Table 33.4). Reduction of simple carbohydrate intake (and increased intake of complex carbohydrate), reduced saturated fat intake, and weight loss are associated with decreased TG levels.

It is important for physicians to know that both a high-fat diet and a high-carbohydrate diet raise TG levels. In fact, a high-carbohydrate diet may be a more important source of hypertriglyceridemia than high fat intake. The best established metabolic disturbance attributable to high dietary sugar intake may be a rise in plasma lipids, not in plasma glucose (Hellerstein, 2002). A rise in TG levels after consuming high carbohydrate is known as *carbohydrate-induced hypertriglyceridemia.* The increase in TG is worse with a high glycemic index diet than with a low glycemic index diet. Therefore,

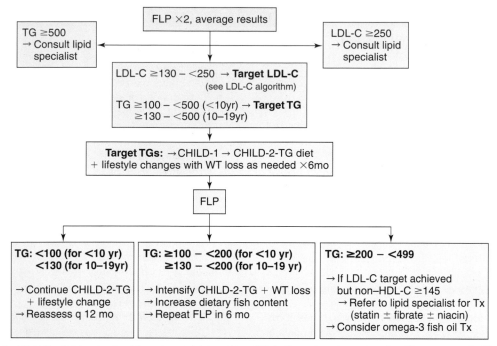

Fig. 33.3 Dyslipidemia algorithm: target triglycerides (TGs). Note that the units of milligrams per deciliter (mg/dL) have been omitted. *CHILD,* Cardiovascular Health Integrated Lifestyle Diet; *FLP,* fasting lipid panel; *LDL-C,* low-density lipoprotein cholesterol; *WT,* weight. (Modified from Expert Panel on Integrated Guidelines for Cardiovascular Health and Risk Reduction in Children and Adolescents: Summary report, *Pediatrics* 128[suppl]:S213–S256, 2011.)

all refined carbohydrate foods such as sugary drinks, cookies, ice cream, and desserts, should be avoided and complex carbohydrates such as whole-grain products should be consumed more often.

2. Lifestyle changes with increased physical activity (at least 30 minutes of moderate-intensity exercise 5 days a week) and weight control help reduce TG levels. Exercise also helps decrease LDL-C and increase HDL-C.

3. Increasing dietary fish (to increase omega-3 fatty acids) may be effective.
   a. Children with increased TG levels (100–200 mg/dL) after a trial of lifestyle and diet management with CHILD-2-TG should increase dietary fish consumption.
   b. Children with fasting TG levels of 200 to 499 mg/dL and non-HDL levels of greater than 145 mg/dL, after a trial of lifestyle and diet management with CHILD-2-TG and increased fish intake, may be considered for fish oil supplementation.

Omega-3 fatty acids in fish oils lower plasma TGs levels by inhibiting the synthesis of VLDL-C and TGs in the liver. They also have antithrombotic properties. A review of human studies (Harris, 1997) concluded that approximately 4 g/day of omega-3 fatty acids reduced serum TG concentrations by 25% to 30%, increased LDL-C levels by 5% to 10%, and increased HDL-C levels by 1% to 3%. Total cholesterol was not significantly affected by omega-3 fatty acids. A prescription omega-3 fatty acid product (e.g., Omacor) 4 g/day and 8 g/day may be used. (Most fish oil capsules contain omega-3 fatty content, only one third of that contained in Omacor.)

4. Children with average fasting TG levels of 500 mg/dL or above or any single measurement of 1000 mg/dL or above should be treated in conjunction with a lipid specialist. For these patients, in addition to the dietary management with CHILD-2-TG and fish oil, use of fibrate or niacin should be considered to prevent pancreatitis (see later discussion for other lipid-lowering drugs, fibrates, and niacin).

Fibrates have the effect of both lowering TGs and raising HDL-C. Side effects seen in adults include myalgia, myositis, myopathy, rhabdomyolysis, liver toxicity, gallstones, and glucose intolerance. Safety and efficacy data in children are limited. Therefore, CK level and liver enzymes should be monitored every 3 months.

Niacin is the best known drug that raises HDL-C, but it also reduces TG levels. Adverse effects of niacin include liver toxicity, GI tract upset, and facial flushing. Less commonly seen side effects are hyperuricemia and glucose intolerance. Extended-release preparations produce less flushing, but they are more likely to produce liver toxicity. Niacin is rarely used to treat the pediatric population because of reported poor tolerance and the potential for very serious adverse effects. Liver transaminases should be checked every 3 months.

LOW HIGH-DENSITY LIPOPROTEIN LEVEL

Low levels of HDL-C represent a major CV risk factor. Despite the presence of desirable total cholesterol levels, patients with low HDL-C may be at very high risk of developing a subsequent CV event. In the Framingham study, approximately 50% of primary myocardial infarctions occurred in subjects with total cholesterol levels of 250 mg/dL, and 20% of them had desirable cholesterol levels (200 mg/dL). In the Helsinki Heart Study, HDL-C elevation independently reduced CV event rate. An increase in HDL-C is associated with a reduction in the CV events. It is estimated that a rise of 1 mg/dL in HDL lowers the risk of fatal MI by about 3%.

High-density lipoprotein cholesterol has a number of antiatherogenic effects. The best known of these relates to the ability of HDL-C to promote the efflux of cholesterol from macrophages in the arterial wall through reverse cholesterol transport. Other antiatherogenic potentials of HDL-C include antioxidant, antithrombotic, and antiinflammatory effects.

Low HDL level is defined as less than 40 mg/dL in adolescent boys and girls. In adults, low level is defined as less than 40 mg/dL in men and less than 50 mg/dL in women.

The primary approach in managing low levels of HDL-C is lifestyle change and diet therapy. Drugs used for this condition (niacin, fibrates) have unacceptable side effects. The following has been suggested for adult patients with low levels of HDL-C (Ashen et al, 2005; others).

1. Lifestyle change is the best way to deal with low levels of HDL-C. Regular exercise (30 minutes of brisk aerobic exercise every day or every other day) is recommended. Weight control (and quitting smoking) is equally important.
2. Dietary intervention
   a. A diet low in saturated fat and rich in the polyunsaturated fatty acids is recommended. This is because the most effective way to reduce CV risk in patients with low HDL levels is to maintain low LDL-C levels, not because it raises HDL levels.
   b. Omega-3 fatty acids may help raise HDL levels.
   c. Restrict consumption of high glycemic index foods. Consumption of carbohydrates, especially simple carbohydrates, is associated with low HDL levels. Some studies have found that a low-carbohydrate diet can raise HDL levels.
   d. Mild to moderate consumption of alcohol (1–2 drinks a day) in adults resulted in a rise of 4 mg/dL (not for those with liver or addiction problems).
3. Current pharmacologic options for adults include nicotinic acid (niacin), fibrates, and statins, but none is without major adverse effects. The use of drug should be considered only when all nonpharmacologic measures do not achieve the goal of raising HDL-C level in pediatric patients.

- Among these medications, niacin (nicotinic acid or vitamin B$_3$) is known to be the most effective medication for raising HDL-C (raising HDL level by 20%–35%). However, niacin is rarely used in the pediatric population because of the potential for very serious adverse effects.

One of the major adverse effects of niacin is severe flushing. Flushing is a major reason people stop taking the medication. The flushing problem has been substantially reduced by the development of a newer extended-release formulation of niacin (Niaspan), but it is more likely to increase liver toxicity. Flushing (which may involve prostaglandin D2) can be blocked by taking 300 mg of aspirin half an hour before taking niacin.
- Fibrate therapy is also effective, producing an average increase of 10% to 25%.
- Statins are the least effective of the three drug classes in raising HDL levels (by 2%–15%).
- When used in combination, low-dose statins and high-dose niacin have been shown to produce benefits of 21% to 26%.

ELEVATED TRIGLYCERIDE AND LOW HIGH-DENSITY LIPOPROTEIN

A subgroup of patients with a combination of elevated TG and low HDL-C needs special attention. This combination of dyslipidemia is typically seen in patients with obesity, the metabolic syndrome, and diabetes and in some patients with FCH. Although LDL-C may not be elevated, this phenotype is usually associated with small, dense LDL particles, which are much more atherogenic than large LDL particles.

For this subgroup of patients, the following are recommended.

1. Lifestyle change, in particular with adequate exercise, is probably the most important approach for this subgroup of patients.
2. Low-carbohydrate and low-fat diets. Low glycemic index diets appear to be more beneficial to these patients than low-fat diets, which are traditionally known to lower LDL levels.
3. Cholesterol-lowering drugs that impact small, dense LDL are nicotinic acid and the fibric acid derivatives in adult patients. No consensus guidelines exist for pediatric patients. Of note is that the statin drugs do not appear to affect particle composition, although they lower LDL concentration.

34

Pediatric Preventive Cardiology

OUTLINE

Atherosclerotic cardiovascular disease (CVD) is a major cause of morbidity and mortality and is responsible for more than 50% of all the deaths in the United States and other Western countries. The best and longest known risk factor for coronary artery disease (CAD) is hypercholesterolemia. Other types of dyslipidemia, obesity, smoking, hypertension, and diabetes mellitus are among the known cardiovascular (CV) risk factors. Although most of the clinical burden of CVD occurs in adulthood, these risk factors can develop during childhood and adolescence. In fact, there is now clear evidence that atherosclerosis begins during childhood. To reduce CV death, we need to turn our attention to preventing and correcting these risk factors before adulthood, when atherosclerotic processes may have progressed too far to be reversible by therapy.

Unfortunately, the importance of preventing heart disease in the pediatric population is not well perceived by pediatricians and pediatric cardiologists. When pediatricians and pediatric cardiologists are asked about heart disease in children, they think about congenital heart disease (CHD). Although CHD is associated with the highest mortality rate of any congenital defects, only 0.4% of death from CVDs is caused by congenital heart defects in the United States. The great majority of CV death is from CAD (54%), stroke (18%), congestive heart failure (6%), and hypertension (5%) (Lauer et al, 2006). Therefore, preventive cardiology is and should be pediatric domain. The primary purpose of this chapter is to raise physicians' attention to the emerging importance of practicing medicine to prevent future CVD (and type II diabetes) during childhood.

This chapter discusses the following topics in the order listed below. Hypertension and dyslipidemia, two other important CV risk factors, are discussed in earlier chapters (Chapters 28 and 33, respectively).

1. Evidence of childhood onset of atherosclerotic heart disease
2. Identification of standard CV risk factors
3. Metabolic syndrome in children
4. Lipid screening for dyslipidemia with newly recommended guidelines
5. Diagnosis and principles of management of childhood obesity
6. Strategies for smoke cessation
7. The summary table of the American Heart Association (AHA) Guidelines on practice of pediatric preventive cardiology

CHILDHOOD ONSET OF CORONARY ARTERY DISEASE

Atherosclerotic lesions start to develop in early childhood and progress to irreversible lesions in adolescence and adulthood. The strongest evidence of childhood onset of CAD comes from the Bogalusa Heart Study (Berenson et al, 1998) and the Pathological Determinants of Atherosclerosis in Youth (PDAY) Research Group (Strong et al, 1995; McGill et al, 2002). Autopsy studies of the aorta and coronary arteries in the youth after unexpected deaths in the Bogalusa Heart Study and in the study by the PDAY Research Group have found that atherosclerosis originates in childhood, with a rapid increase in the prevalence of coronary pathology during adolescence and young adulthood.

These studies have found the following.

1. Fatty streak, the earliest lesion of the atherosclerosis, occurred by 5 to 8 years of age, and fibrous plaque, the advanced lesion, appeared in the coronary arteries in subjects in their late teens.
2. Fibrous plaque was found in more than 30% of 16- to 20 year-olds, and the prevalence of the lesion reached nearly 70% by age 26 to 39 years.
3. The extent of pathological changes in the aorta and coronary arteries increased with age, and so did the number of

BOX 34.1 Major Risk Factors for Coronary Heart Disease

- Family history of premature coronary heart disease, cerebrovascular, or occlusive peripheral vascular disease (with onset before age 55 yr for men and 65 yr for women in parents or grandparents)
- Hypercholesterolemia
- Low levels (<40 mg/100 mL)
- Hypertension (BP >140/90 mm Hg or taking antihypertensive medication)
- Cigarette smoking
- Diabetes mellitus (regarded as a coronary heart disease risk equivalent)

BP, Blood pressure; *HDL,* high-density lipoprotein.
Modified from Summary of the Third Report of the National Cholesterol Education Program (NCEP) Expert Panel on Detection, Education, and Treatment of High Blood Cholesterol in Adults (Adult Treatment Panel III) final report, *Circulation* 106:3143–3421, 2002.

known CV risk factors that the individual had at the time of death.

Therefore, one strategy of reducing CAD in adults would be to prevent or correct CV risk factors in children and adolescents.

CARDIOVASCULAR RISK FACTORS

Box 34.1 lists major risk factors for CVD, according to the Third Report of the National Cholesterol Education Program (NCEP) (*Circulation*, 2002). CV risk factors include positive family history of coronary heart disease, smoking, high levels of cholesterol, hypertension, being overweight, smoking, and diabetic or prediabetic states. These risk factors are all associated with an increased prevalence and extent of atherosclerosis. Obtaining a history of these CV risk factors should be a routine process in the practice of medicine.

A family history of premature CAD in the first-degree relatives (parents and siblings) has been found to be the single best predictor of CV risk for adults. For children, however, family history includes the first- *and* second-degree relatives (including parents, siblings, grandparents, or blood-related aunts and uncles) who have or had CAD before age 55 years for boys and before age 60 years for girls. The reason that the second-degree relatives are included in family history for children is because some children's parents are too young to have developed clinical CAD when their children are examined.

The prevalence of obesity has increased rapidly in recent decades, which is now known to be an independent risk factor for CVD and diabetes. Obese individuals have increased prevalence of clustering of multiple CV risk factors, called the metabolic syndrome, that lead to increased incidence of both type 2 diabetes and CV events (see later).

Metabolic Syndrome

Recent studies have shown that obesity is a risk factor for CAD independently of the standard risk factors, probably through the emerging risk factors. The emerging risk factors,

which are commonly found in obese persons, include atherogenic dyslipidemia (also known as *"lipid triad"* consisting of raised level of triglycerides [TGs]; small, dense low-density lipoprotein [LDL] particles; and low levels of high-density lipoprotein cholesterol [HDL-C]), insulin resistance (hyperinsulinemia), a proinflammatory state (elevation of serum high-sensitivity C-reactive protein), and a prothrombotic state (increased amount of plasminogen activator inhibitor-1 [PAI-1]). The cluster of these risk factors occurring in one person is known as "the metabolic syndrome."

In the metabolic syndrome, LDL-C levels may not be elevated, but apoprotein B and small, dense LDL particles are elevated. The smallest particles in the LDL fraction are known to have the greatest atherogenicity (see Chapter 33 for further discussion). This syndrome occurs more commonly in individuals with abdominal (visceral) obesity. The exact mechanism for the role of visceral adiposity is not completely understood, but it appears to be closely related to insulin resistance. It has been assumed that obese adipose tissue releases an excess of fatty acids and cytokines that induce insulin resistance. With increasing adiposity, the lipid triad becomes more pronounced. Hispanics and South Asians seem to be particularly susceptible to the syndrome. Black men have a lower frequency of the syndrome than do white men, likely because of a lower prevalence of atherogenic dyslipidemia.

Clinically identifiable components of the metabolic syndrome for adults are listed in Table 34.1. The presence of at least three of the risk factors is required to make the diagnosis of the metabolic syndrome in adults, according to the AHA/National Heart Lung and Blood Institute (NHLBI) scientific statement (Grundy et al, 2005), but the International Diabetes Federation recommend obesity plus at least two of remaining four criteria (Alberti et al, 2006). Evidence has supported that waist circumference (WC; reflecting visceral adiposity) is a better predictor of CVD than body mass index (BMI). Although LDL-C may not be elevated, small, dense LDL particles present in this syndrome are highly atherogenic. Other components of metabolic syndrome, such as proinflammatory and prothrombotic states, are not routinely measured in clinical practice. C-reactive protein of 3 mg/L or greater may be significant in adults.

Several definitions for use in the clinical setting for diagnosis of the metabolic syndrome in children exist. One in particular, Cook and coworkers' (2003) definition, includes TGs of 110 mg/dL or greater and fasting glucose of 110 mg/dL or greater. On the other hand, the International Diabetes Federation (Zimmet, 2007) has proposed different cutoff points for these two, 150 mg/dL or greater for TGs and 100 mg/dL or greater for fasting glucose. The TG level of 150 mg/dL is more appropriate according to a more recent National Health and Nutrition Examination Survey data (collected between 1988 and 2002); the 90th percentile of TG is much higher than 110 mg/dL (Jolliffe, 2006). Note that the new values for TGs and fasting glucose proposed by the International Diabetes Federation are the same as in adults (see Table 34.1). According to the recommendation of the International Diabetes Federation, obesity and the presence of at least two

TABLE 34.1   Definitions of the Metabolic Syndrome in Adults and in Children and Adolescents

	Adults[a]	Children and Adolescents[b]
Obesity (WC)	Men: WC ≥40 in (102 cm) Women: WC ≥35 in (88 cm)	WC ≥90th percentile or adult cutoff point
Triglycerides	≥150 mg/dL	≥150 mg/dL
HDL-C	Men <40 mg/dL Women <50 mg/dL	≤40 mg/dL
Hypertension	≥130/85 mm Hg	Systolic ≥130/diastolic ≥85 mm Hg
Elevated fasting glucose	≥100 mg/dL	≥100 mg/dL
Defining criteria	≥3 criteria (AHA/NHLBI Consensus Statement)[a] or Obesity + ≥2 remaining 4 criteria[c]	Obesity + ≥2 remaining 4 criteria[b]

[a]Grundy SM, Cleeman JI, Daniels SR, et al: Diagnosis and management of the metabolic syndrome: an American Heart Association/National Heart, Lung, and Blood Institute scientific statement: executive summary, *Circulation* 112(17):2735–2752, 2005.
[b]Zimmet P, Alberti G, Kaufman F, et al: International Diabetes Federation Task Force on Epidemiology and Prevention of Diabetes. The metabolic syndrome in children and adolescents, *Lancet* 369(9579):2059–2061, 2007.
[c]Alberti KG, Zimmer P, Shaw J: Metabolic syndrome–a new world-wide definition. A Consensus Statement from the International Diabetes Federation, *Diabetes Med* 23(5):469–480, 2006.
AHA, American Heart Association; *BMI,* body mass index; *BP,* blood pressure; *HDL-C,* high-density lipoprotein cholesterol; *NHLBI,* National Heart, Lung, and Blood Institute; *WC,* waist circumference.

of the remaining four criteria are required to make the diagnosis of the metabolic syndrome in children (see Table 34.1). It is important to note that LDL cholesterol (LDL-C) levels may not be elevated, but it is because the LDL is mostly made up of small, dense LDL particles, which are much more atherogenic than large LDL particles. The prevalence of the metabolic syndrome in adolescents has been reported to be about 4%, but it increases to 30% to 50% in overweight adolescents (Singh, 2006).

As in adults, WC is preferable to BMI for children as well, which represents abdominal (visceral or central) obesity. Ethnicity and gender specific WC percentiles are now available for children (Fernandez et al, 2004), and they are presented in Appendix C (Tables C.1 to C.3). There are significant differences in WC according to ethnicity and gender. In general, Mexican American boys and girls have higher WCs than other ethnic groups. Note that the 75th percentiles of WC of African American and Mexican American girls 16 and 17 years old exceed the WC values of 88 cm (35 inches) identified as the cutoff point for increased risk of obesity-related comorbidities in adult women.

Comorbidities of metabolic syndrome include (1) nonalcoholic fatty liver disease (NAFLD), (2) polycystic ovary syndrome (PCOS) in females, (3) obstructive sleep apnea (OSA), and (4) mental health disorders (Magge et al, 2017). NAFLD is defined by having liver fat greater than 5% liver weight (not caused by alcohol consumption) and is strongly associated with insulin resistance. NAFLD can be screened by measuring aspartate aminotransferase and alanine aminotransferase in overweight and obese children. PCOS is characterized by hyperandrogenism, menstrual irregularities or ovulatory dysfunction, and polycystic ovaries. OSA occurs because of enlarged soft tissues in and around the airway as well as decreased lung volumes because of increased abdominal fat. Treatment of OSA improves multiple components of metabolic syndrome, such as blood pressure, lipids, and glucose

control. Obesity and type 2 diabetes mellitus are associated with worse mental health, including increased risk for anxiety and depression.

The mainstay of the treatment of the metabolic syndrome for both adults and children is weight control through dietary intervention and promotion of active lifestyle to achieve and maintain optimum weight, normal blood pressure, and normal lipid profile for age. Decreased obesity also results in decreases in insulin resistance and inflammatory markers. The principles of managing obesity are presented in the section on obesity in this chapter. In addition, each component of the syndrome present should be treated aggressively because the presence of the syndrome indicates a higher risk for CVDs and diabetes. Treatment of dyslipidemias is presented in some detail in the section of dyslipidemia. Treatment of insulin resistance involves lifestyle modification only (Magge et al, 2017). Although some studies have revealed beneficial effects of metformin on BMI, total cholesterol (TC) levels, fasting plasma glucose, and insulin resistance (Yanovski et al, 2011), metformin is not currently recommended for treatment of insulin resistance.

There appears to be a difference in susceptibility to different risk factors for different populations when they gain weight (Grundy, 2002). For example:

1. The white population of European origin appears to be more predisposed to atherogenic dyslipidemia than other populations when they gain weight.
2. Blacks of African origin are prone to hypertension when they gain weight; they also appear to be susceptible to type 2 diabetes. On the other hand, they develop less atherogenic dyslipidemia than do whites with the same degree of weight gain.
3. Native Americans and Hispanics are especially susceptible to type 2 diabetes but less likely to develop hypertension than are blacks.

4. People of South and Southeast Asia also have a high frequency of insulin resistance and type 2 diabetes. They appear more susceptible to CAD than are East Asians.

Lipid Screening for Dyslipidemia

Dyslipidemia including high levels of LDL-C, elevated TGs, and low levels of HDL-C are the best known, long established risk factors for CAD. Therefore, it is natural to detect (and treat) patients with dyslipidemia as the most important approach to preventing CV events.

In the past, the NCEP Expert Panel (1991) as well as the American Academy of Pediatrics (AAP) (Daniels, 2008) recommended *selective* screening of children based on the family history of premature CV disease. This selective screening was somewhat controversial because several studies published in the pediatric literature have indicated that about 50% of children with high LDL levels will be missed by following this recommendation. A major reason for this is that there is no reliable family history available on adopted children and because parents of children (and some grandparents) are still too young to have experienced premature coronary heart disease. Universal screening should theoretically detect all children with high LDL-C levels, but no pediatric organizations have recommended universal screening.

Current Recommendations

In 2011, however, the Expert Panel on Integrated Guidelines for Cardiovascular Health and Risk Reduction in Children and Adolescents convened by the NHLBI made major changes in the recommendations (*Pediatrics*, 2011) (Table 34.2).

1. A universal screening for children between the ages of 9 and 11 years (late childhood)
2. An additional universal screening between the ages of 17 and 21 years
3. Selective screening for children in other age groups who have certain CV risk factors (see below).

The reasons for choosing the age 9 to 11 years are that there is the strongest statistical correlation between results in late childhood (around 10 years of age) and in the adult life and that cholesterol levels decrease as much as 10% to 20% during puberty. The Expert Panel thought that, in the absence of clinical or historic marker, identification of lipid disorders that predispose to accelerated atherosclerosis requires universal lipid assessment. Age-specific descriptions of the recommended screening are shown in Table 34.2.

In this recommendation, either nonfasting lipid profile (non-FLP) or fasting lipid panel (FLP) is acceptable. Non-FLP is more convenient because it can be obtained at the time of office visit without fasting. In this case, non–HDL-C is calculated from the nonfasting blood samples (by subtracting HDL-C from TC) because non–HDL-C has been shown to be as powerful a predictor of atherosclerosis as any other lipoprotein cholesterol measurement in children and adolescents. If non–HDL-C is abnormal (≥145 mg/dL), then two FLP measurements are obtained.

For children who belong to other age groups that do not require universal screening (i.e., ages 2-8 and 12-16 years),

selective screening is recommended, as young as 2 years of age, if they have one of the following risk factors. For selective screening, FLP is measured and the average of two measurements is used.

1. Positive family history (Box 34.2)
2. Parent(s) with TC ≥240 mg/dL or known dyslipidemia
3. Child who has moderate- to high-level *risk factors*, such as diabetes, hypertension, BMI ≥85th percentile, or smokes cigarettes (see Box 34.2 for details)
4. Child who has a moderate- or high-risk *special risk condition,* such as diabetes, chronic renal disease, posttransplant patients, Kawasaki's disease, HIV infection, nephritic syndrome, and others (see Box 34.2 for details)

What To Do with the Results of the Screening

1. When NFLP is obtained, an abnormal level of non–HDL-C is 145 mg/dL or greater. In this case, one needs to obtain two FLPs to get LDL-C and TG levels. The average of the two LDL-C and TG levels determine what steps to take.
2. Abnormal levels of LDL-C and TG levels that need attention are as follows. These children with abnormal levels need to be treated (see Management later).
   LDL-C >130 mg/dL
   TGs >100 mg/dL for children younger than 10 years
   >130 mg/dL for 10- to 19-year-old patients

Management Plans

Management plans for children with dyslipidemia are presented in detail in Chapter 33.

1. For children with LDL-C greater than 130 mg/dL, dietary management and lifestyle change are recommended. The first step is to use the Cardiovascular Health Integrated Lifestyle Diet (CHILD)-1 for 3 to 6 months. If CHILD-1 is ineffective, CHILD-2 is used for 3 to 6 months. If unsuccessful in lowering LDL-C levels by dietary management, the use of lipid-lowering drugs (statins) is considered (see Fig. 33.2 in Chapter 33).
2. For high levels of TG, dietary therapy is used as the primary tool. Continued use of CHILD-2-TG diet, weight control efforts, reduction of sugar consumption, and increased consumption of fish (or omega-3 fish oil) are added to the effort (see Fig. 33.3 in Chapter 33).
3. Children with LDL-C of 250 mg/dL or greater and those with TGs of 500 mg/dL or greater should be referred to lipid specialists.

Obesity

Information provided in this section is only provided to assist health care providers in making a diagnosis of overweight and obesity, recognizing complications of obesity, providing the basic knowledge needed in patient counseling, and helping them with appropriate time for referral to a weight management specialist. This section is not meant to describe in detail treatment of obesity; successful treatment of obesity requires special skills and facilities with availability of a multidisciplinary team consisting of registered dietitians, specialized nurses, psychologists, and

TABLE 34.2	**Recommendations for Lipid Assessment According to Age Group**
Age Group	**Recommendation**
<2 yr	No lipid screening
2–8 yr	No routine lipid screening Measure FLP twice and average the result if any of the following applies: • Positive family history (see Box 34.2) • Parent with TC ≥240 mg/dL or known dyslipidemia • Child has diabetes, hypertension, BMI ≥95th percentile, or smokes cigarettes • Child has a moderate- or high-risk medical condition (see Box 34.2) Interpret the results according to Table 33.3.

9–11 yr	**Universal screening** (by either non-FLP or FLP)
	• **Non-FLP:** Calculate non–HDL-C
	  • [Non–HDL-C = TC – HDL-C]
	  • If non–HDL-C ≥145 mg/dL or HDL <40 mg/dL, measure FLP twice and average results.
	OR
	• FLP
	  • If LDL-C ≥130 mg/dL, non–HDL-C ≥145 mg/dL, HDL-C <40 mg/dL, or TGs ≥100 mg/dL if <10 yr; or ≥130 mg/dL if ≥10 yr
	Repeat FLP and average results.
	Interpret the result according to Table 33.3.

12–16 yr	No routine lipid screening Measure FLP twice and average results if any of the following applies: • Positive family history (see Box 34.2) • Parent with TC ≥240 mg/dL or known dyslipidemia • Child has diabetes, hypertension, BMI ≥85th percentile, or smokes cigarettes • Child has a moderate- or high-risk medical condition (see Box 34.2) Interpret the results according to Table 33.3.
17–21 yr	Universal screening once in this time period (by either non-FPL or FLP) For 17–19 yr: • Non-FLP and calculate non–HDL-C If non–HDL-C ≥145 mg/dL or HDL <40 mg/dL, measure FLP twice and average results. OR • FLP If LDL-C ≥130 mg/dL, non–HDL-C ≥145 mg/dL, HDL-C <40 mg/dL, or TGs ≥130 mg/dL: Repeat FLP and average results. Interpret the result according to Table 33.3. For 20–21 yr: • Non-FLP and calculate non–HDL-C If non–HDL-C ≥190 mg/dL or HDL-C <40 mg/dL, measure FLP twice and average results. OR • FLP If LDL-C ≥160 mg/dL, non–HDL-C ≥190 mg/dL, HDL-C <40 mg/dL, or TGS ≥150 mg/dL: Repeat FLP and average results. Interpret the result according to Table 33.4.

BMI, Body mass index; *FLP,* fasting lipid panel; *HDL-C,* high-density lipoprotein cholesterol; *LDL-C,* low-density lipoprotein cholesterol; *non-FLP,* nonfasting lipid profile; *TC,* total cholesterol; *TG,* triglyceride.
From Expert Panel on Integrated Guidelines for Cardiovascular Health and Risk Reduction in Children and Adolescents: summary report, *Pediatrics* 128:S213–S256, 2011.

exercise specialists. Such specialized programs are costly and, unfortunately, are insufficient in number.

Definition and Classification

The BMI (weight in kilograms divided by square of the height in meters [kg/m^2]) is a simple, valid measure of relative weight and is recommended in clinical diagnosis of overweight states. In adults, obesity is present when BMI is greater than 30, and overweight is present when BMI is between 25.0 and 29.9.

For children, statistical definition of overweight is used.
• Children whose BMI is between the 85th and 95th percentiles are "overweight."

• Children whose BMI is at or greater than the 95th percentile are "obese."
• Children whose BMI is greater the 99th percentile are "severely obese."

Age- and gender-specific BMI percentile curves for the US pediatric population have been published by the Centers for Disease Control and Prevention (CDC) (see Appendix C, Figs. C.1 and C.2). A large BMI does not always indicate an increase in body fat; lean muscular individuals may have a large BMI. Percent body fat may be more accurate in determining obesity than BMI, but the method of determining body fat is cumbersome and is not routinely used in clinical practice.

BOX 34.2 Cardiovascular Risk Factor Categories

Positive Family History

Parent, grandparent, aunt, uncle, or sibling with MI; angina; CABG, stent, or angioplasty; or sudden cardiac death (at <55 yr for men, <65 yr for women)

Risk Factors

High-level risk factors:

- Hypertension that requires drug therapy (BP ≥99th percentile + 5 mm Hg)
- Current cigarette smoker
- BMI ≥97th percentile
- Presence of high-risk conditions, including diabetes mellitus (see later)
  Moderate-level risk factors:
- Hypertension that does not require drug therapy
- BMI at the ≥95th percentile <97th percentile
- HDL-C <40 mg/dL
- Presence of moderate-risk conditions (see later)

Special Risk Medical Conditions

High-risk conditions:

- Type 1 and 2 diabetes mellitus
- CKD, ESRD, post renal transplant
- Post-orthotopic heart transplant
- Kawasaki's disease with current aneurysm
  Moderate-risk conditions:
- Kawasaki's disease with regressed coronary aneurysm
- Chronic inflammatory disease (SLE, JRA)
- HIV infection
- Nephrotic syndrome

BMI, Body mass index; *CABG*, coronary artery bypass graft; *CKD*, chronic kidney disease; *ESRD*, end-stage renal disease; *HDL-C*, high-density lipoprotein cholesterol; *JRA*, juvenile rheumatoid arthritis; *MI*, myocardial infarction; *SLE*, systemic lupus erythematosus; *TC*, total cholesterol.
From Expert Panel on Integrated Guidelines for Cardiovascular Health and Risk Reduction in Children and Adolescents: summary report, *Pediatrics* 128:S213–S256, 2011.

Prevalence

Obesity is one of the most pressing public health issues today in the United States. Between 1980 and 2002, obesity prevalence doubled in adults and tripled in children and adolescents aged 6 to 19 years (Hedley et al, 2004). According to the recent national statistics (from the National Health and Nutrition Examination Survey conducted in 2011 and 2012), 16.9% of children and adolescents (2–19 years old) and 34.9% of adults in the United States are obese. In addition, approximately 32% of children and adolescents are either overweight or obese (Ogden et al, 2014). Therefore, nearly half of all American children and adolescents are either overweight or obese.

Pathogenesis

The pathogenesis of obesity may be, in part, inherited, but genetics alone cannot account for the rapid increases in overweight in the US population. Environmental factors appear

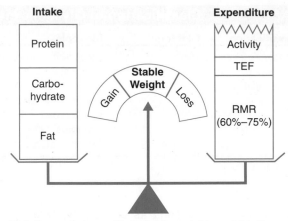

Fig. 34.1 Energy balance. To maintain a stable weight, the energy intake (protein, carbohydrate, and fat) of a person should be equal to the energy expenditure, which is composed of resting metabolic rate (RMR), the thermic effect of food (TEF), and expenditure associated with physical activities. When intake is greater than expenditure, weight gain will result; when expenditure of energy is greater than the intake, weight loss may result.

importantly related to the recent rise in the prevalence of obesity in this country. Increased consumption of calorie-dense food and a decrease in physical activity and an increased time spent on TV and video games may be causally related to the increasing prevalence of obesity seen in children and adolescents (Gortmaker et al, 1996). In recent decades, the role of high–glycemic index (GI) food has emerged as an important cause of weight gain.

Concept of Energy Balance

The concept of energy balance applies to the pathogenesis of obesity (Fig. 34.1). When energy intake exceeds energy expenditure on a chronic basis, obesity results. When energy intake is less than energy expenditure, weight loss may result. All energy intake comes from ingestion of macronutrients. Whereas the caloric value of fat is 9 kcal/g, that of protein and carbohydrate (CHO) is 4 kcal/g; this is an important reason for recommending reduced fat intake to control weight. A large portion of energy expenditure is the resting metabolic rate (RMR), accounting 60% to 75% of energy expenditure. Approximately 10% of energy expenditure is dissipated through the thermic effect of food (TEF), which is mainly the result of the energy cost of nutrient absorption, processing, and storage. Energy expenditure resulting from physical activity is relatively small, accounting for only 10% to 15% of the total energy expenditure. This component is least affected by genetics, and it varies greatly from individual to individual depending on the level of physical activities. The level of energy expenditure from RMR and TEF may be predominantly determined by genetic factors.

By measure, 3500 calories is equivalent to 1 lb. A relatively small positive energy balance can lead to significant weight gain over time. For example, an excess intake of only 100 calories per day will lead to a 10-lb weight gain over 1 year.

TABLE 34.3	Classification of Glycemic Index and Examples	
Classification	GI Range	Examples
Low GI	≤55	Most fruits and vegetables (except potatoes), whole-grain products, legumes, whole-grains, nuts and seeds, and fructose
Medium GI	56–69	Whole-wheat products, stone-ground breads, whole-grain cereals, table sugars, some brown rice, sweet potato, corn taco shells, and some cakes and cookies
High GI	≥70	White bread, baked potatoes, some processed cereals, most white rice, cornflakes, most muffins, honey, some cookies and cakes, most food made with enriched white flour, watermelon, and glucose

GI, Glycemic index.

High Glycemic Index Food as a Cause of Obesity and Increased Cardiovascular Risks

Beside the traditional concept of energy balance in the pathogenesis of obesity as discussed, the consumption of high-GI food has emerged as an important cause of obesity in recent decades. This concept needs to be discussed in some detail.

Several decades ago, the US government, the AHA, and other scientific organizations recommended that people eat low-fat diets to reduce weight gain and improve CV health. However, low-fat diets have not had much effect on obesity rate. Even though mean fat intake in the United States has decreased since the 1960s (from 42% to 34% of dietary energy), the prevalence of obesity has risen in the past several decades. During this period, people were eating low-fat, high-CHO diets. On the other hand, low-CHO diet (with more protein and fat), such as the Atkins diet, became popular, appearing to be effective in terms of weight reduction. Researchers started finding out that high CHO portion in the diet was responsible for weight gain. It turned out that the CHO consumed by people on low-fat diets were mostly refined and high in sugar content (i.e., high-GI food) (Ludwig et al, 1999; Brand-Miller et al, 2002). Consumption of high-GI food results in hormonal and metabolic changes that can cause weight gain (as discussed later). A brief review of the concept of the GI and glycemic load (GL) follows.

Glycemic Index. The **glycemic index**, first described by Dr. David J. Jenkins of the University of Toronto and his colleagues in 1981, is the number given to a food based on how quickly a CHO diet is digested and absorbed into the bloodstream (Jenkins et al, 1981). Even with equal amounts of total CHO, some foods cause a higher and quicker rise in blood sugar than others. After ingestion of enough food to provide 50 g of a particular CHO, blood glucose levels are determined and plotted every 15 minutes for the first hour and every 30 minutes for the second hour (for a total of 2 hours). The area under the resulting curve is calculated. The same is done after ingestion of 50 g of glucose, and the area under the curve is again calculated. The area under the curve for a particular food and that for glucose are then compared with the index of pure glucose set at 100.

The GI is classified into three categories: low (a GI of ≤55), medium (or intermediate) (a GI of 55–69), and high (a GI of ≥70). Examples of low-, medium-, and high-GI food are shown in Table 34.3.

Here is some general information about the GI of various foods:

- In general, fruits, vegetables (except potatoes), and legumes have a low GI, and sweets, refined-grain products (e.g., white bread), and potatoes have a high GI.
- The presence of fat lowers the GI. A baked potato has a GI of 85, but fried potatoes (French fries) have a GI of 75.
- The presence of soluble dietary fiber lowers the GI. Whole-wheat breads with higher amounts of fiber generally have a lower GI than white breads.
- The way food is prepared can change its GI. A boiled potato has a GI of 56, steamed potatoes have a GI of 65, and a microwaved potato has a GI of 82.
- The ripeness of fruit increases the GI. Whereas the GI of underripe bananas is 30, that of overripe bananas is 52.
- Organic acids or their salts (e.g., adding vinegar) lower the GI.

Glycemic Load. One criticism of the GI is that it tells only how rapidly 50 g of CHO in a particular food turns into blood sugar, but it does not tell how much of that CHO is in a serving of a particular food. The GL is a new way of assessing the impact of CHO consumption that takes into account serving size. For example, although candies have a high GI, eating a single piece of candy, which contains a small fraction of 50 g, will result in a relatively small glycemic response. Thus, the GL of the candy is not high. The CHO in watermelon has a high GI (72), but watermelon's GL is low (4 from 120 g of watermelon). A GL of a typical serving of food is the product of the amount of available CHO in that serving and the GI of the food (calculated by the amount of CHO contained in a specified serving size of the food × the GI of that food ÷ 100).

The GL is categorized as follows.

- High: a GL of ≥20 points
- Medium: a GL of 11 to 19 points
- Low: a GL of ≤10 points

The higher the food's GL, the greater the expected elevation in blood glucose after consumption. A diet with a low GL has been linked to a lower risk of heart disease. A diet low in CHO automatically has a low GL. Almost all food with a low GI has a low GL. Table 34.4 shows the GI and GL of selected food. A more complete list of GI is periodically published by the American Society for Clinical Nutrition. The official website for GI is http://www.ajcn.org/content/76/1/5.full.

TABLE 34.4	Glycemic Index and Glycemic Load for Selected Foods[a]				
Food	GI	GL[b]	Food	GI	GL[b]
Instant rice	91	24.8 (110 g)	Banana	53	13.3 (170 g)
Baked potato	85	20.3 (110 g)	Corn tortilla	52	12 (50 g)
Cornflakes	81	21 (30 g)	Wheat breads	50	10 (30 g)
French fries	75	22 (150 g)	Brown rice	50	16 (150 g)
Bagel, white	72	25 (70 g)	Orange	48	5 (120 g)
Carrot	71	3.6 (55 g)	Spaghetti	41	16.4 (55 g)
White bread	70	21.0 (2 slices)	Apple	36	8.1 (170 g)
Rye bread	65	19.5 (2 slices)	Lentils	29	5.7 (110 g)
Coca-Cola	63	16 (250 g)	Milk	27	3.2 (225 mL)
Sweet corn	60	11 (80 g)	Peanuts	14	0.7 (30 g)

[a]From various sources.
[b]The numbers in the parentheses indicate the amount of the food consumed.
GI, Glycemic index; *GL*, glycemic load.

How may high-GI food contribute to weight gain and increase CV risk? Figure 34.2 shows the data reported by Dr. David S. Ludwig and his colleagues (1999) on hormonal and metabolic changes after ingestion of high- and low-GI diets in adolescents. Two important differences observed in blood *glucose* and serum *fatty acid* levels may offer partial explanation for weight gain after consumption of high-GI food (see later). In addition, consuming high-GI food may also increase CV risk factors.

Consumption of high-GI food resulted in the following changes in hormone levels and blood chemistry (see Fig. 34.2).

- Blood levels of *glucose* and *insulin* rose rapidly to much higher levels and stayed elevated for a longer period of time (>3 hours) than seen in the low-GI food group, which may predispose one to the development of diabetes.
- Low glucose levels seen 4 hours after eating high-GI food (reactive hypoglycemia) may trigger hunger sensations and lead to overeating, resulting in weight gain.
- Lower levels of serum *fatty acid* seen (2 hours after eating) may mean that insulin forced fat cells to take in fatty acids or a low level of glucagon impaired the breakdown of lipids (lipolysis) in the fat cells. The combined action of high insulin and low glucagon may be fat accumulation and preservation, resulting in weight gain.
- A higher level of growth hormone after eating a high-GI food (not shown in Fig. 34.2) may also promote weight gain.
- High-GI food produces undesirable metabolic effects similar to those seen in metabolic syndrome, thus increasing CV risks. The changes include raising blood TG levels, raising LDL-C, and lowering levels of HDL-C.

Why is low-GI food good for your health?. Consumption of low-GI food has been shown to have the following benefits, opposite to those described for high-GI food:

- No reactive hypoglycemia is seen, so people feel fuller, and hunger pangs are delayed.
- The levels of glucose and insulin are much lower, reducing the risk of developing diabetes.

- Serum fatty acid levels remain higher, which may mean that lipids are not forced into the body cell or that high levels of glucagon made the cells break down fats and made more fatty acids available for the energy system.
- Serum *growth hormone* levels do not rise after low-GI food, not promoting weight gain.
- The prevalence of metabolic syndrome is lower in people eating low-GI food, reducing the risk of heart disease and stroke (by reducing TGs and LDL-C levels, increasing HDL-C, and reducing plasminogen activator inhibitor).

Health Consequences of Obesity

A number of disease states are associated with obesity in adults, which are not only risk factors for heart disease and diabetes but also responsible for significant health care costs: approximately 5% of total health care costs (>$100 billion) can be attributed to obesity. Common conditions associated with adult obesity include hyperlipidemia, heart disease, hypertension, type 2 diabetes, stroke, and osteoarthritis. Obesity also increases the prevalence of some cancers, gallbladder disease, sleep disorders, gout, and mood disorders.

Health consequences of obesity in children are somewhat different from those seen in obese adults (Dietz,1998).

1. Common medical consequences of obesity
   a. CV risk factors (data from Becque, 1998; Srinivasan et al, 1999)
      1) Hypercholesterolemia: 31%
      2) Hypertriglyceridemia: 64%
      3) Low HDL-C: 64%
   b. Glucose intolerance is linked to the recent increase in the prevalence of type 2 diabetes in children.
   c. Hypertension is present in 10% to 30% of overweight children.
   d. Asthma is more common in obese children and is more difficult to control than in nonobese children.
   e. Acanthosis nigricans (~25%), an indication of hyperinsulinemia
   f. Hepatic steatosis (fatty degeneration) with elevated liver enzymes (seen in >10% of overweight children), cholelithiasis (caused by increased cholesterol

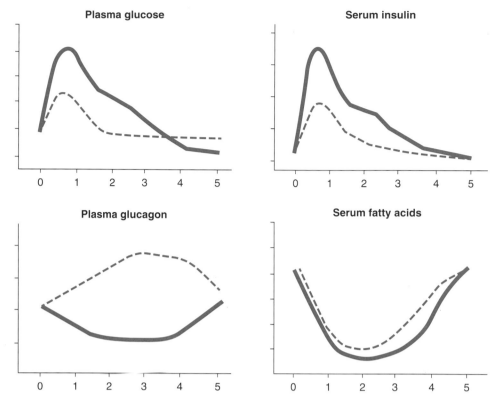

Fig. 34.2 Comparison of hormonal and metabolic changes following ingestion of high–glycemic index (GI) and low-GI food in adolescents. *Thick lines* represent the high-GI food group, and *thin broken lines* represent the low-GI food group. (Redrawn from Ludwig DS, Majzoub JA, Al-Zahrani A, Dallal GE, Blanco I, Roberts SB: High glycemic index foods, overeating, and obesity, *Pediatrics* 103(3):E26, 1999.)

synthesis), and cholecystitis (occurring more often with weight reduction)

2. Less common medical consequences of obesity
   a. Pseudotumor cerebri (with manifestations of headache, visual impairment or blindness, papilledema, occurring before adolescence) requires aggressive treatment. About 50% of children with the condition are obese.
   b. Sleep apnea occurs in fewer than 7% of obese children. This requires an aggressive treatment, including tonsillectomy and adenoidectomy or weight reduction.
   c. Orthopedic complications. Blount disease (bowing of the tibia and femur with resulting overgrowth of the medial aspect of the proximal tibial metaphysis) or slipped capital femoral epiphysis
   d. Polycystic ovary disease: Menstrual abnormalities and hirsutism in association with obesity, acanthosis, hyperinsulinemia, hyperandrogenemia suggest this condition.
3. Psychosocial consequences
   a. Early discrimination (in childhood)
   b. Negative self-esteem (in adolescence)
   c. Inappropriate expectation to be more mature because of their large size. This may lead to frustration, a sense of failure, and social isolation.
   d. Learning difficulties
   e. Eating disorders (in white girls)

Evaluation of Obese Children

1. Physicians should consider identifiable underlying causes of obesity, such as genetic or endocrine disorders
   a. Genetic causes. Prader-Willi, Bardet-Biedl, and Alström syndrome all have severe early onset of obesity. Most of the genetic conditions associated with obesity have in common mental retardation and short stature, and often with dysmorphic features.
   b. Endocrine abnormalities, such as hypothyroidism, Cushing syndrome, and generalized hypothalamic dysfunction, should be considered. Children with hypothyroidism and cortisol excess have short stature and delayed puberty rather than tall stature and early puberty seen in most obese children. When questions arise, determination of free thyroxine and thyroid-stimulating hormone and 24-hour urinary free cortisol or diurnal salivary cortisol levels should clarify the questions.
2. Check for the presence of other risk factors for CVD, diabetes, or metabolic syndrome (see Tables 34.1 and 34.2).
   a. Blood pressure measurement
   b. Lipoprotein analysis, fasting insulin, and blood glucose
   c. Glycosylated hemoglobin (HbA_{1C}) may also be useful.
3. Search for possible obesity-related complications by history and physical examination, such as those listed below.
   a. Acanthosis nigricans is associated with hyperinsulinemia and a higher risk of developing type 2 diabetes.

b. Thyroid enlargement may be associated with hypothyroidism.

c. History of nighttime snoring, breathing difficulties, or daytime somnolence may indicate OSA or obesity hypoventilation syndrome.

d. Hip or knee pain may be manifestations of slipped capital femoral epiphysis.

e. Abdominal pain or tenderness may be associated with gallbladder disease.

f. Headaches and blurred optic disk margins may indicate pseudotumor cerebri.

g. Hepatomegaly may be associated with hepatic steatosis.

h. Oligomenorrhea, amenorrhea, striae, or hirsutism may indicate polycystic ovary disease or Cushing's syndrome.

i. Signs of depression, bulimia nervosa, binge-eating disorder, or other serious psychological disorders require further evaluation and treatment by a child psychiatrist or psychologist.

Management

All successful pediatric weight management programs include four components: (1) dietary component, (2) exercise, (3) behavior modification, and (4) family component. Among these, dietary intervention and regular exercise combined are the cornerstones of the weight management. Only through behavior modification can long-term healthy eating and activity patterns be established; attempts at using diet and exercise for quick weight loss usually fail. Without involvement of the parents and family, behavior modification of children and adolescents is difficult to achieve. Currently, there are no pharmacologic agents that are shown to be safe and effective for long-term weight management in children and adolescents. Presently, the Food and Drug Administration has approved two drugs, sibutramine (Meridia) and orlistat (Xenical), which may be used for treating severely obese children. Consultations with registered dietitians, psychologists, and exercise specialists may be sought, or a referral to a multidisciplinary weight management programs may become necessary.

Assessment of usual diet and activity patterns of overweight children and adolescents is important. Selected questions (or assessments) and appropriate counseling are listed next.

Dietary Component

1. The following questions are helpful in assessing dietary habits of the child and family.
   a. How often vegetables and fruits are eaten as main meal or snack
   b. How often high calorie drinks (soda pops, fruit punches, fruit juices, and so on) are consumed
   c. Number and types of fast food eaten per week
   d. How often the child eats fish, chicken, and red meats
   e. Type of milk, bread, and butter consumed
   f. How often fried foods are eaten in a week
2. The counseling should include at least the following.

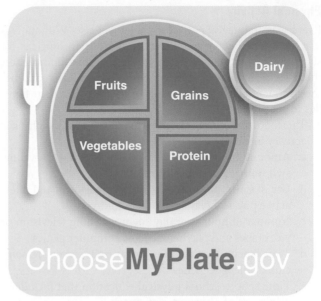

Fig. 34.3 MyPlate, the new food guide system. (Source: UDS Department of Agriculture: USDA's MyPlate. Available at: http://www.choosemyplate.gov/images/MyPlateImages/JPG/myplate_green.jpg.)

a. The diet of choice is a diet low in saturated fat and cholesterol that includes 5 or more daily servings of vegetables and fruits and 6 to 11 servings of whole-grain and other complex CHO foods.

b. Low-GI diets may be more effective than low-fat diets in reducing weight and improving CV risks (as discussed in an earlier section).

c. A new Food Guide System, MyPlate, should be introduced (Fig. 34.3). Half of a plate is filled with fruits and vegetables, a quadrant with grains (bread, wheat, rice, and so on), and the last with protein (meat, poultry, fish, soy, and so on).

d. To help people better understand what constitutes healthy habits for controlling obesity, some simple guidelines have been developed, such as the "5-2-1-0" message (which includes physical activity). This message developed by the New Hampshire Health Department has been endorsed by the AAP as a basic healthy lifestyle counseling tool. The message is simple to understand and remember and can be given in a few minutes. The 5-2-1-0 message stands for:

- 5: Eat at least 5 servings of fruits and vegetables most days.
- 2: Limit screen time to 2 hours or less daily.
- 1: Participate in at least 1 or more hours of physical activity every day.
- 0: Encourage no soda and sugar-sweetened drinks. Instead, drink water and low-fat or fat-free milk.

3. Physicians may consider using the following as handout materials for counseling.
   a. Table C.4 in Appendix C (specific food to choose and to decrease)
   b. Boxes C.1 (dietary strategies) and C.2 (tips for parents) in Appendix C

Physical Activity

Exercise is an integral part of management also. Without regular exercise, dietary modification alone is insufficient for successful weight management. Physicians should first assess the level of physical activity of overweight children and use their influential position to counsel children and their families to adopt healthy lifestyles.

1. The following questions are useful in assessing physical activity in children.
   a. Amount of time regularly spent walking, bicycling, swimming, and in backyard play
   b. Use of stairs, playgrounds, and gymnasiums, and interactive physical play with other children
   c. Number of hours per day spent watching television or videotapes and playing video or computer games
   d. Time spent participating organized sports, lessons, clubs, or league games
   e. Time sent in school physical education that includes a minimum of 30 minutes of exercise
   f. Participation in household chores
   g. Positive role modeling for a physically active lifestyle by parents and other caretakers
2. Physician's counseling and education should include the following areas.
   a. Physicians should formally address the subject of exercise, emphasizing the health benefits of regular physical activity, which include:
      1) Helping weight control by lowering level of weight gain
      2) Metabolic benefits, including improved glucose tolerance and insulin sensitivity, reduction in very-low-density lipoprotein cholesterol (VLDL-C), and rise in HDL-C levels
      3) Lowering of blood pressure
      4) Improving psychological well-being
      5) Predisposition to increased physical activity in adulthood.
   b. Children should participate in at least 30 minutes of moderate physical activity at least 4 or more days of the week, preferably every day.
   c. Parents should be encouraged to help their children reduce excessive time spent on sedentary behaviors such as watching television and videotapes, playing on a computer, listening to music, and talking on the phone. TV sets should be removed from the child's bedroom.
   d. More physical activity should be part of their lifestyle, such as walking or biking to school instead of driving, skating, stairs instead of elevators, and helping with active chores inside and outside of the house.
   e. Teach parents the importance of being role models for active lifestyle and providing children with opportunities for increased physical activity.

Behavior Modification

Behavior modification is essential for permanent changes in dietary and exercise habits.

1. Promotion of long-term permanent changes in behavior patterns, rather than short-term diet or exercise program for rapid weight loss, should be the goal of the treatment.
2. Emphasis should be on small and gradual behavior changes.

Early Intervention and Family Involvement

Physicians should also talk about the importance of early intervention (beginning before adolescence) and family involvement for successful weight management.

1. The importance of early intervention includes:
   a. Many lifestyle habits (eating and exercise habits) are established early in childhood. Parents have much control of their children's behaviors in the early school years.
   b. There is a tracking of CV risk factors from childhood to adulthood. About 80% of obese adolescents became obese adults. When established, obesity is difficult to cure.
2. Family involvement is very important in pediatric weight management programs.
   a. Willingness on the part of both child and family to participate and involvement of the entire family and other caregivers are important.
   b. Parents need to learn certain skills and commit themselves to the program.
      1) Parent role modeling of healthful dietary and activity habits
      2) Understanding the new food guide system (MyPlate)
      3) Ability to read food labels
      4) Understanding the benefits of low-GI food and of reducing consumption of high-GI food and drinks
      5) Appropriate ways of praising and rewarding good progress
      6) Changes in family environment, such as removing high-calorie food, reducing the number of meals eaten outside of the home, serving portion controlled meals to the child, promoting active lifestyles and discouraging sedentary lifestyle, and so on
      7) Inclusion of activities to help families monitor their eating and physical activity behaviors and establishing formal routine exercise program at a scheduled time each day or evening
   c. There are not enough weight management centers available to take care of all overweight children, and they are also expensive. Physicians may suggest motivated parents to read a book written specifically for them, such as those listed below and many others. This is a good way to have parents get deeply involved in the project.

Helping Your Overweight Child: A Family Guide by Caroline J. Cederquist, MD

Helping Your Overweight Child: A Do-It-Yourself Guide by Myung K. Park, MD

If Your Child is Overweight: A Guide for Parents by Susan M. Kosharek

Big Kids: A Parents' Guide to Weight Control for Children by Gregory A. Archer

Primary emphasis in weight control efforts should be the lifestyle change; the weight loss itself is of secondary importance. Active lifestyle improves risk factors even when weight loss is minimal. When a weight-loss goal is set, it should be realistic and should not attempt to fully normalize weight. In children without complications of obesity, maintenance of the current weight or modest weight loss, while children continue to grow in height, reduces their degree of overweight. Children with complications of obesity (e.g., hypertension, hyperlipidemias, insulin resistance, hepatic steatosis) should attempt to lose weight to correct these complications.

Cigarette Smoking

Cigarette smoking has been called the chief single preventable cause of death in our society and one of the most important public health issues of our time, costing more than $167 billion a year. Cigarette smoking is a powerful independent risk factor for myocardial infarction, sudden death, and peripheral vascular disease, in addition to being a major cause of lung cancer. Even passive exposure to smoke causes alterations in the risk factors in children.

Prevalence

Overall, cigarette smoking among American adults (aged ≥18 years) declined from 20.9% in 2005 to 15.5% in 2016. Yet nearly 38 million American adults smoke cigarettes ("every day" or "some days"). An estimated 5.6 million children aged younger than 18 years who are living today will eventually die from smoking-related disease unless current rates are reversed.

Some recent statistics on the prevalence of smoking among the youth are presented below based on reports from the CDC and other sources.

1. In 2016, 20.2% of high school students reported current use of any tobacco product; e-cigarettes were the most commonly used tobacco product (11.3%) followed by cigarettes (8.0%) and cigars (7.7%) (Jamal et al, 2017).
2. Among middle school students, 7.2% reported current use of any tobacco product; e-cigarettes were the most commonly used tobacco product (4.3%) followed by cigarettes (3.2%) and cigars (2.2%) (Jamal et al, 2017).
3. Among college students, 33% are current users of tobacco products, and nearly 50% used tobacco products in the past year (Rigotti et al, 2000).
4. Tobacco use was significantly higher among white students than black students.
5. Nearly 90% of adult smokers began smoking at or before age 18 years. Two-thirds of adult smokers became every-day smokers at or before age 18 years.
6. There were smokers in the household in 72% of middle school student smokers and in 58% among high school student smokers.
7. Nearly 50% of middle school student smokers and 62% of high school student smokers reported a desire to stop

smoking cigarettes, and most of them had made at least one cessation attempt during the previous 12 months. On the other hand, among students who had never smoked cigarettes, 21% of middle school students and 23% of high school students were susceptible to initiating cigarette smoking in the next year.

Pathophysiologic Effects of Smoking. The following are some pathophysiologic effects of smoking on the CV system (Lu et al, 2004), all of which appear likely to be involved in accelerating atherosclerosis in the coronary artery and peripheral arteries or increasing the probability of thrombosis (with potential for stroke). Physicians could use this information in counseling sessions with smokers.

1. Smoking causes atherogenic dyslipidemia. It increases levels of LDL-C and VLDL-C and TGs and lowers HDL-C levels. These effects are greater in children and adolescents than those seen in adults. Even passive smoking lowers HDL-C.
2. Smoking contributes to a prothrombotic predisposition.
   a. It increases levels of fibrinogen, factor VII, and other factors involved in the fibrin clotting cascade and decreases the concentration of plasminogen.
   b. It activates platelets, increasing their ability to adhere to the vessel wall.
3. Smoking increases blood viscosity by increasing hemoglobin levels (through carbon monoxide–induced increase in carboxyhemoglobin) and by an elevation of plasma fibrinogen levels.
4. Smoking accelerates atherosclerotic process by
   a. Increasing monocyte adhesion to endothelial cell (the initial step in atherogenesis)
   b. Decreasing nitric oxide synthesis (with resulting endothelial dysfunction)
   c. Decreasing synthesis of prostacyclin
5. Smoking causes peripheral arterial disease through endothelial dysfunction.
6. Smoking raises blood pressure transiently, raises heart rate, and increases myocardial contractility and myocardial oxygen consumption (by stimulation of the sympathetic nervous system).

Psychosociology of Smoking. Physicians should be aware of the psychosociology of initiating smoking to help prevent smoking in children.

1. Most smoking starts during adolescence. The high-risk period is the transition from elementary school to middle school and first and second years of middle school. This should be the target age group to counsel individually or through school systems.
2. Known predictors of smoking include peer influence (the most important), family members who smoke (siblings and parents), less educated parents, being a more independent and rebellious child, and having less academic success.
3. Cited reasons for starting to smoke include wanting to fit into a group, to lose weight, and to appear more mature.

Management

Physicians and health care professionals should assess the status of smoking, provide smoking prevention messages, help counsel parents and children about smoking cessation, and encourage school and community antismoking efforts.

1. Physician should assess the status of smoking during office visits.
   a. Smoking history should be obtained in all children older than 8 years of age during routine health assessments and updated. History regarding any siblings and friends who smoke should also be obtained.
   b. For current smokers, onset of smoking; number and type of cigarette smoked per day, week, or month; and whether they want to quit smoking and need help to quit the habit.
   c. Smoking history should also be obtained for parents and be updated.
2. Parents who smoke should be encouraged to quit. Physicians should emphasize adverse effects of passive smoking on their children and to be a role model for their children. Physicians should refer parent smokers to community smoking cessation programs.
3. Physicians' offices should be nonsmoking environments (without ashtrays), and antismoking posters, pamphlets, and videos in the waiting room may be productive.
4. Counseling techniques may vary with the age of the child.
   a. For elementary school children, antismoking message at each well-child assessment may counterbalance any negative pro-smoking influences exerted by friends or family. Emphasize the harmful physical consequences of smoking and the addictive nature of cigarettes. Parental assistance in the child's cessation of smoking should also be sought.
   a. For adolescents, emphasis should be on current negative physiological and social effects of smoking than long-term health consequence. Adolescents understand the health consequences of smoking but see them as remote and irrelevant. More immediate negative effects include bad breath, smelling like smoke, yellow-stained fingers, smell from clothing and hair, increasing heart rate and blood pressure, lack of stamina for sports, shortness of breath, and so on.
5. Some adolescents quit smoking on the advice of their physicians, and cessation message as brief as 3 minutes may be effective. Many adolescents require repeated efforts to quit smoking. Physicians should also encourage activities that tend to preclude cigarette smoking, such as regular physical activity and a variety of school and after-school activities.

Pharmacologic Approach. Currently, there is insufficient evidence for the effectiveness of pharmacologic treatments with youth smokers. The available experimental studies of youth cessation intervention find that behavioral interventions increase the chances of youth smokers achieving successful cessation.

For established adult smokers, if counseling is ineffective, physicians may try nicotine replacement and bupropion to help them quit smoking.

1. Nicotine replacement (by nicotine polacrilex gum or transdermal patch) delivers less nicotine than does cigarette smoking, which delivers bolus of nicotine. It also eliminates carbon monoxide inhalation.
2. Bupropion, an antidepressant, stimulates dopamine release and curbs the severe withdrawal symptoms of smoking cessation.
3. Other medications, such as varenicline and clonidine, have mixed reviews on beneficial effects and side effects in adults, but they are not approved for use in children and adolescents.

Practice of Preventive Cardiology

The primary mission of pediatrics has been prevention of disease and ensuring normal growth and development. It is natural for pediatricians to pay attention to early detection of children at risk of developing CVD (and type 2 diabetes) and provide counseling, intervention, and treatment whenever possible.

Acquisition of behaviors associated with risk factors occurs in childhood, such as dietary habits, physical activity behaviors, and the use of tobacco. Intervention to reduce the risk factors in childhood has been successful with low-calorie diets, smoking prevention, increasing physical activities, and family-based weight control programs. This is because some risk factors are detectable, modifiable, or treatable.

1. Family history of CVD is very important in assessing a child's risk of developing CAD later in life. Although it is not modifiable, its presence is a marker for a high risk of heart disease. A history of premature CAD in the first- or second-degree relatives (parents, grandparents, blood-related aunts and uncles, or siblings) before age 55 years for boys and before age 60 years for girls should prompt physicians to check on other risk factors.
2. Hypercholesterolemia is one of the major risk factors which are identifiable and treatable.
3. Hypertension is also an identifiable and treatable risk factor (see Chapter 28).
4. Other risk factors, such as smoking, consumption of atherogenic diets, and physical inactivity, are all modifiable by parental education and behavior changes.
5. Obesity is easily detectable. Although treatment of obesity can be frustrating to both the patients and physicians, education of parents and patients and behavior modification can be productive.
6. Inclusion of HbA_{1C} should be considered in the screening protocol to detect diabetic or prediabetic state.

The AHA has published a guideline for the prevention of CVD. Table 34.5 is a handy summary that presents goals and recommendations for reducing risks in children and adolescents for future CVD.

TABLE 34.5 Summary Guidelines for Preventive Pediatric Cardiology

Risk Identification	TREATMENT GOALS	Recommendations
Blood Cholesterol Total cholesterol: >170 mg/dL is borderline >200 mg/dL is elevated LDL-C: >110 mg/dL is borderline >130 mg/dL is elevated	**Goals** LDL-C <130 mg/dL (<110 mg/dL is even better) For patients with diabetes, LDL-C <100 mg/dL	If LDL-C is above goals, initiate additional therapeutic lifestyle changes, including diet (<7% of calories from saturated fat; <200 mg cholesterol per day) in conjunction with a trained dietitian. Consider LDL-lowering dietary options (increase soluble fiber by using age [in years] plus 5 to 10 g up to age 15 yr, when the total remains at 25 g per day) in conjunction with a trained dietitian. Emphasize weight management and increased physical activity. If LDL-C is persistently above goals, evaluate for secondary causes (TSH, LFT, renal function tests, urinalysis). Consider pharmacologic therapy for individuals with LDL >190 mg/dL with no other risk factors for CVD or >160 mg/dL with other risk factors present (BP elevation, diabetes, obesity, strong family history of premature CVD) (see Fig. 33.2). Pharmacologic intervention for dyslipidemia should be accomplished in collaboration with a physician experienced in treatment of disorders of cholesterol in pediatric patients.
Other Lipids and Lipoprotein TGs: >100 mg/dL is elevated for <10 yr >130 mg/dL is elevated for >10 yr HDL-C: <40 mg/dL is reduced	**Goals** Fasting TGs <75 mg/dL for <10 yr <90 mg/dL for >10 yr HDL-C >40 mg/dL	Elevated fasting TG and reduced HDL-C are often seen in the context of overweight with insulin resistance. Therapeutic lifestyle change should include weight management with appropriate energy intake and expenditure. Decrease intake of simple sugars. If fasting TGs are persistently elevated, evaluate for secondary causes such as diabetes, thyroid disease, renal disease, and alcohol abuse. No pharmacologic interventions are recommended in children for isolated elevation of fasting TG unless this is very marked. Treatment may be initiated at TG >400 mg/dL to protect against postprandial TG of 1000 mg/dL or greater, which may be associated with an increased risk of pancreatitis.
Blood Pressure Systolic and diastolic BP >95th percentile for age, sex, and height percentile	**Goal** Systolic and diastolic BP <90th percentile for age, sex, and height	Promote achievement of appropriate weight. Reduce sodium in the diet. Emphasize increased consumption of fruits and vegetables. If BP is persistently above the 95th percentile, consider possible secondary causes (e.g., renal disease, coarctation of the aorta). Consider pharmacologic therapy for individuals above the 95th percentile if lifestyle modification brings no improvement and there is evidence of target organ changes (LVH, microalbuminuria, retinal vascular abnormalities). Start BP medication individualized to other patient requirements and characteristics (e.g., age, race, need for drugs with specific benefits). Pharmacologic management of hypertension should be accomplished in collaboration with a physician experienced in pediatric hypertension.
Weight BMI 85th–95th percentile is overweight >95th percentile is obese	**Goal** Achieve and maintain BMI <95th percentile for age and sex	For children who are overweight (>85th percentile) or obese (>95th percentile), a weight management program should be initiated with appropriate energy balance achieved through changes in diet and physical activity. Use the "5-2-1-0" message and MyPlate for education and counseling. For children of normal height, a secondary cause of obesity is unlikely. Weight management should be directed at all family members who are overweight, using a family-centered, behavioral management approach. Weight management should be done in collaboration with a trained dietitian.
Diabetes Fasting plasma glucose: ≥126 mg/dL	**Goals** Near-normal fasting plasma glucose (<120 mg/dL) Near normal HgA1$_c$ (<7%)	Management of type 1 and type 2 diabetes in children and adolescents should be accomplished in collaboration with a pediatric endocrinologist. For type 2 diabetes, the first step is weight management with improved diet and exercise. Because of risk for accelerated vascular disease, other risk factors (e.g., BP, lipid abnormalities) should be treated more aggressively in patients with diabetes.
Cigarette smoking	**Goal** Complete cessation of smoking for children and parents who smoke	Advise every tobacco user (parents and children) to quit and be prepared to provide assistance with this (counseling or referral to develop a plan for quitting using available community resources to help with smoking cessation).

BMI, Body mass index; *BP*, blood pressure; *CVD*, cardiovascular disease; *HDL-C*, high-density lipoprotein cholesterol; *LDL-C*, low-density lipoprotein cholesterol; *LFT*, liver function test; *LVH*, left ventricular hypertrophy; *TG*, triglycerides; *TSH*, thyroid-stimulating hormone.
Modified from Kavey RW, Daniels SR, Lauer RM, et al: American Heart Association guidelines for primary prevention of atherosclerotic cardiovascular disease beginning in childhood, *Circulation* 107:1562–1566, 2003.

35

Athletes with Cardiac Problems

Competitive athletes are those who participate in an organized team or individual sport that requires regular competition against others. This definition is most easily applied to high school, college, and professional sports. Athletic competitions substantially increase the sympathetic drive, and the resulting increase in catecholamine levels increases blood pressure (BP), heart rate, and myocardial contractility, thereby increasing myocardial oxygen demand. The increase in sympathetic tone can cause arrhythmias and may aggravate existing myocardial ischemia. An athlete with a cardiac problem is at an increased risk of developing serious morbidity and even sudden death during athletic competition compared with nonathletes with similar cardiac problems.

Almost all US states require some type of preparticipation screening of participants in organized sports. The most important reason to screen for heart disease is to prevent sudden unexpected death. Heart disease may also lead to sudden incapacity, which may result in injuries, and preexisting heart disease may be exacerbated by exercise. There are also legal and insurance requirements.

Most physicians encounter this issue in association with high school and college sports; therefore, physicians should be aware of cardiac conditions that may cause problems and have the knowledge base required to accomplish a physician's role in school sports clearance. In addition, physicians should have a general understanding of the eligibility guidelines and the participation eligibility for patients with specific cardiovascular (CV) conditions.

The recommendations presented are mostly from American Heart Association (AHA) and American College of Cardiology (ACC) Scientific Statement. Eligibility and Disqualification Recommendations for Competitive Athletes with Cardiovascular Abnormalities, consisting of nine Task Forces (*Circulation*,

2015), and some are from the 36th Bethesda conference published in 2005 (36th Bethesda conference 2005). The following major areas will be presented, some in a table format for easy access of information.

1. Causes of sudden expected death
2. AHA/ACC 14-element screening procedure (of 2014)
3. Classification of sports according to the type and intensity to help physicians select allowable types of sports
4. Participation eligibility for athletes with different types of CV problems, presented in a table form for easy access of information
5. Guidelines for athletes with hypertension

SUDDEN UNEXPECTED DEATH IN YOUNG ATHLETES

Sudden unexpected death in young athletes is estimated to occur in about 1 per 200,000 high school sports participants per academic year. Most cases of unexpected sudden death in athletes are caused by unrecognized cardiovascular disease (CVD). Although rare, when a sudden unexpected death of an athlete due to a cardiac condition occurs, the public becomes disbelieving, suspicious, and even angry. Sometimes these feelings have been directed at the physicians involved. It is therefore important for primary care physicians to have a good understanding of cardiac conditions that can result in sudden death in order to reduce that possibility and to know their responsibilities in recommending sports clearance.

Among a variety of congenital or acquired heart diseases that can cause sudden death during athletic competition, hypertrophic cardiomyopathy (HCM) and coronary artery anomalies or diseases are the two most important groups,

TABLE 35.1 Cardiovascular Causes of Sudden Death in Young Athletes (n = 690)

Cause	Proportion of All Causes (%)
Hypertrophic cardiomyopathy	36
Coronary artery anomalies	17
Possible hypertrophic cardiomyopathy[a]	8
Myocarditis	6
Arrhythmogenic right ventricular cardiomyopathy	4
Ion channel disease	4
Mitral valve prolapse	3
Bridged left anterior descending coronary artery	3
Atherosclerotic coronary artery disease	3
Aortic rupture	3
Aortic stenosis	2
Dilated cardiomyopathy	2
Wolff-Parkinson-White syndrome	2
Others	5

[a]Finding suggestive but not diagnostic of hypertrophic cardiomyopathy.

From Balady GJ, Ades PA: Exercise and sports cardiology. In Bonow RO, Mann DJ, Zipes DP, Libby P (eds): *Braunwald's Heart Disease*, ed 9, Philadelphia, 2012, Saunders. Adapt AHA's Table from Circulation.2007;115:1643-1655, Page 1646

accounting for nearly two thirds of the cases. Table 35.1 shows previously implicated diseases for sudden cardiac death, which is derived from 690 cases of CV causes of sudden death (Maron et al, 2009).

1. **HCM.** The single most common CV abnormality among the causes of sudden death in young athletes is HCM (36%) and its variants (8%), accounting for nearly half of the cases (see Table 35.1).
2. **Congenital anomalies and acquired diseases of the coronary arteries** are the next important group of causes of sudden death, accounting for nearly 25%, including congenital anomalies of the coronary artery and acquired coronary artery diseases such as atherosclerotic coronary artery disease or coronary artery stenosis resulting from Kawasaki's disease.
3. **Myocarditis.** Sudden cardiac death has been reported at rest and during exercise with both acute and chronic myocarditis (up to 6% of sudden death) by way of ventricular arrhythmias.
4. **Cardiac arrhythmias** (from long QT syndrome, Wolff-Parkinson-White [WPW] syndrome, sinus node dysfunction, arrhythmogenic right ventricular dysplasia [ARVD]) are rare causes of sudden death.
5. **Other rare causes** of sudden death in athletes include severe obstructive lesions (e.g., aortic stenosis [AS], pulmonary stenosis [PS]), Marfan's syndrome (from ruptured aortic aneurysm), mitral valve prolapse (MVP), dilated cardiomyopathy, primary pulmonary hypertension (PH), unexpected blow to the chest (by such objects as a baseball or hockey puck, termed *commotio cordis*), sarcoidosis, and sickle cell trait.

Some patients die while they are sedentary or during mild exertion, but many collapse during or just after vigorous physical activity. On occasion, athletes may die suddenly without evidence of structural heart disease on autopsy. In such instances, it may be due to a noncardiac cause such as drug abuse.

PREPARTICIPATION SCREENING

The objective of preparticipation screening is to detect "silent" CVD that can cause sudden cardiac death, which is caused by a ventricular tachyarrhythmia, with the exception of Marfan's syndrome and related disorders (aortic dissection or rupture). There are, however, no cost-effective practical guidelines for the screening that have been proved to be effective in identifying the potential candidates for sudden death at this time. Prospective CV screening of a large athletic population is impractical. The total number of competitive athletes in the United States may be in the range of 8 to 10 million. Even with the use of specialized tools available to cardiologists, complete prevention of such death is nearly impossible, given the rarity of some of the causes of sudden expected death. Consequently, medical clearance for sports does not necessarily imply the absence of CVD or complete protection from sudden death.

Recommended screening for US high school and college athletes is confined to history-taking and physical examination, which is known to be limited in its power to consistently identify important CV abnormalities. The AHA and ACC in 2014 have reaffirmed the AHA's earlier recommendations (of 1997 and 2007) of using its 14-element (formerly 12-point) screening procedure as shown in Box 35.1. As can be seen, 10 of the 14 points are related to the history, and the remaining 4 are physical examination. The history portion has been expanded and improved since the earlier 12-point screening procedure.

There have been controversies regarding inclusion of electrocardiography (ECG) as part of screening of competitive athletes. A report from the Veneto region of north eastern Italy reported an impressive reduction in sudden death among young competitive athletes by inclusion of ECG in the initial screening. This report prompted the European Society of Cardiology (ESC) to make a recommendation of mandatory ECG screening for athletes in other countries. However, none of the 51 European countries accepted the ESC recommendation.

It is doubtful that similar beneficial effects of inclusion of ECG in the screening reported in Italy would result in the United States. A possible partial explanation for that may lie in the enormous differences in the size and similarity of the population and the most common cause of sudden death in the two countries. Italy has one fifth of the US population with genetically similar subset of population and arrhythmogenic right ventricular cardiomyopathy (ARVC) is the most common cause of sudden death event. On the other hand, the United States is much more diverse ethnically and racially, and HCM is the most common cause of sudden death among athletes.

BOX 35.1 The 14-Element American Heart Association Recommendations for Preparticipation Cardiovascular Screening of Competitive Athletes

Medical History*
Personal History

1. Chest pain/discomfort/tightness/pressure to exertion
2. Unexplained syncope/near syncope†
3. Excessive and unexplained dyspnea/fatigue or palpitations, associated with exercise
4. Prior recognition of heart murmur
5. Elevated systemic blood pressure
6. Prior restriction from participation in sports
7. Prior testing for the heart, ordered by a physician

Family History

8. Premature death (sudden and unexpected, or otherwise) before 50 yr of age attributable to heart disease in ≥1 relative
9. Disability from heart disease in close relative <50 yr of age
10. Hypertrophic or dilated cardiomyopathy, long-QT syndrome, or other ion channelopathies, Marfan syndrome, or clinically significant arrhythmias, specific knowledge of genetic cardiac conditions in family members.

Physical Examination

11. Heart murmur‡
12. Femoral pulse to exclude aortic coarctation
13. Physical stigmata of Marfan syndrome
14. Brachial artery blood pressure (sitting position)§

---

*Parental verification is recommended for high school and middle school athletes.
†Judged not to be of neurocardiogenic (vasovagal) origin, of particular concern when occurring during or after physical exertion.
‡Refers to heart murmurs judged likely to be organic and unlikely to be innocent; auscultation should be performed with the patient in both the supine and standing positions (or with Valsalva maneuver), specifically to identify murmurs of dynamic left ventricular outflow tract obstruction.
§ Preferably taken in both arms.
BP, Blood pressure.
Modified by the American Heart Association with permission from Maron BJ, Friedman RA, Kligfield P, et al: Assessment of the 12-lead ECG as a screening test for detection of cardiovascular disease in healthy general population of young people (12–25 years of age). A scientific statement from the American Heart Association and the American College of Cardiology, *Circulation* 130(18):1617–1624, 2014.

The AHA and ACC believe that the cost of doing ECGs versus the yield is prohibitive, and further, the costs of evaluating false-positive ECG will be too great to make this practice cost effective. There are an estimated near 10 million competitive young athletes to screen. The conservative overall cost for such a program would be at least $2 billion per year to start and somewhat less annually thereafter. It is doubtful such large-scale screening initiatives are feasible or cost effective under the current US health care infrastructure.

Therefore, the position of the AHA and ACC has not changed, and in fact they have published a Scientific Statement jointly in 2014 not to include ECG in the initial screening of young competitive athletes (Maron et al, 2014). The ECG will be used only for patients who are found to be suspicious of having potentially lethal CVD based on the 14-element screening.

History and Physical Examination

Although simple history and physical examination can raise the suspicion of CVD in some at-risk athletes, they do not have sufficient power to guarantee detection of many critical CV abnormalities. However, the AHA's screening method has the capability of raising the clinical suspicion of several CV abnormalities.

Personal History

1. History of chest pain, discomfort, tightness, or pressure to exertion
2. Unexplained syncope or near syncope, except for vasovagal syncope
3. Excessive and unexplained dyspnea or fatigue or palpitation associated with exercise
4. Prior recognition of heart murmur
5. Elevated systemic BP
6. Prior restriction from participation in sports
7. Prior testing for the heart, ordered by a physician

Family History

8. Premature death (sudden and unexpected or otherwise) before 50 years of age attributable to heart disease in one or more relative
9. Disability from heart disease in close relative younger than 50 years of age
10. Hypertrophic or dilated cardiomyopathy, long QT syndrome, or other ion channelopathies, Marfan's syndrome, or clinically significant arrhythmias; specific knowledge of genetic cardiac conditions in family members

Physical Examination

11. Heart murmur (likely to be organic; not likely to be innocent)
12. Femoral pulse to exclude aortic coarctation
13. Physical stigmata of Marfan's syndrome
14. Brachial artery BP (sitting position)

If CV abnormalities are suspected by the AHA's screening procedure, a physician should request specialty consultation or order additional testing. The athlete should be temporarily withdrawn from activities until the issue can be resolved. The utility of ECG and an echocardiographic study are briefly outlined next, although they are not routinely recommended by the AHA.

Electrocardiography

The 12-lead ECG is indicated in patients suspicious of serious CVD raised by the 14-element AHA screening history and physical examination. The ECG is a practical and cost-effective alternative to routine echocardiography. Table 35.2 lists examples of normal and abnormal findings in the ECG screen.

TABLE 35.2 Normal and Abnormal Findings in Electrocardiogram Screening in Athletes

Normal ECG Findings	Abnormal ECG Findings

• Sinus bradycardia (HR >30 beats/min)
• Ectopic atrial rhythm
• Junctional escape
• First-degree AV block
• Mobitz type I second-degree AV block (Wenckebach)
• Isolated incomplete RBBB
• Early repolarization
• Isolated voltage criteria for LVH in the absence of
  • Left axis deviation
  • LAH
  • ST-segment depression
  • T-wave inversion
  • Pathologic Q waves
	• T-wave inversion (in two or more leads V1–V6, II, aVF, or I and aVL)
	• ST depression (≥0.5 mm in two or more leads)
	• Pathologic Q waves (˜3 mm in depth or >4 msec in duration in two or more leads except III and aVR)
	• LBBB
	• Left axis deviation (−30 to −90 degrees)
	• LAH
	• RVH
	• LVH voltage criteria in association with
	  • LAH (or enlargement)
	  • ST-segment depression
	  • T-wave inversion
	• Ventricular preexcitation
	• Sinus bradycardia (HR <30 beats/min)
	• SVT
	• Brugada-like ECG pattern
	• Frequent PVCs (≥two PVCs per 10-second tracing or nonsustained VT)

AV, Atrioventricular; *ECG*, electrocardiogram; *HR*, heart rate; *LAH*, left atrial hypertrophy (or enlargement); *LBBB*, left bundle branch block; *LVH*, left ventricular hypertrophy; *PVC*, premature ventricular contraction; *RAH*, right atrial hypertrophy; *RBBB*, right bundle branch block; *RVH*, right ventricular hypertrophy; *SVT*, supraventricular tachycardia; *VT*, ventricular tachycardia.

Modified from Lisman KA: Electrocardiographic evaluation in athletes and use of the Seattle Criteria to improve specificity, *Methodist DeBakey Cardiovasc J* 2(2):81–85, 2016.

1. The ECG findings are abnormal in up to 75% to 95% of patients with HCM. Common ECG abnormalities in HCM include left ventricular hypertrophy (LVH), ST-T changes, and abnormally deep Q waves (owing to septal hypertrophy) with diminished or absent R waves in the left precordial leads. Occasionally, "giant" negative T waves are seen in the left precordial leads. Cardiac arrhythmias and first-degree atrioventricular (AV) block may be seen occasionally.

2. Coronary artery abnormalities may show ST-T wave abnormalities or abnormal Q waves.

3. It will also identify other abnormalities such as the long QT syndrome (prolonged QTc interval >0.46 sec), Brugada syndrome (right bundle branch block [RBBB] with ST-segment elevation), and other inherited syndromes associated with ventricular arrhythmias.

4. It may also raise suspicion of myocarditis (premature ventricular contractions [PVCs], ST-T changes), or arrhythmogenic right ventricular (RV) cardiomyopathy (by T-wave inversion in leads V1 through V3, tall P waves, decreased RV potentials).

5. However, abnormal ECG findings are seen in about 40% of trained athletes, and this may be the source of confusion. ECG abnormalities seen in trained athletes include increased R- or S-wave voltages, Q-wave and repolarization abnormalities, and frequent or complex ventricular tachyarrhythmias on Holter ECG monitors.

6. On the other hand, normal ECG does not necessarily rule out significant cardiac abnormalities.

Echocardiography

Echocardiographic study is the principal diagnostic imaging modality for clinical identification of HCM and other cardiac abnormalities.

1. HCM can be reliably diagnosed by two-dimensional echocardiography. Diastolic left ventricular (LV) wall thickness of 15 mm or greater (or on occasion, 13 or 14 mm), usually with LV dimension of less than 45 mm, is accepted for the clinical diagnosis of HCM in adults. For children, z-score of 2 or more relative to body surface area is theoretically compatible with the diagnosis. The hearts of some highly trained athletes may show hypertrophy of the LV wall, making the differentiation between the physiologic hypertrophy and HCM difficult. An LV wall thickness of 13 mm or greater is very uncommon in highly trained athletes and is always associated with an enlarged LV cavity (with LV diastolic dimension >54 mm, ranging from 55–63 mm). Therefore, athletes with LV wall thickness greater than 16 mm and a nondilated LV cavity are likely to have HCM (Pelliccia et al, 1991).

2. Echocardiography is also expected to detect other congenital structural abnormalities, such as valvular heart disease (AS, PS), Marfan's syndrome (aortic root dilatation, MVP), myocarditis, and dilated cardiomyopathy (LV dysfunction or enlargement).

3. Definitive diagnosis of congenital coronary artery anomalies may not be accomplished by echo studies; it may require other tests such as computed tomography or coronary angiography.

Although the primary obligation of a physician to the athletes is their best medical interest, the physician must avoid unnecessary exclusion from sports. The physician should seek consultations from a specialist or order additional testing (e.g., ECG, echocardiography) to minimize unnecessary disqualification. The athlete should be temporarily withdrawn from activities until the issue can be resolved. After evaluation by a specialist, if the general physician and the

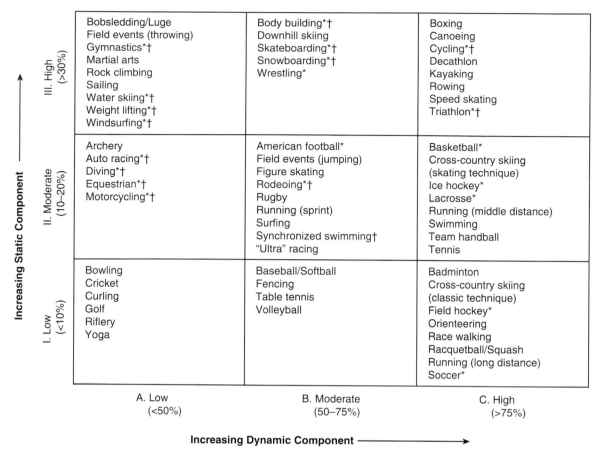

Increasing Static Component

	III. High (>30%)	Bobsledding/Luge Field events (throwing) Gymnastics*† Martial arts Rock climbing Sailing Water skiing*† Weight lifting*† Windsurfing*†	Body building*† Downhill skiing Skateboarding*† Snowboarding*† Wrestling*	Boxing Canoeing Cycling*† Decathlon Kayaking Rowing Speed skating Triathlon*†
	II. Moderate (10–20%)	Archery Auto racing*† Diving*† Equestrian*† Motorcycling*†	American football* Field events (jumping) Figure skating Rodeoing*† Rugby Running (sprint) Surfing Synchronized swimming† "Ultra" racing	Basketball* Cross-country skiing (skating technique) Ice hockey* Lacrosse* Running (middle distance) Swimming Team handball Tennis
	I. Low (<10%)	Bowling Cricket Curling Golf Riflery Yoga	Baseball/Softball Fencing Table tennis Volleyball	Badminton Cross-country skiing (classic technique) Field hockey* Orienteering Race walking Racquetball/Squash Running (long distance) Soccer*
		A. Low (<50%)	B. Moderate (50–75%)	C. High (>75%)

Increasing Dynamic Component ⟶

Fig. 35.1 Classification of sports. Sports in each category are listed in alphabetical order to make them easier to find. *Asterisks* indicate danger of bodily collision. *Daggers* indicate increased risk if syncope occurs. (Modified from Mitchell JH, Haskell W, Snell P, et al: Task Force 8: classification of sports, *J Am Coll Cardiol* 45:1364–1367, 2005. doi:10.1016/j.jacc.2005.02.015.)

specialist both agree that the patient's condition requires disqualification, then they should not hesitate to disqualify the individual from participation. Such decisions, if based on a reasonable preparticipation evaluation, have generally been upheld in court cases. Also, there seems to be little liability risk if an asymptomatic condition is missed.

The physician should resist pressure from competing interests such as the athlete, the family, the coach, and administrative officials of the educational institution. The importance of the player to the team should be a secondary factor; it is the player's safety that should be the primary factor in making recommendations. After a decision has been made, the physician should report only to the patient and his or her parents; the referring doctor; and in some cases, the institutional officials when an institution is paying for the medical evaluation.

CLASSIFICATION OF SPORTS

If CV or other abnormalities are found when evaluating an individual, the next step is to estimate how much physical exercise can be safely tolerated. Depending on the cardiac condition, the athlete may be able to safely engage in less demanding athletic activities. This requires knowledge of the type of exercise the individual will be doing, how much static and dynamic exertion is required, and how vigorous the training program is.

For the purpose of making recommendations on athletes' participation eligibility, the AHA and ACC in 2015 jointly published Scientific Statement on Classification of Sports (Fig. 35.1). Sports are divided into two broad types: dynamic and static, and each sport is categorized by the level of intensity (low, medium, or high). It should not be regarded as a rigid classification but rather a spectrum in which some athletes in the same sport could possibly deserve placement in different categories. Sports can also be classified according to the type and intensity of exercise performed and also with regard to the danger of bodily injury from collision as well as the consequences of syncope.

Dynamic (isotonic) exercise involves changes in muscle length and joint movement with rhythmic contractions that develops relatively small intramuscular force. Dynamic exercise causes a marked increase in oxygen consumption with a substantial increase in cardiac output, heart rate, and stroke volume and a decrease in systemic vascular resistance. The increasing dynamic component is defined in terms of estimated percentage of maximal oxygen uptake ($VO2_{max}$) achieved and results in an increasing cardiac output.

Static (isometric) exercise involves development of relatively large intramuscular force with little or no change in muscle length or joint movement. Static exercise causes a marked increase in systolic, diastolic, and mean arterial pressures. It causes only a small increase in oxygen consumption, cardiac output, and heart rate (and no change in stroke volume). The increasing static component is related to the estimated percentages of maximal voluntary contraction reached and results in an increasing BP. An athlete with a CVD that would preclude a sport that produces a high pressure load on the LV may be advised to avoid sports classified as IIIA, IIIB, and IIIC.

Thus, dynamic exercise primarily causes a volume load on the LV, whereas static exercise causes a pressure load. Most of sports activities are a combination of static and dynamic exercises.

ELIGIBILITY DETERMINATION OF ATHLETES WITH CARDIOVASCULAR DISEASES

For the purpose of eligibility recommendations for athletes with CV abnormalities, recommendations for each specific condition are presented in a table format for easy access of information.

1. Acyanotic congenital heart defects (Table 35.3)
2. Cyanotic congenital heart defects (Table 35.4)
3. Miscellaneous cardiac conditions (Table 35.5)
4. Valvular heart disease
5. Cardiomyopathy, pericarditis, and other select CVDs (Table 35.6)
6. Cardiac arrhythmias
7. AV or intraventricular block
8. Systemic hypertension

Most of the recommendations are excerpts from the AHA/ACCF Scientific Statement of 2015. These recommendations apply to athletes in high school and college. For middle school and elementary school children, less strict restriction may apply because of less strenuous training and sports activities. However, these guidelines are still useful in making final recommendations for this group of athletes as well.

It should be noted that beta-blockers that are used to treat certain heart conditions and arrhythmias are expressly banned in sports such as riflery (class IA) and archery (class IIA) in which the athlete would benefit from a slow heart rate. In these sports, beta-blockers are banned substances, so that putting athletes on beta-blockers would risk them having positive drug test results.

Acyanotic Congenital Heart Defects

The participation eligibility of athletes with acyanotic heart diseases (which include left-to-right shunt lesions and obstructive lesions) is importantly determined by the level of pulmonary artery (PA) systolic pressure and the status of LV systolic function. Note that pressure levels shown are those obtained in the cardiac catheterization laboratory (i.e., peak-to-peak pressure gradient); Doppler-derived pressure gradients are higher than these (see Chapter 29).

Elevated PA pressure or LV systolic dysfunction are major determinants of allowing or restricting participation in competitive sports. PH is defined as a mean PA pressure of 25 mm Hg or greater. Normal LV systolic function is ejection fraction (EF) of greater than 60%.

1. Mean PA pressure:
   a. Athletes with the mean PA pressure less than 25 mm Hg can participate in all competitive sports.
   b. Athletes with the mean PA pressure of 25 mm Hg or greater, regardless of the associated lesions, are restricted from all competitive sports, with the possible exception of low-intensity class IA sports.
2. LV systolic function:
   a. Athletes with normal or near normal LV systolic function (EF >50%) can participate in all sports.
   b. Athletes with mildly diminished LV function (EF 40%–50%) can participate in low- and medium-intensity static and dynamic sports (classes IA, IB, IIA, and IIB).
   c. Athletes with moderate to severely diminished LV function (EF <40%) should be restricted from all competitive sports, with the possible exception of low-intensity class IA sports.

Detailed participation recommendations for specific left-right shunt lesion and obstructive lesion are presented in Table 35.3.

Cyanotic Congenital Heart Defects

All patients with cyanotic heart defects, unrepaired or postoperative, should undergo evaluation, including clinical assessment, ECG, imaging assessment of ventricular function, and exercise stress test (EST). Detailed recommendations are provided for specific cyanotic heart defects in Table 35.4.

Other Miscellaneous Cardiac Conditions

Included in this category are congenital coronary artery anomalies, myocardial bridging, Kawasaki's disease, MVP, and Marfan's syndrome. Their participation recommendations are summarized in Table 35.5.

Valvular Heart Diseases

The severity of the valvular lesion determines the eligibility of participation in competitive sports.

1. With mild valvular lesions (e.g., mitral stenosis [MS], mitral regurgitation [MR], atrial stenosis, and atrial regurgitation), participation in all competitive sports is allowed.
2. With moderate valvular lesions, participation is limited to low to moderate-intensity sports.
3. With severe obstructive lesions such as atrial stenosis, participation in competitive sports is not permitted.
4. With valvular lesions that produce significant PH, no participation in competitive sports is permitted.
5. For patients with prosthetic valve and taking warfarin, no sports involving the risk of bodily contact are allowed.

Detailed participation recommendations for specific valvular heart disease presented below are based on the

TABLE 35.3   Participation Recommendations for Acyanotic Congenital Heart Defects

Heart Defects	Clinical Status	Can participate in:
ASD, untreated	Small ASD with no PH	All sports
	Moderate to large ASD with no PH	All sports
	Large ASD with PH (cyanosis)	Only low-intensity class IA sports
	ASD with associated PVOD	No competitive sports (with possible exception of class IA sports)
ASD, closed by surgery or device	Postclosure ASD in the absence of PH, myocardial dysfunction, or arrhythmias	All sports (3–6 mo after closure)
	Athletes with PH, arrhythmias, or myocardial dysfunction	Low-intensity class IA sports
VSD, untreated	Small or restrictive VSD with normal heart size and no PH	All sports
	Large hemodynamically significant VSD	Only low-intensity class IA sports
VSD, closed by surgery or device	Asymptomatic, no or small residual defect, and no evidence of PH, arrhythmias, or ventricular dysfunction	All sports (3–6 mo after closure)
	Persistent PH	Class IA sports only
	With symptomatic atrial or ventricular tachycardia or second- or third-degree AV block	No competitive sports until further evaluation by an electrophysiologist
	With mild to moderate PH or ventricular dysfunction	No competitive sports (with possible exception of low-intensity class IA sports)
PDA, untreated	Small PDA, normal PA pressure, normal LA and LV size	All competitive sports
	Moderate to large PDA and persistent PH	Class IA sports only
	Moderate or large PDA with LV enlargement	No competitive sports until surgical or interventional closure
PDA, closed by surgery or device	Asymptomatic, with no PH and no LV enlargement	All sports (after 3 mo)
	Residual PH	No competitive sports (with possible exception of class IA sports)
PS, untreated	Mild PS and normal RV function	All competitive sports (annual reevaluation needed)
	Moderate PS (peak Doppler gradient 40–60 mm Hg) and severe PS (peak gradient >60 mm Hg)	Class IA and IB
PS, treated	No or mild residual PS (Doppler gradient <40 mm Hg)	All competitive sports (2–4 wk after balloon or 3 mo after surgery)
	Severe PR with marked RV enlargement	Class IA and IB
AS, untreated	Mild AS	All competitive sports
	Moderate AS (peak Doppler gradient 40–70 mm Hg)	Class IA, IB, and IIA
	Severe AS (peak Doppler gradient >70 mm Hg)	Only low-intensity class IA
AS, treated by surgery or balloon	Residual mild, moderate, or severe AS	Same as untreated AS
	Moderate to severe AR	See Table 34.5 recommendations
COA, untreated	Mild COA (no aortic root dilatation, normal EST, arm to leg SP gradient at rest <20 mm Hg, and arm SP ≤95th percentile)	All competitive sports
	Arm to leg SP gradient >20 mm Hg, exercise-induced hypertension (>95th percentile), or significant ascending aortic dilatation	Only low-intensity class IA sports
COA, treated by surgery or balloon	Arm-to-leg SP gradient <20 mm Hg at rest, normal EST with no significant dilatation of the ascending aorta, no aneurysm at the coarctation site, and no significant aortic valve disease	All competitive sports with the exception of classes IIIA, IIIB, and IIIC, as well as sports that pose a danger of bodily collision
	Significant aortic dilatation or aneurysm formation	Only in low-intensity class IA and IB sports

AR, Aortic regurgitation; *AS,* aortic (valve) stenosis; *ASD,* atrial septal defect; *AV,* atrioventricular; *COA,* coarctation of the aorta; *EST,* exercise stress test; *PA,* pulmonary artery; *PDA,* patent ductus arteriosus; *PH,* pulmonary hypertension; *PR,* pulmonary regurgitation; *PS,* pulmonary (valve) stenosis; *PVOD,* pulmonary vascular obstructive disease; *RV,* right ventricle; *PVS,* pulmonary vascular resistance; *SP,* systolic pressure; *VSD,* ventricular septal defect.

Modified from Van Hare GF, Ackerman MJ, Evangelista J, et al: Eligibility and disqualification recommendations for competitive athletes with cardiovascular abnormalities: Task Force 4: congenital heart disease, *Circulation* 132:e281–291, 2015.

TABLE 35.4 Participation Recommendations for Cyanotic Congenital Heart Defects

Heart Defects	Clinical Status	Can participate in:
Cyanotic CHD, unoperated	Clinically stable without symptoms of heart failure	Only class IA sport
TOF, postoperative	Excellent repair without significant LV dysfunction (EF >50%), arrhythmias, or outflow tract obstruction	Moderate- to high-intensity sports (class II to III)
	Must undergo EST without evidence of exercise-induced arrhythmias, hypotension, ischemia, or other concerning medical symptoms	
	Residual problems with severe LV dysfunction (EF <40%), severe outflow tract obstruction, or recurrent or uncontrolled atrial or ventricular arrhythmias	Restricted from all competitive sports (with possible exception of class IA sports)
TGA, post–atrial switch (Mustard or Senning)	Athletes without significant arrhythmias, ventricular dysfunction, exercise intolerance, or exercise-induced ischemia	Low- and moderate-intensity competitive sports (classes IA, IB, IIA and IIB)
	Athletes with severe systemic RV dysfunction, severe RVOT obstruction, or recurrent or uncontrolled atrial or ventricular arrhythmias	No competitive sports (with possible exception of low-intensity class IA sports)
TGA, post–arterial switch operation	Athletes with no cardiac symptoms, normal ventricular function, and no tachyarrhythmias	All competitive sports
	Athletes with more than mild hemodynamic abnormalities or ventricular dysfunction but with normal EST	Low- and moderate-static or low-dynamic sports (classes IA, IB, IC, and IIA)
	Athletes with evidence of coronary ischemia	No competitive sports
Congenitally corrected TGA	Athletes without significant arrhythmias, ventricular dysfunction, exercise intolerance, or exercise-induced ischemia	Low- and moderate-intensity competitive sports (classes IA and IB)
	Asymptomatic athletes without abnormalities on clinical evaluation	Moderate- to high-intensity competitive sports (classes II and IIIB or IIIC)
	Athletes with severe clinical systemic RV dysfunction, severe RVOT obstruction, or recurrent or uncontrolled atrial or ventricular arrhythmias	No competitive sports (with possible exception of class IA)
Fontan operation, postoperative	No symptoms of heart failure or significantly abnormal intravascular hemodynamics	Low-intensity class IA sports
	Normal EST without evidence of exercise-induced arrhythmias, hypotension, ischemia, or other concerning clinical symptoms	Consider on an individual basis
Ebstein's anomaly	Mild Ebstein's anomaly (with no cyanosis, less than moderate TR, normal RV size, no evidence of atrial or ventricular arrhythmias)	All competitive sports
	Severe TR but without evidence of arrhythmias on ambulatory ECG monitoring	Only in low-intensity class IA sports

CHD, Congenital heart defect; ECG, electrocardiogram; EF, ejection fraction; EST, exercise stress test; LV, left ventricle; RV, right ventricle; RVOT, right ventricular outflow tract; TGA, transposition of the great arteries; TR, tricuspid regurgitation; TOF, tetralogy of Fallot.

recommendations in the AHA/ACC Scientific Statement (2014), which are primarily for adult patients (Bonow et al, 2015).

1. AS
   a. Athletes with mild AS (mean gradient <20 mm Hg) can participate in all competitive sports.
   b. Athletes with moderate AS (mean gradient 20–40 mm Hg) with EST performed to the level comparable to a competitive sport without symptoms, ST depression, or ventricular arrhythmias and with normal BP response can participate in low and moderate static or dynamic sports (IA, IB, and IIA).
   c. Athletes with severe AS (mean gradient >40 mm Hg), asymptomatic or symptomatic, should not participate in competitive sports (with the possible exception of class IA sports).

2. Aortic regurgitation (AR)

   a. Athletes with mild or moderate AR (with normal left ventricular ejection fraction [LVEF] and slight or no left ventricular enlargement) and normal EST can participate in all competitive sports.
   b. Athletes with mild to moderate AR (with moderate left ventricular enlargement) but with good EST to the level of that sports with no symptom or ventricular arrhythmia can participate in all competitive sports.
   c. Athletes with severe AR with normal exercise tolerance can participate in all competitive sports.
   d. Athletes with AR and significant dilatation of the proximal ascending aorta of 41 to 45 mm can participate in sports with low risk of bodily contact.
   e. Athletes with severe AR with symptoms, LVEF less than 50%, or dilated LV should not participate in competitive sports.

3. MS
   a. Athletes with mild MS in sinus rhythm may participate in all competitive sports.
   b. Athletes with severe MS in either sinus rhythm or atrial fibrillation should not participate in competitive sports, with the possible exception of class IA.
   c. Athletes with MS of any severity who are in atrial fibrillation or have a history of atrial fibrillation who are taking anticoagulation therapy should not engage in any competitive sports involving the risk of bodily contact.
4. MR
   a. Athletes with mild to moderate MR who are in sinus rhythm with normal LV size and function and with normal PA pressure can participate in all competitive sports.
   b. Athletes with moderate MR in sinus rhythm with normal LV systolic function and mild LV enlargement can participate in all competitive sports.
   c. Athletes with severe MR in sinus rhythm with normal LV systolic function and mild LV enlargement can participate in low-intensity and some moderate-intensity sports (classes IA, IIA, and IB).
   d. Athletes with MR and definite LV enlargement, PH, or any degree of LV systolic dysfunction should not participate in any competitive sports, with the possible exception of low-intensity class IA sports.
5. After cardiac valve surgery
   a. Athletes with aortic or mitral bioprosthetic valves, not on anticoagulant agents, who have normal valvular function and normal LV function can participate in low-intensity and some moderate-intensity competitive sports (classes IA, IB, IC, and IIA).
   b. Athletes with aortic or mitral mechanical prosthetic valves, taking anticoagulant agents, with normal valvular function and normal LV function can participate in low-intensity competitive sports if there is low likelihood of bodily contact (classes IA, IB, and IIA).
   c. Athletes with MS who have undergone successful percutaneous mitral balloon valvotomy or surgical commissurotomy can participate in competitive sports based on the residual severity of the MS or MS and PA pressure at rest and with exercise.

Cardiomyopathy, Pericarditis, and Other Myocardial Diseases

The following are general statements regarding participation recommendations for myocarditis, pericarditis, and cardiomyopathies.

1. Athletes who have either confirmed or probable diagnosis of HCM or ARVD are excluded from most competitive sports, with the possible exception of class IA sports.
2. Athletes with myocarditis or pericarditis of any cause should be excluded from all competitive sports during acute phase. After complete recovery from these illnesses, they may gradually participate in sports.
3. Athletes with Marfan's syndrome can participate only in class IA or IB sports.

4. Athletes with MVP who have any symptoms or abnormalities in ECG, LV function, or arrhythmias are permitted to participate only in low-intensity sports.
5. Athletes with myocardial bridging without ischemia at rest and during exercise may participate in all sports.

Detailed participation recommendations for specific myocardial and pericardial diseases are presented in Table 35.6.

ATHLETES WITH ARRHYTHMIAS AND CONDUCTION DISTURBANCES

Although sudden unexpected death in young athletes is rare, a significant portion of these deaths occurs in relation to exercise, probably related to cardiac arrhythmias. Cardiac arrhythmias occurring while playing sports, however, manifest more often with syncope or near syncope than sudden death. A cardiac arrhythmia should be considered a possible cause of syncope, particularly when it occurs during or immediately after exercise, and a thorough evaluation is required. Although syncope may signal the presence of a serious cardiac problem, it may also be caused by a benign mechanism such as vasovagal syncope, which is a common finding in highly trained athletes. However, the diagnosis of such a benign mechanism should not be made without first excluding underlying structural disease or electrical disorders (see Chapter 31).

Arrhythmias may be associated with a variety of structural heart disease. In the absence of identifiable structural abnormalities of the heart, they may be caused by primary electrical disorders, such as supraventricular tachycardia (SVT) associated with WPW preexcitation or ventricular tachycardia (VT) secondary to long QT syndrome. A number of stimulant-containing drinks that are popular among young athletes can trigger certain arrhythmias. Abuse of drugs such as cocaine or ephedra can precipitate life-threatening arrhythmias.

Young athletes with an arrhythmia who are permitted to engage in athletic activities should be reevaluated at 6- to 12-month intervals to determine whether the training process affected the arrhythmia. Follow-up evaluation should be done to check on compliance of antiarrhythmic drugs. Use of certain drugs, such as β-adrenergic blocking agents, is banned in some competitive sports, such as archery and riflery, in which athletes benefit from slow heart rates.

Diagnostic Workup

In general, all athletes with possible cardiac arrhythmias being considered for athletic activity should have a careful history and cardiac examination, a 12-lead ECG, and echocardiogram. In most cases, a 24-hour Holter recording and EST are also indicated.

History

The screening questionnaires recommended by the ANA (see Box 34.1) are useful starting points in eligibility evaluation. However, review of an athlete's medical history and careful cardiac examination are often negative. The following are

TABLE 35.5 Participation Recommendations for Miscellaneous Conditions

Heart Condition	Clinical Status	Can participate in:
Congenital CA anomalies	CA arising from wrong sinus, passing between great arteries, before surgery	Exclusion from all competitive sports
	Postsurgery: without ischemia, ventricular dysfunction or arrhythmias during maximal EST	All competitive sports 3 mo after successful surgery
Myocardial bridging	Myocardial bridging without evidence of myocardial ischemia at rest or during exercise	All competitive sports
	Myocardial bridging with objective evidence of myocardial ischemia or prior MI	Class IA sports only
	Asymptomatic athletes who had surgical resection or stenting for myocardial bridging should undergo EST; if the EST is normal 6 months after the procedure	All competitive sports
Kawasaki's disease	No CA abnormalities or transient CA ectasia resolving during the convalescent phase	All competitive sports (after 6–8 wk)
	Regressed aneurysm, with no evidence of exercise-induced ischemia by EST with myocardial perfusion scan	All competitive sports
	Isolated small-to medium-sized aneurysm in one or more CAs (but with normal LV function, no exercise-induced ischemia or arrhythmia)	Classes IA, IB, IIA, and IIB sports (EST every 1–2 yr)
	One or more large CA aneurysms or multiple or complex aneurysm, with or without obstruction to coronary blood flow, with normal LV function, and no exercise-induced arrhythmias	Class IA and IIA sports
	Recent MI or revascularization	No competitive sports for 6–8 wks
	1. Those with normal LV function and EST, no reversible ischemia on myocardial perfusion scan, no exercise-induced arrhythmia	1. Class IA and IB sports
	2. Those with LVEF <40%, exercise intolerance, or exercise-induced ventricular arrhythmia	2. No competitive sports
	Patients with CA lesions and taking warfarin or aspirin	No competitive sports
MVP	Athletes with MVP without any of the following features:	All competitive sports
	• Prior syncope judged to be caused by arrhythmia	
	• Sustained or nonsustained SVT and/or complex VT on ambulatory ECG	
	• Severe MR	
	• LV systolic dysfunction (EF <50%)	
	• Prior embolic event	
	• FH of MVP-related sudden death	
	Athletes with MVP with any of the aforementioned features	Class IA sports only
Marfan syndrome	If patients with Marfan syndrome do not have the following:	Class IA and IIA sports (repeat echo every 6 mo to measure aortic root dimension)
	• Aortic root dilatation (≥2 SD from the mean in children; ≥40 mm in adults)	
	• Moderate to severe MR	
	• FH of dissection or sudden death	
	Athletes with aortic root dilatation (≥40 mm), prior aortic root reconstruction, moderate to severe MR, FH of dissection or sudden death	Class IA sports only

CA, Coronary artery; *EF,* ejection fraction; *EST,* exercise stress test; *FH,* family history; *LV,* left ventricle; *LVEF,* left ventricular ejection fraction; *MI,* myocardial infarction; *MR,* mitral regurgitation; *MVP,* mitral valve prolapse; *SD,* standard deviation; *SVT,* supraventricular tachycardia; *VT,* ventricular tachycardia.
Modified from Graham TP, et al: 36th Bethesda Conference: Eligibility Recommendations for Competitive Athletes with Cardiovascular Abnormalities. Task Force 2: congenital heart disease, *J Am Coll Cardiol* 45:1326–1333, 2005, and from Thompson PD, Balady GJ, Chaitman BR, et al: Task Force 6: coronary artery disease, *J Am Coll Cardiol* 45:1348–1353, 2005.

some important history, which should prompt one to consider the possibility of arrhythmia in an athlete.

- History of syncope, near syncope, dizziness or light-headedness, seizures, palpitation, chest pain, or pallor
- History of known heart disease (congenital or acquired) and medications or surgery for it
- Family history of arrhythmias or sudden death
- Certain medications or drugs of abuse (e.g., tricyclic antidepressant, inhalants, or cocaine)

Physical Examination. Physical examination may reveal irregularity of heart rate but regular heart rate on examination does not rule out arrhythmias.

Recording of Electrocardiogram. Normal ambulatory ECG monitor does not provide absolute safety or absence of arrhythmias because arrhythmias are commonly evanescent, often disappearing unpredictably for long periods of time in some cases.

Although most high school and college athletes are not fully trained athletes, it is important to understand the range

TABLE 35.6   Participation Recommendations for Cardiomyopathy, Myocarditis, Pericarditis, and Other Selected Cardiovascular Diseases

Heart Condition	Clinical Status	Can participate in:
HCM[a]	Genotype-positive HCM patients, without evidence of LVH by echo, and in the absence of FH of HCM-related sudden death	May participate in competitive sports
	Probable or definite diagnosis of HCM (regardless of age, gender, symptoms, LVOT obstruction, prior drug treatment, or ICD)	Should not participate in most competitive sports (with the possible exception of class IA sports)
Arrhythmogenic RV dysplasia	Definite, borderline, or even possible diagnosis of the disease	No competitive sports, with the possible exception of class IA sports
DCM, restrictive cardiomyopathy, and infiltrative cardiomyopathies	Symptomatic patients with one of these diagnoses	Exclude from all competitive sports, with the possible exception of low-intensity class IA sports
Myocarditis	Probable or definite active myocarditis	No competitive sports
	When all of the following are met, 3–6 mo after the initial illness: • Normal LV systolic function • No serum markers of myocardial injury, inflammation, and heart failure • No arrhythmias on Holter monitor and graded exercise ECGs	Reasonable to resume training and competition
Pericarditis	Acute pericarditis, regardless of etiology	No competitive sports during the acute phase
	Complete recovery from acute pericarditis (no evidence of active disease, no effusion by echo, normal serum markers of inflammation)	Return to full activity
	Chronic pericarditis resulting in constrictive pericarditis	No competitive sports

[a]Treatment with beta-blockers or implantable cardioverter–defibrillator (ICD) in patients with hypertrophic cardiomyopathy (HCM) for the sole purpose of permitting sport participation is not acceptable.
DCM, Dilated cardiomyopathy; *EF,* ejection fraction; *EST,* exercise stress testing; *FH,* family history; *LV,* left ventricle; *LVH,* left ventricular hypertrophy; *LVOT,* left ventricular outflow tract; *MI,* myocardial infarction; *MR,* mitral regurgitation; *MVP,* mitral valve prolapse; *RV,* right ventricle; *SD,* standard deviation; *SVT,* supraventricular tachycardia; *VT,* ventricular tachycardia.
Modified from Graham TP, et al: 36th Bethesda Conference: Eligibility Recommendations for Competitive Athletes with Cardiovascular Abnormalities. Task Force 2: congenital heart disease, *J Am Coll Cardiol* 45:1326–1333, 2005, and from Thompson PD, Balady GJ, Chaitman BR, et al: Task Force 6: coronary artery disease, *J Am Coll Cardiol* 45:1348–1353, 2005.

of normal heart rate and rhythm for the trained athlete recorded on 24-hour Holter ECG recordings.

1. Heart rates of 25 beats/min and sinus pauses greater than 2 seconds may be found.
2. Mobitz type I second-degree AV block and single uniform PVCs each may occur in about 40% of trained athletes.
3. Complex ventricular arrhythmias (including multiform PVCs, couplets, and nonsustained VT) are rarely present without adverse clinical events (Marion et al, 2006).

Exercise Stress Test. An EST is often needed to document appearance or disappearance of arrhythmias with exercise. Arrhythmias that disappear or reduce in their frequency during exercise are usually benign. Those that appear with exercise or those that increase their frequency are more significant. EST may be indicated to document the efficacy of medical treatment or ablation of arrhythmias.

Eligibility Recommendations for Cardiac Arrhythmias

The following are general statements regarding participation eligibility for athletes with cardiac arrhythmias who are asymptomatic and do not have underlying structural heart disease. There are subsets of athletes with additional issues, such as symptoms or underlying heart disease, who need a full evaluation with EST, electrophysiological study (EPS), or both before eligibility for participation in sport activities can be decided. Some of them may require pacemaker or implantable cardioverter implanted. Detailed participation recommendations are available for these athletes in a recent AHA/ACC Scientific Statement (Zipes et al, 2014).

1. The presence of a symptomatic cardiac arrhythmia requires exclusion from physical activity until this problem can be adequately evaluated and controlled by a cardiologist or an electrophysiologist.
2. Asymptomatic athletes with sinus bradycardia, sinus exit block, sinus pauses, and sinus arrhythmia can participate in all competitive sports.
2. Sinus arrhythmias and premature atrial contractions (PACs) are benign if the heart is structurally normal; they can participate in all competitive sports.
3. Asymptomatic athletes with atrial flutter or fibrillation and structurally normal heart may participate in competitive sports when the arrhythmias are fully under control either by medication or ablation.
4. Athletes with SVT and structurally normal heart may participate in all competitive sports when the SVT is in full control with medication or after successful ablation.

5. For athletes with structurally normal heart, who have PVCs or more complex arrhythmias, an exercise stress test is a useful technique. If the PVCs disappear when the heart rate reaches 140 to 150 beats/min, the PVCs are benign, and full participation may be permitted.

6. Athletes with VT who had successful treatment to prevent recurrence of the arrhythmias may participate in sports, provided that VT is not inducible by EST or EPS.

7. Asymptomatic adult athletes with WPW preexcitation with no history of SVT may participate in all competitive sports after risk stratification by exercise stress testing, but children with the same diagnosis require more in-depth evaluation.

8. Athletes with long QT syndrome can only participate in class IA sports.

9. Athletes with catecholaminergic polymorphic ventricular tachycardia (CPVT) can only participate in class IA sports.

10. Athletes who had a successful ablation for any of the arrhythmias may participate in all competitive sports after verification of the success by appropriate tests.

11. Athletes with implantable cardioverter–defibrillator may participate in class IA sports if they are free of ventricular flutter or ventricular fibrillation requiring device therapy for 3 months. Participation in sports with higher component than class IA may be considered if the athlete is free of ventricular flutter or fibrillation requiring device therapy for 3 months.

Eligibility Recommendations for Atrioventricular Block and Intraventricular Blocks

The following are general statements regarding asymptomatic athletes' participation eligibility. There are subsets of athletes with additional issues or problems in each category for whom a different level of sport category may apply. These subsets of athletes need to be fully investigated and treated before eligibility for participation in sport activities can be decided. Some of them may require pacemaker implantation. Detailed participation recommendations are available in a recent AHA/ACC Scientific Statement (Zipes et al, 2015).

1. Asymptomatic athletes with first-degree AV block and structurally normal hearts can participate in all competitive sports.

2. Asymptomatic patients with Wenckebach AV block (Mobitz type 1 second-degree AV block) with improvement in conduction with exercise or recovery can participate in all competitive sports.

3. Athletes with Mobitz type 2 second-degree AV block or complete heart block usually require pacemaker implantation before being permitted to participate in any sports.

4. Asymptomatic athletes without heart disease who have a junctional escape rhythm with normal QRS duration and resting ventricular rate greater than 40 beats/min that increase appropriately with exertion can participate in all competitive sports.

5. Athletes with acquired complete heart block should have a permanent pacemaker placed regardless of symptoms, type of structural heart disease, and exercise capacity.

6. Asymptomatic athletes with RBBB or left bundle branch block (LBBB) who do not have ventricular arrhythmias or develop AV block during exercise can participate in all sports. However, patients with LBBB who have an abnormal prolongation of HV interval on EPS should receive pacemaker.

7. Athletes with permanent pacemakers
   a. Athletes who are completely pacemaker dependent should not engage in sports in which there is a risk of collision.
   b. Athletes who are not pacemaker dependent may participate in sports with a risk of collision or trauma if they understand and accept the risk of damage to the pacemaker system.
   c. For athletes with permanent pacemakers, protective equipment should be considered for participation in contact sports that have the potential to damage the implanted device.

ATHLETES WITH SYSTEMIC HYPERTENSION

Reports of cerebrovascular accident during maximal exercise have raised concerns that the rise in BP accompanying strenuous activity may cause harm. However, changes in BP depend on the type of exercise in which they are engaged. For example:

1. Dynamic exercise causes a substantial increase in systolic pressure, heart rate, stroke volume, and cardiac output. A moderate increase in mean arterial pressure and a decrease in diastolic pressure occur, with a marked decrease in total peripheral resistance.

2. Static exercise, in contrast, causes a small increase in cardiac output and heart rate and no change in stroke volume. There are marked increases in systolic, diastolic, and mean arterial pressures and no appreciable change in total peripheral resistance.

Correct diagnosis of hypertension is very important before recommending restrictions. On each occasion, two or more BP readings should be taken, and when the readings vary by greater than 5 mm Hg, additional readings should be taken until two consecutive readings are close. When the initial office BP readings are high, an out-of-office measurement of BP may be needed to exclude "white-coat" hypertension. The diagnosis of hypertension should be made only after several elevated BP are obtained on separate occasions. When the diagnosis of hypertension is confirmed, an evaluation including a history, thorough physical examination, and appropriate laboratory test should be performed (see Chapter 28).

The following are recommendations by the AHA/ACC Scientific Statement (2014) (Black et al, 2015).

1. Athletes with elevated BP (formerly prehypertension) (BP levels between the 90th and 95th percentiles or >120/80 mm Hg)
   a. May participate in physical activity but should be encouraged to modify lifestyle
   b. If prehypertension persists, echo studies are done to see if there is LVH (beyond that seen with "athletes' heart").

c. If LVH is present, athletic participation is limited until BP is normalized by appropriate drug therapy.

2. Athletes with stage 1 hypertension (BP levels between the 95th and 95th percentiles + 12 mm Hg; or 130/80–139/89 mm Hg), in the absence of target organ damage, may participate in any competitive sports.

3. Athletes with stage 2 hypertension (BP levels >95th percentile + 10 mm Hg or >140/90 mm Hg), even in the absence of target organ damage (e.g., LVH), should be restricted, particularly from high-static sports (e.g., weightlifting, boxing, and wrestling), until hypertension is controlled by either lifestyle modification or drug therapy.

All drugs being taken must be registered with appropriate governing bodies to obtain a therapeutic exemption. When hypertension coexists with another CVD, eligibility for participation in competitive sports is usually based on the type and severity of the associated condition.

With respect to the treatment of hypertension, beta-blockers are not banned for most sports, including football and basketball, but they are banned for riflery or archery. However, athletes with essential hypertension do not tolerate beta-blockers well because they reduce their maximum performance. Therefore, one should avoid treating hypertensive athletes with beta-blockers. Instead, angiotensin-converting enzyme (ACE) inhibitors or calcium channel blockers are preferred. One should be aware of potential teratogenic effects of ACE inhibitors if taken during pregnancy.

Cardiac Transplantation

Lower and Shumway at Stanford University performed the first successful orthotopic heart transplantation in a dog in 1960. Barnard in South Africa unexpectedly performed the first successful human heart transplantation in 1966. This was followed by an explosive interest in heart transplantation but almost uniformly poor results because of organ rejection. Introduction of cyclosporine in 1980 markedly improved the results of adult heart transplantation. This success has extended to pediatric patients, and the first infant cardiac transplantation was carried out by Bailey at Loma Linda University in 1985. Although some ethical and medical issues exist, cardiac transplantation will continue to contribute to the treatment of children with some heart diseases.

Physicians may have a chance to participate in the care of cardiac transplant recipients. Therefore, practitioners should have some basic knowledge on the topic, and that is the aim of this chapter. A number of complex issues involved in the steps before the transplant and a long posttransplant management to prevent rejection and infection need to be known to physicians. This chapter is not intended to review up-to-date advances in the transplantation or to provide detailed management guidelines on transplant patients. Cardiac transplantation is done by transplantation centers with a multidisciplinary team of professionals and supporting staff and they are primarily responsible for follow-up of their posttransplant patients according to the management protocol established by the center. Management protocols may be quite different from one transplantation center to another.

INDICATIONS

Pediatric heart transplantation is a treatment option for children with intractable heart failure or congenital heart diseases (CHDs) not amenable to surgical palliation. Several decades ago, when the surgical mortality rate was very high, hypoplastic left heart syndrome (HLHS) was a major indication for heart transplantation. With improved surgical outcome, HLHS is no longer considered a major indication for heart transplantation.

The majority of pediatric transplant patients are those with pre- and postoperative complex CHDs and those with cardiomyopathies. In infants younger than 12 months of age, who account for about 23% of pediatric cardiac transplantation, HLHS is still the most common indication followed by dilated cardiomyopathy. In older children, cardiomyopathies (dilated, hypertrophic, and restrictive) account for about 60% of the cases. Most of the other indications for the transplant are patients who had surgical repairs, including Fontan operation, for complex CHDs (e.g., single ventricle, atrioventricular canal defect, truncus arteriosus, L-transposition of the great arteries). Rarely, patients with unresectable cardiac tumor are candidates for transplantation. Significant cardiac allograft vasculopathy and chronic graft dysfunction of a previous heart transplant are rare indications for heart transplantation.

SELECTION OF THE RECIPIENT

Careful selection of appropriate recipients remains the most important determinant of a favorable outcome. Multidisciplinary evaluation of the recipient includes assessment of cardiopulmonary, renal, hepatic, neurologic, and infectious disease status and socioeconomic assessment. In general, the recipient should satisfy the following selection criteria:

1. Terminal heart disease with death expected within 6 to 12 months

2. The presence of adequate dimension of hilar pulmonary arteries (PAs). If the pulmonary vascular resistance (PVR) is high or if severe hypoplasia or stenosis of the PAs is present, the patient may be a candidate for heart and lung transplantation.
3. Other general requirements
   a. Normal function or reversible dysfunction of the kidneys and liver
   b. Lack of systemic infection
   c. Malignancy under complete remission for longer than 1 year
   d. Lack of systemic disease (e.g., diabetes and degenerative neuromuscular disease) that would limit recovery or survival
   e. Lack of drug addiction
   f. Lack of mental deficiency
4. Equally important for successful pediatric heart transplantation are a family history of stability, past history of compliance, and evidence of strong motivation for the transplant as assessed by physicians and social workers. The child and parents should demonstrate sufficient responsibility, resources, and psychological strength to cope with multiple outpatient clinic visits, routine endomyocardial biopsy, and a lifetime of vigilance of the immunosuppressed state.
5. Unique to pediatric transplantation is the requirement of a reliable caregiver for the recipient child. The caregiver identified need not be a parent but must have legal responsibility for total care and be prepared to deal with the strict medical regimen required.
   Cardiac transplantation is contraindicated:
1. If PVR is 6 Wood units/m^2 or greater and/or
2. Transpulmonary gradient (TPG = PA pressure – PA wedge pressure) is 15 mm Hg or greater, which does not respond to vasodilators

After the decision has been made for heart transplantation and after complete multidisciplinary evaluation, the patient is placed on the cardiac transplantation waiting list (to the United Network of Organ Sharing [UNOS] and the Regional Organ Bank). Each listing is specific for ABO blood type and the recipient's weight.

EVALUATION AND MANAGEMENT OF THE CARDIAC DONOR

1. The cardiac donor must meet the legal definition of *brain death*. Most neonatal donors are victims of sudden infant death syndrome or birth asphyxia. Most older children donors are victims of car accidents or violence.
2. The screening of the donor is accomplished in three phases.
   a. Primary screening is done by organ procurement specialists to obtain information on body size, ABO blood type, serologic data on hepatitis B and human immunodeficiency virus (HIV), cause of death, clinical course, and routine laboratory data.
   b. Secondary screening is performed by cardiac surgeons or cardiologists, who pay attention to the extent of other (especially thoracic) injuries, the extent of treatment required to sustain acceptable hemodynamic status, electrocardiogram (ECG), chest radiographs, arterial blood gas analysis, and echocardiogram.
   c. Tertiary screening is inspection of the heart by a "harvesting" surgeon to ensure that there is no evidence of a palpable thrill over the heart and great arteries, obvious arteriosclerotic heart disease, or myocardial contusion.
3. Donor heart should have:
   a. No evidence of cardiac abnormalities by echocardiography, ECG, or myocardial enzyme tests
   b. Left ventricular (LV) fractional shortening greater than 28%, regardless of inotropic support
4. Specific compatibility should exist between the donor and recipient in three aspects:
   a. ABO blood group compatibility
   b. The donor's body weight should be within 20% of the recipient's weight; a larger donor heart is better tolerated than a smaller one.
   c. The donor should be within close geographic range so that the donor heart can be harvested, transported, and implanted within 4 hours (≤9 hours for infants).
5. Medical management of donor heart before transplantation: The donor should be managed in the intensive care unit with routine monitoring. The systolic blood pressure should be maintained in the normal range (>100 mg Hg for adults). Inotropic support and fluid resuscitation may be necessary. Normal serum electrolyte levels, acid–base balance, and oxygenation should be maintained. The hematocrit should be above 30%.

INFORMED CONSENT FROM THE FAMILY AND RECIPIENT

The public often misunderstands what transplantation can accomplish. The recipient and parents must fully understand the short- and long-term implications of transplantation by knowing the following facts, which are not well publicized:
1. Unlike most cardiac surgeries, cardiac transplantation is not a cure for the condition for which it is being considered. It can be viewed as another medical problem that will require *lifelong* medical attention, including frequent hospital visits or admissions for noninvasive and invasive procedures, frequent adjustments of immunosuppressive and antibiotic medications, varying degrees of limitations in activity, and adjustments in lifestyle.
2. There is always a threat of rejection and infection throughout the patient's life. Even with full compliance, rejection can occur, resulting in death or a need for retransplantation.
3. The heart received will not last for an indefinite period; it will eventually develop allograft coronary artery disease (CAD), requiring consideration of retransplantation.
4. Immunosuppressive therapy may cause malignancies (especially lymphoma in children) and an increased risk of infection.
5. Lifelong medical attention will place a tremendous financial, emotional, and social burden on the family. A dysfunctional family could result.

OPERATIVE TECHNIQUE

There are currently two surgical techniques used in cardiac transplantation: the right atrial (RA) technique and the bicaval technique. The latter is a more recent technique and has become more popular than the former.

In RA cardiac transplantation, when the native heart is explanted, the posterior walls of both atria of the recipient heart are left in place and are anastomosed to the donor heart. End-to-end anastomoses are also made between the donor and recipient aortas and PAs (Fig. 36.1). This technique is similar to those described by Lower and Shumway in 1960. The hospital mortality rate is 10% to 15%.

A modification of the above, called "bicaval" cardiac transplantation, has become popular in some institutions (Fig. 36.2). In this technique, the RA is also explanted from the recipient, leaving only the posterior wall of the left atrium (LA) with four pulmonary veins attached. Anastomoses are made between the venae cavae, the aorta, the PA, and the LA.

For patients with HLHS who are placed on a transplantation algorithm, it is necessary to keep the ductus arteriosus open and to increase the size of the interatrial communication. A hybrid procedure as described under HLHS (in Chapter 14) may be used as a bridge to cardiac transplantation, in which an endovascular stent is placed in the closing ductus to keep the ductus open and PA branches are banded to control

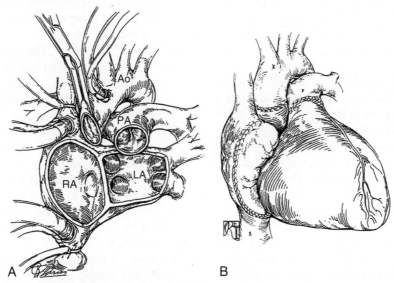

Fig. 36.1 "Right atrial" (RA) technique of cardiac transplantation. **A,** The recipient cardiectomy has been completed, leaving the anastomosis to be performed in the following sequence: (1) left atrium (LA), (2) aorta (Ao), (3) RA, and (4) pulmonary artery (PA). **B,** The completed transplant. (From Backer CL, Mavroudis C: Pediatric transplantation, part A: heart transplantation. In Stuart FP, Abecassis MM, Kaufman DB [eds]: *Organ Transplantation*, Georgetown, TX, 2000, Landes Bioscience.)

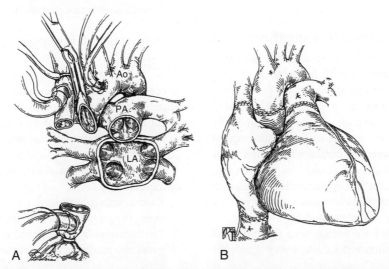

Fig. 36.2 "Bicaval" technique of cardiac transplantation. **A,** The recipient cardiectomy has been completed. Note that the entire right atrium has been removed. The sequence of the anastomosis is (1) left atrium (LA), (2) aorta (Ao), (3) inferior vena cava, (4) pulmonary artery (PA), and (5) superior vena cava. **B,** The completed transplant. (From Backer CL, Mavroudis C: Pediatric transplantation, part A: heart transplantation. In Stuart FP, Abecassis MM, Kaufman DB [eds]: *Organ Transplantation*, Georgetown, TX, 2000, Landes Bioscience.)

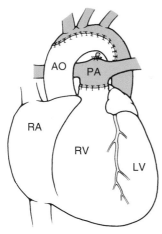

Fig. 36.3 Modification of heart transplantation surgery for hypoplastic left heart syndrome. *AO,* Aorta; *LV,* left ventricle; *PA,* pulmonary artery; *RA,* right atrium; *RV,* right ventricle.

pulmonary blood flow (see Fig. 14.49). Blade atrial septostomy followed by balloon dilatation is performed to increase the size of the interatrial communication.

For most babies with HLHS, the donor cardiectomy is modified in that the entire aortic arch is harvested well beyond the insertion of the ligamentum arteriosus to augment the ascending aorta and aortic arch, such as those shown in Fig. 36.3.

POSTTRANSPLANT MANAGEMENT

This section is not meant to describe how to take care of patients after heart transplantation. Medical professionals and support staff of the transplantation center are the providers of appropriate care for these children. This section is intended to show what is involved in the proper care of posttransplant patients for physicians who may become involved in their care. Very close follow-ups are required by frequent clinic visits and a number of investigations to detect possible rejection or infection.

Frequency of Clinic Visits and Investigations

The early postoperative period is the period of highest risk and requires a very close follow-up with frequent clinic visits and laboratory tests and other investigations. In general, the frequency of clinic visits and investigation is most intense in the first year after the transplant, and it decreases gradually thereafter. The following is an excerpt of the posttransplant follow-up plans of a transplantation center, which shows how complex and tedious the plan is. It should be pointed out, however, that each institution has a detailed management plan established by the transplantation team, which may be somewhat different from the one presented here.

1. Office visit twice weekly for 6 weeks; then monthly visit for the first year. It is then reduced to every 3 months thereafter.
2. Echocardiography study is done twice weekly for 4 weeks; then reduced to monthly to coincide with the clinic visit.
3. ECG is done monthly for 3 months, then every 3 months for the first year, and then every 6 months thereafter.

4. Chest radiography is performed monthly for 3 months, at 12 months, and then annually.
5. Blood levels of immunosuppressive agents are obtained twice weekly for 2 weeks, weekly for 4 weeks, monthly for the first year, and then every 3 months thereafter. See a later section for target trough levels of each immunosuppressive agent.
6. Complete blood count and platelets are obtained every 2 weeks, then monthly for the first year, and then every 3 months thereafter.
7. Cytomegalovirus (CMV) immunoglobulin titer is assessed at 6 and 12 months and then annually until conversion. Epstein-Barr virus (EBV) polymerase chain reaction is assessed every 3 months. HIV and the surface antigen of the hepatitis B virus (HBsAg) tests are obtained at 6 months.
8. Isotopic glomerular filtration rate is assessed at 3 and 12 months and every year thereafter for patients who received transplant during infancy. For those who received transplant after infancy, it is assessed every 2 years.
9. Renal ultrasonography is performed at 3 and 12 months and every other year thereafter.
10. Endomyocardial biopsy is obtained annually for newborns and children 2 years or younger. For children 2 to 8 years of age, it is obtained at 1, 3, and 12 months and annually thereafter. For children 9 years of age and older, it is obtained at 1, 2, 3, 6, and 12 months and annually thereafter.
11. Coronary angiography is performed annually starting at the first anniversary of transplantation.
12. Intravascular echocardiography is performed at age 6 years and every other year thereafter.
13. All routine vaccinations, except for live virus vaccines (e.g., oral polio, varicella, and measles–mumps–rubella vaccines) should be administered, starting as early as 6 weeks after transplantation.

OVERVIEW OF IMMUNOSUPPRESSIVE THERAPY

Successful immunosuppression depends on a delicate balance between suppression of the host mechanisms that would reject the foreign graft and preservation of the mechanisms of the immune response that protect against bacterial, fungal, and viral invasion.

The so-called triple-drug therapy consists of three classes of medications.
1. Calcineurin inhibitors (e.g., cyclosporine [Neoral], tacrolimus [Prograf, FK506]) inhibit T-cell activation.
2. Corticosteroids (methylprednisolone or prednisone) suppress cell-mediated immunity as well as the humoral immunity.
3. Antiproliferative agents (e.g., azathioprine [Imuran], mycophenolate mofetil [CellCept]) prevent rejection by interfering with purine synthesis, resulting in antiproliferative effects on T and B cells.

TABLE 36.1 **Dosages of Immunosuppressive Agents**

Drug	Preoperative	Early Postoperative Dosage	Late Postoperative Dosage
Cyclosporine[a]	10 mg/kg IV	0.5–1 mg/kg/day IV	3–6 mg/kg/day PO[a]
Methylprednisolone	10 mg/kg IV	2 mg/kg IV q8h × 3	
Prednisone		1 mg/kg/day PO	Taper to 0.2 mg/kg/day PO by 3 mo; stop by 6 mo
Azathioprine		1–2 mg/kg PO or IV	1–2 mg/kg/day (adjust according to WBC count)

[a]Adjust cyclosporine dosage by orally (PO) twice-a day dosing (or q8h dosing for infants younger than 6 mo of age) to maintain target trough level as follows:

0–3 mo postoperatively: 300 ng/mL
3–12 mo postoperatively: 200–250 ng/mL
>12 mo postoperatively: 150–200 ng/mL
IV, Intravenous; *q,* every; *WBC,* white blood cell.
Modified from Canter CE: Pediatric cardiac transplantation. In Moller JH, Hoffman JIE (eds): *Pediatric Cardiovascular Medicine,* New York, 2000, Churchill Livingstone, pp 942–952.

Calcineurin Inhibitors

Cyclosporine

Cyclosporine is the most commonly used agent for maintenance therapy. The first dose of cyclosporine (10 mg/kg) is administered before surgery because it may be most effective when given before the antigenic challenge (Table 36.1). Target trough levels of cyclosporine are as follows: 250 to 300 ng/mL for 6 months, 200 to 250 ng/mL for 6 to 12 months, and 125 to 150 ng/mL thereafter. Cyclosporine is continued for as long as the patient lives.

The drug's primary toxic effects are hypertension and associated renal insufficiency. Other side effects of the drug include hyperlipidemia, hirsutism, gingival hyperplasia, and facial dysmorphism (with widening of the nose, thickening of the nares and lips, and prominence of the supraorbital ridge and eyebrows).

Tacrolimus

Tacrolimus (Prograf), a newer agent in the same class as cyclosporine, is being used increasingly by some centers as a primary calcineurin agent. It has remarkably lower rates of hypertension and hyperlipidemia and does not cause hirsutism, gingival hyperplasia, or the facial dysmorphism associated with cyclosporine.

Corticosteroids

Methylprednisolone (10 mg/kg for children) is administered intravenously (IV) as the sternotomy is made. After cardiopulmonary bypass has been discontinued, a 2-mg/kg IV dose is given every 8 hours, totaling three doses. After 24 hours, prednisone is administered in high doses (1 mg/kg per day by mouth). After about 3 weeks, the dose is tapered to 0.2 mg/kg per day by 3 months after surgery (see Table 36.1). Further tapering or discontinuation depends on the institution's protocol and the presence or absence of rejection. Some centers discontinue it after 6 months, particularly in neonates and infants. Most centers aim to establish a steroid-free regimen in selected patients by 1 year after the transplantation to minimize the risk of steroid-associated morbidity.

Antiproliferative Agents

Azathioprine

Azathioprine is given immediately after the transplantation surgery. The starting dose is 1 to 2 mg/kg per day to produce a peripheral white blood cell count around 5000/mm³. If the count falls below 4000/mm³, the drug is reduced, or it is stopped if the reduction is severe (see Table 36.1). The major toxicity of azathioprine is bone marrow depression and less frequently hepatotoxicity. The drug is generally continued indefinitely.

Mycophenolate Mofetil

Mycophenolate mofetil (CellCept) is an antiproliferative agent and has largely replaced azathioprine. A clinical study has demonstrated a lower rate of rejection rates than azathioprine when used with cyclosporine and corticosteroids. This agent also allowed reduction of the dosage of cyclosporine and tacrolimus, which may potentially reduce the side effects of these drugs. The dosage is 600 mg/m²/dose orally twice a day. Its side effects include gastrointestinal (GI) symptoms (in 30%), bone marrow suppression (anemia), hypertension, headache, fever, and increased risk of developing lymphomas or other malignancies.

EARLY POSTTRANSPLANTATION FOLLOW-UP

The highest risk of dying is in the first 6 months after transplantation. In the early postoperative period, acute graft dysfunction and technical issues account for more than 50% of the deaths. The two most common causes of death in the early posttransplant period are acute rejection (26%) and infection (16%).

Acute Rejection

Identification

1. Subtle symptoms may be the only indication of the beginning of a rejection episode. These symptoms include unexplained fever, tachycardia, fatigue, shortness of breath, joint pain, and personality changes.
2. Echocardiographic techniques rely on a physiologic abnormality of the rejecting heart (myocardial edema or decreased LV contractility) (see a later section for further discussion).

TABLE 36.2   International Society for Heart and Lung Transplantation Cardiac Biopsy Grading Scheme for the Diagnosis of Acute Cellular Rejection

Grade	Description
0R	No rejection
1R	Interstitial and/or perivascular infiltrate with up to one focus of myocyte damage
2R	Two or more foci of infiltrate associated myocyte damage
3R	Diffuse infiltrate with multifocal myocyte damage ± edema, ± hemorrhage, ± vasculitis

From Stewart S, Winters GL, Fishbein MC, et al: Revision of the 1990 working formulation for the standardization of nomenclature in the diagnosis of heart rejection, *J Heart Lung Transplant* 24:1710-1720, 2005.

3. Endomyocardial biopsy remains the most important method for identifying acute rejection. The endomyocardial biopsy is graded according to the International Society of Heart and Lung Transplantation (ISHLT) scale (2005) (Table 36.2).

Treatment

Rejection treatment depends on the grade of rejection. Generally, specific antirejection therapy is initiated only for moderate or severe rejection (≥grade 2R).

1. Methylprednisolone (1000 mg for adults; 15 mg/kg for children weighing <50 kg) given IV or prednisone (100 mg for adults) given orally for 3 days is followed by tapering to the baseline dose over the next 2 weeks.
2. If rejection does not respond to steroids or if hemodynamic compromise occurs, antithymocyte sera such as antithymocyte globulin (ATG) or the monoclonal antibody to T3 lymphocytes (OKT3) are used for 5 or 10 days, respectively.
3. If all measures prove ineffective, retransplantation is considered.

Infection

Immunosuppressive medications used to prevent allograft rejection increase the risk of infection. There are two peak incidences for infection after transplantation.

1. An "early" infection, occurring within the first month of transplantation, is dominated by nosocomial, often catheter-related, infection caused by *Staphylococcus* spp. and gram-negative organisms.
2. A "late" infection, occurring within 2 to 5 months, is caused by opportunistic infections from organisms such as CMV, *Pneumocystis* spp., and fungal pathogens (see later section). The lung is the most common site of infection in heart transplant recipients followed by the blood, urine, GI tract, and sternal wound.

Late Posttransplantation Follow-up

Late follow-up examinations are intended to detect rejection, infection, and the side effects of immunosuppression.

Infection and rejection remain the most common causes of death after heart transplantation. For those who survive beyond 1 year after transplantation, acute rejection (30%), allograft vasculopathy (24%), and infection (12%) account for most of the deaths. Graft failure, lymphoma, and CAD are responsible for the remaining deaths.

Rejection

Although the risk of rejection is greatest in the first 3 months after transplantation, continued surveillance for rejection is necessary. A high index of suspicion is necessary to detect rejection because many rejections occur without symptoms. Endomyocardial biopsy at regular intervals is required to detect rejection.

1. Clinically evident cardiac dysfunction or congestive heart failure (CHF) is usually absent. Nonspecific clinical signs and symptoms (e.g., fever, tachycardia, malaise, personality changes, gallop rhythm, arrhythmias, hypotension) may be the only indications of rejection. These symptoms are often caused by infection rather than rejection. Decreased ECG voltages and decreased ventricular function (by echocardiography) are late signs of acute rejection.
2. Some centers have used serial echocardiography to assess rejection, but this method has not been universally accepted.
3. Endomyocardial biopsies are the criterion standard and are graded according to the criteria of the ISHLT, with treatment generally occurring only for biopsy samples that demonstrate a 2R or greater histology. Patients with no or mild rejection (grade 0R or 1R) on the biopsy receive no change in drug dosage.

Infection

Infection is a common cause of death and is probably related to the immunosuppressive therapy. Infection after the immediate posttransplantation period is caused by opportunistic infective agents such as CMV, *Pneumocystis* organisms, and fungi. The average mortality rate from infection is about 12%; that of fungal infection is about 36%. The lung is the most commonly infected organ; the mortality rate of patients with infected lungs is 22%. CMV remains the most common single infection, but the specific antiviral agent for CMV, ganciclovir, does not appear to reduce the incidence of primary CMV infection. The efficacy of pyrimethamine and trimethoprim–sulfamethoxazole has been proved for the prophylaxis of toxoplasmosis and *Pneumocystis* infection, respectively. The risk-to-benefit ratio of using influenza vaccines after transplantation remains controversial.

Most researchers agree that children receiving immunosuppressive therapy, as well as their siblings, should not receive all live vaccines, including varicella, measles, mumps, rubella, and oral polio. Because of their immunosuppressed status, there is an increased risk that these patients will develop active disease from the vaccine strains.

Allograft Coronary Artery Disease

An unusual, accelerated form of CAD, probably an immune-mediated disease, is the third most common cause of death after infection and rejection. CAD is the major determinant of long-term survival. Virtually all adult patients have some histopathologic evidence of CAD by 1 year after transplantation. It may occur in up to 40% of transplanted hearts in 3 years and in more than 50% in 5 years. This disease also occurs in pediatric patients, perhaps to a lesser degree, but 28% of pediatric patients surviving 6 months to 6 years after transplantation develop CAD.

Most patients with transplanted, denervated hearts fail to experience typical chest pain. Life-threatening ventricular arrhythmias, CHF, silent myocardial infarction, and sudden death may result. Coronary angiography (or computed tomography [CT] coronary angiography) is necessary to diagnose the disease. The unique angiographic hallmark of this disease is diffuse, concentric, longitudinal, and rapid pruning and obliteration of distal branch vessels. Many centers recommend performing the first coronary angiography (or CT coronary angiography) within 2 to 4 weeks of transplantation to obtain a baseline; some centers also recommend performing an exercise stress test, if appropriate for the patient's age, and coronary angiography (or CT coronary angiography) 1 year after transplantation to evaluate graft function and to detect premature and aggressive coronary atherosclerosis. The only effective treatment of allograft CAD is retransplantation.

Side Effects of Immunosuppression

1. Cyclosporine. Hypertension and renal toxicity are common side effects, and malignancies are rare side effects of cyclosporine therapy. Less severe adverse side effects of the drug include reversible hepatotoxicity, fluid retention, hirsutism, gum hypertrophy, and GI symptoms. Rarely (10% of patients), lymphoma develops with a larger dose of the drug.
2. Hypertension occurs in 50% to 90% of heart transplant recipients who take cyclosporine. The mechanisms of cyclosporine-associated hypertension include nephrotoxicity, increased sympathetic tone, volume expansion, increased endothelin levels, and stimulation of the renin–angiotensin system. Calcium channel blockers, angiotensin-converting enzyme inhibitors, and beta- and alpha-blockers have been used with varying degrees of success.
3. Another side effect of chronic immunosuppressive treatment is the development of malignant neoplasms, occurring in 1% to 2% of patients each year, or 12.5% during a mean follow-up period of 50 months. A unique form of lymphoma, *posttransplant lymphoproliferative disease,* is the most common tumor reported (80%) with cyclosporine-based immunosuppression; it occurs more frequently in young patients. Most of these tumors are thought to be the result of EBV infection. The use of OKT3 and ATG, as well as higher initial doses of cyclosporine and prednisone, appears to increase the risk of posttransplant lymphoproliferative disease. About 40% of patients respond to a reduction in immunotherapy, but chemotherapy and radiation therapy may be needed.
4. Corticosteroids. Growth retardation may occur with large doses of steroids. The dosage of steroids is kept at a minimum, or steroids are not given at all.
5. Azathioprine may produce bone marrow depression (e.g., thrombocytopenia, leukocytopenia, anemia), alopecia, and GI symptoms. Cutaneous malignancy (squamous cell and basal cell carcinoma) is the most common tumor associated with the use of azathioprine, perhaps related to the drug's enhanced photosensitivity. The mortality rate from posttransplant tumors is high (38%).

PHYSIOLOGY OF THE TRANSPLANTED HEART

In following posttransplantation patients, physicians should first be aware of the unique physiology of the transplanted heart, which responds differently to exercise and to certain medications. The transplanted heart remains largely, but not entirely, denervated throughout the life of the recipient.

1. The response of the transplanted heart to exercise or stress is less than normal but adequate for most activities. With exercise, the heart rate accelerates slowly, and it parallels the rise in circulating catecholamine levels.
2. Most patients with denervated hearts experience no chest pain even with significant CAD.
3. Transplant recipients are supersensitive to catecholamines, in part because of the upregulation of beta-adrenergic receptors and in part because of a loss of norepinephrine uptake in sympathetic neurons.
4. Coronary vasodilator response may be abnormal if allograft CAD has developed.

PROGNOSIS

Recent data from the ISHLT Registry (2009) revealed that the overall 20-year survival rate for all pediatric heart transplant recipients is 40%. The 1-, 5-, and 10-year survival rates are 80%, 68%, and 58%, respectively. Another recent study (Zuppen et al, 2009) reported similar overall survival rates of 85% at 1 year, 75% at 5 years, and 65% at 10 years. Newborns and infants appear to have better survival rates after transplantation; the 5-year actuarial survival rate is 80%.

Miscellaneous

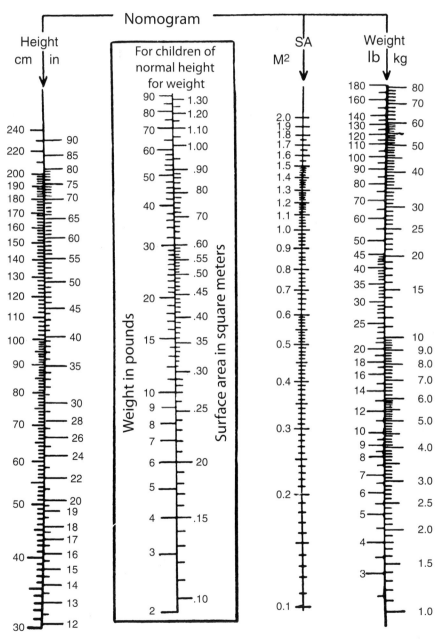

Fig. A.1 Body surface area nomogram.

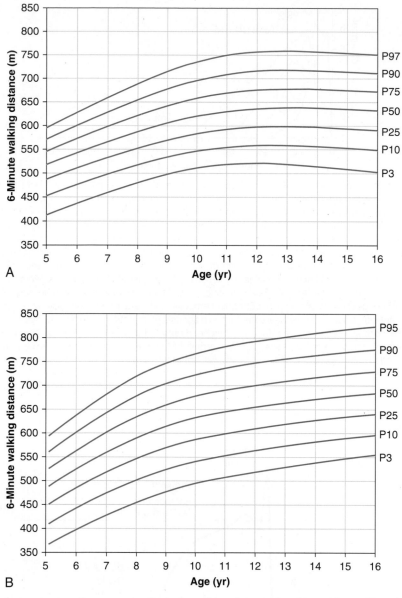

Fig. A.2 Reference percentile curves for 6-minute walking distance for girls and boys. (From Ulrich S, Hildebrand FF, Treder U, et al: Reference values for the 6-minute walk test in healthy children and adolescents in Switzerland, *BMC Pulmonary Med* 13:49, 2013.)

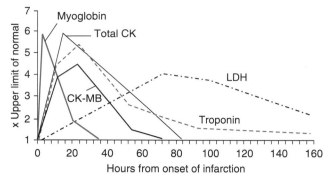

Fig. A.3 Time course of elevation of selected serum markers after acute myocardial infarction in an adult. This figure summarizes the relative timing, rate of rise, peak values, and duration of elevation above the upper limit of normal for the serum markers. Myoglobin (MB) rises quickly soon after the onset of infarction, but it is not specific for cardiac muscle; it may also come from skeletal muscles. Total creatine kinase (CK) rises within 4 to 8 hours, reaches a peak at 24 hours, and declines to normal levels within 2 to 3 days. There are three isoenzymes (BB, MM, and MB) of CK identified by electrophoresis. The CK-MB isoenzyme occurs primarily in cardiac muscles, the BB enzyme occurs primarily in the brain and kidneys, and the MM isoenzyme occurs in cardiac and skeletal muscles. Lactate dehydrogenase (LDH) elevation occurs several days after the onset of myocardial infarction. False elevation of LDH occurs in patients with hemolysis, leukemia, liver disease or congestion, renal disease, pulmonary embolism, skeletal muscle disease, shock, and myocarditis. Cardiac-specific troponin I may be useful for the diagnosis of infarction even 3 to 4 days after the event. In children, the normal value of cardiac troponin I has been reported to be 2 ng/mL or less, and it is frequently below the level of detection for the assay. (From Antman EM: General hospital management. In Julian DG, Braunwald E [eds]: *Management of Acute Myocardial Infarction*, London, 1994, WB Saunders, p. 63.)

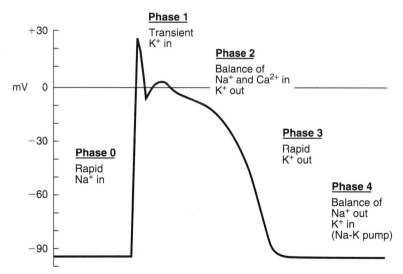

Fig. A.4 Action potential of human ventricular myocyte of subepicardial origin.
- Phase 0 (rapid depolarization) is the result of sudden increase in membrane conductance to Na^+ iron.
- Phase 1 (early rapid repolarization) is due to transient outward K^+ current.
- Phase 2 (plateau) is maintained by the competition between outward current carried by K^+ and Cl^- ions and inward current carried by Ca^{2+} ions.
- Phase 3 (final rapid repolarization) is due to activation of repolarizing outward K^+ current.
- Phase 4 (the resting potential or diastolic depolarization) is caused by the Na-K pump that maintains high K^+ concentration and low intracellular Na^+ concentration by pumping K^+ inward and Na^+ outward.

TABLE A.1   Recurrence Risks Given One Sibling Who Has a Cardiovascular Anomaly

Anomaly	Suggested Risk (%)
Ventricular septal defect	3.0
Patent ductus arteriosus	3.0
Atrial septal defect	2.5
Tetralogy of Fallot	2.5
Pulmonary stenosis	2.0
Coarctation of the aorta	2.0
Aortic stenosis	2.0
Transposition of the great arteries	1.5
Atrioventricular canal (complete endocardial cushion defect)	2.0
Endocardial fibroelastosis	4.0
Tricuspid atresia	1.0
Ebstein's anomaly	1.0
Persistent truncus arteriosus	1.0
Pulmonary atresia	1.0
Hypoplastic left heart syndrome	2.0

Modified from Nora JJ, Nora AH: The evaluation of specific genetic and environmental counseling in congenital heart diseases, *Circulation* 57:205–213, 1978.

TABLE A.2   Affected Offspring Given One Parent With a Congenital Heart Defect

Defect	Mother Affected (%)	Father Affected (%)
Aortic stenosis	13.0–18.0	3.0
Atrial septal defect	4.0–4.5	1.5
Atrioventricular canal (complete endocardial cushion defect)	14.0	1.0
Coarctation of the aorta	4.0	2.0
Patent ductus arteriosus	3.5–4.0	2.5
Pulmonary stenosis	4.0–6.5	2.0
Tetralogy of Fallot	6.0–10.0	1.5
Ventricular septal defect	6.0	2.0

From Nora JJ, Nora AH: Maternal transmission of congenital heart disease: new recurrence risk figures and the questions of cytoplasmic inheritance and vulnerability to teratogens, *Am J Cardiol* 59:459–463, 1987.

TABLE A.3   New York Heart Association Functional Classification[a]

Class	Impairment
I	The patient has the disease, but the condition is asymptomatic.
II	The patient experiences symptoms with moderate activity.
III	The patient has symptoms with mild activity.
IV	The patient's condition is symptomatic at rest.

[a]This is a classification of functional impairment in exercise capacity based on symptoms of dyspnea and fatigue. It is simple and useful in the evaluation of cardiac patients.

TABLE A.4   Summary of Antiarrhythmic Agents

Class	Mechanism of Action	Examples	Remarks
I	Sodium channel blockers Delays phase 0 of the action potential and slows conduction velocity in the tissue		Has a significant proarrhythmic effect
IA	Slows the rate of rise of phase 0 and prolongs the refractory period	Quinidine Procainamide	Major effect on QTc and QRS prolongation
IB	Minimal effect on phase 0 and refractory period	Lidocaine Mexiletine	Least proarrhythmic among class I agents
IC	Marked depression in conduction velocity with minimal effects on refractoriness	Flecainide Propafenone	Major effect on PR and QRS duration
II	Beta-blockers	Propranolol ($\beta_1 + \beta_2$) Atenolol (β_1) Nadolol ($\beta_1 + \beta_2$) Esmolol (β_1)	Minor effects on ECG
III	K-channel blockers Delaying repolarization	Amiodarone Sotalol Dofetilide Ibutilide	Has a significant proarrhythmia Major effect on QT prolongation
IV	Calcium channel blockers (slows inward Ca^{2+} current) Slows conduction velocity and increases refractoriness in the AV node	Verapamil Diltiazem	Minor effects on ECG

AV, Atrioventricular; ECG, electrocardiogram.

TABLE A.5   Effects Of Antiarrhythmic Agents on the Electrocardiogram

Class	Drug	PR	QRS	QT
I				
IA	Quinidine	±	↑↑	↑↑↑
	Procainamide	±	↑	↑↑
IB	Lidocaine	±	±	±
	Mexiletine	±	±	±
IC	Flecainide	↑↑	↑↑	↑
	Propafenone	↑↑	↑↑	±
III	Amiodarone	Acute effect ± Chronic effect ↑	Acute effect ± Chronic effect ↑	Acute effect ± Chronic effect ↑↑↑
	Sotalol	↑	±	↑↑↑
	Dofetilide	±	±	↑↑↑
	Ibutilide	±	±	↑↑↑

Modified from Fischbach PS: Pharmacology of antiarrhythmic agents. In Macdonald Dick II (ed): *Clinical Cardiac Electrophysiology in the Young*, New York, 2010, Springer.

TABLE A.6 Oxygen Consumption Per Body Surface Area[a]

Age (yr)	HEART RATE (BEATS/MIN)												
	50	60	70	80	90	100	110	120	130	140	150	160	170
MALE PATIENTS													
3				155	159	163	167	171	175	178	182	186	190
4			149	152	156	160	163	168	171	175	179	182	186
6		141	144	148	151	155	159	162	167	171	174	178	181
8		136	141	145	148	152	156	159	163	167	171	175	178
10	130	134	139	142	146	149	153	157	160	165	169	172	176
12	128	132	136	140	144	147	151	155	158	162	167	170	174
14	127	130	134	137	142	146	149	153	157	160	165	169	172
16	125	129	132	136	141	144	148	152	155	159	162	167	
18	124	127	131	135	139	143	147	150	154	157	161	166	
20	123	126	130	134	137	142	145	149	153	156	160	165	
25	120	124	127	131	135	139	143	147	150	154	157		
30	118	122	125	129	133	136	141	145	148	152	155		
35	116	120	124	127	131	135	139	143	147	150			
40	115	119	122	126	130	133	137	141	145	149			
FEMALE PATIENTS													
3				150	153	157	161	165	169	172	176	180	183
4			141	145	149	152	156	159	163	168	171	175	179
6		130	134	137	142	146	149	153	156	160	165	168	172
8		125	129	133	136	141	144	148	152	155	159	163	167
10	118	122	125	129	133	136	141	144	148	152	155	159	163
12	115	119	122	126	130	133	137	141	145	149	152	156	160
14	112	116	120	123	127	131	134	133	143	146	150	153	157
16	109	114	118	121	125	128	132	136	140	144	148	151	
18	107	111	116	119	123	127	130	134	137	142	146	149	
20	106	109	114	118	121	125	128	132	136	140	144	148	
25	102	106	109	114	118	121	125	128	132	136	140		
30	99	103	106	110	115	118	122	125	129	133	136		
35	97	100	104	107	111	116	119	123	127	130			
50	94	98	102	105	109	112	117	121	124	128			

[a]In (mL/min)/m^2.
From LaFarge CG, Miettinen OS: The estimation of oxygen consumption, *Cardiovasc Res* 4:23, 1970.

Blood Pressure Values

TABLE B.1   Blood Pressure Levels for Boys by Age and Height Percentile (NHBPEP)

Age	BP Percentile	SYSTOLIC BP (MM HG) PERCENTILE OF HEIGHT							DIASTOLIC BP (MM HG) PERCENTILE OF HEIGHT						
		5th	10th	25th	50th	75th	90th	95th	5th	10th	25th	50th	75th	90th	95th
1	50th	80	81	83	85	87	88	89	34	35	36	37	38	39	39
	90th	94	95	97	99	100	102	103	49	50	51	52	53	53	54
	95th	98	99	101	103	104	106	106	54	54	55	56	57	58	58
	99th	105	106	108	110	112	113	114	61	62	63	64	65	66	66
2	50th	84	85	87	88	90	92	92	39	40	41	42	43	44	44
	90th	97	99	100	102	104	105	106	54	55	56	57	58	58	59
	95th	101	102	104	106	108	109	110	59	59	60	61	62	63	63
	99th	109	110	111	113	115	117	117	66	67	68	69	70	71	71
3	50th	86	87	89	91	93	94	95	44	44	45	46	47	48	48
	90th	100	101	103	105	107	108	109	59	59	60	61	62	63	63
	95th	104	105	107	109	110	112	113	63	63	64	65	66	67	67
	99th	111	112	114	116	118	119	120	71	71	72	73	74	75	75
4	50th	88	89	91	93	95	96	97	47	48	49	50	51	51	52
	90th	102	103	105	107	109	110	111	62	63	64	65	66	66	67
	95th	106	107	109	111	112	114	115	66	67	68	69	70	71	71
	99th	113	114	116	118	120	121	122	74	75	76	77	78	78	79
5	50th	90	91	93	95	96	98	98	50	51	52	53	54	55	55
	90th	104	105	106	108	110	111	112	65	66	67	68	69	69	70
	95th	108	109	110	112	114	115	116	69	70	71	72	73	74	74
	99th	115	116	118	120	121	123	123	77	78	79	80	81	81	82
6	50th	91	92	94	96	98	99	100	53	53	54	55	56	57	57
	90th	105	106	108	110	111	113	113	68	68	69	70	71	72	72
	95th	109	110	112	114	115	117	117	72	72	73	74	75	76	76
	99th	116	117	119	121	123	124	125	80	80	81	82	83	84	84
7	50th	92	94	95	97	99	100	101	55	55	56	57	58	59	59
	90th	106	107	109	111	113	114	115	70	70	71	72	73	74	74
	95th	110	111	113	115	117	118	119	74	74	75	76	77	78	78
	99th	117	118	120	122	124	125	126	82	82	83	84	85	86	86
8	50th	94	95	97	99	100	102	102	56	57	58	59	60	60	61
	90th	107	109	110	112	114	115	116	71	72	72	73	74	75	76
	95th	111	112	114	116	118	119	120	75	76	77	78	79	79	80
	99th	119	120	122	123	125	127	127	83	84	85	86	87	87	88
9	50th	95	96	98	100	102	103	104	57	58	59	60	61	61	62
	90th	109	110	112	114	115	117	118	72	73	74	75	76	76	77
	95th	113	114	116	118	119	121	121	76	77	78	79	80	81	81
	99th	120	121	123	125	127	128	129	84	85	86	87	88	88	89
10	50th	97	98	100	102	103	105	106	58	59	60	61	61	62	63
	90th	111	112	114	115	117	119	119	73	73	74	75	76	77	78
	95th	115	116	117	119	121	122	123	77	78	79	80	81	81	82
	99th	122	123	125	127	128	130	130	85	86	86	88	88	89	90
11	50th	99	100	102	104	105	107	107	59	59	60	61	62	63	63
	90th	113	114	115	117	119	120	121	74	74	75	76	77	78	78
	95th	117	118	119	121	123	124	125	78	78	79	80	81	82	82
	99th	124	125	127	129	130	132	132	86	86	87	88	89	90	90

Continued

TABLE B.1   Blood Pressure Levels for Boys by Age and Height Percentile (NHBPEP)—cont'd

| | | SYSTOLIC BP (MM HG) | | | | | | | DIASTOLIC BP (MM HG) | | | | | | |
| | | PERCENTILE OF HEIGHT | | | | | | | PERCENTILE OF HEIGHT | | | | | | |
Age	BP Percentile	5th	10th	25th	50th	75th	90th	95th	5th	10th	25th	50th	75th	90th	95th
12	50th	101	102	104	106	108	109	110	59	60	61	62	63	63	64
	90th	115	116	118	120	121	123	123	74	75	75	76	77	78	79
	95th	119	120	122	123	125	127	127	78	79	80	81	82	82	83
	99th	126	127	129	131	133	134	135	86	87	88	89	90	90	91
13	50th	104	105	106	108	110	111	112	60	60	61	62	63	64	64
	90th	117	118	120	122	124	125	126	75	75	76	77	78	79	79
	95th	121	122	124	126	128	129	130	79	79	80	81	82	83	83
	99th	128	130	131	133	135	136	137	87	87	88	89	90	91	91
14	50th	106	107	109	111	113	114	115	60	61	62	63	64	65	65
	90th	120	121	123	125	126	128	128	75	76	77	78	79	79	80
	95th	124	125	127	128	130	132	132	80	80	81	82	83	84	84
	99th	131	132	134	136	138	139	140	87	88	89	90	91	92	92
15	50th	109	110	112	113	115	117	117	61	62	63	64	65	66	66
	90th	122	124	125	127	129	130	131	76	77	78	79	80	80	81
	95th	126	127	129	131	133	134	135	81	81	82	83	84	85	85
	99th	134	135	136	138	140	142	142	88	89	90	91	92	93	93
16	50th	111	112	114	116	118	119	120	63	63	64	65	66	67	67
	90th	125	126	128	130	131	133	134	78	78	79	80	81	82	82
	95th	129	130	132	134	135	137	137	82	83	83	84	85	86	87
	99th	136	137	139	141	143	144	145	90	90	91	92	93	94	94
17	50th	114	115	116	118	120	121	122	65	66	66	67	68	69	70
	90th	127	128	130	132	134	135	136	80	80	81	82	83	84	84
	95th	131	132	134	136	138	139	140	84	85	86	87	87	88	89
	99th	139	140	141	143	145	146	147	92	93	93	94	95	96	97

BP, Blood pressure; *NHBPEP,* National High Blood Pressure Education Program.
From The Fourth Report on the Diagnosis, Evaluation, and Treatment of High Blood Pressure in Children and Adolescents: National High Blood Pressure Education Program Working Group on High Blood Pressure in Children and Adolescents, *Pediatrics* 114:555–576, 2004.

TABLE B.2   Blood Pressure Levels for Girls by Age and Height Percentile (NHBPEP)

| | | SYSTOLIC BP (MM HG) | | | | | | | DIASTOLIC BP (MM HG) | | | | | | |
| | | PERCENTILE OF HEIGHT | | | | | | | PERCENTILE OF HEIGHT | | | | | | |
Age	BP Percentile	5th	10th	25th	50th	75th	90th	95th	5th	10th	25th	50th	75th	90th	95th
1	50th	83	84	85	86	88	89	90	38	39	39	40	41	41	42
	90th	97	97	98	100	101	102	103	52	53	53	54	55	55	56
	95th	100	101	102	104	105	106	107	56	57	57	58	59	59	60
	99th	108	108	109	111	112	113	114	64	64	65	65	66	67	67
2	50th	85	85	87	88	89	91	91	43	44	44	45	46	46	47
	90th	98	99	100	101	103	104	105	57	58	58	59	60	61	61
	95th	102	103	104	105	107	108	109	61	62	62	63	64	65	65
	99th	109	110	111	112	114	115	116	69	69	70	70	71.	72	72
3	50th	86	87	88	89	91	92	93	47	48	48	49	50	50	51
	90th	100	100	102	103	104	106	106	61	62	62	63	64	64	65
	95th	104	104	105	107	108	109	110	65	66	66	67	68	68	69
	99th	111	111	113	114	115	116	117	73	73	74	74	75	76	76
4	50th	88	88	90	91	92	94	94	50	50	51	52	52	53	54
	90th	101	102	103	104	106	107	108	64	64	65	66	67	67	68
	95th	105	106	107	108	110	111	112	68	68	69	70	71	71	72
	99th	112	113	114	115	117	118	119	76	76	76	77	78	79	79
5	50th	89	90	91	93	94	95	96	52	53	53	54	55	55	56
	90th	103	103	105	106	107	109	109	66	67	67	68	69	69	70
	95th	107	107	108	110	111	112	113	70	71	71	72	73	73	74
	99th	114	114	116	117	118	120	120	78	78	79	79	80	81	81

TABLE B.2   Blood Pressure Levels for Girls by Age and Height Percentile (NHBPEP)—cont'd

| | | SYSTOLIC BP (MM HG) | | | | | | | DIASTOLIC BP (MM HG) | | | | | | |
| | | PERCENTILE OF HEIGHT | | | | | | | PERCENTILE OF HEIGHT | | | | | | |
Age	BP Percentile	5th	10th	25th	50th	75th	90th	95th	5th	10th	25th	50th	75th	90th	95th
6	50th	91	92	93	94	96	97	98	54	54	55	56	56	57	58
	90th	104	105	106	108	109	110	111	68	68	69	70	70	71	72
	95th	108	109	110	111	113	114	115	72	72	73	74	74	75	76
	99th	115	116	117	119	120	121	122	80	80	80	81	82	83	83
7	50th	93	93	95	96	97	99	99	55	56	56	57	58	58	59
	90th	106	107	108	109	111	112	113	69	70	70	71	72	72	73
	95th	110	111	112	113	115	116	116	73	74	74	75	76	76	77
	99th	117	118	119	120	122	123	124	81	81	82	82	83	84	84
8	50th	95	95	96	98	99	100	101	57	57	57	58	59	60	60
	90th	108	109	110	111	113	114	114	71	71	71	72	73	74	74
	95th	112	112	114	115	116	118	118	75	75	75	76	77	78	78
	99th	119	120	121	122	123	125	125	82	82	83	83	84	85	86
9	50th	96	97	98	100	101	102	103	58	58	58	59	60	61	61
	90th	110	110	112	113	114	116	116	72	72	72	73	74	75	75
	95th	114	114	115	117	118	119	120	76	76	76	77	78	79	79
	99th	121	121	123	124	125	127	127	83	83	84	84	85	86	87
10	50th	98	99	100	102	103	104	105	59	59	59	60	61	62	62
	90th	112	112	114	115	116	118	118	73	73	73	74	75	76	76
	95th	116	116	117	119	120	121	122	77	77	77	78	79	80	80
	99th	123	123	125	126	127	129	129	84	84	85	86	86	87	88
11	50th	100	101	102	103	105	106	107	60	60	60	61.	62	63	63
	90th	114	114	116	117	118	119	120	74	74	74	75	76	77	77
	95th	118	118	119	121	122	123	124	78	78	78	79	80	81	81
	99th	125	125	126	128	129	130	131	85	85	86	87	87	88	89
12	50th	102	103	104	105	107	108	109	61	61	61	62	63	64	64
	90th	116	116	117	119	120	121	122	75	75	75	76	77	78	78
	95th	119	120	121	123	124	125	126	79	79	79	80	81	82	82
	99th	127	127	128	130	131	132	133	86	86	87	88	88	89	90
13	50th	104	105	106	107	109	110	110	62	62	62	63	64	65	65
	90th	117	118	119	121	122	123	124	76	76	76	77	78	79	79
	95th	121	122	123	124	126	127	128	80	80	80	81	82	83	83
	99th	128	129	130	132	133	134	135	87	87	88	89	89	90	91
14	50th	106	106	107	109	110	111	112	63	63	63	64	65	66	66
	90th	119	120	121	122	124	125	125	77	77	77	78	79	80	80
	95th	123	123	125	126	127	129	129	81	81	81	82	83	84	84
	99th	130	131	132	133	135	136	136	88	88	89	90	90	91	92
15	50th	107	108	109	110	111	113	113	64	64	64	65	66	67	67
	90th	120	121	122	123	125	126	127	78	78	78	79	80	81	81
	95th	124	125	126	127	129	130	131	82	82	82	83	84	85	85
	99th	131	132	133	134	136	137	138	89	89	90	91	91	92	93
16	50th	108	108	110	111	112	114	114	64	64	65	66	66	67	68
	90th	121	122	123	124	126	127	128	78	78	79	80	81	81	82
	95th	125	126	127	128	130	131	132	82	82	83	84	85	85	86
	99th	132	133	134	135	137	138	139	90	90	90	91	92	93	93
17	50th	108	109	110	111	113	114	115	64	65	65	66	67	67	68
	90th	122	122	123	125	126	127	128	78	79	79	80	81	81.	82
	95th	125	126	127	129	130	131	132	82	83	83	84	85	85	86
	99th	133	133	134	136	137	138	139	90	90	91	91	92	93	93

BP, Blood pressure; NHBPEP, National High Blood Pressure Education Program.
From The Fourth Report on the Diagnosis, Evaluation, and Treatment of High Blood Pressure in Children and Adolescents: National High Blood Pressure Education Program Working Group on High Blood Pressure in Children and Adolescents, *Pediatrics* 114:555–576, 2004.

TABLE B.3   Auscultatory Blood Pressure Values for Boys 5 to 17 Years Old (San Antonio Children's Blood Pressure Study)

Age (yr)	5th	10th	25th	Mean	75th	90th	95th	99th[a]
SYSTOLIC BLOOD PRESSURE								
5	78	81	87	92	98	103	106	112
6	81	84	89	95	100	105	108	114
7	82	85	90	96	102	107	110	116
8	83	86	92	97	103	108	111	117
9	85	88	93	99	104	109	113	118
10	86	89	95	100	106	111	114	120
11	88	91	97	102	108	113	116	122
12	91	94	99	105	111	116	119	125
13	94	97	102	108	113	118	122	127
14	96	99	105	110	116	121	122	130
15	99	102	107	113	118	124	127	132
16	100	103	108	114	120	125	128	134
17	100	103	109	114	120	125	128	134
DIASTOLIC BLOOD PRESSURE (K5)								
5	34	37	43	49	55	60	63	70
6	38	41	47	53	59	64	67	73
7	40	44	49	55	61	66	70	76
8	42	45	50	56	62	68	71	77
9	42	45	51	57	63	68	71	77
10	42	45	51	57	63	68	71	77
11	42	45	51	57	63	68	71	77
12	42	45	50	56	62	68	71	77
13	42	45	51	56	62	68	71	77
14	42	45	51	57	63	68	71	77
15	43	46	51	57	63	69	72	78
16	45	48	53	59	65	71	74	80
17	47	51	56	62	68	73	77	83

*[a]The 99th percentile values were added after publication.

K5, Korotkoff phase 5.

Data presented in graphic form in Park MK, Menard SW, Yuan C: Comparison of blood pressure in children from three ethnic groups, *Am J Cardiol* 87:1305–1308, 2001.

TABLE B.4   Auscultatory Blood Pressure Values for Girls 5 to 17 Years Old (San Antonio Children's Blood Pressure Study)

				PERCENTILE				
Age (yr)	5th	10th	25th	Mean	75th	90th	95th	99th[a]
SYSTOLIC BLOOD PRESSURE								
5	79	82	87	92	97	102	105	110
6	80	83	88	93	98	103	106	111
7	81	84	89	94	99	104	107	112
8	83	86	91	96	101	106	109	114
9	85	88	93	98	103	108	111	116
10	87	90	95	100	105	110	113	118
11	89	92	97	102	107	112	115	120
12	91	94	98	104	109	113	116	122
13	92	95	100	105	110	115	118	123
14	93	96	101	106	111	116	119	124
15	94	97	101	107	112	117	119	125
16	94	97	102	107	112	117	120	125
17	95	98	103	108	113	118	121	126
DIASTOLIC BLOOD PRESSURE (K5)								
5	35	38	44	49	55	60	63	69
6	38	41	47	52	58	63	66	72
7	40	41	49	54	60	65	68	74
8	42	45	50	56	61	67	70	75
9	43	46	51	56	62	67	70	76
10	43	46	51	57	63	68	71	77
11	43	46	51	57	63	68	71	77
12	43	46	52	57	63	68	71	77
13	43	47	52	57	63	68	71	77
14	44	47	52	58	63	68	72	77
15	44	47	52	58	64	69	72	78
16	45	48	53	59	64	69	73	78
17	46	49	54	59	65	70	73	79

[a]The 99th percentile values were added after publication.

K5, Korotkoff phase 5.

Data presented in graphic form in Park MK, Menard SW, Yuan C: Comparison of blood pressure in children from three ethnic groups, *Am J Cardiol* 87:1305–1308, 2001.

TABLE B.5 DINAMAP (Model 1846) Blood Pressure Percentiles for Neonates to 5-Year-Old Children

	PERCENTILE						
Age	**5th**	**10th**	**25th**	**Mean**	**75th**	**90th**	**95th**
SYSTOLIC BLOOD PRESSURE							
1–3 days	52	56	58	65	71	74	77
2–3 wk	62	66	71	78	84	89	92
1–5 mo	76	79	88	94	102	106	111
6–11 mo	79	84	88	94	99	104	109
1 yr	80	84	89	94	99	104	108
2 yr	82	85	91	95	101	106	109
3 yr	84	87	92	98	103	108	112
4 yr	86	90	95	100	105	110	114
5 yr	89	93	96	102	107	113	116
DIASTOLIC BLOOD PRESSURE							
1–3 days	31	33	37	41	45	50	52
2–3 wk	31	37	42	47	63	58	61
1–5 mo	45	48	53	59	64	71	75
6–11 mo	41	44	52	57	63	67	69
1 yr	44	48	52	57	73	67	69
2 yr	45	47	52	56	61	65	68
3 yr	44	47	52	56	61	65	69
4 yr	44	48	52	56	61	65	68
5 yr	44	48	53	57	62	66	68

Data presented in graphic form in Park MK, Menard SM: Normative oscillometric BP values in the first 5 years in an office setting, *Arch J Dis Child* 143:860–864, 1989.

TABLE B.6 DINAMAP (Model 8100) Blood Pressure Percentile for Boys 5 to 17 Years Old (San Antonio Children's Blood Pressure Study)

	PERCENTILES							
Age (yr)	5th	10th	25th	Mean	75th	90th	95th	99th[a]
SYSTOLIC BLOOD PRESSURE								
5	90	93	98	104	110	115	118	124
6	92	95	100	106	112	117	120	126
7	93	96	102	107	113	118	121	127
8	94	97	103	108	114	119	123	128
9	95	99	104	110	115	121	124	130
10	97	100	105	110	117	122	125	131
11	99	102	107	113	119	124	127	133
12	101	104	109	115	121	126	129	135
13	104	107	112	118	123	129	132	138
14	106	109	114	120	126	131	134	140
15	108	111	116	122	128	133	136	141
16	109	112	117	123	128	134	137	143
17	109	112	117	123	129	134	137	143
DIASTOLIC BLOOD PRESSURE								
5	46	49	53	58	63	68	71	76
6	47	49	54	59	64	68	71	76
7	47	50	54	59	64	69	72	77
8	48	51	55	60	65	70	72	78
9	49	51	56	61	66	70	73	78
10	49	52	56	61	66	71	74	79
11	49	52	57	62	67	71	74	79
12	50	52	57	62	67	71	74	79
13	50	52	57	62	67	71	74	79
14	50	52	57	62	67	72	74	79
15	50	52	57	62	67	72	74	79
16	50	53	57	62	67	72	74	80
17	50	53	57	62	67	72	75	80

[a]The 99th percentile values were added after submission of the manuscript.

From Park MK, Menard SW, Schoolfield J: Oscillometric blood pressure standards for children, *Pediatr Cardiol* 26(5):601–607, 2005.

TABLE B.7   DINAMAP (Model 8100) Blood Pressure Percentile for Girls 5 to 17 Years Old (San Antonio Children's 5 To 17 Years Old Study)

Age (yr)	5th	10th	25th	Mean	75th	90th	95th	99th[a]
SYSTOLIC BLOOD PRESSURE								
5	90	93	98	103	109	114	117	122
6	91	94	99	1043	110	115	118	123
7	92	95	100	106	111	116	119	125
8	94	97	102	107	113	118	121	126
9	95	98	103	109	114	119	122	128
10	97	100	105	110	116	121	124	129
11	98	101	106	112	117	122	125	131
12	100	103	107	113	118	123	126	132
13	101	104	109	114	120	125	128	133
14	102	104	109	115	120	125	128	134
15	102	105	110	115	121	126	129	134
16	102	105	110	115	121	126	129	134
17	102	105	110	115	121	126	129	134
DIASTOLIC BLOOD PRESSURE								
5	46	48	53	59	64	68	71	76
6	47	49	54	59	64	68	71	76
7	47	50	54	60	65	69	72	77
8	48	50	55	60	65	70	73	78
9	49	51	55	61	66	70	73	78
10	49	51	56	61	66	71	74	79
11	49	52	56	62	67	71	74	79
12	50	52	57	62	67	71	74	79
13	50	53	57	62	67	71	74	79
14	50	53	58	62	67	72	74	79
15	50	54	58	62	67	72	74	79
16	50	54	58	62	67	72	74	80
17	50	54	58	62	67	72	75	80

[a]The 99th percentile values were added after submission of the manuscript.
From Park MK, Menard SW, Schoolfield J: Oscillometric blood pressure standards for children, *Pediatr Cardiol* 26(5):601–607, 2005.

TABLE B.8   Normal Values for Ambulatory Blood Pressure for Healthy Boys by Age

BP Percentile	AGE (YR)											
	5	6	7	8	9	10	11	12	13	14	15	16
24-HOUR SBP												
50th	105	106	106	107	108	109	110	113	115	118	121	123
75th	109	110	111	112	113	114	116	118	121	124	127	129
90th	113	115	116	117	118	119	121	124	126	129	132	135
95th	116	118	119	120	121	123	125	127	130	133	136	138
99th	123	1241	125	127	128	129	131	134	137	140	142	145
DAYTIME SBP												
50th	111	112	112	112	113	113	1159	117	120	122	125	128
75th	116	116	117	117	118	119	1201	123	126	129	132	135
90th	120	121	122	122	123	124	126	128	131	134	137	140
95th	123	124	125	125	126	127	129	132	135	138	141	144
99th	129	130	131	132	132	134	136	139	142	144	147	150
NIGHTTIME SBP												
50th	95	96	96	97	97	98	99	101	103	106	108	111
75th	99	100	101	102	103	104	105	107	109	112	114	117
90th	103	105	106	108	109	110	111	113	115	118	120	123
95th	106	108	110	111	112	113	115	116	119	121	123	126
99th	112	115	117	118	120	121	122	123	126	128	130	132
24H DBP												
50th	65	66	66	66	67	67	67	67	67	68	68	69
75th	69	69	70	70	70	70	71	71	71	71	72	72
90th	72	73	73	73	73	73	74	74	74	75	75	76
95th	74	75	75	75	75	75	76	76	76	77	77	78
99th	79	79	79	79	79	79	79	80	80-	80	81	81
DAYTIME DBP												
50th	72	72	73	73	72	72	72	72	72	73	73	74
75th	76	76	76	76	76	76	76	76	76	77	77	78
90th	79	79	80	80	80	80	80	80	80	80	81	81
95th	81	81	82	82	82	82	82	82	82	82	83	84
99th	85	84	85	86	85	85	85	85	86	86	87	88
NIGHTTIME DBP												
50th	55	55	55	56	56	56	56	56	56	56	57	57
75th	59	59	60	60	60	60	60	60	60	61	61	61
90th	62	63	64	64	64	64	64	64	64	64	64	64
95th	65	66	67	67	67	67	67	67	67	67	66	66
99th	72	73	74	74	73	73	72	71	71	71	71	70
24-HOUR MAP												
50th	77	78	79	79	80	80	81	82	83	84	85	86
75th	81	82	83	83	84	84	85	86	86	88	89	91
90th	86	86	87	87	88	88	89	90	91	92	93	94
95th	88	89	90	90	90	91	91	92	93	94	95	96
99th	94	95	95	95	96	96	96	92	97	97	98	99

Continued

TABLE B.8   Normal Values for Ambulatory Blood Pressure for Healthy Boys by Age—cont'd

DAYTIME MAP

50th	84	84	85	85	85	85	85	86	87	88	89	91
75th	88	88	89	89	89	90	90	91	92	93	94	96
90th	91	92	93	93	94	94	94	95	96	97	98	100
95th	94	95	95	96	96	96	97	97	98	99	101	102
99th	98	99	100	101	101	101	101	102	102	103	105	106

NIGHTTIME MAP

50th	67	68	69	69	70	70	71	71	72	73	74	75
75th	71	72	73	74	74	75	75	76	76	77	78	79
90th	75	76	77	78	79	79	79	80	80	81	81	82
95th	78	79	80	81	82	82	82	82	83	83	83	83
99th	84	86	86	88	88	88	87	87	87	87	87	86

DBP, Diastolic blood pressure; *MAP*, mean arterial pressure; *SBP*, systolic blood pressure.
Modified from Wühl E, Witte K, Soergel M, et al: Distribution of 24-h ambulatory blood pressure in children: normalized reference values and role of body dimension, *J Hypertens* 20:1995–2007, 2002.

TABLE B.9   Normal Values for Ambulatory Blood Pressure for Healthy Girls by Age[a]

BP Percentile	AGE (YR)											
	5	6	7	8	9	10	11	12	13	14	15	16
24-HOUR SBP												
50th	103	104	105	107	108	109	110	111	112	113	114	115
75th	108	109	110	112	113	114	115	116	117	118	118	119
90th	112	114	115	116	117	118	119	120	121	122	123	123
95th	114	116	118	119	120	121	122	123	124	125	125	126
99th	120	122	123	124	126	127	128	128	129	130	130	130
DAYTIME SBP												
50th	108	110	111	112	112	113	114	115	116	118	119	120
75th	114	115	116	117	118	119	120	121	122	123	124	124
90th	118	120	121	122	122	123	124	125	126	127	128	129
95th	121	122	123	124	125	126	127	128	129	130	130	131
99th	126	127	128	130	131	132	133	134	135	135	135	135
NIGHTTIME SBP												
50th	95	96	96	97	98	98	99	100	101	101	102	103
75th	100	101	102	103	103	104	105	105	106	106	107	107
90th	105	106	107	108	109	110	110	110	111	111	111	111
95th	108	110	111	112	112	113	114	114	114	114	114	114
99th	115	116	117	118	119	120	120	120	119	119	118	118
24-HOUR DBP												
50th	66	66	66	66	66	66	66	67	67	67	678	68
75th	69	69	69	69	70	70	70	70	71	71	71	71
90th	72	72	72	72	73	73	73	74	74	74	75	75
95th	74	74	74	74	74	75	75	76	76	76	77	77
99th	78	78	78	78	78	78	78	79	80	80	80	81
DAYTIME DBP												
50th	73	73	72	72	72	72	72	72	72	73	73	74
75th	77	77	76	76	76	76	76	76	77	77	77	77
90th	80	80	80	80	80	79	79	80	80	80	80	80
95th	82	82	82	82	82	81	81	82	82	82	82	82

TABLE B.9   Normal Values for Ambulatory Blood Pressure for Healthy Girls by Age[a]—cont'd

DAYTIME DBP

99th	86	86	86	86	85	85	85	85	86	86	86	85

NIGHTTIME DBP

50th	55	56	56	55	55	55	54	54	54	55	55	55
75th	61	61	60	60	59	59	59	59	59	59	59	59
90th	66	65	65	64	64	64	63	63	63	63	63	63
95th	69	68	67	67	67	67	66	65	66	65	65	65
99th	74	74	73	72	72	72	72	71	71	71	70	70

24H MAP

50th	78	78	78	79	79	80	80	81	82	82	83	83
75th	81	82	82	83	83	83	84	85	85	86	87	87
90th	85	85	85	86	86	87	87	88	89	89	90	91
95th	87	87	87	88	88	88	89	90	91	91	92	92
99th	91	91	91	91	91	92	92	93	94	94	95	95

DAYTIME MAP

50th	84	83	84	84	84	84	85	85	86	87	87	88
75th	88	88	88	88	88	89	89	89	90	91	91	92
90th	92	92	92	92	92	92	92	93	94	94	95	95
95th	95	95	94	94	94	94	94	95	96	96	97	97
99th	99	99	99	98	98	98	98	99	99	100	100	101

NIGHTTIME MAP

50th	69	69	69	69	69	69	69	70	70	71	71	72
75th	73	73	73	73	73	74	74	74	75	75	75	76
90th	77	77	77	77	77	78	78	78	78	79	79	79
95th	79	79	80	80	80	80	80	80	81	81	81	81
99th	84	84	84	84	85	85	85	85	85	85	85	85

[a]Numbers have been rounded off to the nearest whole number.

DBP, Diastolic blood pressure; *MAP,* mean arterial pressure; *SBP,* systolic blood pressure.

Modified from Wühl E, Witte K, Soergel M, et al: Distribution of 24-h ambulatory blood pressure in children: normalized reference values and role of body dimension, *J Hypertens* 20:1995–2007, 2002.

Cardiovascular Risk Factors

TABLE C.1 Estimated Value for Percentile Regression of Waist Circumference[a] for European American Children and Adolescents According to Sex

Age (yr)	PERCENTILE FOR BOYS (CM)					PERCENTILE FOR GIRLS (CM)				
	10th	25th	50th	75th	90th	10th	25th	50th	75th	90th
2	42.9	46.9	47.1	48.6	50.6	43.1	45.1	47.4	49.6	52.5
3	44.7	48.8	49.2	51.2	54.0	44.7	46.8	49.3	51.9	55.4
4	46.5	50.6	51.3	53.8	57.4	46.3	48.5	51.2	54.2	58.2
5	48.3	52.5	53.3	56.5	60.8	47.9	50.2	53.1	56.5	61.1
6	50.1	54.3	55.4	59.1	64.2	49.5	51.8	55.0	58.8	64.0
7	46.5	50.6	51.3	53.8	57.4	46.3	48.5	51.2	54.2	58.2
8	48.3	52.5	53.3	56.5	60.8	47.9	50.2	53.1	56.5	61.1
9	50.1	54.3	55.4	59.1	64.2	49.5	51.8	55.0	58.8	64.0
10	46.5	50.6	51.3	53.8	57.4	46.3	48.5	51.2	54.2	58.2
11	59.1	63.6	65.8	72.2	81.1	57.5	60.2	64.4	70.3	78.3
12	60.9	65.5	67.9	74.9	84.5	59.1	61.9	66.3	72.6	81.2
13	62.7	67.4	70.0	77.5	87.9	60.7	63.6	68.2	74.9	84.1
14	64.5	69.2	72.1	80.1	91.3	62.3	65.3	70.1	77.2	86.9
15	66.3	71.1	74.1	82.8	94.7	63.9	67.0	72.0	79.5	89.8
16	68.1	72.9	76.2	85.4	98.1	65.5	68.6	73.9	81.8	92.7
17	69.9	74.8	78.3	88.0	101.5	67.1	70.3	75.8	84.1	95.5
18	71.7	76.7	80.4	90.6	104.9	68.7	72.0	77.7	86.4	98.4

[a]Waist circumference was measured with a tape at just above the uppermost lateral border of the right ileum at the end of normal expiration. From Fernandez JR, Redden DT, Pietrobelli A, Allison DB: Waist circumference percentiles in nationally representative samples of African-American, European-American, and Mexican-American children and adolescents, *J Pediatr* 145:439–444, 2004.

TABLE C.2 Estimated Value for Percentile Regression of Waist Circumference[a] for African American Children and Adolescents According to Sex

Age (yr)	PERCENTILE FOR BOYS (CM)					PERCENTILE FOR GIRLS (CM)				
	10th	25th	50th	75th	90th	10th	25th	50th	75th	90th
2	43.2	44.6	46.4	48.5	50.0	43.0	44.6	46.0	47.7	50.1
3	44.8	46.3	48.3	50.7	53.2	44.6	46.3	48.1	50.6	53.8
4	46.3	48.0	50.1	52.9	56.4	46.1	48.0	50.2	53.4	57.5
5	47.9	49.7	52.0	55.1	59.6	47.7	49.7	52.3	56.2	61.1
6	49.4	51.4	53.9	57.3	62.8	49.2	51.4	54.5	59.0	64.8
7	51.0	53.1	55.7	59.5	66.1	50.8	53.2	56.6	61.8	68.5
8	52.5	54.8	57.6	61.7	69.3	52.4	54.9	58.7	64.7	72.2
9	54.1	56.4	59.4	63.9	72.5	53.9	56.6	60.9	67.5	75.8
10	55.6	58.1	61.3	66.1	75.7	55.5	58.3	63.0	70.3	79.5
11	57.2	59.8	63.2	68.3	78.9	57.0	60.0	65.1	73.1	83.2
12	58.7	61.5	65.0	70.5	82.1	58.6	61.7	67.3	75.9	86.9
13	60.3	63.2	66.9	72.7	85.3	60.2	63.4	69.4	78.8	90.5
14	61.8	64.9	68.7	74.9	88.5	61.7	65.1	71.5	81.6	94.2
15	63.4	66.6	70.6	77.1	91.7	63.3	66.8	73.6	84.4	97.9
16	64.9	68.3	72.5	79.3	94.9	64.8	68.5	75.8	87.2	101.6

continued

TABLE C.2 Estimated Value for Percentile Regression of Waist Circumference[a] for African American Children and Adolescents According to Sex—cont'd

	PERCENTILE FOR BOYS (CM)					PERCENTILE FOR GIRLS (CM)				
Age (yr)	10th	25th	50th	75th	90th	10th	25th	50th	75th	90th
17	66.5	70.0	74.3	81.5	98.2	66.4	70.3	77.9	90.0	105.2
18	68.0	71.7	76.2	83.7	101.4	68.0	72.0	80.0	92.9	108.9

[a]Waist circumference was measured with a tape at just above the uppermost lateral border of the right ileum at the end of normal expiration.
From Fernandez JR, Redden DT, Pietrobelli A, Allison DB: Waist circumference percentiles in nationally representative samples of African-American, European-American, and Mexican-American children and adolescents, *J Pediatr* 145:439–444, 2004.

TABLE C.3 Estimated Value for Percentile Regression of Waist Circumference[a] for Mexican American Children and Adolescents According to Sex

	PERCENTILE FOR BOYS (CM)					PERCENTILE FOR GIRLS (CM)				
Age (yr)	10th	25th	50th	75th	90th	10th	25th	50th	75th	90th
2	44.4	45.6	47.6	49.8	53.2	44.5	45.7	48.0	50.0	53.5
3	46.1	47.5	49.8	52.5	56.7	46.0	47.4	50.1	52.6	56.7
4	47.8	49.4	52.0	55.3	60.2	47.5	49.2	52.2	55.2	59.9
5	49.5	51.3	54.2	58.0	63.6	49.0	51.0	54.2	57.8	63.0
6	51.2	53.2	56.3	60.7	67.1	50.5	52.7	56.3	60.4	66.2
7	52.9	55.1	58.5	63.4	70.6	52.0	54.5	58.4	63.0	69.4
8	54.6	57.0	60.7	66.2	74.1	53.5	56.3	60.4	65.6	72.6
9	56.3	58.9	62.9	68.9	77.6	55.0	58.0	62.5	68.2	75.8
10	58.0	60.8	65.1	71.6	81.0	56.5	59.8	64.6	70.8	78.9
11	59.7	62.7	67.2	74.4	84.5	58.1	61.6	66.6	73.4	82.1
12	61.4	64.6	69.4	77.1	88.0	59.6	63.4	68.7	76.0	85.3
13	63.1	66.5	71.6	79.8	91.5	61.1	65.1	70.8	78.6	88.5
14	64.8	68.4	73.8	82.6	95.0	62.6	66.9	72.9	81.2	91.7
15	66.5	70.3	76.0	85.3	98.4	64.1	68.7	74.9	83.8	94.8
16	68.2	72.2	78.1	88.0	101.9	65.6	70.4	77.0	86.4	98.0
17	69.9	74.1	80.3	90.7	105.4	67.1	72.2	79.1	89.0	101.2
18	71.6	76.0	82.5	93.5	108.9	68.6	74.0	81.1	91.6	104.4

[a]Waist circumference was measured with a tape at just above the uppermost lateral border of the right ileum at the end of normal expiration.
From Fernandez JR, Redden DT, Pietrobelli A, Allison DB: Waist circumference percentiles in nationally representative samples of African-American, European-American, and Mexican-American children and adolescents, *J Pediatr* 145:439–444, 2004.

TABLE C.4 Foods to Choose and Decrease for the Step-One[a] and Step-Two Diets

Foods to Choose	Foods to Decrease
MEAT, POULTRY, AND FISH	
Beef, pork, lamb—lean cuts well trimmed before cooking	Beef, pork, lamb—regular ground beef, fatty cuts, spare ribs, organ meats, sausage, regular luncheon meats, wieners, bacon
Poultry without skin	Poultry with skin, dried chicken
Fish, shellfish	Fried fish, fried shellfish
Processed meat—prepared from lean meat (e.g., turkey, ham, tuna wieners)	Regular luncheon meats (e.g., bologna, salami, sausage, wieners)
EGGS	
Egg whites (two whites equal one whole egg in recipes), cholesterol-free egg substitute	Egg yolks (if more than four per week on step one or if more than two per week on step two); includes eggs used in cooking
DAIRY PRODUCTS	
Milk—skim or 1% fat (fluid, powdered, evaporated), buttermilk	Whole milk (fluid, evaporated, condensed), 2% low-fat milk, imitation milk
Yogurt—nonfat or low-fat yogurt or yogurt beverages	Whole-milk yogurt, whole-milk yogurt beverages
Cheese—low-fat natural or processed cheese (part-skim mozzarella, ricotta) with no more than 6 g of fat per ounce on step one or 2 g of fat per ounce on step two	Regular cheese (American, blue, Brie, cheddar, Colby, Edam, Monterey Jack, whole-milk mozzarella, Parmesan, Swiss), cream cheese, Neufchâtel cheese
Cottage cheese—low fat, nonfat, or dry curd (0%–2% fat)	Cottage cheese (4% fat)
Frozen dairy dessert—ice milk, frozen yogurt (low fat or nonfat)	Ice cream
	Cream, half and half, whipping cream, nondairy creamer, whipped topping, sour cream

TABLE C.4 Foods to Choose and Decrease for the Step-One[a] and Step-Two Diets—cont'd

FATS AND OILS

Unsaturated oils—safflower, sunflower, corn, soybean, cottonseed, canola, olive, peanut	Coconut oil, palm kernel oil, palm oil
Margarine—made from unsaturated oils previously listed, light or diet margarine	Butter, lard, shortening, bacon fat
Salad dressings—made with unsaturated oils previously listed, low fat or oil free	Dressing made with egg yolk, cheese, sour cream, whole milk
Seeds and nuts—peanut butter, other nut butters	Coconut
Cocoa powder	Chocolate

BREADS AND CEREALS

Breads—whole-grain bread, hamburger and hot dog buns, corn tortillas	Bread in which eggs are a major ingredient, croissants
Cereals—oat, wheat, corn, multigrain	Granola made with coconut
Pasta	Egg noodles and pasta containing egg yolk
Rice	
Dry beans and peas	
Crackers—low-fat animal type, graham, saltine	High-fat crackers
Homemade baked goods using unsaturated oil, skim or 1% milk, and egg substitute—quick breads, biscuits, cornbread muffins, bran muffins, pancakes, waffles	Commercially baked pastries, muffins, biscuits
Soup—chicken or beef noodle, minestrone, tomato, vegetarian, potato	Soup containing whole milk, cream, meat fat, poultry fat, or poultry skin

VEGETABLES

Fresh, frozen, or canned vegetables	Vegetables prepared with butter, cheese, or cream sauce
Fruits	
Fruit—fresh, frozen, canned, or dried	Fried fruit or fruit served with butter or cream sauce
Fruit juice—fresh, frozen, or canned	
Sweets and modified-fat desserts	
Beverages—fruit-flavored drinks, lemonade, fruit punch	
Sweets—sugar, syrup, honey, jam, preserves, candy made without fat (candy corn, gumdrops, hard candy), fruit-flavored gelatin	Candy made with chocolate, coconut oil, palm kernel oil, palm oil
Frozen desserts—sherbet, sorbet, fruit ice, popsicles	Ice cream and frozen treats made with ice cream
Cookies, cake, pie, pudding—prepared with egg whites, egg substitute, skim milk or 1% milk, and unsaturated oil or margarine; gingersnaps; fig bar cookies; angel food cake	Commercially baked pies, cakes, doughnuts, high-fat cookies, cream pies

[a]The step one diet has the same nutrient recommendations as the eating pattern recommended for the general population.

From National Cholesterol Education Program: Report of the Expert Panel on Blood Cholesterol Levels in Children and Adolescents, *NIH Publication* No. 91-2732, September 1991.

Box C.1 American Heart Association's Pediatric Dietary Strategies for Individuals Aged Older Than 2 Years: Recommendations to All Patients and Families

- Balance dietary calories with physical activity to maintain normal growth.
- Have 60 minutes of moderate to vigorous play or physical activity daily.
- Eat vegetables and fruits daily, limit juice intake.
- Use vegetable oil and soft margarines low in saturated fat and trans-fatty acids instead of butter or most other animal fats in the diet.
- Eat whole-grain breads and cereals rather than refined grain products.
- Reduce the intake of sugar-sweetened beverages and foods.
- Use nonfat (skim) or low fat milk and dairy products daily.
- Eat more fish, especially oily fish, broiled or baked.
- Reduce salt intake, including salt from processed foods.

From Gidding SS, Dennison BA, Birch LL, et al; American Heart Association; American Academy of Pediatrics: Dietary recommendations for children and adolescents: a guide for practitioners, *Pediatrics* 117:544–559, 2006.

BOX C.2 Tips for Parents to Implement American Heart Association Pediatric Dietary Guidelines

- Reduce added sugars, including sugar-sweetened drinks and juices.
- Use canola, soybean, corn oil, safflower oil, or other unsaturated oils in place of solid fats during food preparation.
- Use recommended portion size on food labels when preparing and serving food.
- Use fresh, frozen, and canned vegetables and fruits and serve at every meal; be careful with added sauces and sugar.
- Introduce and regularly serve fish as an entrée.
- Remove the skin from poultry before eating.
- Use only lean cuts of meat and reduced-fat meat products.
- Limit high-calorie sauces such as Alfredo, cream sauces, cheese sauces, and hollandaise sauce.
- Eat whole-grain breads and cereals rather than refined products; read labels and ensure that "whole grain" is the first ingredient on the food label of these products.
- Eat more legumes (beans) and tofu in place of meat for some entrées.
- Breads, breakfast cereals, and prepared foods, including soups, may be high in salt and sugar; read food labels for content and choose high-fiber, low-salt, low sugar alternatives.

From Gidding SS, Dennison BA, Birch LL, et al; American Heart Association; American Academy of Pediatrics: Dietary recommendations for children and adolescents: a guide for practitioners, *Pediatrics* 117:544–559, 2006.

CDC Growth Charts: United States

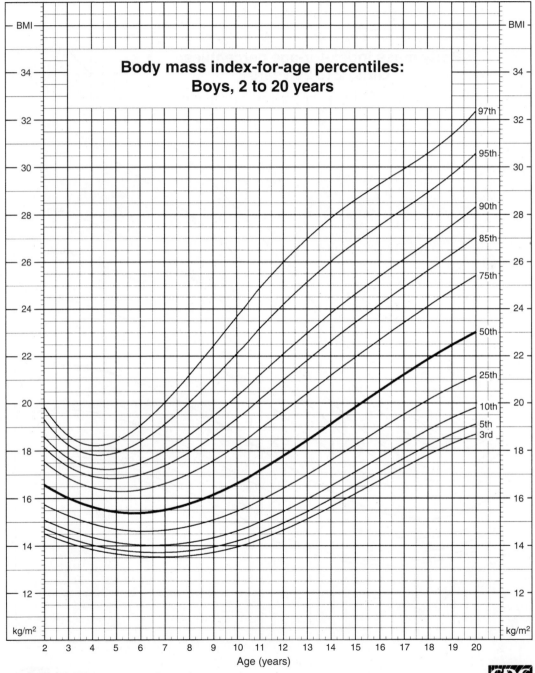

Body mass index-for-age percentiles:
Boys, 2 to 20 years

Published May 30, 2000.
SOURCE: Developed by the National Center for Health Statistics in collaboration with
the National Center for Chronic Disease Prevention and Health Promotion (2000).

SAFER·HEALTHIER·PEOPLE™

Fig. C.1 Centers for Disease Control and Prevention (CDC) body mass index percentile curves for boys 2 to 20 years old.

CDC Growth Charts: United States

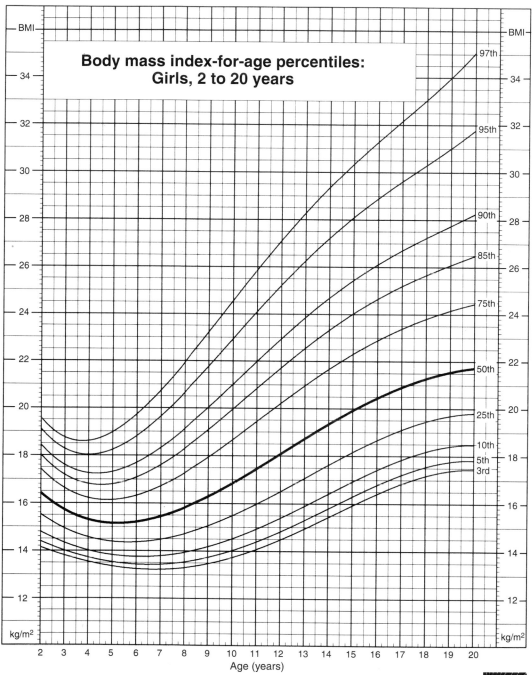

Body mass index-for-age percentiles:
Girls, 2 to 20 years

Published May 30, 2000.
SOURCE: Developed by the National Center for Health Statistics in collaboration with
the National Center for Chronic Disease Prevention and Health Promotion (2000).

Fig. C.2 Centers for Disease Control and Prevention (CDC) body mass index percentile curves for girls 2 to 20 years old.

Normal Echocardiographic Values

TABLE D.1 Two-Dimensional Echocardiography-Derived M-Mode Measurements of the Left Ventricular Dimension and Wall Thickness: Mean (-2 SD to +2 SD)[a]

Echo Views	BSA	0.2	0.3	0.4	0.5	0.6	0.7	0.8	0.9	1.0	1.2	1.4	1.6	1.8	2.0	2.2
RV	LV EDD	19.5 (15.5–23.0)	23.0 (19.0–27.0)	26.0 (22.0–30.5)	29.5 (24.5–34.0)	31.5 (27.0–36.5)	33.5 (29.0–38.5)	35.5 (30.5–41.0)	37.5 (32.0–43.0)	39.5 (33.5–45.0)	42.0 (36.0–48.0)	45.0 (38.5–51.0)	47.0 (40.5–54.0)	49.5 (42.5–57.0)	51.5 (44.0–60.0)	53.5 (45.5–62.0)
LV	IVS (D)	4.5 (3.0–5.5)	5.0 (3.5–6.0)	5.0 (4.0–6.5)	5.5 (4.0–7.0)	6.0 (4.5–7.5)	6.0 (4.5–8.0)	6.5 (4.5–8.5)	7.0 (5.0–9.0)	7.0 (5.0–9.5)	8.0 (5.5–10.0)	8.5 (6.0–11.0)	9.0 (6.0–12.0)	9.5 (6.5–12.5)	10.5 (7.0–13.5)	11.0 (7.5–14.5)
	LVPW (D)	4.0 (3.0–5.0)	4.5 (3.0–5.5)	4.5 (3.5–6.0)	5.0 (3.5–6.5)	5.5 (4.0–7.0)	6.0 (4.0–7.5)	6.0 (4.5–8.0)	6.5 (4.5–8.0)	7.0 (5.0–8.5)	7.5 (5.5–9.5)	8.0 (5.5–10.0)	8.5 (6.0–11.0)	9.0 (6.5–11.5)	9.5 (7.0–12.0)	10.0 (7.5–13.0)
RV	LV ESD	12.0 (8.0–15.0)	15.0 (11.5–18.0)	17.0 (13.5–20.0)	18.5 (15.0–22.5)	20.0 (16.5–24.5)	21.5 (17.5–26.0)	23.0 (18.5–28.0)	24.0 (19.5–29.0)	25.5 (20.5–31.0)	28.0 (22.0–33.5)	29.5 (23.5–35.5)	31.5 (24.5–37.5)	33.0 (25.5–39.5)	34.5 (26.5–41.5)	36.0 (27.5–43.0)
LV	IVS (S)	6.5 (5.0–8.0)	7.0 (5.5–9.0)	7.5 (6.0–9.5)	8.0 (6.0–10.0)	8.5 (6.5–10.5)	9.0 (7.0–11.0)	9.5 (7.5–11.5)	9.5 (7.5–12.0)	10.0 (8.0–12.5)	10.5 (8.0–13.5)	11.5 (9.0–14.5)	12.0 (9.0–15.5)	12.5 (9.5–16.5)	13.5 (10.0–18.0)	14.0 (10.0–19.0)
	LVPW (S)	6.5 (5.5–8.0)	7.0 (6.0–8.5)	8.0 (6.5–9.5)	9.0 (7.0–10.5)	9.5 (7.5–11.0)	10.0 (8.0–12.0)	10.5 (8.5–12.5)	11.5 (9.0–13.5)	11.5 (9.0–14.0)	12.5 (10.0–15.0)	13.0 (10.5–16.0)	14.0 (11.0–17.5)	14.5 (11.0–18.5)	15.0 (11.5–19.5)	16.0 (12.0–20.0)

[a]Values are rounded off to the nearest 0.5 mm.

AO, Aorta; AV, atrioventricular; BSA, body surface area; IVS (D), interventricular septal thickness, end diastolic; IVS (S), interventricular septal thickness, end systolic; LA, left atrium; LV, left ventricle; LVEDD, left ventricular end-diastolic dimension; LVESD, left ventricular end-systolic dimension; LVPW (D), left ventricular posterior wall thickness, end diastolic; LVPW (S), left ventricular posterior wall thickness, end systolic; RV, right ventricular; SD, standard deviation.

Values have been derived from graphic data of Lai WW, Mertens LL, Coher MS, Geva T (eds): Appendix 1. In Echocardiography in Pediatric and Congenital Heart Disease, Oxford, UK, 2010, Wiley-Blackwell.

TABLE D.2   **Stand-Alone M-Mode Echocardiographic Measurements: Right Ventricle, Aorta, and Left Atrium by Body Surface Area: Mean (90% Tolerance Limits) (in mm)[a]**

Echo Views	BSA	0.2	0.3	0.4	0.5	0.6	0.7	0.8	0.9	1.0	1.2	1.4	1.6	1.8	2.0
RV (diastolic)		7 (0–16)	9.5 (0–17)	10 (0–17)	10 (2.5–18)	11 (3–19)	12 (3.5–21)	13 (4–22)	14 (4.5–23)	14 (5–24)	16 (6–26)	18 (6.5–29)	20 (7–32)	22 (7.5–35)	23 (8–42)
LV															
Aorta (diastolic)		10 (6–14)	12 (7.5–16)	13 (9–17.5)	14 (9.5–19)	15 (10.5–21)	16 (11.5–22)	17 (12.5–24)	18 (13–24.5)	19 (13.5–25)	21 (14.5–27)	22 (15.5–29)	23 (16–30.5)	24 (16–32)	24 (16–33)
LA (systolic)		13 (6–20)	16 (8–23)	18 (9–25)	19 (11–27)	20 (12–29)	22 (13–31)	23 (14–33)	24 (15–34)	26 (16–35)	27 (17–38)	28 (17–40)	29 (18–42)	29 (18–43)	30 (18–44)

[a]Values rounded off to the nearest 0.5 mm for measurements <10 mm and to the nearest 1 mm for measurements ≥10 mm.

BSA, Body surface area; LA, left atrium; RV, right ventricle.

Values have been derived from graphic data of Roge CL, Silverman NH, Hart PA, Ray RM: Cardiac structure growth pattern determined by echocardiography, *Circulation* 57:285–290, 1978.

TABLE D.3   Two-Dimensional Echocardiographic Measurements of Aortic Root and Aorta: Mean (-2 SD To +2 SD) (in mm)[a]

Echo Views	BSA	0.2	0.3	0.4	0.5	0.6	0.7	0.8	0.9	1.0	1.2	1.4	1.6	1.8	2.0	2.2
	Aortic annulus	7.0 (5.5–9.0)	8.5 (7.0–10.0)	10.0 (8.0–12.0)	11.0 (9.0–13.5)	12.0 (10.0–14.5)	13.5 (11.0–15.5)	14.0 (11.5–16.5)	15.0 (12.5–17.5)	15.5 (13.9–18.5)	17.5 (14.5–20.5)	18.5 (15.0–22.0)	20.0 (16.0–23.5)	21.0 (17.0–25.0)	22.0 (18.0–26.0)	23.0 (18.5–27.5)
	Sinus of Valsalva	9.5 (7.0–12.0)	11.5 (9.0–14.0)	13.0 (10.0–16.0)	14.5 (11.5–17.5)	16.0 (13.0–19.5)	17.5 (14.0–21.0)	18.5 (15.5–22.05)	19.5 (15.5–23.5)	20.5 (16–25.0)	22.0 (18.0–27.0)	24.0 (19.0–30.0)	25.5 (20.0–31.5)	27.0 (21.0–33.5)	28.5 (22.0–35.5)	30.5 (23.0–38.5)
	Sinotubular junction	8.0 (6.0–10.0)	10.0 (7.5–12.0)	11.0 (9.0–13.5)	12.5 (10.0–15.0)	14.0 (11.0–16.5)	15.0 (12.0–18.0)	16.0 (12.5–19.0)	16.5 (13.0–20.5)	17.5 (14.0–21.5)	19.5 (15.5–24.0)	21.0 (16.5–26.0)	22.0 (17.0–27.5)	24.0 (18.0–29.0)	25.0 (19.0–31.0)	26.0 (20.0–32.0)
	Ascending aorta	8.0 (5.5–11.0)	10.0 (7.0–13.0)	11.5 (8.5–15.0)	13.0 (10.0–16.0)	14.5 (11.0–17.5)	15.5 (12.0–19.0)	16.5 (13.0–20.5)	17.5 (14.0–21.5)	18.5 (14.5–23.0)	20.5 (15.5–25.5)	22.0 (16.5–27.5)	24.0 (18.0–29.5)	25.5 (19.0–31.0)	26.5 (20.0–33.0)	28.0 (21.0–35.0)
	Transverse aorta	6.5 (4.0–8.5)	8.0 (5.5–10.0)	9.5 (8.0–13.0)	10.5 (8.0–13.0)	11.5 (9.0–14.5)	12.5 (9.5–15.5)	13.0 (10.0–17.0)	14.0 (11.0–18.0)	15.0 (11.5–19.0)	17.0 (12.5–20.5)	18.0 (14.0–22.0)	19.5 (15.0–24.0)	20.5 (15.5–25.5)	21.5 (16.0–27.0)	22.5 (17.0–28.5)
	Aortic isthmus	5.5 (3.0–7.5)	6.5 (4.0–9.0)	7.5 (5.0–10.0)	8.5 (6.0–11.0)	9.5 (6.5–12.5)	10.5 (7.0–13.5)	11.0 (7.5–14.5)	12.0 (8.0–15.5)	12.5 (8.5–16.0)	13.5 (9.5–17.5)	15.0 (10.0–19.5)	16.0 (10.5–21.0)	17.0 (11.0–22.0)	17.5 (11.5–23.5)	18.0 (12.0–25.0)

[a]Values are rounded off to the nearest 0.5 mm.

BSA, Body surface area; SD, standard deviation.

Values have been derived from graphic data of Lai WW, Mertens LL, Cohen MS, Geva T (eds): Appendix 1. In *Echocardiography in Pediatric and Congenital Heart Disease*, Oxford, UK, 2010, Wiley-Blackwell.

TABLE D.4 **Two-Dimensional Echocardiographic Measurements of the Pulmonary Valve and Pulmonary Arteries (in mm): Mean (-2 SD to +2 SD)[a]**

Echo Views	BSA	0.2	0.3	0.4	0.5	0.6	0.7	0.8	0.9	1.0	1.2	1.4	1.6	1.8	2.0	2.2
	Pulmonary annulus	8.5 (6.0–10.5)	10.0 (8.0–12.5)	11.5 (9.0–14.0)	13.0 (10.0–16.0)	14.0 (11.0–17.5)	15.5 (11.5–19.0)	16.5 (12.0–20.5)	17.5 (13.0–21.5)	18.5 (13.5–23.0)	20.0 (15.0–25.0)	22.0 (16.0–27.5)	23.5 (17.0–29.0)	25.0 (18.0–30.5)	26.0 (19.0–33.0)	27.0 (19.5–34.0)
	Main PA	7.5 (5.0–10.0)	9.0 (6.5–12.0)	10.5 (7.5–14.0)	12.0 (9.0–15.0)	13.0 (9.5–16.5)	14.0 (10.0–17.5)	15.0 (11.0–18.5)	16.0 (11.5–20.0)	17.0 (12.0–21.0)	18.5 (13.5–23.0)	20.0 (14.5–25.5)	21.0 (15.0–28.0)	22.5 (16.0–30.0)	24.0 (16.5–32.0)	25.0 (17.0–33.0)
	Right PA	5.0 (3.5–7.0)	6.0 (4.5–8.0)	7.0 (5.0–9.0)	8.0 (5.5–10.0)	9.0 (6.0–11.0)	9.5 (6.5–12.0)	10.0 (7.0–13.0)	10.5 (7.5–13.5)	11.0 (8.0–14.0)	12.5 (9.0–16.0)	13.0 (9.5–17.5)	14.0 (10.0–18.5)	15.0 (10.5–20.0)	15.5 (10.5–21.0)	16.5 (11.0–22.0)
	Left PA	4.5 (3.0–6.5)	5.5 (4.0–7.5)	6.5 (4.5–8.5)	7.5 (5.0–9.5)	8.0 (5.5–10.5)	9.0 (6.0–11.0)	9.5 (6.5–12.0)	10.0 (7.0–13.0)	10.5 (7.5–14.0)	11.5 (8.0–15.5)	12.5 (8.5–16.5)	13.5 (9.0–18.0)	14.0 (9.0–19.0)	15.0 (9.5–20.0)	15.5 (10.0–21.0)

[a]Values are rounded off to the nearest 0.5 mm.

BSA, Body surface area; PA, pulmonary artery; SD, standard deviation.

Values have been derived from graphic data of Lai WW, Mertens LL, Cohen MS, Geva T (eds): Appendix 1. In *Echocardiography in Pediatric and Congenital Heart Disease*, Oxford, UK, 2010, Wiley-Blackwell.

TABLE D.5   Two-Dimensional Echocardiographic Measurements of Atrioventricular Valves (in mm): Mean (-2 SD to +2 SD)[a]

Echo Views		BSA	0.2	0.3	0.4	0.5	0.6	0.7	0.8	0.9	1.0	1.2	1.4	1.6	1.8	2.0	2.2
	Mitral (apical-four chamber)		10.0 (8.0–12.0)	12.5 (9.5–15.0)	13.5 (10.5–17.5)	15.1 (12.0–19.0)	17.0 (12.5–21.0)	18.0 (13.5–22.5)	19.0 (14.5–24.0)	20.5 (15.0–25.5)	22.0 (15.5–27.5)	23.5 (16.5–30.0)	25.0 (17.5–33.0)	27.0 (18.0–35.5)	28.0 (18.5–37.5)	29.5 (19.0–40.0)	31.0 (19.0–42.0)
	Tricuspid (apical-four chamber)		11.0 (7.5–14.0)	13.0 (8.5–17.0)	15.0 (10.5–18.5)	17.0 (12.0–20.5)	18.0 (13.0–22.5)	19.0 (14.0–23.5)	20.0 (15.0–25.0)	21.5 (16.0–27.5)	22.5 (17.0–28.0)	24.0 (18.0–30.5)	26.5 (19.0–33.0)	28.0 (20.5–35.0)	29.5 (21.5–37.5)	31.0 (22.5–39.5)	32.5 (23.5–42.0)
	Mitral (parasternal-long)		10.0 (7.5–12.5)	11.5 (9.0–15.0)	13.0 (10.0–16.0)	14.5 (11.0–18.0)	16.0 (12.0–19.5)	17.0 (12.5–21.0)	18.0 (13.0–22.5)	19.0 (14.0–23.0)	20.0 (15.0–25.0)	22.0 (16.0–27.5)	23.0 (17.0–30.0)	25.0 (18.0–32.0)	26.0 (18.5–34.5)	28.0 (19.0–37.0)	29.0 (20.0–39.0)
	Tricuspid (RV inflow view)		10.5 (7.5–13.0)	12.5 (9.0–15.5)	14.5 (10.5–17.5)	15.5 (12.5–19.5)	17.5 (13.0–22.0)	18.5 (14.0–23.0)	20.0 (15.0–25.0)	21.5 (16.0–27.0)	22.0 (17.0–28.0)	23.5 (17.5–30.5)	25.5 (18.5–33.0)	27.5 (19.5–35.5)	29.0 (20.5–38.0)	30.5 (21.5–40.0)	32.5 (22.5–42.5)

[a]Values are rounded off to the nearest 0.5 mm.

BSA, Body surface area; RV, right ventricular; SD, standard deviation.

Values have been derived from graphic data of Lai WW, Mertens LL, Cohen MS, Geva T (eds): Appendix 1. In Echocardiography in Pediatric and Congenital Heart Disease, Oxford, UK, 2010, Wiley-Blackwell.

TABLE D.6   Two-Dimensional Echocardiographic Measurements of Mean and Prediction Limits for 2 and 3 Standard Deviations for Major Coronary Artery Segments[a]

Echo Views		BSA	0.2	0.3	0.4	0.5	0.6	0.7	0.8	1.0	1.2	1.4	1.6	1.8	2.0
	LAD	Mean	1.2	1.4	1.6	1.8	1.9	2.0	2.2	2.3	2.5	2.7	2.8	2.9	3.0
		Mean + 2 SD	1.5	1.8	2.1	2.3	2.5	2.7	2.8	3.0	3.3	3.5	3.7	4.0	4.2
		Mean + 3 SD	1.7	2.0	2.3	2.5	2.8	3.0	3.2	3.4	3.8	4.0	4.3	4.5	4.7
	RCA	Mean	1.3	1.4	1.6	1.7	1.8	2.0	2.1	2.3	2.5	2.7	2.8	3.0	3.2
		Mean + 2 SD	1.9	2.1	2.3	2.4	2.6	2.7	2.8	3.1	3.4	3.6	3.8	4.0	4.3
		Mean + 3 SD	2.2	2.4	2.6	2.8	3.0	3.1	3.3	3.5	3.8	4.1	4.3	4.5	4.8
	LMCA	Mean	1.7	1.9	2.1	2.3	2.4	2.5	2.7	2.9	3.1	3.3	3.4	3.6	3.7
		Mean + 2 SD	2.3	2.6	2.8	3.0	3.3	3.4	3.6	3.9	4.2	4.4	4.6	4.8	5.1
		Mean + 3 SD	2.7	3.0	3.2	3.4	3.7	3.9	4.0	4.3	4.7	4.9	5.2	5.5	5.8

[a]Measurements are made from inner edge to inner edge. Values are rounded off to the nearest 0.1 mm.
BSA, Body surface area; LCA, left anterior descending coronary artery; LMCA, left main coronary artery; RCA, right coronary artery; SD, standard deviation.
Values are from graphic data of Kurotobi S, Nagai T, Kawakami N, Sano T: Coronary diameter in normal infants, children and patients with Kawasaki disease, Pediatr Int 44:1–4, 2002.

TABLE D.7 Left Ventricular Mass and Left Ventricular Mass Index by M-Mode Echocardiography

Boys

Age	Left Ventricular Mass (g)				Left Ventricular Mass Index (g/m$^{2.7}$)			
	50th Percentile	90th Percentile	95th Percentile	Maximum	50th Percentile	90th Percentile	95th Percentile	Maximum
<6 mo	10.94	16.28	17.60	21.18	56.44	75.72	80.10	83.00
6 mo ≤2 yr	23.88	32.47	33.70	36.32	44.95	61.27	68.60	74.75
2 ≤4 yr	33.32	45.48	48.4	58.13	39.50	48.74	52.40	77.07
4 ≤6 yr	45.49	59.26	63.20	83.51	36.96	45.12	48.10	57.25
6 ≤8 yr	51.73	70.48	77.40	97.29	32.79	40.18	44.60	59.47
8 ≤10 yr	62.09	84.61	91.10	122.0	29.11	38.25	41.00	53.19
10 ≤12 yr	74.10	105.3	111.0	124.7	28.18	36.42	38.20	43.05
12 ≤14 yr	97.76	138.1	150.0	202.3	28.8	39.08	41.40	47.75
14 ≤16 yr	125.7	167.2	181.0	212.0	28.77	38.47	40.50	46.01
≥16 yr	131.5	183.1	204.0	256.7	29.0	37.73	39.4	46.33

Girls

Age	Left Ventricular Mass (g)				Left Ventricular Mass Index (g/m$^{2.7}$)			
	50th Percentile	90th Percentile	95th Percentile	Maximum	50th Percentile	90th Percentile	95th Percentile	Maximum
<6 mo	11.15	16.05	16.50	28.74	55.38	73.47	85.60	109.2
6 mo ≤2 yr	22.25	31.98	34.60	35.98	42.04	52.86	57.10	61.06
2 ≤4 yr	33.38	43.88	46.10	50.98	37.88	47.65	55.30	66.58
4 ≤6 yr	39.67	50.38	57.30	76.64	32.29	43.47	44.30	59.25
6 ≤8 yr	48.38	65.54	72.10	89.30	29.71	37.73	43.50	54.76
8 ≤10 yr	54.76	75.49	83.60	91.82	26.63	34.30	36.00	44.35
10 ≤12 yr	71.66	98.00	102.0	149.1	26.11	330.5	35.70	44.88
12 ≤14 yr	92.36	119.8	128.0	165.9	26.68	34.65	38.20	43.59
14 ≤16 yr	98.73	130.0	143.0	235.0	26.51	34.89	36.90	54.33
≥16 yr	101.6	139.5	154.0	201.4	26.35	37.93	40.00	50.74

From Khoury PR, Mitsnefes M, Daniels SR, Kimball TR: Age-specific reference intervals for indexed left ventricular mass in children, *J Am Soc Echocardiogr* 22:709–714, 2009.

TABLE D.8   Left Ventricular Mass Using the 5/6AL by Body Surface Area: Mean (-2 SD to +2 SD)[a]

BSA	0.3	0.4	0.5	0.6	0.7	0.8	0.9	1.0	1.1	1.2
LV mass	13 (9–20)	19 (12–28)	24 (16–36)	31 (20–44)	37 (25–53)	44 (30–62)	51 (36–71)	60 (40–80)	66 (47–92)	72 (52–102)
BSA	**1.3**	**1.4**	**1.5**	**1.6**	**1.7**	**1.8**	**1.9**	**2.0**	**2.1**	**2.2**
LV mass	80 (58–112)	91 (64–123)	102 (70–136)	110 (77–144)	120 (83–154)	130 (90–166)	138 (100–178)	148 (108–190)	158 (114–202)	166 (122–212)

[a]Values are rounded off to the nearest 1 gram.

BSA, Body surface area; *LV,* left ventricular; *SD,* standard deviation.

Values have been derived from graphic data of Lai WW, Mertens LL, Cohen MS, Geva T (eds): Figure left ventricular mass using the 5/6 × area × length algorithm (5/6AL) versus body surface area from *Echocardiography in Pediatric and Congenital Heart Disease*, Oxford, UK, 2010, Wiley-Blackwell.

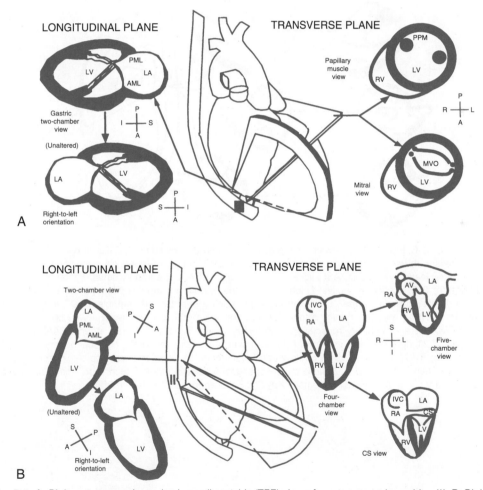

Fig. D.1 A, Biplane transesophageal echocardiographic (TEE) views from transgastric position III. **B,** Biplane TEE views at midesophageal position II.

Continued

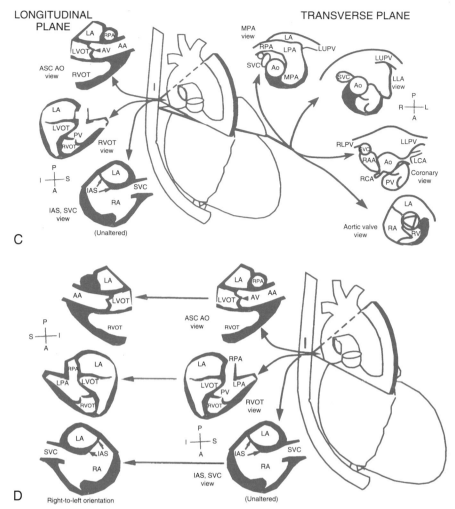

Fig. D.1, cont'd C, Biplane TEE views from the base of the heart at position I. **D,** Basal views of the heart and great vessels with use of the longitudinal plane probe at position I. *A,* Anterior; *AA,* ascending aorta; *AML,* anterior mitral leaflet; *AO,* aorta; *ASC,* ascending; *AV,* aortic valve; *CS,* coronary sinus; *I,* inferior; *IAS,* inter-atrial septum; *IVC,* inferior vena cava; *L,* left; *LA,* left atrium; *LAA,* left atrial appendage; *LCA,* left coronary artery; *LPA,* left pulmonary artery; *LUPV,* left upper pulmonary vein; *LV,* left ventricle; *LVOT,* left ventricular outflow tract; *MPA,* main pulmonary artery; *MVO,* mitral valve orifice; *P,* posterior; *PML,* posterior mitral leaflet; *PPM,* posterior papillary muscle; *PV,* pulmonary valve; *R,* right; *RA,* right atrium; *RAA,* right atrial appendage; *RCA,* right coronary artery; *RLPV,* right lower pulmonary vein; *RPA,* right pulmonary artery; *RV,* right ventricle; *RVOT,* right ventricular outflow tract; *S,* superior; *SVC,* superior vena cava. (From Bansal RC, Shakudo M, Shah PM, Shah PM: Biplane transesophageal echocardiography: technique, image orientation, and preliminary experience in 131 patients, *J Am Soc Echocardiogr* 3:348–366, 1990.)

Drugs Used in Pediatric Cardiology

TABLE E.1   Dosages of Drugs Used in Pediatric Cardiology

Drug	Route and Dosage	Toxicity or Side Effects	How Supplied
Acetaminophen (Tylenol, paracetamol)	*For PDA closure in premature infants:* IV or PO: 15 mg/kg q6hr for 3–7 days Or 20 mg/kg loading dose followed by 7.5 mg/kg q6hr for 3–7 days (Treatment duration is guided by echocardiographic findings)	Increase in ALT, AST, hepatotoxicity Rare: Stevens-Johnson Syndrome, toxic epidermal necrolysis, acute generalized exanthematous pustulosis	Inj: 10 mg/mL Susp: 32 mg/mL
Acetazolamide (Diamox) (carbonic anhydrase inhibitor, diuretic)	*Children:* IV, PO: 5 mg/kg/dose QD–QOD *Adults:* IV, PO: 250–375 mg/dose QD–QOD	GI irritation, paresthesia, sedation, hypokalemia, acidosis, reduced urate secretion, aplastic anemia, polyuria, renal calculi Contraindications: hepatic failure, severe renal failure, sulfonamide hypersensitivity	Tabs: 125, 250 mg Susp: 25, 50 mg/mL Caps: sustained release: 500 mg Inj: 500 mg/5 mL
Acetylsalicylic acid (aspirin)	*Children and adults:* **Antiplatelet therapy:** PO: 3–5 mg/kg QD **Antipyretic/analgesic:** PO, PR: 10–15 mg/kg/dose, q4–6 hr (Max, 4 g/24 hr) **Antiinflammatory:** PO: 80–100 mg/kg/24 hr TID–QID	Rash, nausea, hepatotoxicity, GI bleeding, bronchospasm, GI distress, tinnitus Contraindications: hepatic failure, bleeding disorder, hypersensitivity, children <16 yr old with chickenpox or flu symptoms (because of the association with Reye's syndrome)	Tabs: 325, 500 mg Tabs, enteric coated: 81,165, 325, 500, 650 mg Tabs, chewable: 81 mg Supp: 60, 80, 120, 125, 200, 300, 325, 600, 650 mg, and 1.2 g
Adenosine (Adenocard) (antiarrhythmic)	*For SVT:* *Children and adults:* IV: 100–200 mcg/kg Repeat q1–2 min, with increment of 50 mcg/kg, to maximum of 250 mcg/kg (Max single dose, 12 mg)	Bronchospasm, chest pain, transient asystole, bradycardia and tachycardia Transient AV block in atrial flutter or fibrillation (±)	Inj: 3 mg/mL (2, 5 mL)
Amiodarone (Cordarone) (class III antiarrhythmic)	*Children:* IV (in emergency situation): *Loading:* 5 mg/kg, slow infusion over 30 min followed by infusion of 7 mcg/kg/min (which is calculated to deliver 10 mg/kg/24 hr); switch to oral maintenance dose as soon as clinical condition permits PO: 10–20 mg/kg/24 hr (*infants*) or 10 mg/kg/24 hr (*children and adolescents*) in two doses for 5–14 days, followed by maintenance dose of 5–7 mg/kg once a day [*Therapeutic level:* 0.5–2.5 mg/L] *Adults:* PO: *Loading:* 800–1600 mg QD for 1–3 wk; then reduce to 600–800 mg QD for 1 mo *Maintenance:* 200–400 mg QD	Progressive dyspnea and cough (pulmonary fibrosis), worsening of arrhythmias, hepatotoxicity, nausea and vomiting, corneal microdeposits, hypotension, heart block, ataxia, hypo- or hyperthyroidism, photosensitivity Contraindications: AV block, sinus node dysfunction, sinus bradycardia	Tabs: 200, 400 mg Susp: 5 mg/mL Inj: 50 mg/mL

Continued

TABLE E.1   Dosages of Drugs Used in Pediatric Cardiology—cont'd

Drug	Route and Dosage	Toxicity or Side Effects	How Supplied
Amlodipine (Norvasc) (CCB, antihypertensive)	*For hypertension:* *Children:* PO: Initial 0.1 mg/kg/dose QD–BID; may be increased gradually to a max of 0.6 mg/kg/24 hr *Adults:* PO: 5–10 mg/dose QD (Max, 10 mg/24 hr)	Edema, dizziness, flushing, palpitation, headache, fatigue, nausea, abdominal pain, somnolence	Tabs: 2.5, 5, 10 mg Susp: 1 mg/mL
Amrinone (Inocor) (noncatecholamine inotropic agent with vasodilator effects)	*Children* IV: *Loading:* 0.5 mg/kg over 2–3 min in ½ NS (not D_5W) *Maintenance:* 5–20 mcg/kg/min *Adults:* IV: *Loading:* 0.75 mg/kg over 2–3 min *Maintenance:* 5–10 mcg/kg/min	Thrombocytopenia, hypotension, tachyarrhythmia, hepatotoxicity, nausea and vomiting, fever	Inj: 5 mg/mL (20 mL)
Atenolol (Tenormin) (β_1-adrenoceptor blocker, antihypertensive, antiarrhythmic)	*Children:* PO: 1–2 mg/kg/dose QD *Adults:* PO: 25–100 mg/dose QD for 1–2 wk (alone or with diuretic for hypertension); may increase to 200 mg QD	CNS symptoms (dizziness, tiredness, depression), bradycardia, postural hypotension, nausea and vomiting, rash, blood dyscrasias (agranulocytosis, purpura)	Tabs: 25, 50, 100 mg Susp: 2 mg/mL Inj: 0.5 mg/mL (10 mL)
Atorvastatin (Lipitor) (antilipemic, "statin", HMG-CoA reductase inhibitor)	*Children:* PO: Starting dose, 10 mg QD for 4–6 wk; increase to 20 mg QD and 40 mg QD as needed (Adult max dose, 80 mg/24 hr)	Headache, constipation, diarrhea, elevated liver enzymes, rhabdomyolysis, myopathy	Tabs: 10, 20, 40, 80 mg
Azathioprine (Imuran, Azasan) (immunosuppressant)	*Children:* IV, PO: *Initial:* 3–5 mg/kg/24 hr QD *Maintenance:* 1–3 mg/kg/24 hr (to produce WBC count ~5000/mm³); may be reduced if WBC count falls below 4000/mm³	Bone marrow suppression (leukopenia, thrombocytopenia, anemia), GI symptoms (nausea and vomiting)	Tabs: 25, 50, 75, 100 mg Susp: 50 mg/mL Inj: 100 mg powder for reconst
Bosentan (Tracleer) (nonselective endothelin receptor blocker)	*For pulmonary hypertension:* *Children:* PO: *<20 kg:* 31.25 mg BID *20–40 kg:* 62.5 mg BID *>40 kg:* 125 mg BID *Adults:* PO: 125 mg BID	Liver dysfunction, decrease in hemoglobin, fluid retention, heart failure, headache	Tabs: 62.5, 125 mg
Bumetanide (Bumex) (loop diuretic)	*Children:* PO, IM, IV: >6 mo: 0.015–0.1 mg/kg/dose QD–QOD *Adults:* PO: 0.5–2 mg/dose QD–BID IV: 0.5–1 mg over 1–2 min, q2–3 hr PRN (Max, 10 mg/24 hr)	Hypotension, cramps, dizziness, headache, electrolyte losses (hypokalemia, hypocalcemia, hyponatremia, hypochloremia), metabolic alkalosis	Tabs: 0.5, 1, 2 mg Inj: 0.25 mg/mL
Calcium glubionate (Neo-Calglucon 6.4% elemental calcium) (calcium supplement)	*For neonatal hypocalcemia:* PO: 1200 mg/kg/24 hr, q4–6 hr *Maintenance:* *Infants and children:* PO: 600–2000 mg/kg/24 hr QID (Max, 9 g/24 hr) *Adults:* PO: 6–18 g/24 hr QID	GI irritation, diarrhea, dizziness, headache Best absorbed when given before meals	Syrup: 1.8 g/5 mL (480 mL) (1.2 mEq Ca/mL)

TABLE E.1   Dosages of Drugs Used in Pediatric Cardiology—cont'd

Drug	Route and Dosage	Toxicity or Side Effects	How Supplied
Captopril (Capoten) (ACE inhibitor, antihypertensive, vasodilator)	*Neonates:* PO: 0.1–0.4 mg/kg/24 hr TID–QID *Infants:* PO: Initially 0.15–0.3 mg/kg/dose QD–QID; titrate upward if needed (Max, 6 mg/kg/24 hr) *Children:* PO: Initially 0.3–0.5 mg/kg/dose TID; titrate upward if needed (Max, 6 mg/kg/24 hr BID–QID) *Adolescents and adults:* PO: Initially 12.5–25 mg/dose BID–TID; increase weekly if needed by 25 mg/dose to max dose, 450 mg/24 hr (Adjust dose with renal failure)	Neutropenia or agranulocytosis, proteinuria, hypotension and tachycardia, rash, taste impairment, hyperkalemia Evidence of fetal risk if given during second and third trimesters (same with all other ACE inhibitors)	Tabs: 12.5, 25, 50, 100 mg Susp: 0.75, 1 mg/mL
Carnitine (Carnitor)	*Children:* PO: 50–100 mg/kg/24 hr BID–TID; increase slowly as needed (Max, 3 g/24 hr) *Adults:* PO: 330 mg–1 g/dose BID–TID IV (*child and adult*): 50 mg/kg as loading dose; then 50 mg/kg/24 hr, q4–6 hr	Nausea and vomiting, abdominal cramps, diarrhea, seizure	Tabs: 330, 500 mg Caps: 250 mg Oral sol: 100 mg/mL (118 mL) Inj: 200 mg/mL (5 mL)
Carvedilol (Coreg, Coreg CR) (nonselective α- and β-adrenergic blocker)	*Children:* PO: Initial 0.09 mg/kg/dose BID; increase gradually to 0.36 and 0.75 mg/kg as tolerated to adult max dose, 50 mg/24 hr *Adults:* PO: 3.125 mg BID for 2 wk; increase slowly to a max dose of 25 mg BID as needed (for heart failure) (Max, 25 mg BID for <85 kg; 50 mg BID for >85 kg)	Dizziness, hypotension, headache, diarrhea, rarely AV block	Tabs: 3.125, 6.125, 12.5, 25 mg Tabs, extended release: 10, 20, 40, 80 mg
Chloral hydrate (Noctec, Aquachloral) (sedative, hypnotic)	**As sedative:** *Children:* PO, PR: 25–50 mg/kg/dose q6–8 hr Sedation for procedures: 25–100 mg (Max dose, 2 g) *Adults:* PO, PR: 250 mg/dose q8 hr **As hypnotic:** *Adults:* PO, PR: 500–2000 mg/dose	Mucous membrane irritation (laryngospasm if aspirated), GI irritation, excitement or delirium, hypotension Contraindicated in hepatic and renal impairment	Caps: 500 mg Syrup: 250, 500 mg/5 mL Supp: 324, 500, 648 mg
Chlorothiazide (Diuril) (diuretic)	*Children:* PO: 20–40 mg/kg/24 hr BID IV: 2–8 mg/kg/24 hr BID *Adults:* PO, IV: 250–2000 mg/dose QD–BID	Hypercalcemia, hyperbilirubinemia, hyperglycemia, hyperuricemia, hypochloremic alkalosis, hypokalemia, hyponatremia, prerenal azotemia, hyperlipidemia, rarely pancreatitis, blood dyscrasias, allergic reactions	Tabs: 250, 500 mg Susp: 250 mg/5 mL (237 mL) Inj: 500 mg powder for reconst with 18 mL of sterile water
Cholestyramine (Questran, Prevalite) (antilipemic, bile acid sequestrant)	*Children:* PO: 250–1500 mg/kg/24 hr BID–QID *Adults:* PO: *Starting:* 1 packet (or scoopful) of Questran powder or Questran Light 1–2 times/day *Maintenance:* 2–4 packets or scoopfuls/24 hr in 2 doses (or 1–6 doses) (Max, 6 packets/24 hr)	Constipation and other GI symptoms, bleeding, hyperchloremic acidosis	Packet of 9-g Questran powder or 5-g Questran Light, each packet containing 4 g of anhydrous cholestyramine resin

Continued

TABLE E.1   Dosages of Drugs Used in Pediatric Cardiology—cont'd

Drug	Route and Dosage	Toxicity or Side Effects	How Supplied
Clofibrate (Atromid-S) (antilipemic, triglyceride-lowering agent)	*Children:* PO: 0.5–1.5 mg/24 hr BID–TID *Adults:* PO: *Initial and maintenance:* 2 g/24 hr BID–TID	Nausea and other GI symptoms (vomiting, diarrhea, flatulence), headache, dizziness, fatigue, rash, blood dyscrasias, myalgia, arthralgia, hepatic dysfunction	Caps: 500 mg
Clopidogrel (Plavix) (antiplatelet)	*Children:* PO: 1 mg/kg/24 hr to max (adult dose) of 75 mg/24 hr *Adults:* PO: 75 mg/dose QD	Bleeding, especially when used with aspirin, neutropenia or agranulocytosis, abdominal pain constipation, rash, syncope, palpitation	Tabs: 75 mg
Colestipol (Colestid) (antilipemic, bile acid sequestrant)	*Children:* PO: 300–1500 mg/24 hr in 2–4 doses *Adults:* PO: *Starting dose:* 5 g 1–2 times/24 hr; increment of 5 g q1–2 mo *Maintenance:* 5–30 g/24 hr BID–QID (mix with 3–6 oz water or another fluid)	Constipation and other GI symptoms (abdominal distention, flatulence, nausea and vomiting, diarrhea), rarely rash, muscle and joint pain, headache, dizziness	Packet: 5 g
Cyclosporine, cyclosporine microemulsion (Sandimmune, Gengraf, Neoral) (immunosuppressant)	*Children:* PO: 15 mg/kg as a single dose given 4–12 hr pretransplant; give same daily dose for 1–2 wk posttransplant; then reduce by 5% per wk to 5–10 mg/kg/24 hr QD–BID [*Therapeutic level:* 100–300 ng/mL] IV: 5–6 mg/kg as a single dose given 4–12 hr pretransplant; administer over 2–6 hr; give same dose posttransplant until patient able to tolerate oral form	Nephrotoxicity, tremor, hypertension, less commonly hepatotoxicity, hyperlipidemia, hirsutism, gum hypertrophy, rarely lymphoma, hypomagnesemia	Oral sol: 100 mg/mL (50 mL) Neoral sol: 100 mg/mL (50 mL) Caps: 25, 50, 100 mg Neoral caps: 25, 100 mg Inj: 50 mg/mL
Diazoxide (Hyperstat IV, Proglycem) (Antihypertensive, peripheral vasodilator)	*For hypertensive crisis:* *Children and adults:* IV: 1–3 mg/kg (max, 150 mg single dose); repeat q5–15 min; titrate to desired effect	Hypotension, transient hyperglycemia, nausea and vomiting, sodium retention (CHF±)	Inj: 15 mg/mL
Digoxin (Lanoxin, Digitek) (cardiac glycoside, antiarrhythmic, inotrope)	*Children:* PO: *Total digitalizing dose:* Premature infant: 20 mcg/kg; Full term newborn: 30 mcg/kg; Child 1 mo–2 yr: 40–50 mcg/kg; Child >2–10 yr: 30–40 mcg/kg; >10 yr and <100 kg: 10–15 mcg/kg PO: *Maintenance:* 25%–30% of TDD/24 hr BID IV: 75%–80% of PO dose *Adults:* PO: *Loading:* 8–12 mcg/kg *Maintenance:* 0.10–0.25 mg/24 hr [*Therapeutic level:* 0.8–2 ng/mL]	AV conduction disturbances, arrhythmias, nausea and vomiting	Elixir: 50 mcg/mL (60 mL) Tabs: 125, 250, mcg Caps: 50, 100, 200 mcg Inj: 100, 250 mcg/mL
Digoxin immune Fab (Digibind, Digifab) (antidigoxin antibody)	*Infants and children:* IV: 1 vial (40 mg) dissolved in 4 mL H₂O over 30 min *Adults:* IV: 4 vials (240 mg)	Allergic reaction (rare), hypokalemia, rapid AV conduction in atrial flutter	Inj: 38, 40 mg powder for reconst

TABLE E.1   Dosages of Drugs Used in Pediatric Cardiology—cont'd

Drug	Route and Dosage	Toxicity or Side Effects	How Supplied
Diltiazem (Cardizem, Cardizem SR, Cardizem CD, Dilacor XR, Tiazac) (CCB, antihypertensive)	*Children:* PO: 1.5–2 mg/kg/24 hr TID–QID (Max, 3.5 mg/kg/24 hr) *Adolescents:* Immediate release: PO: 30–120 mg/dose TID–QID; usual range, 180–360 mg/24 hr Extended release: PO: 120–300 mg/24 hr QD–BID (BID dosing with Cardizem SR; QD dosing with Cardizem CD, Dilacor XR, and Tiazac)	Dizziness, headache, edema, nausea and vomiting, heart block, and arrhythmias Contraindicated in second- and third-degree AV block, sinus node dysfunction, acute MI with pulmonary congestion Maximum antihypertensive effect seen within 2 weeks	Tabs: 30, 60, 90, 120 mg Tabs, extended release: 120, 180, 240, 300, 360, 420 mg Caps, extended release: 60, 90, 120, 180, 240, 300, 360, 420 mg Inj: 5 mg/mL (5, 10 mL)
Dipyridamole (Persantine) (antiplatelet)	*Children:* PO: 2–6 mg/kg/24 hr TID *Adults:* PO: 75–100 mg QID (As an adjunct to warfarin therapy; not to use with aspirin)	Vasodilation, rarely dizziness, angina	Tabs: 25, 50, 75 mg
Disopyramide (Norpace) (class IA antiarrhythmic)	*Children:* PO: <1 yr: 10–30 mg/kg/24 hr, q6 hr 1–4 yr: 10–20 mg/kg/24 hr, q6 hr 4–12 yr: 10–15 mg/kg/24 hr, q6 hr 12–18 yr: 6–15 mg/kg/24 hr, q6 hr (q4 hr dosing when using regular caps) *Adults:* PO: 150 mg/dose q6 hr or 300 mg (extended release) q12 hr (Max, 1.6 g/24 hr) [*Therapeutic level:* 3–7 mg/L]	Heart failure or hypotension, anticholinergic effects (urinary retention, dry mouth, constipation), nausea and vomiting, hypoglycemia	Caps: 100, 150 mg Caps, CR: 100, 150 mg Susp: 1 mg/mL, 10 mg/mL
Dobutamine (Dobutrex) (β-adrenergic stimulator)	*Children:* IV infusion: 2.5–15 mcg/kg/min in D_5W or NS (incompatible with alkali solution) (Max, 40 mcg/kg/min) *Adults:* IV infusion: 2.5–10 mcg/kg/min (Max, 40 mcg/kg/min)	Tachyarrhythmias, hypertension, nausea and vomiting, headache Contraindicated in HOCM and atrial flutter or fibrillation	Inj: 12.5 mg/mL (20 mL)
Dopamine (Intropin, Dopastat) (natural catecholamine inotropic agent)	*Children:* IV: Effects are dose dependent: 2–5 mcg/kg/min—increases RBF and urine output (minimum effects on heart rate and cardiac output) 5–15 mcg/kg/min—increases heart rate, cardiac contractility, and cardiac output >20 mcg/kg/min—α-adrenergic effects with decreased RBF (±) (Incompatible with alkali solution)	Tachyarrhythmias, nausea and vomiting, hypotension or hypertension, extravasation (tissue necrosis [treat with local infiltration of phentolamine])	Inj: 40, 80, 160 mg/mL (5, 10, 20 mL)
Enalapril, enalaprilat (Vasotec) (ACE inhibitor, vasodilator)	*Children:* PO: 0.1 mg/kg/dose QD or BID Increase PRN over 2 wk (Max, 0.5 mg/kg/24 hr) *Adults:* *For CHF:* PO: Start with 2.5 mg QD or BID (Usual range, 5–20 mg/24 hr) *For hypertension:* PO: Start with 5 mg QD (Usual dose, 10–40 mg/24 hr)	Hypotension, dizziness, fatigue, headache, rash, diminishing taste, neutropenia, hyperkalemia, chronic cough Evidence of fetal risk if given during second and third trimesters (same with all other ACE inhibitors)	Tabs: 2.5, 5, 10, 20 mg (Enalapril) Oral susp: 1 mg/mL Inj: 1.25 mg/mL (enalaprilat)

Continued

TABLE E.1 Dosages of Drugs Used in Pediatric Cardiology—cont'd

Drug	Route and Dosage	Toxicity or Side Effects	How Supplied
Enoxaparin (Lovenox) (LMWH, anticoagulant)	*For DVT treatment:* *Infants <2 mo:* SC: 1.5 mg/kg/dose, q12 hr *Infants ≥2 mo to adults:* SC: 1 mg/kg/dose, q12 hr (Adjust dose to achieve target anti–factor Xa levels of 0.5–1 units/mL) *For DVT prophylaxis:* *Infants <2 mo:* SC: 1 mg/kg/dose q12 hr *Infants ≥2 mo up to 18 yr:* SC: 0.5 mg/kg/dose q12 hr *Adults:* SC: 30 mg BID for 7–10 days	Bleeding Contraindicated in major bleeding and drug-induced thrombocytopenia Protamine sulfate is the antidote; 1 mg of protamine sulfate neutralizes 1 mg of enoxaparin	Inj: 100 mg/mL (3 mL)
Epinephrine (Adrenalin) (α-, β₁, and β₂-adrenergic stimulator)	*For asystole and bradycardia:* *Children:* IV/ET: 0.1–0.3 mL/kg of 1:10,000 sol (or 0.01–0.03 mg/kg) q3–5 min *For circulatory shock or heart failure:* *Children:* IV: 0.1–1 mcg/kg/min; titrate to effect	Tachyarrhythmias, hypertension, nausea and vomiting, headache, tissue necrosis (±)	Inj: 0.1 mg/mL (1:10,000 sol, 10 mL prefilled syringe) 1 mg/mL (1:1000 sol, 1, 30 mL)
Esmolol (Brevibloc) (β₁-selective adrenergic blocking agent, antihypertensive, class II antiarrhythmic)	*Children:* *Loading:* IV:100–500 mcg/kg over 1 min *Maintenance:* IV: 25–100 mcg/kg/min; increase by 25–50 mcg/kg to a maximum of 300 mcg/kg/min (Usual maintenance dose, 50–500 mcg/kg/min)	Bronchospasm, CHF, hypotension, nausea and vomiting	Inj: 10, 20, 250 mg/mL
Ethacrynic acid (Edecrin) (loop diuretic)	*Children:* PO: 1 mg/kg/dose QD–TID (Max, 3 mg/kg/24 hr) IV: 1 mg/kg/dose *Adults:* PO: 50–100 mg QD (Max, 400 mg) IV: 0.5–1 mg/kg/dose or 50 mg/dose	Dehydration, hypokalemia, prerenal azotemia, hyperuricemia, eighth cranial nerve damage (deafness), abnormal LFT, agranulocytosis or thrombocytopenia, GI irritation, rash	Tabs: 25 mg Inj: 50 mg vial for recons with 50 mL of D₅W
Flecainide (Tambocor) (class IC antiarrhythmic)	*For sustained VT:* *Children:* PO: Initial 1–3 mg/kg/24 hr, q8 hr (Usual range, 3–6 g/kg/24 hr, q8 hr) Monitor serum level to adjust dose if needed *Adults:* PO: 100 mg/dose BID; may increase by 50 mg q12 hr q4 days to max dose of 600 mg/24 hr [*Therapeutic level: 0.2–1 mg/L*]	Worsening of HF, bradycardia, AV block, dizziness, blurred vision, dyspnea, nausea, headache, increased PR and QRS duration	Tabs: 50, 100, 150 mg Susp: 5, 20 mg/mL
Fludrocortisone acetate (Florinef, Fluohydrisone) (corticosteroid)	*For syncopal episodes:* *Children:* PO: 0.1 mg/dose QD *Adults:* PO: 0.2 mg/dose QD	Hypertension, hypokalemia, acne, rash, bruising, headache, GI ulcers, and growth suppression Weight gain (1–2 kg in 2–3 wk)	Tabs: 0.1 mg
Furosemide (Lasix, Furosemide) (loop diuretic)	*Children:* IV: 0.5–2 mg/kg/dose BID–QID PO: 1–2 mg/kg/dose QD–TID (Max, 6 mg/kg/dose) *Adults:* IV, PO: 20–80 mg/24 hr BID–QID	Hypokalemia, hyperuricemia, prerenal azotemia, ototoxicity, rarely bloody dyscrasias, rash	Oral liquid: 10 mg/mL, 40 mg/5 mL Tabs: 20, 40, 80 mg Inj: 10 mg/mL

TABLE E.1 **Dosages of Drugs Used in Pediatric Cardiology—cont'd**

Drug	Route and Dosage	Toxicity or Side Effects	How Supplied
Heparin (anticoagulant)	*Infants and children:* IV: *Initial:* 50 U/kg IV bolus *Maintenance:* 10–25 U/kg/hr or 50–100 U/kg q4 hr (Adjust dose to give APTT 1.5–2.5 times control, 6–8 hr after IV infusion [or 3.5–4 hr after intermittent injection]) *Adults:* IV: *Initial:* 10,000 U IV injection *Maintenance:* 5000–10,000 U q4–6 hr IV drip: *Initial dose:* 5000 U followed by 20,000–40,000 U/24 hr	Bleeding Antidote: protamine sulfate (1 mg per 100 U heparin in previous 4 hr)	Inj: 1000, 2000, 2500, 5000, 7500, 10,000, 20,000, 40,000 U/mL
Hydralazine (Apresoline) (peripheral vasodilator, antihypertensive)	*For hypertensive crisis:* *Children:* IM, IV: 0.15–0.2 mg/kg/dose; may be repeated q4–6 hr (Max, 20 mg/dose) *Adults:* IM, IV: 20–40 mg/dose; repeat q4–6 hr PRN *For chronic hypertension:* *Children:* PO: 0.75–3 mg/kg/24 hr BID–QID *Adults:* PO: Start with 10 mg 4 times/24 hr for 3–4 days; increase to 25 mg/dose QID for 3–4 days; then up to 50 mg QID	Hypotension, tachycardia and palpitation, lupus-like syndrome with prolonged use (fever, arthralgia, splenomegaly and positive LE-cell preparation), blood dyscrasias	Tabs: 10, 25, 50, 100 mg Oral liquid: 1.25, 2, 4 mg/mL Inj: 20 mg/mL
Hydrochlorothiazide (HydroDIURIL, Esidrix, Hydro-Par, Oretic) (thiazide diuretic)	*Children:* PO: 2–4 mg/kg/24 hr BID (Max, 100 mg/24 hr) *Adults:* PO: 25–100 mg/24 hr QD–BID (Max, 200 mg/24 hr)	Same as for chlorothiazide	Tabs: 25, 50, 100 mg Caps: 12.5 mg Sol: 10 mg/mL (500 mL)
Ibuprofen (NeoProfen) (NSAID)	*For PDA closure in premature infants:* *Neonates ≤32 weeks (500–1500 g):* IV: Initial dose 10 mg/kg followed by two doses of 5 mg/kg after 24 and 48 hr (Hold second and third dose if urine output is <0.6 mL/kg/hr)	Sepsis, anemia, interventricular hemorrhage, apnea, GI disorders, renal impairment Contraindicated in interventricular hemorrhage, thrombocytopenia, necrotizing enterocolitis, significant renal dysfunction	Inj: 17.1 mg/mL ibuprofen lysine equivalent to 10 mg/mL of ibuprofen (2 mL)
Inamrinone (Inocor) (phosphodiesterase type III inhibitor)	*Children:* IV: *Loading:* 0.75 mg/kg over 2–3 min *Maintenance:* 5–10 mcg/kg/min *Adults:* IV: *Loading:* 0.75 mg/kg over 2–3 min *Maintenance:* 5–10 mcg/kg/min	Thrombocytopenia, hypotension, tachyarrhythmias, hepatotoxicity, nausea and vomiting, fever	Inj: 5 mg/mL (20 mL)
Indomethacin (Indocin) (NSAID, antipyretic agent, PG synthesis inhibitor)	*For PDA closure in premature infants:* IV: *<48 hr:* 0.2, 0.1, and 0.1 mg/kg/dose, q12–24 hr *2–7 days:* 0.2, 0.2, and 0.2 mg/kg/dose, q12–24 hr *>7 days:* 0.2, 0.25, and 0.25 mg/kg/dose, q12–24 hr	GI or other bleeding, GI disturbances, renal impairment, electrolyte disturbances (↓ Na, ↑ K levels)	Vials: 1 mg
Isoproterenol (Isuprel) (β_1- and β_2-adrenergic agonist)	*Children:* IV: 0.1–2 mcg/kg/min, titrated to desired effect *Adults:* IV: 2–20 mcg/min, titrated to desired effect (incompatible with alkali solution)	Similar to epinephrine	Inj: 0.2 mg/mL (1, 5, 10 mL)

Continued

TABLE E.1   Dosages of Drugs Used in Pediatric Cardiology—cont'd

Drug	Route and Dosage	Toxicity or Side Effects	How Supplied
Ketamine (Ketalar) (general anesthetic)	*For cyanotic spells:* *Infants:* IM: 2–3 mg/kg Repeat smaller doses q30 min PRN IV: 1–3 mg/kg/dose over 60 sec Repeat smaller doses q30 min PRN	Hypertension or tachycardia, respiratory depression or apnea, CNS symptoms (dreamlike state, confusion, agitation)	Inj: 10, 50, 100 mg/mL
Labetalol (Normodyne, Trandate) (α- and β-adrenergic antagonist)	*Children:* PO: Initial 4 mg/kg/24 hr BID (Max, 40 mg/kg/24 hr) IV: (for hypertensive emergency) Initial 0.2–1 mg/kg/dose q10 min PRN (Max, 20 mg/dose)	Orthostatic hypotension, edema, CHF, bradycardia Contraindicated in asthma	Tabs: 100, 200, 300 mg Susp: 10, 40 mg/mL Inj: 5 mg/mL (20, 40 mL)
Lidocaine (Xylocaine) (class IB antiarrhythmic)	*Children:* IV: *Loading:* 1 mg/kg/dose slow IV, q5–10 min PRN *Maintenance:* 30 mcg/kg/min (Range 20–50 mcg/kg/min) *Adults:* IV: *Loading:* 1 mg/kg/dose q5 min *Maintenance:* 1–4 mg/min [*Therapeutic level:* 1.5–5 mg/L]	Seizure, respiratory depression, CNS symptoms (anxiety, euphoria or drowsiness), arrhythmias, hypotension or shock	Inj: 0.5%, 1%, 1.5%, 2%, 4%, 10%, 20% (1% = 10 mg/mL)
Lisinopril (Zestril, Prinivil) (ACE inhibitor, antihypertensive)	*For hypertension:* *Children ≥6 yr:* PO: Initial 0.07 mg/kg/24 hr (max initial dose is 5 mg/24 hr); increase dose at 1- to 2-week intervals (Max, 0.6 mg/kg/day or 40 mg/24 hr) *Adults:* PO: Initial 10 mg QD; may increase upward as needed to max dose of 80 mg/24 hr	Dry nonproductive cough, rash, hypotension, hyperkalemia, angioedema, rarely bone marrow depression Evidence of fetal risk if given during second and third trimesters (same with all other ACE inhibitors)	Tabs: 2.5, 5, 10, 20, 30, 40 mg
Losartan (Cozaar) (angiotensin II receptor blocker)	*For hypertension:* *Children ≥6 yr:* PO: 0.7 mg/kg/24 hr QD–BID (Max, 50 mg/24 hr) *Adults:* PO: Initial dose 50 mg QD (Max, 100 mg QD)	Hypotension, dizziness, nasal congestion, muscle cramps Evidence of fetal risk if given during second and third trimesters	Tabs: 25, 50, 100 mg
Lovastatin (Mevacor) (antilipemic, HMG-CoA reductase inhibitor)	*Adolescents:* PO: Starting dose, 10 mg/24 hr QD for 6–8 wk; increase to 20 mg/24 hr for 8 wk; then increase to 40 mg/24 hr for 8 wk *Adults:* PO: Starting dose, 20 mg/day QD–BID (range 40–80 mg/24 hr) (Max dose with concurrent amiodarone or verapamil use is 40 mg/24 hr)	Mild GI symptoms, myositis syndrome, elevated transaminase levels, increased CK levels	Tabs: 10, 20, 40 mg
Methyldopa (Aldomet) (antihypertensive)	*For hypertensive crisis:* *Children:* IV: Start at 2–4 mg/kg/dose q6–8 hr (Max dose, 65 mg/kg/24 hr or 3 g/24 hr, whichever is less) *Adults:* IV: 250–500 mg q6 hr (Max, 1 g q6 hr) *For hypertension:* *Children:* PO: 10 mg/kg/24 hr BID–QID May be increased or decreased (Max dose, 65 mg/kg/24 hr or 3 g/24 hr, whichever is less) *Adults:* PO: 250 mg/dose BID–TID for 2 days May be increased or decreased q2 days. (Usual dose: 0.5–2 g/24 hr BID–QID) (Max, 3 g/24 hr)	Sedation, orthostatic hypotension and bradycardia, lupus-like syndrome, Coombs (+) hemolytic anemia and leukopenia, hepatitis or cirrhosis, colitis, impotence	Inj: 50 mg/mL (5 mL) Susp: 50 mg/mL Tabs: 250, 500 mg

TABLE E.1	Dosages of Drugs Used in Pediatric Cardiology—cont'd		
Drug	**Route and Dosage**	**Toxicity or Side Effects**	**How Supplied**
Metoprolol (Lopressor) (β-adrenoceptor blocker)	*Children >2 yr:* PO: Initially 0.1–0.2 mg/kg/dose BID; gradually increase to 1–3 mg/kg/24 hr *Adults:* PO: Initially 100 mg/24 hr QD–TID May increase to 450 mg/24 hr BID–TID (Usual dose, 100–450 mg/24 hr) (Usually used with hydrochlorothiazide 25–100 mg/24 hr)	CNS symptoms (dizziness, tiredness, depression), bronchospasm, bradycardia, diarrhea, nausea and vomiting, abdominal pain	Tabs: 25, 50, 100 mg Tabs, extended release: 25, 50, 100, 200 mg
Metolazone (Zaroxolyn, Diulo, Mykrox) (thiazide-like diuretic)	*Children:* PO: 0.2–0.4 mg/kg/24 hr QD–BID *Adults:* PO: For hypertension: 2.5–5 mg QD For edema: 5–20 mg QD	Electrolyte imbalance, GI disturbance, hyperglycemia, bone marrow depression, chills, hyperuricemia, hepatitis, rash May be more effective than thiazide diuretics in impaired renal function	Tabs: 0.5 (Mykrox), 2.5, 5, 10 mg Susp: 1 mg/mL
Mexiletine (Mexitil) (class IB antiarrhythmic)	*Children:* PO: 6–8 mg/kg/24 hr BID–TID for 2–3 days; then 2–5 mg/kg/dose q6–8 hr Increase 1–2 mg/kg/dose q2–3 days until desired effect achieved (with food or antacid) *Adults:* PO: 200 mg q8 hr for 2–3 days Increase to 300–400 mg q8 hr (Usual dose, 200–300 mg q8 hr) [*Therapeutic level:* 0.75–2 mcg/mL]	Nausea and vomiting, CNS symptoms (headache, dizziness, tremor, paresthesia, mood changes), rash, hepatic dysfunction (±)	Caps: 150, 200, 250 mg
Milrinone (Primacor) (phosphodiesterase type III inhibitor)	*Children:* IV: *Loading:* 10–50 mcg/kg over 10 min; then 0.1–1 mcg/kg/min *Adults:* IV: *Loading:* 50 mcg/kg over 10 min 0.5 mcg/kg/min (Range, 0.375–0.75 mcg/kg/min)	Arrhythmias, hypotension, hypokalemia, thrombocytopenia	Inj: 1 mg/mL (5, 10, 20 mL) Inj, premixed in D$_5$W: 200 mcg/mL (100, 200 mL)
Minoxidil (Loniten) (peripheral vasodilator)	*Children <12 yr:* PO: 0.2 mg/kg/24 hr QD–BID initially Increase 0.1–0.2 mg/kg/24 hr q3 days until desired effect achieved (Usual dose, 0.25–1 mg/kg/24 hr QD–BID; max, 50 mg/24 hr) *Children >12 yr and adults:* PO: 5 mg/dose QD initially May be increased to 10, 20, 40 mg QD–BID q3-day interval (Usual dose, 10–40 mg/24 hr QD–BID; max, 100 mg/24 hr)	Reflex tachycardia and fluid retention (used with a beta-blocker and diuretic), pericardial effusion, hypertrichosis, rarely blood dyscrasias (leukopenia, thrombocytopenia)	Tabs: 2.5, 10 mg
Morphine sulfate (narcotic, analgesic)	*Children:* SC, IM, IV: 0.1–0.2 mg/kg/dose q2–4 hr (Max, 15 mg/dose) *Adults:* SC, IM, IV: 2.5–20 mg/dose q2–6 hr PRN	CNS depression, respiratory depression, nausea and vomiting, hypotension, bradycardia	Inj: 0.5, 1, 2, 4, 5, 8, 10, 15, 25, 50 mg/mL
Mycophenolate mofetil (CellCept) (immunosuppressant)	*Children:* PO: 600 mg/m^2/dose BID (Maximum 2000 mg/24 hr) [*Therapeutic level:* 5–7 ng/mL] *Adults:* PO/IV: 2000–3000 g/24 hr BID	Headache, GI symptoms, hypertension, bone marrow suppression (anemia), fever, increased risk of developing lymphomas or other malignancies	Tabs: 500 mg Caps: 250 mg Oral susp: 200 mg/mL Inj: 500 mg

Continued

TABLE E.1 Dosages of Drugs Used in Pediatric Cardiology—cont'd

Drug	Route and Dosage	Toxicity or Side Effects	How Supplied
Nifedipine (Procardia, Adalat) (CCB)	*For hypertrophic cardiomyopathy:* *Children:* PO: 0.5–0.9 mg/kg/24 hr TID–QID *For hypertension:* *Children:* PO: 0.25–0.5 mg/kg/24 hr QD–BID (Max, 3 mg/kg/24 hr up to 120 mg/24 hr) *Adults:* PO: Initially 10 mg/dose TID Titrate up to 20–30 mg/dose TID–QID over 7–14 days (Usual dose, 10–20 mg TID; max dose, 180 mg/24 hr)	Hypotension, peripheral edema, CNS symptoms (headache, dizziness, weakness), nausea	Caps: 10, 20 mg Tabs, sustained release (Adalat CC, Procardia XL): 30, 60, 90 mg
Nitroglycerine (Nitro-Bid, Tridil, Nitrostat) (peripheral vasodilator)	*Children:* IV: 0.5–1 mcg/kg/min Increase 1 mcg/kg/min q20 min to titrate to effect (Max, 6 mcg/kg/min) (Dilute in D_5W or NS with final concentration <400 mcg/mL; light sensitive) *Adults:* IV: Initial dose: 5 mcg/min through infusion pump Increase 5 mcg/min q3–5 min until desired effect achieved	Hypotension, tachycardia, headache, nausea and vomiting	Inj: 0.5, 5 mg/mL Inj, premixed in D_5W: 100, 200, 400 mcg/mL
Nitroprusside (Nipride) (peripheral vasodilator)	*Children:* IV: 0.3–0.5 mcg/kg/min, titrate to effect with BP monitoring (Usual dose, 3–4 mcg/kg/min; max dose, 10 mcg/kg/min) (Dilute stock solution [50 mg] in 250–2000 mL D_5W; light sensitive)	Hypotension, palpitation, and cyanide toxicity (metabolic acidosis earliest and most reliable evidence) Monitor thiocyanate level when used >48 hr and in patients with renal or hepatic dysfunction. Thiocyanate level should be <50 mg/L; cyanate levels >2 mcg/mL are toxic levels	Inj: 25 mg/mL (2 mL) Inj: 50 mg for reconst with 2–3 mL of D_5W
Norepinephrine (Levophed, levarterenol) (α_1- and β_1 adrenoceptor stimulant)	*Children:* IV: 0.1 mcg/kg/min IV infusion initially; increase dose to attain desired effect (Max, 2 mcg/kg/min) *Adults:* IV: Start at 4 mcg/min IV infusion; titrate to effect (Usual dose, range, 8–12 mcg/min)	Hypertension, bradycardia (reflex), arrhythmias, tissue necrosis (treat with phentolamine infiltration)	Inj: 1 mg/mL (4 mL)
Phentolamine (Regitine) (α-adrenoceptor blocker)	*For diagnosis of pheochromocytoma:* *Children:* IM, IV: 0.05–0.1 mg/kg/dose; repeat q5 min until hypertension is controlled; then q2–4 hr PRN *Adults:* IM, IV: 2.5–5 mg/dose; repeat q5 min until hypertension is controlled; then q2–4 hr PRN *For treatment of extravasated α-adrenergic drugs:* SC: Make a solution of 0.5–1 mcg/mL with NS; inject 1–5 mL (in five divided doses) around the site of extravasation (Max, 0.1–0.5 mg/kg or 5 mg total)	Hypotension, tachycardia or arrhythmias, nausea and vomiting	Inj: 5 mg powder for reconst

TABLE E.1 Dosages of Drugs Used in Pediatric Cardiology—cont'd

Drug	Route and Dosage	Toxicity or Side Effects	How Supplied
Phenylephrine (Neo-Synephrine) (α_1-adrenoceptor stimulant)	*For hypotension:* *Children:* IM, SC: 0.1 mg/kg/dose q1–2 hr PRN (Max dose, 5 mg) IV: 5–10 mcg/kg/dose IV bolus q10–15 min or 0.1–0.5 mcg/kg/min *Adults:* IM, SC: 2–5 mg/dose q1–2 hr PRN (Max dose, 5 mg) IV: 0.1–0.5 mg/dose IV bolus q10–15 min PRN Start IV drip at 100–180 mcg/min (Usual maintenance dose, 40–60 mcg/min)	Arrhythmias, hypertension, angina	Inj: 10 mg/mL
Phenytoin (Dilantin) (class IB antiarrhythmic, anticonvulsant)	*Children:* IV: 2–4 mg/kg/dose over 5–10 min followed by PO dose PO: 2–5 mg/kg/24 hr BID–TID [*Therapeutic level:* 5–18 mcg/mL for arrhythmias, 10–20 mcg/mL for seizures] *Adults:* IV: 100 mg q5 min (total 500 mg) PO: 250 mg QID for 1 day, 250 mg/dose BID for 2 days, and 300–400 mg/24 hr QD–QID	Rash, Stevens-Johnson syndrome, CNS symptoms (ataxia, dysarthria), lupus-like syndrome, blood dyscrasias, peripheral neuropathy, gingival hypertrophy	Susp: 125 mg/5 mL (240 mL) Tabs, chewable: 50 mg (Infatab) Caps: 100 mg Caps, extended release: 30, 100, 200, 300 mg Inj: 50 mg/mL
Potassium chloride	*Supplement in diuretic therapy:* *Children:* PO: 1–2 mEq/kg/24 hr TID–QID (or 0.8–1.5 mL 10% potassium chloride/kg/24 hr, or 0.4–0.7 mL 20% potassium chloride/kg/24 hr TID–QID)	GI disturbances, ulcerations, hyperkalemia	Oral sol: 10% (1.3 mEq/mL), 20% (2.7 mEq/mL) Caps, sustained release: 8, 10 mEq Tabs, sustained release: 8, 10, 15, 20 mEq
Potassium gluconate	*Supplement in diuretic therapy:* *Children:* PO: 1–2 mEq/kg/24 hr TID–QID, or 0.8–1.5 mL/kg/24 hr TID–QID	Same as for potassium chloride	Elixir: 1.3 mEq/mL
Pravastatin (Pravachol) (antilipemic, HMG-CoA reductase inhibitor)	*Children (8–13 yr):* PO: Starting dose, 10 mg QD for 4–6 wk Increase to 20 QD as needed *Adolescents (14–18 yr):* PO: 40 mg QD (Adult max dose, 40 mg/day)	Headache, constipation, diarrhea, elevated liver enzymes, rhabdomyolysis, myopathy	Tabs: 10, 20, 40, 80 mg
Prazosin (Minipress) (Postsynaptic α_1-adrenergic blocker, antihypertensive)	*Children:* PO: 5 mcg/kg as a test dose; then 25–150 mcg/kg/24 hr QID *Adults:* PO: 1 mg/dose BID–TID initially Increase to 20 mg/24 hr BID–QID (Usual dose, 6–15 mg/24 hr)	CNS symptoms (dizziness, headache, drowsiness), palpitation, nausea	Caps: 1, 2, 5 mg
Procainamide (Procanbid, Pronestyl) (class IA antiarrhythmic)	*Children:* IV: *Loading:* 2–6 mg/kg/dose over 5 min repeated q10–30 min (Max, 100 mg) *Maintenance:* 20–80 mcg/kg/min (Max, 2 g/24 hr) PO: 15–50 mg/kg/24 hr q3–6 hr (Max, 4 g/24 hr) *Adults:* IV: *Loading:* 50–100 mg/dose q5 min PRN *Maintenance:* 1–6 mg/min PO: Immediate release, 250–500 mg/dose q3–6 hr (sustained release, 500–1000 mg/dose q6 hr) [*Therapeutic level:* 4–10 mcg/mL]	Nausea and vomiting, blood dyscrasias, rash, lupus-like syndrome, hypotension, confusion or disorientation	Tabs, sustained release: 250, 500, 750, 1000 mg Caps: 250, 375, 500 mg Susp: 5, 50, 100 mg/mL Inj: 100, 500 mg/mL

Continued

TABLE E.1   Dosages of Drugs Used in Pediatric Cardiology—cont'd

Drug	Route and Dosage	Toxicity or Side Effects	How Supplied
Propranolol (Inderal) (β-adrenoceptor blocker, class II antiarrhythmic)	*For hypertension:* *Children:* PO: 0.5–1 mg/kg/24 hr BID–QID; may increase q3–5 days (Usual dose, 2–4 mg/kg/24 hr; max dose, 8 mg/kg/24 hr) *For arrhythmias:* *Children:* IV: 0.01–0.15 mg/kg/dose over 10 min; repeat q6–8 hr PRN (Max, 1 mg/dose for infants; 3 mg/dose for children) PO: Start at 0.5–1 mg/kg/24 hr TID–QID; increase dose q3–5 days PRN (Usual dose, 2–4 mg/kg/24 hr; max dose, 16 mg/kg/24 hr) *Adults:* IV: 1 mg/dose q5min (maximum 5 mg) PO: 10–20 mg/dose TID–QID; increase PRN (Usual dose, 40–320 mg/24 hr TID–QID)	Hypotension, syncope, bronchospasm, nausea and vomiting, hypoglycemia, lethargy or depression, heart block	Tabs: 10, 20, 40, 60, 80, 90 mg Caps, extended release: 60, 80, 120, 160 mg Oral sol: 20, 40 mg/5 mL Concentrated sol: 80 mg/mL Inj: 1 mg/mL
Prostaglandin E₁ or alprostadil (Prostin VR, PGE₁) (vasodilator)	*For patency of ductus arteriosus:* IV: Begin infusion at 0.05–0.1 mcg/kg/min When desired effect achieved, reduce to 0.05, 0.025, and 0.01 mcg/kg/min If unresponsive, dose may be increased to 0.4 mcg/kg/min	Apnea, flushing, bradycardia, hypotension, fever	Inj: 500 mcg/mL
Protamine sulfate (heparin antidote)	*Antidote to heparin overdose:* IV: Each 1 mg protamine neutralizes ~100 U heparin given in preceding 3–4 hr; slow IV infusion at rate not exceeding 20 mg/min or 50 mg/10 min (Check APTT)	Hypotension, bradycardia, dyspnea, flushing, coagulation problem	Inj: 10 mg/mL
Quinidine (Cardioquin, Quinidex, Quinaglute) (class IA antiarrhythmic)	*Children:* Test dose for idiosyncrasy: 2 mg/kg once (PO as sulfate; IM/IV as gluconate) Therapeutic dose: IV (as gluconate): 2–10 mg/kg/dose, q3–6 hr PRN PO (as sulfate): 15–60 mg/kg/24 hr, q6 hr *Adults:* Test dose: 200 mg once PO/IM Therapeutic dose: PO (as sulfate, immediate release): 100–600 mg/dose q4–6 hr Begin at 200 mg/dose and titrate to desired effect or PO (sulfate, sustained release): 300–600 mg/dose q8–12 hr PO (as gluconate): 324–972 mg q8–12 hr IM (as gluconate): 400 mg/dose q4–6 hr IV (as gluconate): 200–400 mg/dose, infused at a rate of ≤10 mg/min [*Therapeutic level:* 3–7 mg/L]	Nausea and vomiting, ventricular arrhythmias, prolonged QRS complex, depressed myocardial contractility, blood dyscrasias, symptoms of cinchonism	*Gluconate* (62% quinidine): Tabs, slow release: 324 mg Inj: 80 mg/mL *Sulfate* (83% quinidine): Tabs: 200, 300 mg Tabs, slow release: 300 mg Susp: 10 mg/mL
Sildenafil (Revatio, Viagra) (phosphodiesterase type V inhibitor)	*For pulmonary hypertension:* *Neonates:* PO: 0.25–1 mg/kg/dose BID–QID *Infants and children:* PO: 0.25–1 mg/kg/dose, q4–6 hr *Adults:* PO: 20 mg TID	Hypotension, tachycardia, flushing, headache, rash, nausea, diarrhea, priapism, platelet dysfunction, myalgia, paresthesia, blurred vision, epistaxis, dyspnea Contraindicated in concurrent use of organic nitrates	Tabs: 20, 25, 50, 100 mg

TABLE E.1   Dosages of Drugs Used in Pediatric Cardiology—cont'd

Drug	Route and Dosage	Toxicity or Side Effects	How Supplied
Simvastatin (Zocor) (antilipemic, HMG-CoA reductase inhibitor)	*Children:* PO: Starting dose, 10 mg QD Increment of 10 mg q6–8 wk to max dose, of 40 mg QD as needed (Adult max, 80 mg/24 hr)	Headache, constipation, diarrhea, elevated liver enzymes, rhabdomyolysis, myopathy	Tabs: 5, 10, 20, 40, 80 mg
Sirolimus (Rapamune) (immunosuppressant)	*Children:* PO: *Loading:* 3 mg/m^2 *Maintenance:* 1 mg/m^2/day QD *Adults:* PO: *Loading:* 6 mg *Maintenance:* 2 mg/day QD [*Therapeutic level:* 6–15 ng/mL]	Hypertension, peripheral edema, chest pain, fever, headache, acne, hirsutism, hypercholesterolemia, neurotoxicity, abdominal pain, anemia, pneumonitis	Tabs: 1, 2 mg Oral sol: 1 mg/mL
Sodium polystyrene sulfonate (Kayexalate, Kionex) (potassium-removing resin)	*For hyperkalemia (slowly effective, taking hours to days):* *Children:* PO, NG: 1 g/kg/dose q6 hr PR: 1 g/kg/dose q2–6 hr *Adults:* PO, NG, PR: 15 g QD–QID (Cation exchange resin with practical exchange rates of 1 mEq potassium per 1 g resin) (NOTE: Delivers 1 mEq sodium for each mEq of potassium removed)	Nausea and vomiting, constipation, severe hypokalemia (muscle weakness, confusion [monitor serum potassium levels, ECG]), hypocalcemia or hypernatremia (edema)	Powder: 454, 480 g Susp: 15 g/60 mL
Sotalol (Betapace) (class II and III antiarrhythmic)	*For SVT and VT:* PO: 80–120 mg/m^2/24 hr TID (*infants*) BID (*older children and adults*)	Chest pain, palpitation, hypoglycemia, hypotension, torsades de pointes, nausea and vomiting, abdominal pain, CNS symptoms (depression, weakness, dizziness), bronchospasm, heart block, bradycardia, negative inotropic effects, QT prolongation (Discontinue if QTc >550 msec)	Tabs: 80, 120, 160, 240 mg Syrup: 5 mg/mL
Spironolactone (Aldactone) (potassium-sparing diuretic, aldosterone antagonist)	*Children:* PO: 3 mg/kg/24 hr BID–TID *Adults:* PO: 50–100 mg/24 hr TID–QID (Max, 200 mg/24 hr)	Hyperkalemia (when given with potassium supplements and ACE inhibitors), GI distress, rash, gynecomastia, agranulocytosis Contraindicated in renal failure	Tabs: 25, 50, 100 mg Susp: 1, 2, 2.5, 5, 25 mg/mL
Streptokinase (Streptase, Kabikinase) (thrombolytic enzyme)	*For thrombolysis:* (Use in consultation with a hematologist) *Children:* IV: 3500–4000 U/kg over 30 min followed by 1000–1500 U/kg/hr or 2000 U/kg load over 30 min followed by 2000 U/kg/hr (Duration of infusion based on response but generally does not exceed 3 days; obtain tests at baseline and q4 hr: APTT, TT, fibrinogen, PT, hematocrit, platelet count; APTT and TT should be <two times control)	Potential for allergic reaction with repeated use; premedicate with acetaminophen and antihistamine and repeat q4–6hr	Inj: 250,000, 750,000, 1,500,000 IU powder for reconst
Tacrolimus (Prograf) (immunosuppressant)	*Children and adults:* PO: 0.15–0.4 mg/kg/day BID IV: 0.03–0.15 mg/kg/day continuous infusion [*Therapeutic level:* 5–15 ng/mL]	Hypertension, hypotension, peripheral edema, myocardial hypertrophy, chest pain, fever, headache, encephalopathy, pruritus, hypercholesterolemia, electrolyte imbalance, neurotoxicity, nephrotoxicity, diarrhea, anemia, dyspnea	Caps: 0.5, 1, 5 mg Susp: 0.5 mg/mL Inj: 5 mg/mL (1 mL)

Continued

TABLE E.1	Dosages of Drugs Used in Pediatric Cardiology—cont'd		
Drug	**Route and Dosage**	**Toxicity or Side Effects**	**How Supplied**
Tolazoline (Priscoline) (α-adrenoceptor blocker)	*For neonatal pulmonary hypertension:* IV: *Loading:* 1–2 mg/kg over 10 min *Maintenance:* 1–2 mg/kg/hr	Hypotension and tachycardia, pulmonary hemorrhage, GI bleeding, arrhythmias, thrombocytopenia, leukopenia	Inj: 25 mg/mL
Triamterene (Dyrenium) (potassium-sparing diuretic)	*Children:* PO: 2–4 mg/kg/24 hr QD–BID May increase up to max of 6 mg/kg/24 hr or 300 mg/24 hr *Adults:* PO: 50–100 mg/24 hr QD–BID (Max, 300 mg/24 hr)	Nausea and vomiting, leg cramps, dizziness, hyperuricemia, rash, prerenal azotemia	Caps: 50, 100 mg
Urokinase (Abbokinase) (thrombolytic enzyme)	*For thrombolysis (in vein thrombosis or PE):* (Should be used in consultation with a hematologist) *Children:* IV: *Loading:* 4400 U/kg over 10 min *Maintenance:* 4400 U/kg/hr for 6–12 hr; some patients may require 12–72 hr of therapy (Monitor same laboratory tests as for streptokinase) *For occluded IV catheter clearance:* *Aspiration method:* Use 5000 U/mL concentrate; instill into the catheter a volume equal to the internal volume of catheter over 1–2 min, leave in place for 1–4 hr; then aspirate; may repeat with 10,000 U/mL if no response; do not infuse into the patient *IV infusion method:* 150–200 U/kg/hr in each lumen for 8–48 hr at a rate of at least 20 mL/hr *Adults:* *For PE* IV: Priming dose: 4400 U/kg. IV infusion: 4400 U/kg/hr for 12 hr by infusion pump	Bleeding, allergic reactions, rash, fever and chills, bronchospasm	Inj: 5000 U/mL
Verapamil (Isoptin, Calan) (CCB, class IV antiarrhythmic)	*For dysrhythmia (SVT):* *Children:* IV: 1–15 yr (for SVT): 0.1–0.3 mg/kg over 2 min May repeat same dose in 15 min (Max dose, 5 mg first dose; 10 mg second dose) *Adults:* IV: 5–10 mg, 10 mg second dose *For hypertension:* *Children:* PO: 4–8 mg/kg/24 hr TID *Adults:* PO: 240–480 mg/24 hr TID	Hypotension, bradycardia, cardiac depression	Tabs: 40, 80, 120 mg Tabs, extended release: 120, 180, 240 mg Caps, extended release: 100, 120, 180, 200, 240, 300, 360 mg Susp: 50 mg/mL Inj: 2.5 mg/mL
Vitamin K₁	*Antidote to dicumarol or warfarin:* PO/IM/SC/IV: 2.5–10 mg/dose in one dose for correction of excessive PT from dicumarol or warfarin overdose		Tabs: 5 mg Inj: 2, 10 mg/mL

TABLE E.1 Dosages of Drugs Used in Pediatric Cardiology—cont'd

Drug	Route and Dosage	Toxicity or Side Effects	How Supplied
Warfarin (Coumadin, Safarin) (anticoagulant)	*Children:* PO: *Initial:* 0.1–0.2 mg/kg/dose QD in evening for 2 days (Max dose, 10 mg/dose) (In liver dysfunction, 0.1 mg/kg/day; max, 5 mg/dose) *Maintenance:* 0.1 mg/kg/24H QD (Monitor INR after 5–7 days of new dosage; keep INR at 2.5–3.5 for mechanical prosthetic valve; 2–3 for prophylaxis of DVT, PE) (Heparin preferred initially for rapid anticoagulation; warfarin may be started concomitantly with heparin or may be delayed 3–6 days) *Adults:* PO: *Initial:* 5–15 mg/dose QD for 2–5 days *Maintenance:* 2–10 mg/day (Adjust dosage based on INR)	Bleeding (antidote: vitamin K or fresh-frozen plasma) *Increased PT response:* salicylates, acetaminophen, alcohol, lipid-lowering agents, phenytoin, ibuprofen, some antibiotics *Decreased PT response:* antihistamines, barbiturates, oral contraceptives, vitamin C, diet high in vitamin K Onset of action: 36–72 hr; full effects in 4–5 days Mode of action: inhibits hepatic synthesis of vitamin K–dependent factors (I, VII, IX, X)	Tabs: 1, 2, 2.5, 3, 4, 5, 6, 7.5, 10 mg Inj: 5 mg

ACE, Angiotensin-converting enzyme; *ALT,* alanine aminotransferase; *APTT,* activated partial thromboplastin time; *AST,* aspartate aminotransferase; *AV,* atrioventricular; *BID,* two times a day; *BP,* blood pressure; *Caps,* capsule; *CCB,* calcium channel blocker; *CHF,* congestive heart failure; *CK,* creatine kinase; *CNS,* central nervous system; *CR,* controlled release; *D₅W,* 5% dextrose in water; *DVT,* deep vein thrombosis; *ECG,* electrocardiogram; *ET,* endotracheal; *GI,* gastrointestinal; *HMG-CoA,* 3-hydroxy-3-methylglutaryl coenzyme A; *HOCM,* hypertrophic obstructive cardiomyopathy; *IM,* intramuscular; *Inj,* injection; *INR,* international normalized ratio; *IV,* intravenous; *LE,* lupus erythematosus; *LFT,* liver function test; *max,* maximum; *LMWH,* low-molecular weight heparin; *NE,* norepinephrine; *NG,* nasogastric; *NS,* normal saline; *NSAID,* nonsteroidal antiinflammatory drug; *PDA,* patent ductus arteriosus; *PE,* pulmonary embolism; *PG,* prostaglandin; *PO,* by mouth; *PR,* per rectum; *PRN,* as necessary; *PT,* prothrombin time; *q,* every; *QD,* once a day; *QID,* four times a day; *QOD,* every other day; *RBF,* renal blood flow; *reconst,* reconstitution; *SC,* subcutaneous; *sol,* solution; *Supp,* suppository; *Susp,* suspension; *SVT,* supraventricular tachycardia; *Tabs,* tablet; *TDD,* total digitalizing dose; *TID,* three times a day; *TT,* thrombin time; *WBC,* white blood cell; *(±),* may occur.

GENERAL REFERENCES

Allen HD, Shaddy RE, Penny DJ, Feltes TF, Cetta F. *Moss and Adams' Heart Disease in Infants, Children, and Adolescents, Including the Fetus and Young Adult.* 7th ed. Philadelphia: Wolters Kluwer; 2016.

Armstrong WF, Ryan T. *Feigenbaum's Echocardiography.* 7th ed. Philadelphia: Lippincott Williams & Wilkins; 2010.

Dick II M. *Clinical Electrophysiology in the Young.* 2nd ed. New York: Springer; 2015.

Eidem BW, O'Leary PW, Cetta F. *Echocardiography in Pediatric and Adult Congenital Heart Disease.* 2nd ed. Philadelphia: Wolters Kluwer; 2015.

Jonas RA. *Comprehensive Surgical Management of Congenital Heart Disease.* 2nd ed. Boca Raton, FL: CRP Press; 2014.

Kwiterovich Jr PO. *The Johns Hopkins Textbook of Dyslipidemia.* Philadelphia: Wolters Kluwer; 2010.

Mavroudis C, Backer CL. *Pediatric Cardiac Surgery.* 4th ed. Hoboken, NJ: Wiley-Blackwell; 2013.

Moller JH, Hoffman JIE, Benson DW, Van Hare GF, Wren C. *Pediatric Cardiovascular Medicine.* 2nd ed. New York: Wiley-Blackwell; 2012.

Oh JK, Kane GC, Seward JB, Tajik AJ. *The Echo Manual.* 4th ed. Philadelphia: Wolters Kluwer; 2019.

Park MK, Guntheroth WG. *How to Read Pediatric ECGs.* 4th ed. Philadelphia: Mosby; 2006.

Walsh EP, Saul JP, Triedman JK. *Cardiac Arrhythmias in Children and Young Adults with Congenital Heart Disease.* Philadelphia: Lippincott Williams & Wilkins; 2001.

CHAPTER 1. HISTORY TAKING

Barger AP, Hurley R. Evaluation of the hypercoagulable state. Whom to screen, how to test and treat. *Postgrad Med.* 2000;108(4):5–66.

Copel JA, Kleinman CS. Congenital heart disease and extracardiac anomalies: association and indications for fetal echocardiography. *Am J Obstet Gynecol.* 1986;154:1121–1132.

Greenwood RD, Rosenthal A, Nadas AS. Cardiovascular malformations associated with congenital diaphragmatic hernia. *Pediatrics.* 1976;57:92–97.

Nora JJ. Etiologic aspects of heart disease. In: Adams FH, Emmanouilides GC, Riemenschneider TA, eds. *Moss' Heart Disease in Infants, Children, and Adolescents.* 4th ed. Baltimore: Williams & Wilkins; 1989.

Simeone RM, Devine OJ, Marcinkevage JA, et al. Diabetes and congenital heart defects: a systematic review, meta-analysis, and modeling project. *Am J Prev Med.* 2015;48(2):195–204.

CHAPTER 2. PHYSICAL EXAMINATION

Braunwald E, Perloff JK. Physical examination of the heart and circulation. In: Braunwald E, Zipes DP, Libby P, eds. *Heart Disease.* 6th ed. Philadelphia: WB Saunders; 2001:45–81.

Fyler DC, Nadas AS. History, physical examination, and laboratory tests. In: Fyler DC, ed. *Nadas' Pediatric Cardiology.* St. Louis: Mosby; 1992.

Hammond IW, Urbina EM, Wattigney WA, et al. Comparison of fourth and fifth Korotkoff diastolic blood pressure in 5 to 30 years old individuals. The Bogalusa Heart Study. *Am J Hypertens.* 1995;8:1083–1089.

Kaelber DC, Pickett F. Simple table to identify children and adolescents needing further evaluation of blood pressure. *Pediatrics.* 2009;123(6):e972.

Leatham A. Auscultation of the heart. *Lancet.* 1958;2:757–766.

McDonald-McGinn DM, Emanuel BS, Zackai EH. 22q11.2 deletion syndrome. *GeneReviews.* 2013;28. https://www.ncbi.nlm.nih.gov/books/NBK1523.

The Fourth Report on the Diagnosis, Evaluation, and Treatment of High Blood Pressure in Children and Adolescents. National high blood pressure education program working group on high blood pressure in children and adolescents. *Pediatrics.* 2004;111:555–576.

National High Blood Pressure Education Program Working Group on Hypertension Control in Children and Adolescents. Update on the 1987 Task Force on high blood pressure in children: a working group report from the national high blood pressure education program. *Pediatrics.* 1996;98:649–658.

O'Rourke MF, Blazek JV, Morreels Jr CL, Krovetz LJ. Pressure wave transmission along the human aorta: changes with age and in arterial degenerative disease. *Circ Res.* 1968;23:567–579.

Park MK, Guntheroth WG. Accurate blood pressure measurement in children: a review. *Am J Noninvas Cardiol.* 1989;3:297–309.

Park MK, Guntheroth WG. Direct blood pressure measurement in brachial and femoral arteries in children. *Circulation.* 1970;41:231–237.

Park MK, Kawabori I, Guntheroth WG. Need for an improved standard for blood pressure cuff size. *Clin Pediatr.* 1976;15:784–787.

Park MK, Lee D-H. Normative blood pressure values in the arm and calf in the newborn. *Pediatrics.* 1989;83:240–243.

Park MK, Lee D-H, Johnson GA. Oscillometric blood pressure in the arm, thigh and calf in healthy children and those with aortic coarctation. *Pediatrics.* 1993;91:761–765.

Park MK, Menard SW. Accuracy of blood pressure measurement by the Dinamap monitor in infants and children. *Pediatrics.* 1987;79: 907–914.

Park MK, Menard SW, Schoolfield J. Oscillometric blood pressure standards for children. *Pediatr Cardiol.* 2005;26:601–607.

Park MK, Menard SW, Yuan C. Comparison of auscultatory and oscillometric blood pressure. *Arch Pediatr Adolesc Med.* 2001;155:50–53.

Park MK, Menard SW, Yuan C. Comparison of blood pressure in children from three ethnic groups. *Am J Cardiol.* 2001;87:1305–1308.

Perloff JK. *Physical Examination of the Heart and Circulation.* 3rd ed. Philadelphia: WB Saunders; 2000.

Report of the second task force on blood pressure control in children. *Pediatrics.* 1987;79:1–25.

Rudolph AM. *Congenital Diseases of the Heart: Clinical-Physiologic Considerations in Diagnosis and Management.* St. Louis: Mosby; 1974.

Urbina E, Alpert B, Flynn J, et al. Ambulatory blood pressure monitoring in children and adolescents: recommendations for standard assessment: a scientific statement from the American Heart Association Atherosclerosis, Hypertension, and Obesity In Youth Committee of the Council on Cardiovascular Disease In The Young and the Council for High Blood Pressure Research. *Hypertension.* 2008;52:433–451.

CHAPTER 3. ELECTROCARDIOGRAPHY

Davignon A, Rautaharju P, Boisselle E, et al. Normal ECG standards for infants and children. *Pediatr Cardiol.* 1979/1980;1:133–152.

Park MK, Guntheroth WG. *How to Read Pediatric ECGs.* 4th ed. Philadelphia: Mosby Elsevier; 2006.

Towbin JA, Bricker JT, Garson A. Electrocardiographic criteria for diagnosis of acute myocardial infarction in childhood. *Am J Cardiol.* 1992;69:1545–1548.

CHAPTER 4. CHEST RADIOGRAPHY

Amplatz K. Plain film diagnosis of congenital heart disease. In: Moller JH, Hoffman JIE, eds. *Pediatric Cardiovascular Medicine.* New York: Churchill Livingstone; 2000:143–155.

CHAPTER 5. NONINVASIVE IMAGING TOOLS

Armstrong WF, Ryan T. *Feigenbaum's Echocardiography.* 7th ed. Philadelphia: Lippincott Williams Wilkins; 2010.

Daniels SR, Meyer RA, Liang YC, et al. Echocardiographically determined left ventricular mass index in normal children, adolescents, and young adults. *J Am Coll Cardiol.* 1988;12:703–708.

Nishimura RA, Abel MD, Hatle LK, et al. Assessment of diastolic function of the heart: background and current applications of Doppler echocardiography. II. Clinical studies. *Mayo Clin Proc.* 1989;64:181–204.

Prakash A, Powell AJ, Geva T. Multimodality non-invasive imaging for assessment of congenital heart disease. *Circulation.* 2010;3:112–125.

Rychik J, Ayers N, Cuneo B, et al. American Society of Echocardiography Guidelines and standards for performance of the fetal echocardiography. *J Am Soc Echocardiogr.* 2004;17:803–810.

CHAPTER 6. OTHER NONINVASIVE INVESTIGATION TOOLS

Ahmed F, Kavey R-E, Kveselis DA, et al. Response of non-obese white children to treadmill exercise. *J Pediatr.* 2001;139:284–290.

Biko DM, Collins 2nd RT, Partington SL, et al. Magnetic resonance myocardial perfusion imaging: safety and indications in pediatrics and young adults. *Pediatr Cardiol.* 2018;39(2):275–282.

Chatrath R, Shenoy R, Serratto M, et al. Physical fitness of urban American children. *Pediatr Cardiol.* 2002;23:608–612.

Cumming GR, Everatt D, Hartman L. Bruce treadmill test in children: normal values in a clinic population. *Am J Cardiol.* 1978;41:69–75.

Dickinson DF, Scott O. Ambulatory electrocardiographic monitoring in 100 healthy teenage boys. *Br Heart J.* 1984;51(2):179–183.

Flynn JT, Daniels SR, Hayman LL, et al. Update: ambulatory blood pressure monitoring in children and adolescents. A scientific statement from the American Heart Association. *Hypertension.* 2014;63:1116–1135.

Gibbons RJ, Balady GJ, Bricker JT, Chaitman BR, et al. ACC/AHA 2002 Guideline Update for Exercise Testing. *J Am Coll Cardiol.* 2005;40(8):1531–1540.

Lobodzinski SS, Laks MM. New devices for very long-term ECG monitoring. *Cardiol J.* 2012;19:210–214.

Paridon SM, Alpert BS, Boas SR, Cabrera ME, et al. Clinical stress testing in pediatric age group. A statement from the American Heart Association Council on cardiovascular disease in the young, committee on atherosclerosis, hypertension, and obesity in youth. *Circulation.* 2006;113:1905–1920.

Rowell LB, Brengelmann GL, Blackmon JR, Bruce RA, Murray JA. Disparities between aortic and peripheral pulse pressure induced by upright exercise and vasomotor changes in man. *Circulation.* 1968;37:954–964.

Soergel M, Kirschstein M, Busch C, et al. Oscillometric twenty-four-hour ambulatory blood pressure values in healthy children and adolescents: a multicenter trial including 1141 subjects. *J Pediatr.* 1997;130:178–184.

Sorof J, Portman RJ. Ambulatory blood pressure monitoring in pediatric patients. *J Pediatr.* 2000;165:578–586.

Southall DP, Johnson AM, Shinebourne EA, et al. Frequency and outcome of disorder of cardiac rhythm and conduction in a population of newborn infants. *Pediatrics.* 1981;68:58–66.

Southall DP, Richards J, Mitchell P, et al. Study of cardiac rhythm in healthy newborn infants. *Br Heart J.* 1980;43:14–20.

Southsall DP, Johnston F, Shineborune EA, et al. 14-hour electrocardiographic study of heart rate and rhythm patterns in population of healthy children. *Br Heart J.* 1981;45(3):281–291.

Urbina E, Alpert B, Flynn J, et al. Ambulatory blood pressure monitoring in children and adolescents: recommendations for standard assessment: a scientific statement from the American Heart Association Atherosclerosis, Hypertension, and Obesity In Youth Committee of the Council on Cardiovascular Disease In The Young and the Council For High Blood Pressure Research. *Hypertension.* 2008;52:433–451.

Ulrich S, Hildebrand FF, Treder U, et al. Reference values for the 6-minute walk test in healthy children and adolescents in Switzerland. *MBC Pulmonary Med.* 2013;13:49.

Wühl E, Witte K, Soergel M, et al. German Working Group on Pediatric Hypertension. Distribution of 24-h ambulatory blood pressure in children: normalized reference values and role of body dimensions. *J Hypertens.* 2002;20:1995–2007.

CHAPTER 7. INVASIVE PROCEDURES

Bonhoeffer P, Boudjemline Y, Saliba Z, et al. Percutaneous replacement of pulmonary valve in a right-ventricle to pulmonary-artery prosthetic conduit with valve dysfunction. *Lancet.* 2000;356:1403–1405.

Cassidy SC, Schmidt KG, Van Hare GF, et al. Complications of pediatric cardiac catheterization: a 3-year study. *J Am Coll Cardiol.* 1992;19:1285–1293.

Feltes TF, Bacha E, Beekman RH, Cheatham JP, et al. Indications for cardiac catheterization and intervention in pediatric cardiac disease: a scientific statement from the American Heart Association. *Circulation.* 2011;123:2607–2652.

Holzer R, Cheatham JP. Therapeutic cardiac catherization. In: Allen HD, Shaddy RE, Penny DJ, eds. *Moss and Adams' Heart Disease in Infants, Children, and Adolescents.* 9th ed. Philadelphia: Wolters Kluwer; 2016:467–521.

Lock JE, Keane JF, Mandell VS, et al. Cardiac catheterization. In: Fyler DC, ed. *Nadas' Pediatric Cardiology.* St. Louis: Mosby; 1992.

Mullins CE, Nihil MR. Cardiac catheterization hemodynamics and intervention. In: Moller JH, Hoffman HE, eds. *Pediatric Cardiovascular Medicine.* New York: Churchill Livingstone; 2000:203–215.

CHAPTER 8. FETAL AND PERINATAL CIRCULATION

Guntheroth WG, Kawabori I, Stevenson JG. Physiology of the circulation: fetus, neonate, and child. In: Kelly VC ed. *Practice of Pediatrics*, Vol. 8, Philadelphia: Harper & Row;1982–1983.

Rudolph AM. *Congenital Diseases of the Heart: Clinical-Physiologic Considerations in Diagnosis and Management*. Chicago: Mosby; 1974.

CHAPTERS 9, 10, AND 11. PATHOPHYSIOLOGY OF LEFT-TO-RIGHT SHUNT LESIONS, PATHOPHYSIOLOGY OF OBSTRUCTIVE AND VALVULAR REGURGITANT LESIONS, AND PATHOPHYSIOLOGY OF CYANOTIC CONGENITAL HEART DEFECTS

Chan WD, Chan MM, Chan MM. Pulse oximetry: understanding its basic principles facilitates appreciation of its limitations. *Respir Med*. 2013;107:780–799.

Duc G. Assessment of hypoxia in the newborn: suggestions for a practical approach. *Pediatrics*. 1971;48:469–481.

Francois K. Aortopathy associated with congenital heart disease: a current literature review. *Ann Pediatr Cardiol*. 2015;8:25–36.

Guntheroth WG, Morgan BC, Mullins GL, Baum D. Venous return with knee-chest position and squatting in tetralogy of Fallot. *Am Heart J*. 1968;75:313–318.

Guntheroth WG, Morgan BC, Mullins GL. Physiologic studies of paroxysmal hyperpnea in cyanotic congenital heart disease. *Circulation*. 1965;31:66–76.

Heath D, Edwards JE. The pathology of hypertensive pulmonary vascular disease. *Circulation*. 1958;18:533–547.

King SB, Franch RH. Production of increased right-to-left shunting by rapid heart rates in patients with tetralogy of Fallot. *Circulation*. 1971;44:265–271.

Moller JH, Amplatz K, Edwards JE. *Congenital Heart Disease*. Kalamazoo, MI: Upjohn; 1971.

Rudolph AM. *Congenital Diseases of the Heart*. Chicago: Mosby; 1974.

CHAPTER 12. LEFT-TO-RIGHT SHUNT LESIONS

Atrial Septal Defect

Feltes TF, Bacha E, Beekman III RH, et al. Indications for cardiac catheterization and intervention in pediatric cardiac disease: a scientific statement from the American Heart Association. *Circulation*. 2011;123:2607–2652.

Laussen PC, Bichell DP, McGowan FX, et al. Postoperative recovery in children after minimum versus full length sternotomy. *Ann Thorac Surg*. 2000;69:591–596.

Radzik D, Davignon A, van Doesburg N, et al. Predictive factors for spontaneous closure of atrial septal defect diagnosed in the first 3 months of life. *J Am Coll Cardiol*. 1993;22:851–853.

Rao V, Freedom RM, Black MD. Minimally invasive surgery with cardioscopy for congenital heart defects. *Ann Thorac Surg*. 2000;68:1742–1745.

Shivaprakashas K, Murthy KS, Coelho R, et al. Role of limited posterior thoracotomy for open-heart surgery in the current era. *Ann Thorac Surg*. 1999;68:2310–2313.

Ventricular Septal Defect

Graham Jr TP, Bender HW, Spach MS. Ventricular septal defect. In: Adams FH, Emmanouilides GC, Riemenschneider TA, eds. *Moss' Heart Disease in Infants, Children and Adolescents*. 4th ed. Baltimore: Williams & Wilkins; 1989.

Hoffman JIE, Kaplan S. The incidence of congenital heart disease. *J Am Coll Cardiol*. 2002;39:1890–1900.

Soto B, Becker AE, Moulaezt AH, et al. Classification of ventricular septal defects. *Br Heart J*. 1980;43:332–363.

Van Mill GJ, Moulaert AJ, Harinck E. *Atlas of Two-Dimensional Echocardiography in Congenital Cardiac Defects*. Boston: Martinus Nijhoff; 1983.

McDaniel NL, Gutgessel HP. Ventricular septal defects. In: *Moss and Adams' Heart Disease in Infants, Children and Adolescents*. 6th ed. Philadelphia: Lippincott Williams & Wilkins; 2001.

Patent Ductus Arteriosus

Benitz WE. Committee on Fetus and Newborn: patent ductus arteriosus in preterm infants. *Pediatrics*. 2016;137(1):e20153730.

Feltes TF, Bacha E, Beekman III RH, et al. Indications for cardiac catheterization and intervention in pediatric cardiac disease: a scientific statement from the American Heart Association. *Circulation*. 2011;123:2607–2652.

Hammerman C, Bin-Nun A, Markovitch E, et al. Ductal closure with paracetamol: a surprising new approach to patent ductus arteriosus treatment. *Pediatrics*. 2011;128:c1618–c1621.

Musewe NN, Poppe D, Smallhorn JF, et al. Doppler echocardiographic measurement of pulmonary artery pressure from ductal Doppler velocities in the newborn. *J Am Coll Cardiol*. 1990;15:446–456.

Musewe NN, Smallhorn JF, Benson LN, et al. Validation of Doppler-derived pulmonary arterial pressure in patients with ductus arteriosus under different hemodynamic states. *Circulation*. 1987;76:1081–1091.

Ohlsson A, Shah PS. Paracetamol (acetaminophen) for patent ductus arteriosus in preterm or low birth weight infants. *Cochrane Database Syst Rev*. 2018;4:CD010061.

Pacifici GM. Clinical pharmacology of furosemide in neonates: a review. *Pharmaceuticals*. 2013;6:1094–1129.

Rao PS, Sideris EB, Haddad J, et al. Transcatheter occlusion of patent ductus arteriosus with adjustable buttoned device: initial clinical experience. *Circulation*. 1993;88:1119–1126.

Van Overmeire B, Smets K, Lecoutere D, et al. A comparison of ibuprofen and indomethacin for closure of patent ductus arteriosus. *N Engl J Med*. 2000;343:674–681.

Varvarigou A, Bardin CL, Beharry K, et al. Early ibuprofen administration to prevent patent ductus arteriosus in premature newborn infants. *JAMA*. 1996;275:539–544.

Endocardial Cushion Defect

Anderson RH, Macartney FJ, Shineboume EA, et al. Atrioventricular septal defects. In: Anderson RH, Macartney FJ, Shinebourne EA, et al., eds. *Pediatric Cardiology, New York*. Churchill Livingstone; 1987.

Piccoli GP, Gerlis LM, Wilkinson JL, et al. Morphology and classification of atrioventricular defects. *Br Heart J*. 1979;42:621–632.

Rastelli GC, Kirklin JW, Titus JL. Anatomic observation on complete form of persistent common atrioventricular canal with special reference to atrioventricular valves. *Mayo Clin Proc*. 1966;41:296–308.

Partial Anomalous Pulmonary Venous Return

Ward KE, Mullins CE. Anomalous pulmonary venous connections; pulmonary vein stenosis; atresia of the common pulmonary vein. In: Garson Jr A, Bricker JT, McNamara DG, eds. *The Science and Practice of Pediatric Cardiology.* Philadelphia: Lea & Febiger; 1990.

CHAPTER 13. OBSTRUCTIVE LESIONS

Pulmonary Stenosis.

Feltes TF, Bacha E, Beekman III RH, et al. Indications for cardiac catheterization and intervention in pediatric cardiac disease: a scientific statement from the American Heart Association. *Circulation.* 2011;123:2607–2652.

Stanger P, Cassidy SC, Dried DA, et al. Balloon pulmonary valvuloplasty: results of the valvuloplasty and angioplasty of congenital anomalies registry. *Am J Cardiol.* 1990;65:775–783.

***Aortic* Stenosis**

ACC/AHA 2006 guidelines for the management of patients with valvular heart disease, *Circulation.* 2006; 114(5):e84–231 or *J Am Coll Cardiol* 48(3):e1–148, 2006.

Biner S, Rafique AM, Ray I, Cuk O, Siegel RJ, Tolstrup K. Aortopathy is prevalent in relatives of bicuspid aortic valve patients. *J Am Coll Cardiol.* 2009;53(24):2288–2295.

Feltes TF, Bacha E, Beekman III RH, et al. Indications for cardiac catheterization and intervention in pediatric cardiac disease: a scientific statement from the American Heart Association. *Circulation.* 2011;123:2607–2652.

Geva A, McMahon CJ, Gauvreau K, et al. Risk factors for reoperation after repair of discrete subaortic stenosis in children. *J Am Coll Cardiol.* 2007;50:1498–1504. 2007.

Graham TP, Driscoll DJ, Newburger JW, et al. Task Force 2: Congenital Heart Disease. 36th Bethesda Conference. Eligibility recommendations for competitive athletes with cardiovascular abnormalities. *J Am Coll Cardiol.* 2005;45:1326–1333.

Hoffman JIE, Kaplan S. The incidence of congenital heart disease. *J Am Coll Cardiol.* 2002;39:1890–1900.

Kouchoukos NT, Davila-Roman VG, Spray TL, et al. Replacement of the aortic root with a pulmonary autograft in children and young adults with aortic valve disease. *N Engl J Med.* 1994;330:1–6.

McMahon CJ, Gauvreau K, Edwards JC, Geva T. Risk factors for aortic valve dysfunction in children with discrete subaortic stenosis. *Am J Cardiol.* 2004;94:459–464.

Nishimura RA, Otto CM, Bonow RO, et al. 2014 AHA/ACC guideline for the management of patients with valvular heart disease: a report of the American College of Cardiology/American Heart Association Task Force on Practice Guidelines. *J Am Coll Cardiol.* 2014;63(22):e57–185.

Parry AJ, Kovalchin JP, Suda K, McElhenney DB, et al. Resection of subaortic stenosis; can a more aggressive approach be justified? *Eur J Cardiothorac Surg.* 1999;15:631–638.

Van Son JAM, Schaff HV, Danielson GK, et al. Surgical treatment of discrete and tunnel subaortic stenosis. II. Late survival and risk of reoperation. *Circulation.* 1993;88:159–169.

Wilson WR, Greer GE, Durzinsky DS, Curtis JJ. Ross procedure for complex left ventricular outflow tract obstruction. *J Cardiovasc Surg.* 2000;41:387–392.

Coarctation of the Aorta

Connolly HM, Huston III J, Brown Jr RD, et al. Intracranial aneurysm in patients with coarctation of the aorta: a prospective magnetic resonance angiographic study of 100 patients. *Mayo Clin Proc.* 2003;78:1491–1499.

Cowley CG, Orsmond GS, Feola P, et al. Long-term, randomized comparison of balloon angioplasty and surgery for native coarctation of the aorta in childhood. *Circulation.* 2005;111:3453–3456.

Feltes TF, Bacha E, Beekman III RH, et al. Indications for cardiac catheterization and intervention in pediatric cardiac disease: a scientific statement from the American Heart Association. *Circulation.* 2011;123:2607–2652.

Hellenbrand WE, Allen HD, Golinko RJ, et al. Balloon angioplasty for aortic recoarctation: results of valvuloplasty and angioplasty of congenital anomalies registry. *Am J Cardiol.* 1990;65:793–797.

Ramaciotti C, Chin AJ. Noninvasive diagnosis of coarctation of the aorta in the presence of a patent ductus arteriosus. *Am Heart J.* 1993;125:179–185.

Torok RD, Campbell MJ, Fleming GA, et al. Coarctation of the aorta: management from infancy to adulthood. *Word J Cardiol.* 2015;7:765–775.

CHAPTER 14. CYANOTIC CONGENITAL HEART DEFECTS

Chang RK, Gurvitz M, Rodriguez S. Missed diagnosis of critical congenital heart disease. *Arch Pediatr Adolesc Med.* 2008;162:969–974.

Ewer AK, Martin GR. Newborn pulse oximetry screening: which algorithm is best? *Pediatrics.* 2016;138(5):e20161206.

Mahle WT, Newburger JW, Matherne GP, et al. Role of pulse oximetry in examining newborns for congenital heart disease: a scientific statement from the American Heart Association and American Academy of Pediatrics. *Circulation.* 2009;120:447–458.

Wandler LA, Martin GR. Critical congenital heart disease screening using pulse oximetry: achieving a national approach to screening, education and implementation in the United States. *Intern J Neonatal Screening.* 2017;3(28).

Complete Transposition of the Great Arteries

Blume ED, Altman K, Mayer JE, et al. Evolution of risk factors influencing early mortality of the arterial switch operation. *J Am Coll Cardiol.* 1999;33:1702–1709.

Jex RK, Puga FJ, Julsrud PR, et al. Repair of transposition of the great arteries with intact ventricular septum and left ventricular outflow tract obstruction. *J Thorac Cardiovasc Surg.* 1990;100:682–686.

Jones RA, Giglia TM, Sanders SP, et al. Rapid, two-stage arterial switch for transposition of the great arteries and intact ventricular septum beyond the neonatal period. *Circulation.* 1989;80(suppl I): I-203–I-208.

Kovalchin JP, Allen HD, Cassidy SC, et al. Pulmonary valve eccentricity in D-transposition of the great arteries and implications for the arterial switch operation. *Am J Cardiol.* 1994;73:186–190.

Lupinetti FM, Bove EL, Minich LL, et al. Intermediate-term survival and functional results after arterial repair for transposition of the great arteries. *J Thorac Cardiovasc Surg.* 1992;103:421–427.

Morell VO, Jacobs JP, Quintessenza JA. Aortic translocation in the management of transposition of the great arteries with ventricular septal defect and pulmonary stenosis: results and follow-up. *Ann Thorac Surg.* 2005;79:2089–2093.

Waldeman JD, Lamberti JJ, George L, et al. Experience with Damus procedure. *Circulation*. 1988;78(suppl III): III 32–III-39.

Yacoub M, Bernhard A, Lange P, et al. Clinical and hemodynamic results of the two-stage anatomic correction of simple transposition of the great arteries. *Circulation*. 1980;62(suppl I): I-190–I-196.

Congenitally Corrected Transposition of the Great Arteries

Dabizzi RP, Barletta GA, Caprioli G, et al. Coronary artery anatomy in corrected transposition of the great arteries. *J Am Coll Cardiol*. 1988;12:486–491.

Graham TP, Bernard YD, Mellen BG, et al. Long-term outcome in congenitally corrected transposition of the great arteries. *J Am Coll Cardiol*. 2000;36:255–261.

Lundstrom U, Bull C, Wyse RKH, et al. The natural and "unnatural" history of congenitally corrected transposition. *Am J Cardiol*. 1990;65:1222–1229.

Tetralogy of Fallot

Bonhoeffer P, Boudjemline Y, Saliba Z, et al. Percutaneous replacement of pulmonary valve in a right-ventricle to pulmonary-artery prosthetic conduit with valve dysfunction. *Lancet*. 2000;356:1403–1405.

Geva T. Indications and timing of pulmonary valve replacement after tetralogy of Fallot repair. *Semin Thorac Cardiovasc Surg Pediatr Card Surg Annu*. 2006:11–22.

Geva T. Indications for pulmonary valve replacement in repaired tetralogy of Fallot. The quest continues [editorial]. *Circulation*. 2013;128: 1855–1847.

Gupta A, Odim J, Levi D, Chang R-K, Laks H. Staged repair of pulmonary atresia with ventricular septal defect and major aortopulmonary collateral arteries: experience with 104 patients. *J Thorac Cardiovasc Surg*. 2003;126:1746–1752.

Lakier JB, Stanger P, Heymann MA, et al. Tetralogy of Fallot with absent pulmonary valve: natural history and hemodynamic considerations. *Circulation*. 1974;50:167–175.

Lee C, Kim YM, Lee CH, et al. Outcome of pulmonary valve replacement in 170 patients with chronic pulmonary regurgitation after relief of right ventricular outflow tract obstruction. Implication for optimal timing of pulmonary valve replacement. *J Am Coll Cardiol*. 2012;60:1005–10014.

Need LR, Powell AJ, del Nide P, et al. Coronary echocardiography in tetralogy of Fallot: diagnostic accuracy, resource utilization and surgical implications over 13 years. *J Am Coll Cardiol*. 2000;36:1371–1377.

Puga FJ, Leoni FE, Julsrud PR, et al. Complete repair of pulmonary atresia, ventricular septal defect, and severe peripheral arborization abnormalities of the central pulmonary arteries. *J Thorac Cardiovasc Surg*. 1989;98:1018–1029.

Reddy VM, Liddicoat JR, Hanley FL. Midline one-stage complete unifocalization and repair of pulmonary atresia with ventricular septal defect and major aortopulmonary collaterals. *J Thorac Cardiovasc Surg*. 1995;109:832–844.

Sawatari K, Imai Y, Kurosawa H, et al. Staged operation for pulmonary atresia and ventricular septal defect with major aortopulmonary collateral arteries. *J Thorac Cardiovasc Surg*. 1989;98:738–750.

Watterson KG, Wilkinson JL, Karly TR, Mee RBB. Very small pulmonary arteries: central end-to-side shunt. *Ann Thorac Surg*. 1991;52:1131–1137.

Total Anomalous Pulmonary Venous Return

Lupinetti FM, Kulik TJ, Beekman RH, et al. Correction of total anomalous pulmonary venous connection in infancy. *J Thorac Cardiovasc Surg*. 1993;106:880–885.

Van der Velde ME, Parness IA, Colan SD, et al. Two-dimensional echocardiography in pre- and postoperative management of totally anomalous pulmonary venous connection. *J Am Coll Cardiol*. 1991;18:1746–1751.

Tricuspid Atresia

Backer CL, Deal BJ, Kaushal S, et al. Extracardiac versus intra-atrial lateral tunnel Fontan: extracardiac is better. *Semin Thorac Cardiovasc Surg Pediatr Cardiol Surg Annu*. 2011;14:4–10.

Bridges ND, Mayer JE, Lock JE, et al. Effects of baffle fenestration on outcome of the modified Fontan operation. *Circulation*. 1992;86:1762–1769.

Castaneda AR. From Glenn to Fontan: a continuing evolution. *Circulation*. 1992;86(suppl II): II-80–II-84.

Gentles TL, Mayer Jr JE, Gauvreau K, et al. Fontan operation in five hundred consecutive patients: factors influencing early and late outcome. *J Thorac Cardiovasc Surg*. 1997;114:376–391.

Giannico S, Como A, Marino B, et al. Total extracardiac right heart bypass. *Circulation*. 1992;86(suppl II): II-110–II-117.

Gupta A, Daggett C, Behera S, et al. Risk factors for persistent pleural effusions after the extracardiac Fontan procedure. *J Thorac Cardiovasc Surg*. 2004;127:1664–1669.

Hirsch JC, Goldberg C, Bove EL, et al. Fontan operation in the current era: a 15-year single institution experience. *Ann Surg*. 2008;248(3):402–410.

Hsu DT, Wuaegebeur JM, Ing FF, et al. Outcome after the single-stage, nonfenestrated Fontan procedure. *Circulation*. 1997;96:11-335–11-340.

Johnson JT, Lindsey I, Day RW, et al. Living at altitude adversely affects survival among patients with a Fontan procedure. *J Am Coll Cardiol*. 2013;61:1283–1289.

Kawashima Y, Kitamura S, Matsuda H, et al. Total cavopulmonary shunt operation in complex cardiac anomalies. A new operation. *J Thorac Cardiovasc Surg*. 1984;87(1):74–81.

Kreutzer G, Galindez H, Bono H, et al. An operation for the correction of tricuspid atresia. *J Thorac Cardiovasc Surg*. 1973;66(3):613–621.

McCrindle BW, Manlhiot C, Cochrane A, et al. Factors associated with thrombotic complications after the Fontan procedure. *J Am Coll Cardiol*. 2013;61:346–353.

Mertens L, Hagler DJ, Sauer U, et al. Protein-losing enteropathy after the Fontan operation: an international multicenter study. *J Thorac Cardiovasc Surg*. 1998;115:1063–1073.

Rogers LS, Glatz AC, Ravishankar C, et al. 18 years of the Fontan operation at a single institution. *J Am Coll Cardiol*. 2012;60:1018–1025.

Salvin JW, Scheurer MA, Laussen PC, et al. Factors associated with prolonged recovery after the Fontan operation. *Circulation*. 2008;118:S171–176.

Song JY, Choi JY, Ko JT, et al. Long-term aspirin therapy for hepatopulmonary syndrome. *Pediatrics*. 1996;97:917–920.

Thompson LD, Petrossian E, McElhinney DB, et al. Is it necessary to routinely fenestrate an extracardiac Fontan? *J Am Coll Cardiol*. 1999;34:539–544.

Pulmonary Atresia

Alwi M, Geetha K, Bilkis AA, et al. Pulmonary atresia with intact ventricular septum percutaneous radiofrequency-assisted valvotomy and balloon dilatation versus surgical valvotomy and Blalock-Taussig shunt. *J Am Coll Cardiol*. 2000;35:468–476.

Bull C, de Leval MR, Mercanti C, et al. Pulmonary atresia and intact ventricular septum: a revised classification. *Circulation.* 1982;66:266–280.

Cheung YF, Leung MP, Chau AK. Usefulness of laser-assisted valvotomy with balloon valvoplasty for pulmonary valve atresia with intact ventricular septum. *Am J Cardiol.* 2002;90:438–442.

Feltes TF, Bacha E, Beekman III RH, et al. Indications for cardiac catheterization and intervention in pediatric cardiac disease: a scientific statement from the American Heart Association. *Circulation.* 2011;123:2607–2652.

Hanley FL, Sade RM, Blackstone EH, Kirklin JW, Freedom RM, Nanda NC. Outcomes in neonatal pulmonary atresia with intact ventricular septum: a multi-institutional study. *J Thorac Cardiovasc Surg.* 1993;105:406–427.

Hypoplastic Left Heart Syndrome

Chang AC, Farrell Jr PE, Murdison KA, et al. Hypoplastic left heart syndrome: hemodynamic and angiographic assessment after initial reconstructive surgery and relevance to modified Fontan procedure. *Pediatr Cardiol.* 1991;17:1143–1149.

Douglas WI, Goldberg CS, Mosca RS, Law IH, Bove EL. Hemi-Fontan procedure for hypoplastic left heart syndrome: outcome and suitability for Fontan. *Ann Thorac Surg.* 1999;68:1361–1368.

Galantowicz M, Cheatham JP, Phillips A, et al. Hybrid approach for hypoplastic left heart syndrome: intermediate results after the learning curve. *Ann Thorac Surg.* 2008;85:2063–2071.

Glauser TA, Rorke LB, Weinberg PM, Clancy RR. Congenital brain anomalies associated with the hypoplastic left heart syndrome. *Pediatrics.* 1990;85(6):984–990.

Hirsch JC, Goldberg C, Bove EL, et al. Fontan operation in the current era: a 15-year single institution experience. *Ann Surg.* 2008;248:402–410.

Jacobs ML. Recent innovations in the Norwood sequence of operations. *Cardiol Young.* 2004;14(suppl 1):47–51.

Norwood WI, Lang P, Castaneda AR, et al. Experience with operations for hypoplastic left heart syndrome. *J Thorac Cardiovasc Surg.* 1981;82:511–519.

Ohye RG, Sleeper LA, Mahony L, et al. Comparison of shunt types in the Norwood procedure for single-ventricle lesions. *N Engl J Med.* 2010;362:1980–1992.

Rogers LS, Glatz AC, Ravishankar C, et al. 18 years of the Fontan operation at a single institution. *J Am Coll Cardiol.* 2012;60:1018–1025.

Starnes VA, Griffin ML, Pitlick PT, et al. Current approach to hypoplastic left heart syndrome: palliation, transplantation, or both. *J Thorac Cardiovasc Surg.* 1992;104:189–195.

Ebstein's Anomaly

Cappato R, Schuter M, Weiss C, et al. Radiofrequency current catheter ablation of accessory atrioventricular pathways in Ebstein's anomaly. *Circulation.* 1996;94:376–383.

Carpentier A, Chauvaud S, Mace L, et al. A new reconstructive operation for Ebstein's anomaly of the tricuspid valve. *J Thorac Cardiovasc Surg.* 1988;96:92–101.

Danielson GK, Driscoll DJ, Mair DD, et al. Operative treatment of Ebstein's anomaly. *J Thorac Cardiovasc Surg.* 1992;104:1195–1202.

Shiina A, Sewer JB, Edwards WD, et al. Two-dimensional echocardiographic spectrum of Ebstein's anomaly: detailed anatomic assessment. *J Am Coll Cardiol.* 1984;3:356–370.

Truncus Arteriosus

Lenox CC, Debich DE, Zuberbuhler JR. The role of coronary artery abnormalities in the prognosis of truncus arteriosus. *J Thorac Cardiovasc Surg.* 1992;104:1724–1742.

Spicer RL, Behrendt D, Crowley DC, et al. Repair of truncus arteriosus in neonates with the use of a valveless conduit. *Circulation.* 1984;70(suppl I): I-26–I-29.

Williams JM, de Leeuw M, Black MD, et al. Factors associated with outcomes of persistent truncus arteriosus. *J Am Coll Cardiol.* 1999;34:545–553.

Single Ventricle

Douville EC, Sade RM, Fyfe DA. Hemi-Fontan operation in surgery for single ventricle: a preliminary report. *Ann Thorac Surg.* 1991;51:893–899.

Freedom RM, Benson LN, Smallhorn JF, et al. Subaortic stenosis, the univentricular heart, and banding of the pulmonary artery: an analysis of the courses of 43 patients with univentricular heart palliated by pulmonary artery banding. *Circulation.* 1986;73:758–764.

Newfeld EA, Niakidoh H. Surgical management of subaortic stenosis in patients with a single ventricle and transposition of the great vessels. *Circulation.* 1987;76(suppl III): III-29–III-33.

Sano S, Ishino K, Kawata M, Arai S, Hasahara S, et al. Right ventricle-pulmonary artery shunt in first-stage palliation of hypoplastic left heart syndrome. *J Thorac Cardiovasc Surg.* 2003;126:504–510.

Stein DG, Laks H, Drinkwater DC, et al. Results of total cavopulmonary connection in the treatment of patients with a functional single ventricle. *J Thorac Cardiovasc Surg.* 1991;102:280–287.

Double-Outlet Right Ventricle

Belli E, Serraf A, Lacour-Gayet F, et al. Biventricular repair for double-outlet right ventricle: results and long-term follow-up. *Circulation.* 1998;98:11-360–11-367.

Kirklin JW, Pacifico AD, Blackstone EH, et al. Current risks and protocols for operation for double-outlet right ventricle: derivation from an 18 year experience. *J Thorac Cardiovasc Surg.* 1986;92:913–930.

Sridaromont S, Feldt RH, Ritter DG, et al. Double outlet right ventricle: hemodynamic and anatomic correlation. *Am J Cardiol.* 1976;38:85–94.

Splenic Syndromes

Lamberti JJ, Waldman JD, Mathewson JW, et al. Repair of subdiaphragmatic total anomalous pulmonary venous connection without cardiopulmonary bypass. *J Thorac Cardiovasc Surg.* 1984;88:627–630.

Kimberlin DW, Brady MT, Jackson MA, Long SS, eds. *Red Book: 2018 Report of the Committee on Infectious Disease.* 31th ed. Elk Grove Village, IL: American Academy of Pediatrics; 2018.

Sapire DW, Ho SY, Anderson RH, et al. Diagnosis and significance of atrial isomerism. *Am J Cardiol.* 1986;58:342–346.

Van Mierop LHS, Gessner IH, Schiebler GL. Asplenia and polysplenia syndrome, *Birth Defects. Original Article Series.* 1972;8:36–44.

Persistent Pulmonary Hypertension of Newborn

Abman SH. Neonatal pulmonary hypertension: a physiologic approach to treatment. *Pediatr Pulmonol Suppl.* 2004;26:127–128.

Rudolph AM. High pulmonary vascular resistance after birth. I. Pathophysiologic considerations and etiologic classification. *Clin Pediatr.* 1980;19:585–590.

CHAPTER 15. MISCELLANEOUS CONGENITAL CARDIAC CONDITIONS

Berthet K, Lavergne T, Cohen A, Guize L, et al. Significant association of atrial vulnerability with atrial septal abnormalities in young patients with ischemic stroke of unknown cause. *Stroke.* 2000;31(2):398–403.

Bird LM, Billman GF, Lacro RV, et al. Sudden death in Williams syndrome: report of ten cases. *J Pediatr.* 1996;129:926–931.

Cheng CP, Taur AS, Lee GS, et al. Relative lung perfusion distribution in normal lung scans: observations and clinical implications. *Congenit Heart Dis.* 2006;1(5):210–216.

Collins RT, Aziz PF, Gleason MM, et al. Abnormalities of cardiac repolarization in Williams syndrome. *Am J Cardiol.* 2010;106:1029–1033.

Gao Y, Burrows PE, Benson LN, et al. Scimitar syndrome in infancy. *J Am Coll Cardiol.* 1993;22:873–882.

Goldmuntz E. DiGeorge syndrome: new insights. *Clin Perinatol.* 2005;32:963–978.

Goldstein LB, Adams R, Alberts MJ, Appel LJ, et al. Primary prevention of ischemic stroke: a guideline from the American Heart Association/American Stroke Association Stroke Council: cosponsored by the Atherosclerotic Peripheral Vascular Disease Interdisciplinary Working Group; Cardiovascular Nursing Council; Clinical Cardiology Council; Nutrition, Physical Activity, and Metabolism Council; and the Quality of Care and Outcomes Research Interdisciplinary Working Group. *Circulation.* 2006;113(24):e873–e923.

Grifka RG, O'Laughlin MP, Nihill MR, Mullins CE. Double-transseptal, double-balloon valvuloplasty for congenital mitral stenosis. *Circulation.* 1992;88:123–129.

Guntheroth WG, Schwaegler R, Trent E. Comparative roles of the atrial septal aneurysm versus patient foramen ovale in systemic embolization with inference from neonatal studies. *Am J Cardiol.* 2004;94:1341–1343.

Hirsch R, Landt Y, Porter S, et al. Cardiac troponin I in pediatrics: normal levels and potential use in the assessment of cardiac injury. *J Pediatr.* 1997;130:872–877.

Latson LA, Pierce LR. Congenital and acquired pulmonary vein stenosis. *Circulation.* 2007;115:103–108.

Lucas Jr RV, Krabill KA. Anomalous venous connections, pulmonary and systemic. In: Adams FH, Emmanouilides GC, Riemenschneider TA, eds. *Moss' Heart Disease in Infants, Children, and Adolescents.* 4th ed. Baltimore: Williams & Wilkins; 1989.

Majadidi MK, Zaman MO, Elgendy IY, et al. Cryptogenic stroke and patent foramen ovale. *J Am College Cardiol.* 2018;71:1035–1043.

Mas J-L, Derumeaux G, Guillon B, et al. Patent foramen ovale closure or anticoagulation vs. antiplatelets after stroke. *N Engl J Med.* 2017;377:1011–1021.

Schwill S, Del Prete J, Cooley DA, et al. Two scimitar veins in an adult: repair through a right thoracotomy without cardiopulmonary bypass. *Tex Heart Inst J.* 2010;37:358–360.

Soendergaard LS, Kasner SE, Rhodes JF, et al. Patent foramen ovale closure or antiplatelet therapy for cryptogenic stroke. *N Engl J Med.* 2017;377:1033–1042.

Takeuchi S, Imamura H, Katsumoto K, et al. New surgical method for repair of anomalous left coronary artery from pulmonary artery. *J Thorac Cardiovasc Surg.* 1979;89:7–11.

Tashiro T, Todo K, Haruta Y, et al. Anomalous origin of the left coronary artery from the pulmonary artery. *J Thorac Cardiovasc Surg.* 1993;106:718–722.

Van Son JAM, Danielson GK, Schaff HV, et al. Congenital partial and complete absence of the pericardium. *Mayo Clin Proc.* 1993;68:743–747.

Zhu D, Bryant R, Heinle J, Hihill MR. Isolated cleft of the mitral valve. *Tex Heart Inst J.* 2009;36:553–556.

CHAPTER 16. VASCULAR RING

Hernanz-Schuylman M. Vascular rings: a practical approach to imaging diagnosis. *Pediatr Radiol.* 2005;35:961–979.

Huhta J, Gutgesell H, Latson L, et al. Two-dimensional echocardiographic assessment of the aorta in infants and children with congenital heart disease. *Circulation.* 1984;70:417–424.

Layton KF, Kallmes DF, Cloft HJ, et al. Bovine aortic arch variant in humans: clarification of a common misnomer. *Am J Neuroradiol.* 2006;27:1541–1542.

Shuford WH, Sybers RG. *The Aortic Arch and Its Malformation with Emphasis on the Angiographic Features.* Springfield, IL: Charles C Thomas; 1974.

CHAPTER 17. CHAMBER LOCALIZATION AND CARDIAC MALPOSITION

Huhta JC, Smallhorn IF, Macartney FJ. Two dimensional echocardiographic diagnosis of situs. *Br Heart J.* 1982;48:97–108.

Van Praagh R, Weinberg PM, Foran RB, et al. Malposition of the heart. In: Adams FH, Emmanouilides GC, Riemenschneider TH, eds. *Moss' Heart Disease in Infants, Children, and Adolescents.* 4th ed. Baltimore: Williams & Wilkins; 1989.

CHAPTER 18. PRIMARY MYOCARDIAL DISEASE

Anderson JL, Gilbert EM, O'Connell JB, et al. Long-term (2 year) beneficial effects of beta-adrenergic blockage with bucindolol in patients with idiopathic dilated cardiomyopathy. *J Am Coll Cardiol.* 1991;17:1373–1381.

Curigliano G, Gardinale Suter T, et al. Cardiovascular toxicity induced by chemotherapy, target agents and radiotherapy: ESMO Clinical Practice Guidelines. *Ann Oncol.* 2012;22(suppl 7):vii155–vii166.

Ergul Y, Nishi K, Dermirel A, et al. Left ventricular non-compaction in child and adolescents: clinical features, treatment and follow-up. *Cardiol J.* 2012;18(10):1–9.

Friedman RA, Moak JP, Garson Jr A. Clinical course of idiopathic dilated cardiomyopathy in children. *J Am Coll Cardiol.* 1991;18:152–156.

Helton E, Darragh R, Francis P, et al. Metabolic aspects of myocardial disease and a role for L-carnitine in the treatment of childhood cardiomyopathy. *Pediatrics.* 2000;105:1260–1270.

Iarussi D, Indolfi P, Casale F, et al. Anthracycline-induced cardiotoxicity in children with cancer: strategies for prevention and management. *Paediatr Drugs.* 2005;7:67–76.

Ino T, Benson LN, Freedom RM, et al. Endocardial fibroelastosis: natural history and prognostic risk factors. *Am J Cardiol.* 1988;62:431–434.

Judge DP. Use of genetics in the clinical evaluation of cardiomyopathy. *JAMA.* 2009;302:2471–2476.

Kalay N, Basar E, Ozdogru I, et al. Protective effects of carvedilol against anthracycline-induced cardiomyopathy. *J Am Coll Cardiol.* 2006;48:2258–2262.

Kantor PF, Lougheed J, Dancea A, et al. Presentation, diagnosis, and medical management of heart failure in children: Canadian Cardiovascular Society guidelines. *Can J Cardiol*. 2013;29(2):1535–1552.

Katritsis D, Wilmshurst PT, Wendon JA, et al. Primary restrictive cardiomyopathy: clinical and pathologic characteristics. *J Am Coll Cardiol*. 1991;18:1230–1235.

Lipshultz SE, Miller TL, Lipsitz SR, et al. Continuous versus bolus infusion of doxorubicin in children with ALKL: long-erm cardiac outcomes. *Pediatrics*. 2012;13:1003–1011.

Marcus Fl, Fontaine GH, Guiraudon G, et al. Right ventricular dysplasia: a report of 24 adult cases. *Circulation*. 1982;65:384–398.

Maron BJ, Bonow RO, Cannon III RO, et al. Hypertrophic cardiomyopathy: interrelations of clinical manifestations, pathophysiology, and therapy, I. *N Engl J Med*. 1987;316:780–789.

Maron BJ, Bonow RO, Cannon III RO, et al. Hypertrophic cardiomyopathy: interrelations of clinical manifestations, pathophysiology, and therapy, II. *N Engl J Med*. 1987;316:843–852.

Maron BJ, McKenna WJ, Danielson GK, Shah PM, et al. American College of Cardiology/European Society of Cardiology Clinical Expert Consensus Document on Hypertrophic Cardiomyopathy. *J Am Coll Cardiol*. 2003;42:1687–1713.

Maron BJ, Towbin JA, Thiene G, et al. Contemporary definition and classification of the cardiomyopathies. *Circulation*. 2006;113:1807–1816.

McElhinney DB, Colan SD, Moran AM, Wypij D, et al. Recombinant human growth hormone treatment for dilated cardiomyopathy in children. *Pediatrics*. 2004;114:e452–458.

Ni J, Bowles NE, Kim YH, et al. Viral infection of the myocardium in endocardial fibroelastosis. Molecular evidence for the role of mumps virus as an etiologic agent. *Circulation*. 1997;95:133–139.

Pahl E, Sleeper LA, Canter CE, et al. Incidence of and risk factors for sudden cardiac death in children with dilated cardiomyopathy: a report from the Pediatric Cardiomyopathy Registry. *J Am Coll Cardiol*. 2012;59(6):607–615.

Pelliccia A, Maron BJ, Spataro A, et al. The upper limit of physiologic cardiac hypertrophy in highly trained elite athletes. *N Engl J Med*. 1991;324:295–301.

Shaddy RE. Beta-blocker therapy in young children with congestive heart failure under consideration for heart transplantation. *Am Heart J*. 1998;136:19–21.

Trachtenberg BH, Landy DC, Franco VI, et al. Anthracycline-associated cardiotoxicity in survivors of childhood cancer. *Pediatr Cardiol*. 2011;32:342–353.

Vejpongsa P, Yeh ETH. Prevention of anthracycline-induced cardiotoxicity. *J Am Coll Cardiol*. 2014;64:938–945.

Viollet L, Thrush PT, Flanigan KM, et al. Effects of angiotensin-converting enzyme inhibitors and/or beta blockers on the cardiomyopathy in Duchenne muscular dystrophy. *Am J Cardiol*. 2012;110(1):98–102.

Yetman AT, McCrindle SW, MacDonald C, et al. Myocardial bridging in children with hypertrophic cardiomyopathy—a risk factor for sudden death. *N Engl J Med*. 1998;339:1201–1209.

CHAPTER 19. CARDIOVASCULAR INFECTIONS

Akagi T, Kato H, Inoue O, et al. Valvular heart disease in Kawasaki syndrome: incidence and natural history. *Am Heart J*. 1990;120:366–372.

Baddour LM, Wilson WR, Bayer AS, et al. Infective endocarditis: diagnosis, antimicrobial therapy, and management of complications: a statement for healthcare professionals from the Committee on Rheumatic Fever, Endocarditis, and Kawasaki Disease, Council on Cardiovascular Disease In The Young, and The Councils on Clinical Cardiology, Stroke, and Cardiovascular Surgery and Anesthesia, American Heart Association: Endorsed by The Infectious Diseases Society of America. *Circulation*. 2005;111(23):e394–e433.

Drucker NA, Colan SD, Lewis AB, et al. γ Globulin treatment of acute myocarditis in the pediatric population. *Circulation*. 1994;89:251–257.

Ferrieri P, Gewitz MH, Gerber MA, et al. Unique features of infective endocarditis in childhood. *Pediatrics*. 2002;109:931–943.

Ishii M, Ueno T, Ikeda H, Iemura M, et al. Sequential follow-up results of catheter intervention for coronary artery lesions after Kawasaki disease: quantitative coronary artery angiography and intravascular ultrasound imaging study. *Circulation*. 2002;105(25):3004–3010.

Kato H, Ichinose E, Yoshioka F, et al. Fate of coronary aneurysms in Kawasaki disease: serial coronary angiography and long-term follow-up study. *Am J Cardiol*. 1982;49:1758–1766.

Kurotobi S, Nagai T, Kawakami N, Sano T. Coronary diameter in normal infants, children and patients with Kawasaki disease. *Pediatr Int*. 2002;44:1–4.

Li JS, Sexton DJ, Mick N, et al. Proposed modification to the Duke Criteria for the diagnosis of infective endocarditis. *Clin Infect Dis*. 2000;30:633–638.

McCrindle BW, Rowley AH, Newburger JW, et al. Diagnosis, treatment, and long-term management of Kawasaki disease: a scientific statement for Health Professionals from the American Heart Association. *Circulation*. 2017;135:e927–e999.

Newburger JW, Takahashi M, Beiser AS, et al. A single intravenous infusion of gamma globulin as compared with four infusions in the treatment of acute Kawasaki syndrome. *N Engl J Med*. 1991;324:1633–1639.

Nishimura RA, Carabello BA, Faxon DP, et al. ACC/AHA 2008 Guideline update on Valvular Heart Disease; focused update on infective endocarditis. *Circulation*. 2008;118:887–896.

Nishimura RA, Otto CM, Bonow RO, et al. 2014 AHA/ACC guideline for the management of patients with valvular heart disease: executive summary: a report of the American College of Cardiology/American Heart Association Task Force on Practice Guidelines. *Circulation*. 2014;129(23):2440–2492.

Nishimura RA, Otto CM, Bonow RO, et al. 2017 AHA/ACC focused update of the 2014 AHA/ACC guideline for the management of patients with valvular heart disease: a report of the American College of Cardiology/American Heart Association Task Force on Clinical Practice Guidelines. *Circulation*. 2017;135(25):e1159–e1195.

Shapiro ED. Lyme disease. *Pediatr Rev*. 1998;19:147–154.

Salamat M, Khan MS. Ring calcification of giant coronary artery aneurysm of an 11-year-old child with history of Kawasaki disease. *Pediatr Cardiol*. 2010;31(4):558–559.

Son MBS, Gauvreau K, Ma L, et al. Treatment of Kawasaki disease analysis of 27 US pediatric hospitals from 2001 to 2006. *Pediatrics*. 2009;124:1–8.

Williams RV, Wilke VM, Tani LY, Minich LL. Does Abciximab enhance regression of coronary aneurysms resulting from Kawasaki disease? *Pediatrics*. 2002;109(1):E4.

Wilson W, Taubert KA, Gewitz M, et al. Prevention of infective endocarditis: guidelines from the American Heart Association: A Guideline From The American Heart Association Rheumatic Fever, Endocarditis, and Kawasaki Disease Committee, Council on Cardiovascular Disease In The Young, and The Council on Clinical Cardiology, Council on Cardiovascular Surgery and Anesthesia, and the quality of care and outcomes research interdisciplinary working group. *Circulation*. 2007;116. 1736–54.

CHAPTER 20. ACUTE RHEUMATIC FEVER

Garvey MA, Snider LA, Leitman SF, Werden R, Swedo SE. Treatment of Sydenham's chorea with intravenous immunoglobulin, plasma exchange, or prednisone. *J Child Neurol.* 2005;20(5):424–429.

Gerber MA, Baltimore RS, Eaton CB, et al. Prevention of rheumatic fever and diagnosis and treatment of acute streptococcal pharyngitis: a scientific statement from the American Heart Association Rheumatic Fever, Endocarditis, and Kawasaki Disease Committee of The Council on Cardiovascular Disease In The Young, the interdisciplinary council on functional genomics and translational biology, and the interdisciplinary council on quality of care and outcome research. *Circulation.* 2009;119:1541–1551.

Gewitz MH, Baltimore RS, Tani LY, et al. Revision of the Jones Criteria for the diagnosis of acute rheumatic fever in the era of Doppler echocardiography. A scientific statement from the American Heart Association. *Circulation.* 2015;131:1806–1818.

Parks T, Smeesters PR, Steer AC. Streptococcal skin infection and rheumatic heart disease. *Curr Opin Infect Dis.* 2012;25(2):145–153.

Vijayalakshmi IB, Mathravinda J, Deva ANP. The role of echocardiography in diagnosing carditis in the setting of acute rheumatic fever. *Cardiol Young.* 2005;15:583–588.

Veasy LG, Tani LY. A new loot at acute rheumatic mitral regurgitation. *Cardiol Young.* 2005;15:568–577.

CHAPTER 21. VALVULAR HEART DISEASE

ACC/AHA 2006 guidelines for the management of patients with valvular heart disease. *Circulation.* 2006;114:450–527.

Bisset III GS, Schwartz DC, Meyer RA, et al. Clinical spectrum and long-term follow-up of isolated mitral valve prolapse in 119 children. *Circulation.* 1980;62:423–429.

Levine RA, Stathogiannis E, Newell JB, et al. Reconsideration of echocardiographic standards for mitral valve prolapse: lack of association between leaflet displacement isolated to the apical four chamber view and independent echocardiographic evidence of abnormality. *J Am Coll Cardiol.* 1988;11:1010–1019.

Levine RA, Triulzi MO, Harrigan P, et al. The relationship of mitral annular shape to the diagnosis of mitral valve prolapse. *Circulation.* 1987;75:756–767.

Lock JE, Khalilullah M, Shrivastava S, et al. Percutaneous catheter commissurotomy in rheumatic mitral stenosis. *N Engl J Med.* 1985;313:1515–1518.

Nishimura RA, Otto CM, Bonow RO, et al. 2014 AHA/ACC Guideline for the Management of Patients With Valvular Heart Disease: executive summary: a report of the American College of Cardiology/American Heart Association Task Force on Practice Guidelines. *Circulation.* 2014;129(23):2440–2492.

Smith MS, Doroshow C, Womack WM, et al. Symptomatic mitral valve prolapse in children and adolescents: catecholamines, anxiety, and biofeedback. *Pediatrics.* 1989;84:290–298.

Warth DC, King ME, Cohen JM, et al. Prevalence of mitral valve prolapse in normal children. *J Am Coll Cardiol.* 1985;5:1173–1177.

CHAPTER 22. CARDIAC TUMORS

Becker AE. Primary heart tumors in the pediatric age group: a review of salient pathologic features relevant for clinicians. *Pediatr Cardiol.* 2000;21:317–323.

Bielefeld KJ, Moller JH. Cardiac tumors in infants and children: study of 120 operated patients. *Pediatr Cardiol.* 2013;34(1):125–128.

Ludomirsky A. Cardiac tumors. In: Garson Jr A, Bricker JT, McNamara DG, eds. *The Science and Practice of Pediatric Cardiology.* Philadelphia: Lea & Febiger; 1990.

Nir A, Tajik AJ, Freeman WK, Seward JB, et al. Tuberous sclerosis and cardiac rhabdomyoma. *Am J Cardiol.* 1995;76:419–421.

CHAPTER 23. CARDIAC INVOLVEMENT IN SYSTEMIC DISEASES

Bhakta D, Lowe MR, Groh WJ. Prevalence of structural cardiac abnormalities in patients with myotonic dystrophy type I. *Am Heart J.* 2004;147:224–227.

Bird LM, Billman GF, Lacro RV, et al. Sudden death in Williams syndrome: report of ten cases. *J Pediatr.* 1996;129:926–931.

Bondy CA. Care of girls and women with Turner syndrome: a guideline of the Turner Syndrome Study Group. *J Clin Endocrinol Metab.* 2007;92:10–25.

Collins RT, Aziz PF, Gleason MM, et al. Abnormalities of cardiac repolarization in Williams syndrome. *Am J Cardiol.* 2010;106:1029–1033.

Dangel JH. Cardiovascular change in children with mucopolysaccharide storage diseases and related disorders—clinical and echocardiographic findings in 64 patients. *Eur J Pediatr.* 1998;157:534–538.

Duboc D, Meune C, Lerebours G, Devaux JY, Vaksmann G, Becane HM. Effect of perindopril on the onset and progression of left ventricular dysfunction in Duchenne muscular dystrophy. *J Am Coll Cardiol.* 2005;45(6). 855–757.

Gott VL, Greene PS, Alejo DE, et al. Replacement of the aortic root in patients with Marfan's syndrome. *N Engl J Med.* 1999;340(17):1307–1313.

Jefferies JL, Eidem BW, Belmont JW, et al. Genetic predictors and remodeling of dilated cardiomyopathy in muscular dystrophy. *Circulation.* 2005;112:2799–2804.

Kajimoto H, Ishigaki K, Okumura K, et al. Beta blocker therapy for cardiac dysfunction in patients with muscular dystrophy. *Circ J.* 2006;20:991–994.

Kim SY, Martin N, Hsia EC, et al. Management of aortic disease in Marfan syndrome: a decision analysis. *Arch Intern Med.* 2005;165(7):749–755.

Mohan UR, Hay AA, Cleary MA, et al. Cardiovascular changes in children with mucopolysaccharide disorders. *Act Paediatr.* 2002;91:799–804.

Pierpoint MEM, Moller JH. Cardiac manifestations of systemic disease. In: Adams FH, Emmanouilides GC, Riemenschneider TA, eds. *Moss' Heart Disease in Infants, Children, and Adolescents.* 4th ed. Baltimore: Williams & Wilkins; 1989.

Romano AA, Allanson JE, Dahlgren J, Geib BD, et al. Noonan syndrome: clinical features, diagnosis, and management guidelines. *Pediatrics.* 2010;126:746–759.

Shores J, Berger KR, Murphy EA, et al. Progression of aortic dilatation and the benefit of long-term beta-adrenergic blockade in Marfan's syndrome. *N Engl J Med.* 1994;330:1335–1341.

Tweddell JS, Earing MG, Bartz PJ, et al. Valve-sparing aortic root reconstruction in children, teenagers, and young adults. *Ann Thorac Surg.* 2012;94:587–591.

Viollet L, Thrush PT, Flanigan, et al. Effects of angiotensin-converting enzyme inhibitors and/or beta blockers on the cardiomyopathy in Duchenne muscular dystrophy. *Am J Cardiol.* 2012;110:98–102.

Weidemann F, Rummey C, Bijnens B, et al. The heart in Friedreich ataxia. Definition of cardiomyopathy, disease severity, and correlation with neurological symptoms. *Circulation.* 2012;125:1626–1634.

Yetman AT, Bornemeier RA, McCrindle BW. Usefulness of enalapril versus propranolol or atenolol for prevention of aortic dilation in patients with the Marfan syndrome. *Am J Cardiol.* 2005;95:1125–1127.

CHAPTER 24. CARDIAC ARRHYTHMIAS

Ackerman MJ. The long QT syndrome. *Pediatr Rev.* 1998;19:232–238.

Alexander ME. Ventricular arrhythmias in children and young adults. In: Walsh EP, Saul JP, Triedman JK, eds. *Cardiac Arrhythmias in Children and Young Adults with Congenital Heart Disease.* Philadelphia: Lippicott Williams & Wilkins; 2001:201–234.

Berul CI, Sweeten TL, Dubin AM, et al. Use of the rate-corrected JT interval for prediction of repolarization abnormalities in children. *Am J Cardiol.* 1994;74:1254–1257.

Collins KK, Van Hare GF. Advances in congenital long QT syndrome. *Curr Opin Pediatr.* 2006;18(5):497–502.

Goel AK, Berger S, Pelech A, Dhala A. Implantable cardioverter defibrillator therapy in children with long QT syndrome. *Pediatr Cardiol.* 2004;25:370–378.

Gollob M, Redpath C, Roberts J. The short QT syndrome: proposed diagnostic criteria. *J Am Coll Cardiol.* 2011;57(7):802–812.

Goldberg I, Moss AJ, Zareba W. QT interval: how to measure it and what is "normal. *J Cardiovasc Electrophysiol.* 2006;17:333–336.

Martin AB, Perry JC, Robinson JL, et al. Calculation of QTc duration and variability in the presence of sinus arrhythmia. *Am J Cardiol.* 1995;75:950–952.

Probst V, Denjoy I, Mercegalli P, et al. Clinical aspect and prognosis of Brugada syndrome in children. *Circulation.* 2007;115:2042–2048.

Reynolds JL, Pickoff AS. Accelerated ventricular rhythm in children: a review and report of a case. *Pediatr Cardiol.* 2001;22:23–28.

Schwartz PJ, Crotti L, Insolia R. Long QT syndrome. From genetics to management. *Circ Arrhythm Electrophysiol.* 2012;5:868–877.

Stambler BS, Dorian P, Sagar PT, et al. Etripamil nasal spray for rapid conversion of supraventricular tachycardia to sinus rhythm. *J Am Coll Cardiol.* 2018;72(5):489–497.

Towbin JA, Friedman RA. Long QT syndrome. In: Walsh EP, Seal JP, Triedman JK, eds. *Cardiac Arrhythmias in Children and Young Adults with Congenital Heart Disease.* Philadelphia: Lippincott Williams & Wilkins; 2001:235–270.

CHAPTER 25. DISTURBANCES OF ATRIOVENTRICULAR CONDUCTION

Eronen M, Siren M-K, Ekblad H, et al. Short- and long-term outcome of children with congenital complete heart block diagnosed in utero or as a newborn. *Pediatrics.* 2000;106:86–91.

Ross BA, Gillette PC. Atrioventricular block and bundle branch block. In: Gillette PC, Garson Jr A, eds. *Clinical Pediatric Arrhythmias.* 2nd ed. Philadelphia: WB Saunders; 1999:63–77.

Zuppa AA, Riccardi R, Frezza S, et al. Neonatal lupus: follow-up in infants with anti-SSA/Ro antibodies and review of the literature. *Autoimmun Rev.* 2017;16(4):427–432.

CHAPTER 26. CARDIAC PACEMAKERS AND IMPLANTABLE CARDIOVERTER–DEFIBRILLATORS IN CHILDREN

Bernstein AD, Daubert JC, Fletcher RD, et al. The revised NASPE/BPEG generic code for antibradycardia, adaptive-rate, and multisite pacing. North American Society of Pacing and Electrophysiology/British Pacing and Electrophysiology Group. *Pacing Clin Electrophysiol.* 2002;25:260–264.

Epstein AE, DiMario JP, Ellenbogen KA, et al. 2012ACCF/AHA/HRS focused update incorporated into the ACCF/AHA/HRS 2008 guidelines for device-based therapy of cardiac rhythm abnormalities: a report of American College of Cardiology Foundation/American Heart Association Task Force on Practice Guidelines and the Heart Rhythm Society. *J Am Coll Cardiol.* 2013;61(3):e6–e75.

Friedman RA. Pacemakers in children: medical and surgical aspects. *Tex Heart Inst J.* 1992;19:178–184.

CHAPTER 27. CONGESTIVE HEART FAILURE

Amman M, Graham Jr TP. Guidelines for vasodilator therapy of congestive heart failure in infants and children. *Am J Cardiol.* 1987;113:994–1005.

Auerbach SR, Richmond ME, Lamour JM, et al. BNP levels predict outcome in pediatric heart failure patients. Post hoc analysis of the pediatric carvedilol trial. *Circ Heart Fail.* 2010;3:606–611.

Berman Jr W, Yabek SM, Dillon T, et al. Effects of digoxin in infants with congested circulatory state due to a ventricular septal defect. *N Engl J Med.* 1983;308:363–366.

Braunwald E. Effects of digitalis on the normal and the failing heart. *J Am Coll Cardiol.* 1985;5(suppl A):51A–59A.

Buchhorn R, Bartmus D, Siekmeyer W, et al. Beta-blocker therapy of severe congestive heart failure in infants with left to right shunts. *Am J Cardiol.* 1998;98:1366–1368.

Foerster SR, Canter CE. Pediatric heart failure therapy with β-adrenoceptor antagonist [review]. *Pediatr Drugs.* 2008;10:125–134.

Helton E, Darragh R, Francis P, et al. Metabolic aspects of myocardial disease and a role for L-carnitine in the treatment of childhood cardiomyopathy. *Pediatrics.* 2000;105:1260–1270.

Huong et al, 2013. ***

Montigny M, Davignon A, Fouron J-C, et al. Captopril in infants for congestive heart failure secondary to a large ventricular left-to-right shunt. *Am J Cardiol.* 1989;63:631–633.

Nir A, Nasser N. Clinical value of NT-ProBNT and BNT in pediatric cardiology. *J Card Fail.* 2005;11:S76–S80.

Park MK. The use of digoxin in infants and children with specific emphasis on dosage. *J Pediatr.* 1986;108:871–877.

Shaddy RE, Boucek MM, Hsu DT, et al. Pediatric carvedilol study group. Carvedilol for children and adolescents with heart failure: a randomized controlled trial. *JAMA.* 2007;198:1171–1179.

CHAPTER 28. SYSTEMIC HYPERTENSION

Chobanian AV, Bakris GL, Black HR, et al. The seventh report of the Joint National Committee on Prevention, Detection, Evaluation, and Treatment of High Blood Pressure: the JNC 7 report. *JAMA.* 2003;21:2560–2572.

Daniels SR, Meyer RA, Liang YC, Bove KE. Echocardiographically determined left ventricular mass index in normal children, adolescents, and young adults. *J Am Coll Cardiol.* 1988;12:703–708.

Dart RA, Gollub S, Lazar J, Nair C, et al. Treatment of systemic hypertension in patients with pulmonary disease-COPD and asthma. *Chest*. 2003;123:222–243.

Feig DI, Johnson RJ. Hyperuricemia in childhood primary hypertension. *Hypertension*. 2003;42:247–252.

Flynn JT, Kaelber DC, Barker-Smith CM, et al. Clinical practice guideline for screening and management of high blood pressure in children and adolescents. *Pediatrics*. 2017;140(3):e20171904.

Flynn JT, Newburger JW, Daniels SR, et al. A randomized, placebo-controlled trial of amlodipine in children with hypertension. *J Pediatr*. 2004;145:288–290.

Frolich ED, Labarth DR, Maxwell MH, et al. Recommendations for human blood pressure determination by sphygmomanometers: report of a Special Task Force appointed by the Steering Committee, American Heart Association. *Circulation*. 1988;77:501A–514A.

The Fourth Report on the Diagnosis, Evaluation, and Treatment of High Blood Pressure in Children and Adolescents. National High Blood Pressure Education Program Working Group on High Blood Pressure in Children and Adolescents. *Pediatrics*. 2004;111:555–576.

Ham SW, Kumar SR, Wang BR, et al. Late outcomes of endovascular and open revascularization of non-atherosclerotic renal artery disease. *Arch Surg*. 2010;145(9):832–839.

Hammond IW, Urbina EM, Wattigney WA, Bao W, et al. Comparison of Fourth and Fifth Korotkoff diastolic blood pressures in 5 to 30 year old individuals. The Bogalusa Heart Study. *Am J Hypertens*. 1995;8:1083–1089.

Jago R, Harrell JS, McMurray RG, et al. Prevalence of abnormal lipid and blood pressure values among an ethnically diverse population of eighth grade adolescents and screening implications. *Pediatrics*. 2006;117:2065–2073.

Kaelber DC, Pickett F. Simple table to identify children and adolescents needing further evaluation of blood pressure. *Pediatrics*. 2009;123(6):e972.

Khoury PR, Matsnefes M, Daniels SR, Kimball TR. Age-specific reference intervals for indexed left ventricular mass in children. *J Am Soc Echocardiogr*. 2009;22:709–714.

Park MK, Guntheroth WG. Accurate blood pressure measurement in children: a review. *Am J Noninvas Cardiol*. 1989;3:297–309.

Park MK, Menard SW, Yuan C. Comparison of auscultatory and oscillometric blood pressure. *Arch Pediatr Adolesc Med*. 2001;155:50–53.

Sorof JM, Cardwell G, Franco K, Portman RJ. Ambulatory blood pressure and left ventricular mass index in hypertensive children. *Hypertension*. 2002;39:903–908.

Urbina E, Alpert B, Flynn J, Hayman L, et al. Ambulatory blood pressure monitoring in children and adolescents: recommendations for standard assessment: a scientific statement from the American Heart Association Atherosclerosis, Hypertension, and Obesity In Youth Committee of The Council on Cardiovascular Disease In The Young and The Council For High Blood Pressure Research. *Hypertension*. 2008;52:433–451.

Whelton PK, Carey RM, Aronow WS, et al. 2017 ACC/AHA/AAPA/ABC/ACPM/ AGS/APhA/ASH/ASPC/NMA/PCNA guidelines for the prevention, detection, evaluation, and management of high blood pressure in adults. *J Am Coll Cardiol*. 2018;71:e127–e247.

Wiesen J, Adkins M, Fortune S, et al. Evaluation of pediatric patients with mild-to-moderate hypertension: yield of diagnostic testing. *Pediatrics*. 2008;122(5):e988–993.

Wühl E, Witte K, Soergel M, Mehls O, et al. Distribution of 24-h ambulatory blood pressure in children: normalized reference values and role of body dimensions. *J Hypertens*. 2002;20:1995–2007.

CHAPTER 29. PULMONARY HYPERTENSION

Abman SH, Hansmann G, Archer SL, et al. Pediatric pulmonary hypertension: guidelines from the American Heart Association and American Thoracic Society. *Circulation*. 2015;132:2037–2099.

Albersheim SG, Solimanu AJ, Sharma AK, et al. Randomized, double-blind, controlled trial of long-term diuretic therapy for bronchopulmonary dysplasia. *J Pediatr*. 1989;115:615–620.

Barst RJ, Maislin G, Fishman AF. Vasodilator therapy for primary pulmonary hypertension in children. *Circulation*. 1999;99:1197–1208.

Barst RJ, Ivy D, Dingemanse J, et al. Pharmacokinetics, safety, and efficacy of bosentan in pediatric patients with pulmonary arterial hypertension. *Clin Pharmacol Ther*. 2003;73:372–382.

Barst RJ, Langleben D, Badesch D, Frost A, et al. Treatment of pulmonary arterial hypertension with the selective endothelin-A receptor antagonist sitaxsentan. *J Am Coll Cardiol*. 2006;47:2049–2056.

Dillon PW, Cilley RE, Mauger D, Zachary C, et al. The relationship of pulmonary artery pressure and survival in congenital diaphragmatic hernia. *J Pediatr Surg*. 2004;39:307–312.

Galie N, Humbert M, Vachiery J-L, et al. 2015 ESC/ERS guidelines for the diagnosis and treatment of pulmonary hypertension. *Eur Heart J*. 2016;37:67–119.

Game S. Pulmonary hypertension (grand rounds). *JAMA*. 2000;284:3160–3168.

Gorenflo M, Nelle M, Schnabel PA, Ullmann MV. Pulmonary hypertension in infancy and childhood. *Cardiol Young*. 2003;13:219–227.

Hansmann G. Pulmonary hypertension in infants, children and young adults. *J Am Coll Cardiol*. 2017;69(20):2551–2560.

Humpl T, Reyes JT, Holtby H, Stephens D, et al. Beneficial effect of oral sildenafil therapy on childhood pulmonary arterial hypertension. Twelve-month clinical trial of a single-drug, open-label, pilot study. *Circulation*. 2005;111:3274–3280.

Maiya S, Hislop AA, Flynn Y, Haworth SG. Response to bosentan in children with pulmonary hypertension. *Heart*. 2006;92:664–670.

Oishi P, Datar SA, Fineman JR. Advances in the management of pediatric pulmonary hypertension. *Respir Care*. 2011;56:1314–1340.

Parasuraman S, Walker S, Loudon BL, et al. Assessment of pulmonary artery pressure by echocardiography—a comprehensive review. *Int J Cardiol Heart Vasc*. 2016;12:45–51.

Richardi MK, Knight BP, Martinet FJ, et al. Inhaled nitric oxide in primary pulmonary hypertension: a safe and effective agent for predicting response to nifedipine. *J Am Coll Cardiol*. 1998;32:1068–1073.

Rosenzweig EB, Ivy DD, Widlitz A, Doran A, et al. Effects of long-term bosentan in children with pulmonary arterial hypertension. *J Am Coll Cardiol*. 2005;46(4):697–704.

Steinhorn RH. Pharmacotherapy for pulmonary hypertension. *Pediatr Clin North Am*. 2012;59:1129–1146.

Stevenson JG. Comparison of several noninvasive methods for estimation of pulmonary artery pressure. *J Am Soc Echocardiogr*. 1989;2:157–171.

Takatsuki S, Rosenzweig EB, Xuckerman WQ, et al. Clinical safety, pharmacokinetics, and efficacy of ambrisentan therapy in children with pulmonary arterial hypertension. *Pediatr Pulmonol*. 2013;48(1):27–34.

Tissot C, Dunbar D, Beghetti M. Medical therapy for pediatric pulmonary hypertension. *J Pediatr*. 2010;157:528–532.

Ulrich S, Hildebrand FF, Treder U, et al. Reference values for the 6-minute walk test in healthy children and adolescents in Switzerland. *MBC Pulmonary Med*. 2013;13:49.

CHAPTER 30. THE CHILD WITH CHEST PAIN

Klone RA, Hale S, Alker K, Rezkalla S. The effects of acute and chronic cocaine use on the heart. *Circulation*. 1992;85:407–418.

Massin MM, Bourguignont A, Coremans C, et al. Chest pain in pediatric patients presenting to an emergency department or to a cardiac clinic. *Clin Pediatr*. 2004;43(3):231–238.

McCord J, Ineid J, Hollander JE, et al. Management of cocaine-associated chest pain and myocardial infarction. A scientific statement from the American Heart Association acute cardiac care committee of the Council on Clinical Cardiology. *Circulation*. 2008;117:1897–1907.

Rowe BH, Dulburg CS, Peterson RG, et al. Characteristics of children presenting with chest pain to a pediatric emergency department. *Can Med Assoc J*. 1990;143:388–394.

Saleeb SF, Li WYV, Warren SZ, et al. Effectiveness of screening for life-threatening chest pain in children. *Pediatrics*. 2011;128:e1062–e1068.

Selbst SM. Approach to the child with chest pain. *Pediatr Clin North Am*. 2010;57(6):1221–1234.

Thull-Freedman J. Evaluation of chest pain in the pediatric patients. *Med Clin North Am*. 2010;94:327–347.

CHAPTER 31. SYNCOPE

Blanc JJ, Mansourati J, Maheu B, et al. Reproducibility of a positive passive upright tilt test at a seven-day interval in patients with syncope. *Am J Cardiol*. 1993;72:467–471.

Connolly SJ, Sheldon R, Thorpe KE, et al. Pacemaker therapy for prevention of syncope in patients with recurrent severe vasovagal syncope: Second Vasovagal Pacemaker Study (VPS II): a randomized trial. *JAMA*. 2003;289:2224–2229.

O'Marcaigh AS, MacLellan-Tobert SG, Perter CP. Tilt-table testing and oral metoprolol therapy in young patients with unexplained syncope. *Pediatrics*. 1994;93:278–283.

Ross BA, Saul JP. Management of vasovagal syncope: pharmacologic, nonpharmacologic, or pacing. In: Walsh EP, Saul JP, Triedman JK, eds. *Cardiac Arrhythmias in Children and Young Adults with Congenital Heart Disease*. Philadelphia: Lippincott Williams & Wilkins; 2001.

Salim MA, Ware LE, Barnard M, et al. Syncope recurrence in children: relation to tilt-test results. *Pediatrics*. 1998;102:924–926.

Scott WA. Syncope and the assessment of the autonomic nervous system. In: Allen HD, Gutgesell HP, Clark EB, Driscoll DJ, eds. *Moss and Adams' Heart Disease in Infants, Children, and Adolescents*. 6th ed. Philadelphia: Lippincott Williams & Wilkins; 2001:443–452.

Strickberger SA, Benson W, Biaggioni I, Callans DJ, et al. AHA/ACCF scientific statement on the evaluation of syncope. From the American Heart Association Council on Clinical Cardiology, Cardiovascular Nursing, Cardiovascular Disease In The Young , and Stroke, and The Quality of Care and Outcome Research Interdisciplinary Working Group; and The American College of Cardiology Foundation In Collaboration With The Heart Rhythm Society. *Circulation*. 2006;113:316–327.

Zhang F, Li X, Ochs T, et al. Midregional pro-adrenomedullin as a predictor for thera.peutic response to midodrine hydrochloride in children with postural orthostatic tachycardia syndrome. *J Am Coll Cardiol*. 2012;60:315–320.

CHAPTER 32. PALPITATION

Giala F, Raviele A. Diagnostic management of patients with palpitation of unknown origin. *Ital Heart J*. 2004;5:581–586.

CHAPTER 33. DYSLIPIDEMIA AND OTHER CARDIOVASCULAR RISK FACTORS

Ashen MD, Blumenthal RS. Clinical practice. Low HDL levels. *N Engl J Med*. 2005;353(12):1252–1260.

Daniels SR, Greer FR. the Committee on Nutrition: lipid screening and cardiovascular health in Childhood. *Pediatrics*. 2008;122(1):198–208.

Egan A, Colman E. Weighing the benefits of high-dose simvastatin against the risk of myopathy. *N Engl J Med*. 2011;365:285–287.

Gidding SS, Dennison BA, Birch LL, et al. American Heart Association; American Academy of Pediatrics. Dietary recommendations for children and adolescents: a guide for practitioners. *Pediatrics*. 2006;117:544–559.

Goldfine AB, Kaul S, Hiatt WR. Fibrates in the treatment of dyslipidemia—time for a reassessment. *N Engl J Med*. 2011;356:481–484.

Hellerstein MK. Carbohydrate-induced hypertriglyceridemia: modifying factors and implications for cardiovascular risk. *Curr Opin Lipidol*. 2002;13:33–40.

Holmes KW, Kwiterovich Jr PO. Treatment of dyslipidemia in children and adolescents. *Curr Cardiol Rep*. 2005;7:445–456.

Jolliffe CJ, Jansen I. Distribution of lipoproteins by age and gender and adolescents. *Circulation*. 2006;114:1056–1062.

Kwiterovich Jr PO, Claus S, McCrindle BW. Dyslipidemia in children and adolescents. In: Kwiterovich Jr PO, ed. *The Johns Hopkins Textbook of Dyslipidemia*. Philadelphia: Lippincott Williams & Wilkins; 2010:143–156.

McCrindle BW, Urbina EM, Dennison BA, et al. Drug therapy of high-risk lipid abnormalities in children and adolescents. A scientific statement from the American Heart Association Atherosclerosis, Hypertension, and Obesity In Youth Committee, Council of Cardiovascular Disease In The Young, With The Council on Cardiovascular Nursing. *Circulation*. 2007;115:1948–1967.

Srinivasan SR, Myers L, Berenson GS. Distribution and correlates of non-high-density lipoprotein cholesterol in children. *Pediatrics*. 2002;110(3):e20.

Stein EA, Illingworth DR, Kwiterovich Jr PO, et al. Efficacy and safety of lovastatin in adolescent males with heterozygous familial hypercholesterolemia. *JAMA*. 1999;281:137–144.

Third Report of the National Cholesterol Education Program (NCEP). Expert panel on detection, education, and treatment of high blood cholesterol in adults (adult treatment panel III) final report. *Circulation*. 2002;106:3143–3421.

Wiegman A, Hutten BA, de Groot E, et al. Efficacy and safety of statin therapy in children with familial hypercholesterolemia. *JAMA*. 2004;292:331–337.

CHAPTER 34. PEDIATRIC PREVENTIVE CARDIOLOGY

Cardiovascular Risk Factors and Metabolic syndrome

Alberti KG, Zimmer P, Shaw J. Metabolic syndrome—a new worldwide definition. A consensus statement from the International Diabetes Federation. *Diabetes Med.* 2006;23(5):469-480.

Berenson GS, Srinivasan SR, Bao W, et al. Association between multiple cardiovascular risk factors and atherosclerosis in children and young adults. *N Engl J Med.* 1998;338:1650-1656.

Cook S, Weizman M, Auinger P, Nguyen M, Dietz WH. Prevalence of a metabolic syndrome phenotype in adolescents: findings from the third National Health and Nutrition Examination Survey, 1988-1994. *Arch Pediatr Adolesc Med.* 2003;157:821-827.

Daniels SR, Greer FR. the Committee on Nutrition: lipid screening and cardiovascular health in Childhood. *Pediatrics.* 2008;122(1):198-208.

Expert Panel on Integrated Guidelines for Cardiovascular Health and Risk Reduction in Children and Adolescents. National heart, lung, and blood institute. *Pediatrics.* 2011;128(suppl 5):S213-S256.

Fernandez JR, Redden DT, Pietrobelli A, Allison DB. Waist circumference percentiles in nationally representative samples of African-American, European-American, and Mexican-American children and adolescents. *J Pediatr.* 2004;145:439-444.

Gundy SM. Obesity, metabolic syndrome, and coronary atherosclerosis [editorial]. *Circulation.* 2002;105. 2696-1698.

Grundy SM, Cleeman JI, Daniels SR, et al. Diagnosis and management of the metabolic syndrome: an American Heart Association/National Heart, Lung, and Blood Institute scientific statement: executive summary. *Circulation.* 2005;112(17):2735-2752.

Grundy SM, Hansen B, Smith Jr SC, Cleeman JI, et al. Clinical management of metabolic syndrome. Report of the American Heart Association/National Heart, Lung, and Blood Institute/American Diabetes Association Conference on Scientific Issues Related to Management. *Circulation.* 2004;109:551-556.

Jago R, Harrell JS, McMurray RG, et al. Prevalence of abnormal lipid and blood pressure values among an ethnically diverse population of eighth grade adolescents and screening implications. *Pediatrics.* 2006;117:2065-2073.

Jolliffe CJ, Jansen I. Distribution of lipoproteins by age and gender and adolescents. *Circulation.* 2006;114:1056-1062.

Kavey RW, Daniels SR, Lauer RM, et al. American heart association guidelines for primary prevention of atherosclerotic cardiovascular disease beginning in childhood. *Circulation.* 2003;107:1562-1566.

Magge SN, Goodman E, Armstrong SC. The metabolic syndrome in children and adolescent: shifting the focus to cardiometabolic risk factor clustering, by Committee on Nutrition, Section on Endocrinology and Section of Obesity. *Pediatrics.* 2017;140(2):e20171603.

Ritchie SK, Murphy ECS, Ice C, et al. Universal versus targeted blood cholesterol screening among youth: the CARDIAC Project. *Pediatrics.* 2010;126:260-265.

Singh GK. Metabolic syndrome in children and adolescents. *Curr Treat Options Cardiovasc Med.* 2006;8(5):403-413.

Steiner MJ, Skinner AC, Perrin EM. Fasting might not be necessary before lipid screening: a nationally representative cross-sectional study. *Pediatrics.* 2011;128:463-470.

Zimmet P, Alberti G, Kaufman F, et al. International Diabetes Federation Task Force on Epidemiology and Prevention of Diabetes.

The metabolic syndrome in children and adolescents. *Lancet.* 2007;369(9579):2059-2061.

Obesity

Brand-Miller JC, Holt SHA, Pawlak DB, et al. Glycemic index and obesity. *Am J Clin Nutr.* 2002;76(suppl):2815-2855.

Dietz WH. Health consequences of obesity in youth: childhood predictors of adult disease. *Pediatrics.* 1998;101:518-525.

Gortmaker SL, Must A, Sobol AM, Peterson K, Colditz GA, Dietz WH. Television viewing as a cause of increasing obesity among children in the United States, 1986-1990. *Arch Pediatr Adolesc Med.* 1996;150:356-362.

Hannan WJ, Wrate RM, Cowen SJ, Freeman CP. Body mass index as an estimate of body fat. *Int J Eat Disord.* 1995;18:91-97.

Hubert HB, Fenileib M, McNamara PM, et al. Obesity as an independent risk factor for cardiovascular disease: a 26-year follow-up of participants in the Framingham heart study. *Circulation.* 1983;67:968-977.

Krebs NF, Baker RD, Greer FR, Heyman, et al. Policy Statement. Prevention of pediatric overweight and obesity. Committee on Nutrition. *Pediatrics.* 2003;112:424-430.

Ludwig DS, Mahziyb HA, Al-Zagrabu A, et al. High glycemic index foods, overeating and obesity. *Pediatrics.* 1999;103:E262-E266.

McGill Jr HC, McMahan CA, Herderick EE, et al. Obesity accelerates the progression of coronary atherosclerosis in young men. *Circulation.* 2002;105:2712-2718.

Ogden CL, Carroll MD, Curtin LS, McDowell MA, et al. Prevalence of overweight and obesity in the United States, 1999-2004. *JAMA.* 2006;295:1549-1555.

Ogden CL, Carroll MD, Kit BK, et al. Prevalence of childhood and adult obesity in the United States, 2011-2012. *JAMA.* 2014;311:806-816.

Yanovski JA, Krakoff J, Salaita CG, et al. Effects of Metformin on body weight and body composition in obese insulin-resistant children: a randomized clinical trial. *Diabetes.* 2011;60(2):477-485.

Smoking

Jamal A, Gentzke A, Ju SS, et al. Tobacco use among middle and high school students—United States, 2011-2016. *MMWR Morb Mortal Wkly Rep.* 2017;66(23):597-603.

Lu JT, Creager MA. The relationship of cigarette smoking to peripheral arterial disease. *Rev Cardiovasc Med.* 2004;5(4):189-193.

Marshall L, Schooley M, Ryan H, Cox P, et al. Youth tobacco surveillance, United States; 2001-2002. *MMWR Surveill Summ.* 2006;55(3):1-56.

Rigotti NA, Lee JE, Wechsler H. US colleges students' use of tobacco products: results of a national survey. *JAMA.* 2000;284(6):699-705.

Williams CL, Hayman LL, Daniels SR, et al. Cardiovascular Health in Childhood. A statement for health professionals from the Committee on Atherosclerosis, Hypertension, and Obesity in the Young (AHOY) of the Council on Cardiovascular Disease in the Young, American Heart Association. *Circulation.* 2002;106:143-160.

CHAPTER 35. ATHLETES WITH CARDIAC PROBLEMS

Conference 36th Bethesda. Eligibility recommendations for competitive athletes with cardiovascular abnormalities. *J Am Coll Cardiol.* 2005;45(8):1313-1375.

Black HR, Sica D, Ferdinand K, et al. Eligibility and disqualification recommendations for competitive athletes with cardiovascular abnormalities: Task Force 6: hypertension. *Circulation.* 2015;132:e298–e302.

Bonow RO, Nishimura RA, Thompson PD, et al. Eligibility and disqualification recommendations for competitive athletes with cardiovascular abnormalities: Task Force 5: valvular heart disease. *Circulation.* 2015;132:e292–e297.

Bonow RO, Cheitlin MD. Bethesda Conference Report. Task Force 3: valvular heart disease. *J Am Coll Cardiol.* 2005;45:1334–1340.

Maron BJ. *Sudden Cardiac Death in the Young Athlete and the Preparticipation Cardiovascular Evaluation.* New York: Churchill Livingstone; 2000.

Levine BD, Baggish AL, Kovacs RJ, et al. Eligibility and disqualification recommendations for competitive athletes with cardiovascular abnormalities: Task Force 1: classification of sports: dynamic, static, and impact. *Circulation.* 2015;132:e262–e266.

Lisman KA. Electrocardiographic evaluation in athletes and use of the Seattle Criteria to improve specificity. *Methodist Debakey Cardiovasc J.* 2016;12(2):81–85.

Maron BJ, Ackerman MJ, Towbin JUA. Bethesda Conference Report. Task Force 4: HCM and other cardiomyopathies, mitral valve prolapse, myocarditis, and Marfan syndrome. *J Am Coll Cardiol.* 2005;45:1340–1345.

Maron BJ, Doerer JJ, Haas TS, et al. Sudden deaths in young competitive athletes: analysis of 1866 deaths in the United States. *Circulation.* 2009;119:1085–1092.

Maron BJ, Friedman RA, Kligfield P, et al. Assessment of the 12-lead ECG as a screening test for detection of cardiovascular disease in healthy general population of young people (12–25yerss of age). A scientific statement from the American Heart Association and the American Collee of Cardiology. *Circulation.* 2014;130(18):1617–1624.

Maron BJ, Pelliccia A. The heart of trained athletes: cardiac remodeling and the risks of sports, including sudden death. *Circulation.* 2006;114:1633–1644.

Maron BJ, Shirani J, Poline LC, et al. Sudden death in young competitive athletes: clinical, demographic and pathological profiles. *JAMA.* 1996;276:199–208.

Maron BJ, Udelson JE, Bonow RO, et al. Eligibility and disqualification recommendations for competitive athletes with cardiovascular abnormalities: Task Force 3: hypertrophic cardiomyopathy, arrhythmogenic right ventricular cardiomyopathy and other cardiomyopathies, and myocarditis. *Circulation.* 2015;132:e273–e280.

Pelliccia A, Maron BJ, Spataro A, Proschan MA, Spirito P. The upper limit of physiologic cardiac hypertrophy in highly trained elite athletes. *N Engl J Med.* 1991;324:295–301.

Van Hare GF, Ackerman MJ, Evangelista J, et al. Eligibility and disqualification recommendations for competitive athletes with cardiovascular abnormalities: Task Force 4: congenital heart disease. *Circulation.* 2015;132:e281–291.

Washington RL, Bernhardt DT, Brenner JS, Gomez J, et al. Promotion of healthy weight-control practices in young athletes. *Pediatrics.* 2005;116:1557–1564.

CHAPTER 36. CARDIAC TRANSPLANTATION

Bailey L, Concepcion W, Shattuck H, et al. Method of heart transplantation for treatment of hypoplastic left heart syndrome. *J Thorac Cardiovasc Surg.* 1986;92:1–5.

Bailey LL, Gundry SR, Razzouk AJ, et al. Bless the babies: one hundred fifteen late survivors of heart transplantation during the first year of life. *J Thorac Cardiovasc Surg.* 1993;105:805–815.

Boucek MM, Mathis CM, Boucek RJ, et al. Prospective evaluation of echocardiography for primary rejection surveillance after infant heart transplantation: comparison with endomyocardial biopsy. *J Heart Lung Transplant.* 1994;13:66–73.

Canter CE. Pediatric cardiac transplantation. In: Moller JH, Hoffman RE, eds. *Pediatric Cardiovascular Medicine.* New York: Churchill Livingstone; 2000:942–952.

Dipchand AI. Current state of pediatric cardiac transplantation. *Ann Cardiothorac Surg.* 2018;7(1):31–55.

Gabrys CA. Pediatric cardiac transplants: a clinical update. *J Pediatr Nurs.* 2005;20:139–143.

Kuhn MA, Jutzy KR, Derming DD, et al. The medium-term findings in coronary arteries by intravascular ultrasound in infants and children after heart transplantation. *J Am Coll Cardiol.* 2000;36:250–254.

Pahl E, Fricker FJ, Armitage J, et al. Coronary arteriosclerosis in pediatric heart transplant survivors: limitation of long-term survival. *J Pediatr.* 1990;116:177–183.

Seipelt IM, Crawford SE, Rodgers S, et al. Hypercholesterolemia is common after pediatric heart transplantation: initial experience with pravastatin. *J Heart Lung Transplant.* 2004;23(3):317–322.

Stewart S, Winters GL, Fishbein MC, et al. Revision of the 1990 working formulation for the standardization of nomenclature in the diagnosis of heart rejection. *J Heart Lung Transplant.* 2005;24:1710–1720.

Page numbers followed by '*f*' indicate figures, '*b*' indicate boxes, and '*t*' indicate tables.